W9-CTE-226

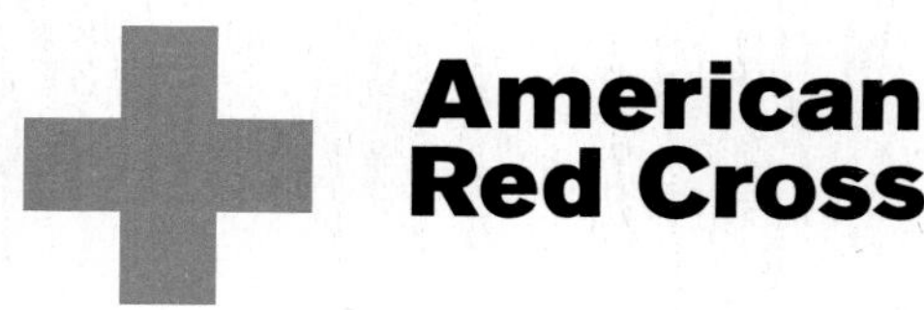

Health and Safety Services

Emergency Response

Important certification information

American Red Cross certificates may be issued upon successful completion of a training program that uses this textbook as an integral part of the course. By itself, the text material does not constitute comprehensive Red Cross training. In order to issue ARC certificates, your instructor must be authorized by the American Red Cross and must follow prescribed policies and procedures. Make certain that you have attended a course authorized by the Red Cross. Ask your instructor about receiving American Red Cross certification, or contact your local chapter for more information.

Liyang Zhou 8/6 — 9/17.

Course Code 3260
Sect 609B04

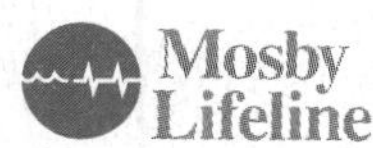

St. Louis Baltimore Boston Carlsbad Chicago Naples New York Philadelphia Portland
London Madrid Mexico City Singapore Sydney Tokyo Toronto Wiesbaden

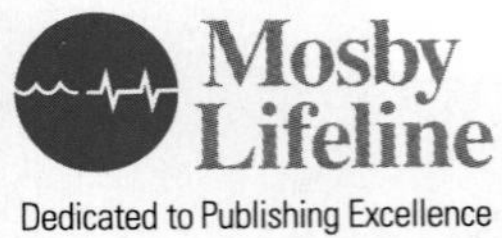

Dedicated to Publishing Excellence

A Times Mirror Company

Copyright © 1997 by The American National Red Cross

All rights reserved. This participant's textbook is an integral part of the American Red Cross Emergency Response course. By itself, it does not constitute complete and comprehensive training. Further, it is not to be construed as an equivalent to Emergency Medical Technician (EMT) training.

The emergency care procedures outlined in this book reflect the standard of knowledge and accepted emergency practices in the United States at the time this book was published. It is the reader's responsibility to stay informed of changes in emergency care procedures.

All rights reserved. No part of this publication may be reproduced, stored in a retrieval system, or transmitted in any form or by any means, electronic, mechanical, photocopying, recording, or otherwise, without prior written permission from the publisher.

Printed in the United States of America

Composition by Progressive Information Technologies
Printing/Binding by The Banta Company

Mosby Lifeline
Mosby–Year Book, Inc.
11830 Westline Industrial Drive
St. Louis, MO 63146

Library of Congress Cataloging in Publication Data

Emergency response / American Red Cross.
p. cm.
Includes bibliographical references and index.
ISBN 0-8151-1260-2 (pbk.)
1. First aid in illness and injury. 2. CPR (First aid)
I. American Red Cross. RC86.7.A476 1997
616.02′5—dc20 96-41118
CIP

96 97 98 99 00 / 9 8 7 6 5 4 3 2 1

This textbook is dedicated to the thousands of first responders who give unselfishly of themselves to save lives.

Acknowledgments

This textbook is the revised edition of American Red Cross Emergency Response program. We have endeavored to revise and polish this text and course through careful consideration to meet the 1995 United States Department of Transportation First Responder: National Standard Curriculum. Many individuals shared in the revision process in various supportive, technical, and creative ways. This revision could not have been developed without the comments of reviewers, the feedback of those who teach the course, and the dedication and support of paid and volunteer staff.

Members of the Development Team at American Red Cross national headquarters who were responsible for designing this course and textbook included: Lawrence D. Newell, EdD, NREMTP, project manager/writer/instructional designer; and S. Elizabeth White, MAEd, ATC, writer/instructional designer/art and design director; Israel M. Zuñiga, development team leader; O. Paul Stearns III, project analyst; Martha F. Beshers, editor; Elaine P. McClatchey and Bob Ogle, feature article writers; Marian F. H. Kirk, artwork and photographic coordinator; Lori M. Compton, AV analyst; Joan Timberlake, assistant editor; and Ella Holloway and Jane Moore, administrative support.

Revised Edition — José V. Salazar, MPH,EMT-P, Project Team Leader; S. Elizabeth White, MAEd, Project Manager; C.P. Dail, Jr., Senior Associate; Thomas A. Bates, EMT-B, Dean Dimke, Michael Espino, Don May, O. Paul Stearns III, Don K. Vardell, MS, Associates; Jane Moore, Specialist; and Betty Williams Butler, Administrative Assistant.

The following American Red Cross national headquarters Health and Safety paid and volunteer staff provided guidance and review for the revised edition: Susan M. Livingstone, Vice President, Health and Safety Sevices; Jean Wagaman, Director, Program and Customer Support; Dana Jessen, Manager, Program and Customer Support; Earl Harbert, Manager, Contracts and Finance; Rhonda Starr, Manager, Educational Development-Aquatics; Karen J. Peterson, PhD, Senior Associate, HIV/AIDS Education; and Linwood Tucker, Risk Management.

The Mosby Lifeline Editorial and Production team included — David T. Culverwell, Senior Vice President; David Dusthimer, Vice President and Publisher; Claire Merrick, Editor in Chief; Ross Goldberg, Editorial Project Manager; Shannon Canty, Project Supervisor; Jerry Wood, Director of Manufacturing; Theresa Fuchs, Manufacturing Manager; Patricia Stinecipher, Special

Product Manager; Elizabeth Rohne Rudder, Design Manager; Douglas Bruce, Director of Editorial, Design, Production, and Manufacturing.

Special thanks go to Martha Beshers, Developmental Editor; Liza Burrill, NREMT-I, Lawrence D. Newell, EdD, NREMT-P, Stephen Marshall, Developmental Writers; Jeffrey B. Hecht, PhD, Objectives and Test Bank Writer; Rick Brady, Photographer and Rolin Graphics, Illustrator.

Guidance and review were also provided by members of the American Red Cross First Aid Advisory Committee:

Ray Cranston, EMT
Committee Chairperson
Commanding Officer
Traffic - Safety Unit Farmington Hills Police - Department
Farmington Hills, Michigan

Frank P. Cooley, EMTP
Subcommittee Chairperson
Coordinator EMS City of Des Moines Fire - Department
Des Moines, Iowa

Pamela D. Alesky, REMT
Health Services Director
Greater Erie County Chapter
American Red Cross
Erie, Pennsylvania

Carol L. Belmont, RN, BES
Consultant Organization Dynamics, Inc.
Burlington, Massachusetts

Ricky Davidson, EMTP
Chief of EMS Shreveport Fire Department
Shreveport, Louisiana

Rodney L. Dennison, EMTP
EMS Program Manager
Texas Department of Health Region I
Temple, Texas

Lance J. Kohn, Sr., EMTP
Coordinator/Senior Instructor
Town of Tonawanda Police Department
Tonawanda, New York

David W. Lewis
Safety Services Director
Dallas Area Chapter
American Red Cross
Dallas, Texas

Rafael A. Ortiz, EMTP
Fire Fighter
Los Angeles County Fire Department
Long Beach, California

External review was provided by the following organizations:

American College of Emergency Physicians — Dallas, Texas
International Association of Fire Fighters — Washington, D.C.
National Association of EMS Physicians — Pittsburgh, Pennsylvania
National Association of Emergency Medical Technicians — Kansas City, Missouri
National Athletic Trainers Association — Dallas, Texas
National Council of State EMS Training Coordinators — Lexington, Kentucky
United States Air Force Pararescue Association — Albuquerque, New Mexico

External review was provided by the following individuals:

Robert S. Behnke, HSD
Professor of Physical Education
Indiana State University Terre
Haute, Indiana

John L. Beckman, EMTP
Fire Fighter
Lincolnwood Fire Department
Lincolnwood, Illinois

Clinton L. Buchanan
Chief, EMS Bureau
Memphis Fire Department
Memphis, Tennessee

John J. Clair
National Ski Patrol System Inc.
Albany, New York

Rod Compton, MEd, ATC
Sports Medicine Director
Assistant Professor
Sports Medicine Division
East Carolina University
Greenville, North Carolina

John Doyle, RN
EMS Coordinator
Victor Valley Community College
Victorville, California

Richard M. Duffy
Director, Occupational Health and Safety
International Association of Fire Fighters, AFLCIO, CLC
Washington, D.C.

Robert Elling, NREMTP
Associate Director
New York State EMS Program
Albany, New York

Technical Sergeant Mark D. Fowler
Pararescue Medical Instructor
USAF Pararescue School
Kirtland AFB, New Mexico

Joseph J. Godek, MS, ATC
West Chester University
West Chester, Pennsylvania

Paul Grace
Coordinator, Sports Medicine
Massachusetts Institute of Technology
Cambridge, Massachusetts

Daniel F. Harshbarger, PA
Baltimore Gas & Electric Company
Baltimore, Maryland

Karla Holmes
National Council of State EMS Training Coordinators
Lexington, Kentucky

Steven A. Meador, MD
Assistant Professor of Medicine
Pennsylvania State University
The Milton S. Hershey Medical Center
Hershey, Pennsylvania

Ray Mitchell
EMS Director
Trenholm State Technical College
Montgomery, Alabama

Lawrence Mottley, MD, FACEP
Senior Medical Advisor, Emergency Services
New York State Department of Health
Attending Physician
Emergency Department
Albany Medical Center
Albany, New York

Major James K. Nickerson
Medical Training Advisor
USAF Pararescue School
Kirtland AFB, New Mexico

Art T. Otto, NREMTP
Operations Manager
Murphy Ambulance Service Inc.
St. Cloud, Minnesota

James O. Page, JD
Publisher
Jems Communications Inc.
Carlsbad, California

S. Scott Polsky, MD, FACEP
Member, ACEP EMS Committee
EMS Director
Akron City Hospital
Akron, Ohio

David C. Pryor, MSM, EMTP
EMS Department Chairperson
Associate Professor Senior
Miami Dade Community College
Miami, Florida

Barbara Reisbach
Coordinator, Public Safety Service
EHOVE Career Center
Vanguard Sentinel JVS
Fremont, Ohio

Matthew M. Rice, MD, JD
Chairman and Program Director
Department of Emergency Medicine
Madigan Army Medical Center
Fort Lewis, Washington

Paul D. Roman, REMT
Chairman, ASTM F30.02.03 Task Group on First Responders
Executive Director
New Jersey EMT Registry
Shrewsbury, New Jersey

Sergeant James Shelly, RN
First Responder Instructor
Baltimore Police Department
Children's Hospital of Baltimore
Baltimore, Maryland

James P. Shinners
Director, Health Services
American Red Cross
St. Paul Area Chapter
St. Paul, Minnesota

Sherman K. Sowby, PhD, CHES
Professor of Health Science
California State University at-Fresno
Fresno, California

Mary Ann Talley
Program Director EMS Education
University of South Alabama
Mobile, Alabama

Bill Vargas
President
USAF Pararescue Association
Albuquerque, New Mexico

Gary W. Waites, EMTP, EMSC
EMS Course Coordinator
College of the Mainland
Emergency Response-Coordinator
Amoco Corporation
Alvin, Texas

Master Sergeant Edward C. Washburn
USAF EMT Program Manager
3790th Medical Service Training Wing
Sheppard AFB, Texas

Gene Weatherall
Chief
Bureau of Emergency Management
Texas Department of Health
Austin, Texas

Katherine H. West, BSN, MSEd, CIC
Consultant
Infection Control/Emerging Concepts Inc.
Springfield, Virginia

Michael D. Zemany, AEMT/3
Deputy Director
North Country Community College
Mt. Lakes Regional EMS Programs
Sarana Lake, New York

Additional assistance was provided by
the Institute of Medicine of the National Academy of Sciences.
Members of a special committee,
the Committee to Advise the American National Red Cross, included:

Paul R. Meyer, Jr., MD
Chairperson Director,
Acute Spine Injury Center
Northwestern Memorial Hospital
Northwestern University Medical School
Chicago, Illinois

George T. Anast, MD
President,
Northern Wisconsin Orthopedic Center
Woodruff, Wisconsin

Harold D. Cross, MD
PROMIS Health Care
Hampden, Maine

Benjamin Honigman, MD
Director,
Emergency Medicine and Trauma
Assistant Professor of Surgery
University of Colorado Medical Center
Denver, Colorado

D. Randy Kuykendall
Operations Supervisor,
Ambulance Department
Memorial General Hospital
Las Cruces, New Mexico

Sylvia H. Micik, MD
Medical Director
North County Health Services
San Marcos, California

John Paraskos, MD
University of Massachusetts Medical School
Director of Noninvasive Lab Division of Cardiovascular Medicine
Worcester, Massachusetts

Frederick P. Rivara, MD, MPH
Director,
Harborview Injury Prevention and Research Center
Harborview Medical Center
Seattle, Washington

Carol W. Runyan, PhD
Associate Director
Injury Prevention Research Center
Research Assistant Professor
School of Public Health
The University of North Carolina
Chapel Hill, North Carolina

John A. Sterba, MD, PhD
Wright State University School of Medicine
Department of Emergency Medicine
Dayton, Ohio

Warren Winkelstein, Jr., MD, MPH
Head, Epidemiology Program School of Public Health University of California at - Berkeley
Berkeley, California

The American Red Cross gratefully acknowledges
the following individuals who assisted
with the field test of this course:

Jay A. Bradley, ATC
School of Physical Education
IUPUI
Indianapolis, Indiana

Liza Burrill, EMT-I
Northeastern New Hampshire EMS
Androscoggin Valley Hospital
Berlin, New Hampshire

David Claxton, EdD
Director, Division of Physical Education
Baylor University
Waco, Texas

Michael Cunningham
Director, Health and Safety
Central North Carolina Chapter American Red Cross
Durham, North Carolina

Doug Darr
Director Division of Emergency Medical Services
Arkansas Department of Health
Little Rock, Arkansas

Mary Celeste Dean
First Aid and CPR Specialist
Oregon Trail Chapter American Red Cross
Portland, Oregon

William E. Hape
National Park Service
Gardinar, Montana

Stan Henderson
Associate Professor
Indiana State University
Terre Haute, Indiana

Tom Lillis
Manager, Training Division
United Airlines
Reston, Virginia

Tim Luloff
City of Des Moines Fire Department
Des Moines, Iowa

Mike Mylar
Safety Division Hewlett Packard
Cupertino, California

Bruce Osman, EMTP
Lineman Detroit Edison Power Company
Detroit, Michigan

Jose Salazar
Specialist, Health and Safety
Greater New York Chapter American Red Cross in Greater New York
New York, New York

Donald S. Walker, EMTP
Mile High Chapter
American Red Cross
Denver, Colorado

Tom Werts
Human Resources Specialist, Recreation
Walt Disney World
Lake Buena Vista, Florida

External review for the revised edition was provided by
the following organizations:

American College of Emergency Physicians — Thornton, Colorado
International Association of Fire Fighters — Washington, D.C.
National Association of EMS Physicians — Milwaukee, Wisconsin
National Council State Emergency Medical Services Training Coordinators, Inc. — Lincoln, Nebraska
National Registry of Emergency Medical Technicians — Columbus, Ohio
National Ski Patrol — St. Paul, Minnesota
Shenandoah Mountain Rescue Group — Sterling, Virginia
Uniformed Services University of the Health Services — Bethesda, Maryland
Wilderness EMS Institute — Pittsburgh, Pennsylvania

External review for the revised edition was provided by the following individuals:

Keith Conover, MD
Medical Director,
Wilderness EMS Institute
Pittsburgh, Pennsylvania

Doug Darr, MS, NREMT-P
Compliance Officer,
Arkansas Emergency Transport
Jacksonville, Arkansas

Phil Dickison,EMT-P
National Registry of EMTs
Columbus, Ohio

Barbara Dodge, BS
Training Coordinator
Nebraska Department of Health
EMS Division
Training Coordinator, Nebraska EMS
National Council State EMS Training Coordinators
Lincoln, Nebraska

Douglas M. Hill, DO, FACEP
Co-Director Emergency Department
North Suburban Medical Center
Board of Directors
American College of Emergency Physicians
Thornton, Colorado

Larry M. Jones, MD, FACS
Director, Trauma Services and Burn Center
Mercy Hospital of Pittsburgh
Pittsburgh, Pennsylvania

Andrew Levinson, MPH
Safety and Health Assistant
International Association of Fire Fighters
Washington, D.C.

Evelyn L. Lewis, MD, MA
Assistant Professor of Family Medicine
Coordinator, Office of Minority Affairs
Uniformed Services University of the Health Services
Bethesda, Maryland

Richard "Chip" Myers, NREMT-P
Alexandria Fire Department
Shenandoah Mountain Rescue Group
Sterling, Virginia

Jeffrey J. Olsen, JD
National Outdoor Emergency Care Supervisor
National Ski Patrol
St. Paul, Minnesota

Jonathan M. Rubin, MD
Assistant Professor of Emergency Medicine,
Medical College of Wisconsin
National Association of EMS Physicians
Milwaukee, Wisonsin

Katherine H. West, BSN, MSEd, CIC
Infection Control Consultant
Infection Control/Emerging Concepts, Inc.
Springfield, Virginia

Additional review of the Oxygen Administration content was provided by:

B. Chris Brewster,
Lifeguard Chief,
San Diego Lifeguard Service
President for the Americas,
International Life Saving Federation
San Diego, California

William H. Clendenen, AB, EMT
Training Coordinator
Divers Alert Network
Durham, North Carolina

Timothy W. Thew
President
Progressive Medical Application Corp.
Berkeley Heights, New Jersey

Kimberly P. Walker, NREMT-P, CHT, MA
Divers Alert Network
Durham, North Carolina

Additional review of the Automated External Defibrillation content was provided by:

James E. Brewer
Director, Research and Regulatory Affairs
SurVivaLink Corporation
Minneapolis, MN

Murray Lorence
Physio Control Corporation
Redmond, WA

Wayne Reval
Director of Marketing, EMS
Zoll Med-Corp
Burlington, Massachusetts

Al Weigel,
Marketing Director
Laerdal Medical Corporation
Wappinger Falls, New York

Contents

Detailed Table of Contents

About This Course

◆ WHY YOU SHOULD TAKE THIS COURSE

It would be ideal if everyone knew what to do when suddenly confronted with an emergency. But that is not reality. Instead, people tend to look to others who are more knowledgeable about what care to provide to an injured or ill person. You, the first responder, are often the first trained person to arrive at the emergency scene. You will be expected to take appropriate action to provide care for injuries or sudden illnesses until more advanced medical personnel arrive. This course prepares you to fulfill this role as a first responder.

◆ HOW YOU WILL LEARN

Course content is presented in various ways. The textbook, which will be assigned reading, contains the information that is discussed in class. Slides, transparencies, and video segments support this information, as do discussions and other class activities. The audiovisuals emphasize the key points you need to remember when making decisions in emergencies and when giving care. They also present skills that you practice in class. Class activities are designed to increase your confidence in your ability to respond to emergencies.

The course design allows you to frequently evaluate your progress in terms of skills competency, knowledge, and decision making. Your ability to correctly perform specific skills described in the textbook will be checked by your instructor during practice sessions.

Your ability to make appropriate decisions when faced with an emergency will be enhanced as you participate in various class activities. Periodically, you will be given situations in the form of scenarios that provide you the opportunity to apply the knowledge and skills you have learned. These scenarios also provide an opportunity to discuss with your instructor and classmates the many different situations that you may encounter in any emergency.

◆ REQUIREMENTS FOR COURSE COMPLETION CERTIFICATE

When this course is taught by a currently authorized American Red Cross instructor, you will be eligible for an American Red Cross course completion certificate. In order for you to receive an American Red Cross course completion certificate, you must —

- Perform specific skills competently and demonstrate the ability to make appropriate decisions for care.

- Pass a final written examination with a score of 80 percent or higher. The final written examination is designed to test your retention and understanding of the course material. You will take this examination at the end of the course. If you do not pass this examination the first time, you may take a second examination.

◆ TEXTBOOK

The textbook has been designed to facilitate your learning and understanding of the material it presents. It includes the following features:

Objectives

At the beginning of each chapter is a list of objectives. Read these objectives carefully and refer back to them from time to time as you read the chapter. The objectives describe what you should be able to do after reading the chapter and participating in class activities. The objectives are seperated into knowledge, attitude, and skill objectives to address the three learning domains.

Knowledge objectives indicate the knowledge that you should obtain from reading the material. Attitude objectives indicate the professional behavior that you should develop as a first responder. Skills objectives indicate the skills you should be able to perform after completing the activities and skill practices for each chapter.

Key Terms

At the beginning of each chapter is a list of defined key terms that you need to know to understand chapter content. Some key terms are listed in more than one chapter because they are essential to your understanding of the material presented in each. The pronunciation of certain medical and anatomical terms is provided, and a pronunciation guide is included in the glossary. In the chapter, key terms are printed in bold italics the first time they are defined or explained.

Enrichment

An Enrichment section appears at the end of most chapters and contains additional information and skills. Certain subjects in each chapter are covered in more depth. Participants are not tested on material in the Enrichment section unless it has been assigned.

Sidebars

Feature articles called sidebars enhance the information in the main body of the text. They appear in most chapters. They present a variety of material ranging from historical information and accounts of actual events to everyday application of the information presented in the main body of the text. You will not be tested on any information presented in these sidebars as part of the American Red Cross course completion requirements.

Tables

Tables are included in many chapters. They concisely summarize important concepts and information and may aid in studying.

You Are the Responder

At the end of each chapter is a section called "You Are the Responder." It contains questions designed to help you evaluate your retention and understanding of the material you have covered up to that point. Completing these questions will help you evaluate your progress and also help you prepare for the final written examination.

Skill Summaries

Skill summaries at the end of certain chapters provide you with an overview of how to perform specific skills described in the chapter. The major steps of each skill are illustrated in photographs. The major steps of each skill are illustrated in photographs.

Appendixes

Two appendixes, located at the end of this textbook, provide additional information on topics first responders will find useful. Appendix A provides information on Automated External Defibrillation (AED). Appendix B is the Healthy Lifestyles Awareness Inventory, which is designed to help you evaluate your present lifestyle and to indicate ways in which you can live a safer, healthier life.

Glossary

The glossary includes definitions of all the key terms and of other words in the text that may be unfamiliar. A pronunciation guide is included in the glossary. All glossary terms appear in the textbook in bold type.

◆ HOW TO USE THIS TEXTBOOK

You should complete the following three steps for each chapter to gain the most from this course:

1. Read the chapter objectives before reading the chapter.
2. As you read the chapter, keep the objectives in mind. When you finish, go back and review the objectives. Check to see that you can meet them without difficulty.
3. Answer the "You Are the Responder" questions after you have read the chapter. If you cannot answer the questions, ask your instructor to help you with concepts with which you are having difficulty.

The Workbook

At the end of each chapter in the textbook, you will find a reference to using the workbook to review chapter content. The workbook is an optional course component containing a summary and an outline of each chapter activity, designed to reinforce understanding and retention of material, and a self test for each chapter. Skill sheets, step-by-step illustrated guides for performing specific skills, are also provided for specific skills taught, such as CPR and splinting. Answers are provided for all activities and self-test questions.

Health Precautions and Guidelines During Training

The American Red Cross has trained millions of people in first aid and CPR (cardiopulmonary resuscitation) using manikins as training aids. According to the Centers for Disease Control (CDC), there has never been a documented case of any disease caused by bacteria, a fungus, or a virus transmitted through the use of training aids such as manikins used for CPR.

The Red Cross follows widely accepted guidelines for cleaning and decontaminating training manikins. **If these guidelines are adhered to, the risk of any kind of disease transmission during training is extremely low.**

To help minimize the risk of disease transmission, you should follow some basic health precautions and guidelines while participating in training. You should take precautions if you have a condition that would increase your risk or other participants' risk of exposure to infections. Request a separate training manikin if you—

- Have an acute condition, such as a cold a sore throat, or cuts or sores on the hands or around your mouth.
- Know you are seropositive (have had a positive blood test) for hepatitis B surface antigen (HBsAg), indicating that you are currently infected with the hepatitis B virus.*
- Know you have a chronic infection indicated by long-term seropositivity (long-term positive blood tests) for the hepatitis B surface antigen (HBsAg)* or a positive blood test for anti-HIV (that is, a positive test for antibodies to HIV, the virus that causes many severe infections including AIDS).
- Have a type of condition that makes you unusually likely to get an infection.

* A person with hepatitis B infection will test positive for the hepatitis B surface antigen (HBsAg). Most persons infected with hepatitis B will get better within a period of time. However, some hepatitis B infections will become chronic and will linger for much longer. These persons will continue to test positive for HBsAg. Their decision to participate in CPR training should be guided by their physician.

After a person has had an acute hepatitis B infection, he or she will no longer test positive for the surface antigen but will test positive for the hepatitis B antibody (anti-HBs). Persons who have been vaccinated for hepatitis B will also test positive for the hepatitis antibody. A positive test for the hepatitis B antibody (anti-HBs) should not be confused with a positive test for the hepatitis B surface antigen (HBsAg).

If you decide you should have your own manikin, ask your instructor if he or she can provide one for you to use. You will not be asked to explain why in your request. The manikin will not be used by anyone else until it has been cleaned according to the recommended end-of-class decontamination procedures. Because the number of manikins available for class use is limited, the more advance notice you give, the more likely it is that you can be provided a separate manikin.

In addition to taking the precautions regarding manikins, you can further protect yourself and other participants from infection by following these guidelines:

- Wash your hands thoroughly before participating in class activities.
- Do not eat, drink, use tobacco products, or chew gum during classes when manikins are used.
- Clean the manikin properly before use. For some manikins, this means vigorously wiping the manikin's face and the inside of its mouth with a clean gauze pad soaked with either a solution of liquid chlorine bleach and water (sodium hypochlorite and water) or rubbing alcohol. For other manikins, it means changing the rubber face. Your instructor will provide you with instructions for cleaning the type of manikin used in your class.
- Follow the guidelines provided by your instructor when practicing skills such as clearing a blocked airway with your finger.

◆ PHYSICAL STRESS AND INJURY

Training in first aid and CPR requires physical activity. If you have a medical condition or disability that will prevent you from taking part in the practice sessions, please let your instructor know.

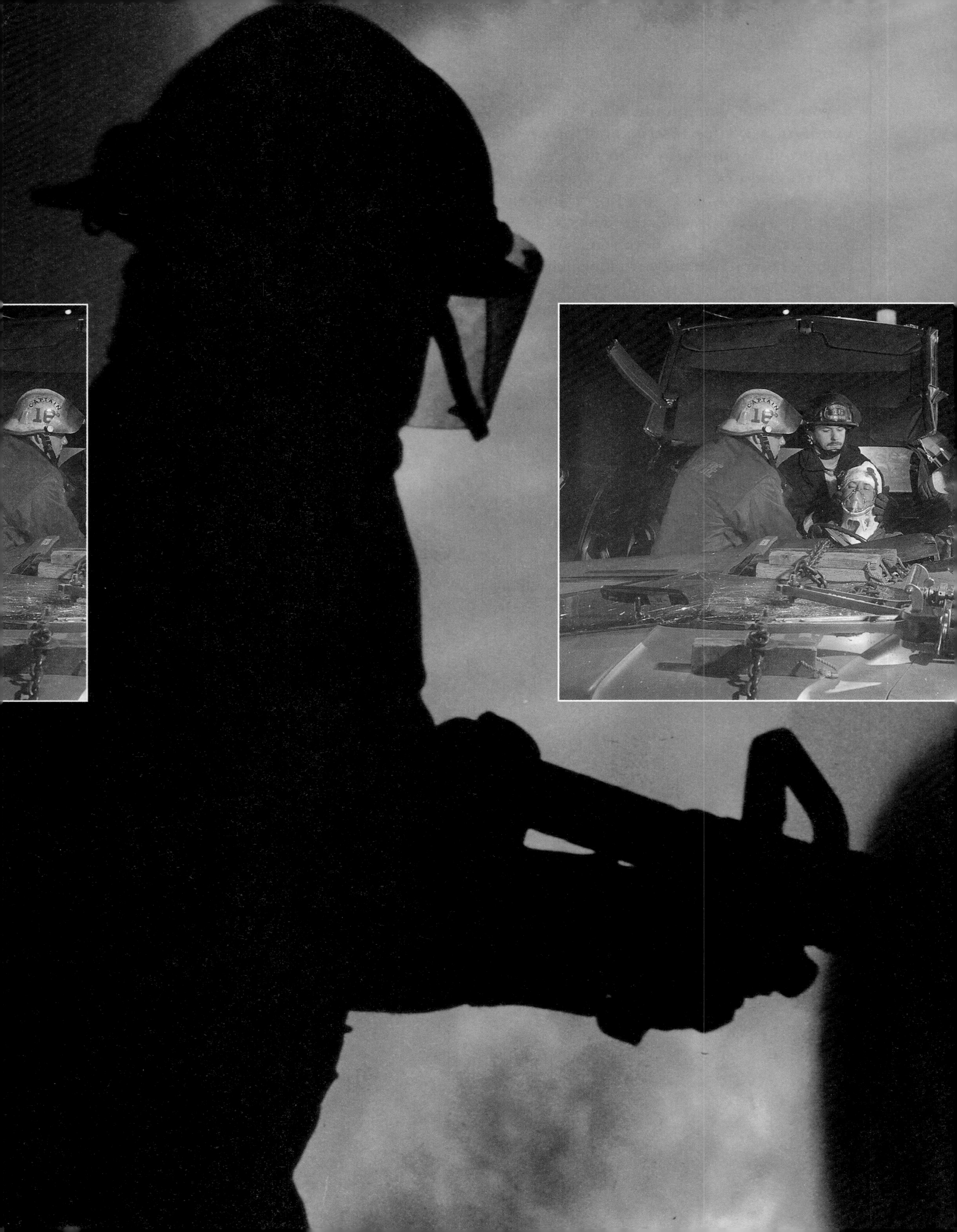
CAPTAIN

Module One

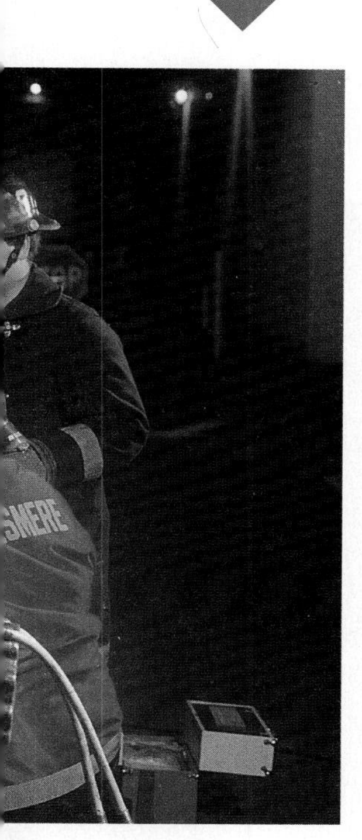

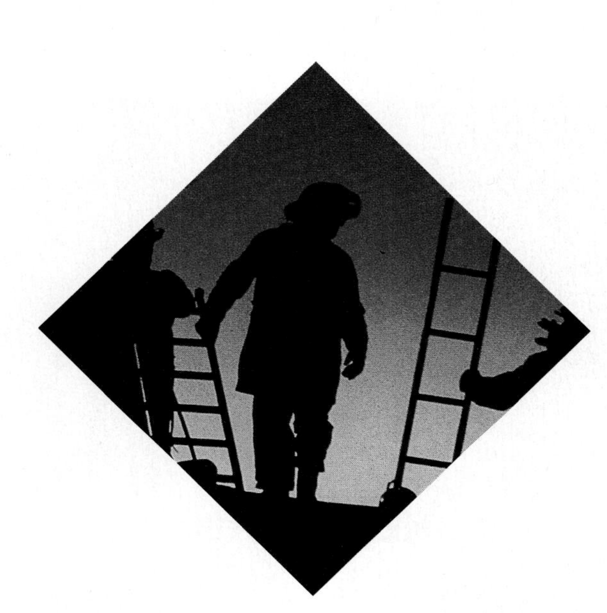

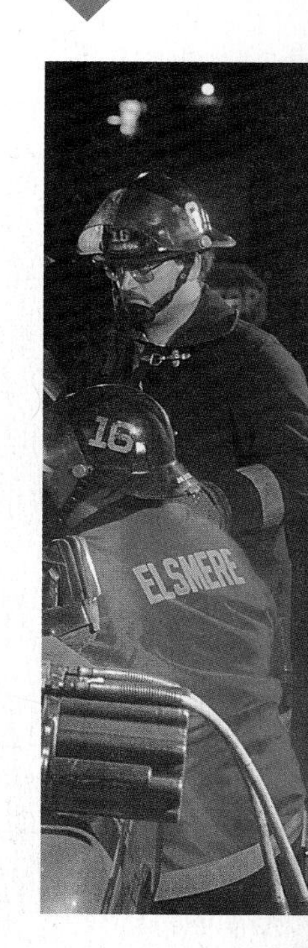

Preparatory

1
The First Responder

2
Well-Being of the First Responder

3
Preventing Disease Transmission

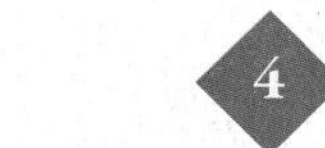
4
Legal and Ethical Issues

5
The Human Body

6
Lifting and Moving

The First Responder

1

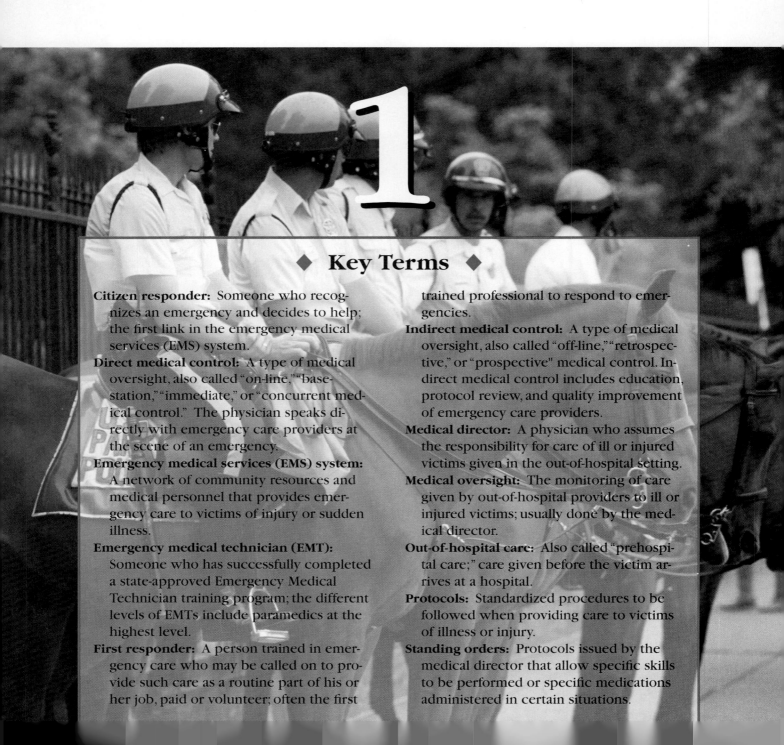

Key Terms

Citizen responder: Someone who recognizes an emergency and decides to help; the first link in the emergency medical services (EMS) system.

Direct medical control: A type of medical oversight, also called "on-line," "base-station," "immediate," or "concurrent medical control." The physician speaks directly with emergency care providers at the scene of an emergency.

Emergency medical services (EMS) system: A network of community resources and medical personnel that provides emergency care to victims of injury or sudden illness.

Emergency medical technician (EMT): Someone who has successfully completed a state-approved Emergency Medical Technician training program; the different levels of EMTs include paramedics at the highest level.

First responder: A person trained in emergency care who may be called on to provide such care as a routine part of his or her job, paid or volunteer; often the first trained professional to respond to emergencies.

Indirect medical control: A type of medical oversight, also called "off-line," "retrospective," or "prospective" medical control. Indirect medical control includes education, protocol review, and quality improvement of emergency care providers.

Medical director: A physician who assumes the responsibility for care of ill or injured victims given in the out-of-hospital setting.

Medical oversight: The monitoring of care given by out-of-hospital providers to ill or injured victims; usually done by the medical director.

Out-of-hospital care: Also called "prehospital care;" care given before the victim arrives at a hospital.

Protocols: Standardized procedures to be followed when providing care to victims of illness or injury.

Standing orders: Protocols issued by the medical director that allow specific skills to be performed or specific medications administered in certain situations.

◆ Knowledge Objectives ◆

After reading this chapter and completing the class activities, you should be able to—

- Define the components of the Emergency Medical Services (EMS) system.
- Describe each link in the chain of survival and how it relates to the EMS system.
- Differentiate between the roles and responsibilities of the first responder and those of other out-of-hospital care providers.
- Explain why the interests of the victim are foremost in making any and all care decisions.
- Define medical oversight and discuss its relationship to first responders.
- Explain the types of medical oversight and how they affect the victim care provided by the first responder.
- Explain the specific statutes and regulations governing the EMS system in your state.

◆ Attitude Objectives ◆

After reading this chapter and completing the class activities, you should be able to—

- Identify with the responsibilities of a first responder in accordance with the standards of an EMS professional.
- Recognize the importance of maintaining a professional appearance when on duty or responding to calls.
- Acknowledge the importance of providing a uniform, high-level standard of care to all victims, regardless of their culture, gender, age, position in society, and income level.
- Appreciate the need to demonstrate a caring attitude toward victims of illness or injury.

◆ INTRODUCTION

As a first responder, you are a key part of the emergency medical services (EMS) system. You provide a link between the first actions of bystanders and more advanced care. A ***first responder*** is a person trained in emergency care, paid or volunteer, who is often summoned to provide initial care in an emergency (Fig. 1-1).

As the first trained professional on the scene, your actions are often critical. They may determine whether a seriously ill or injured person survives.

By taking this course, you will gain the knowledge, skills, and confidence to give appropriate care when you are called to help a victim of injury or sudden illness. You will learn how to assess a victim's condition and how to recognize and care for life-threatening

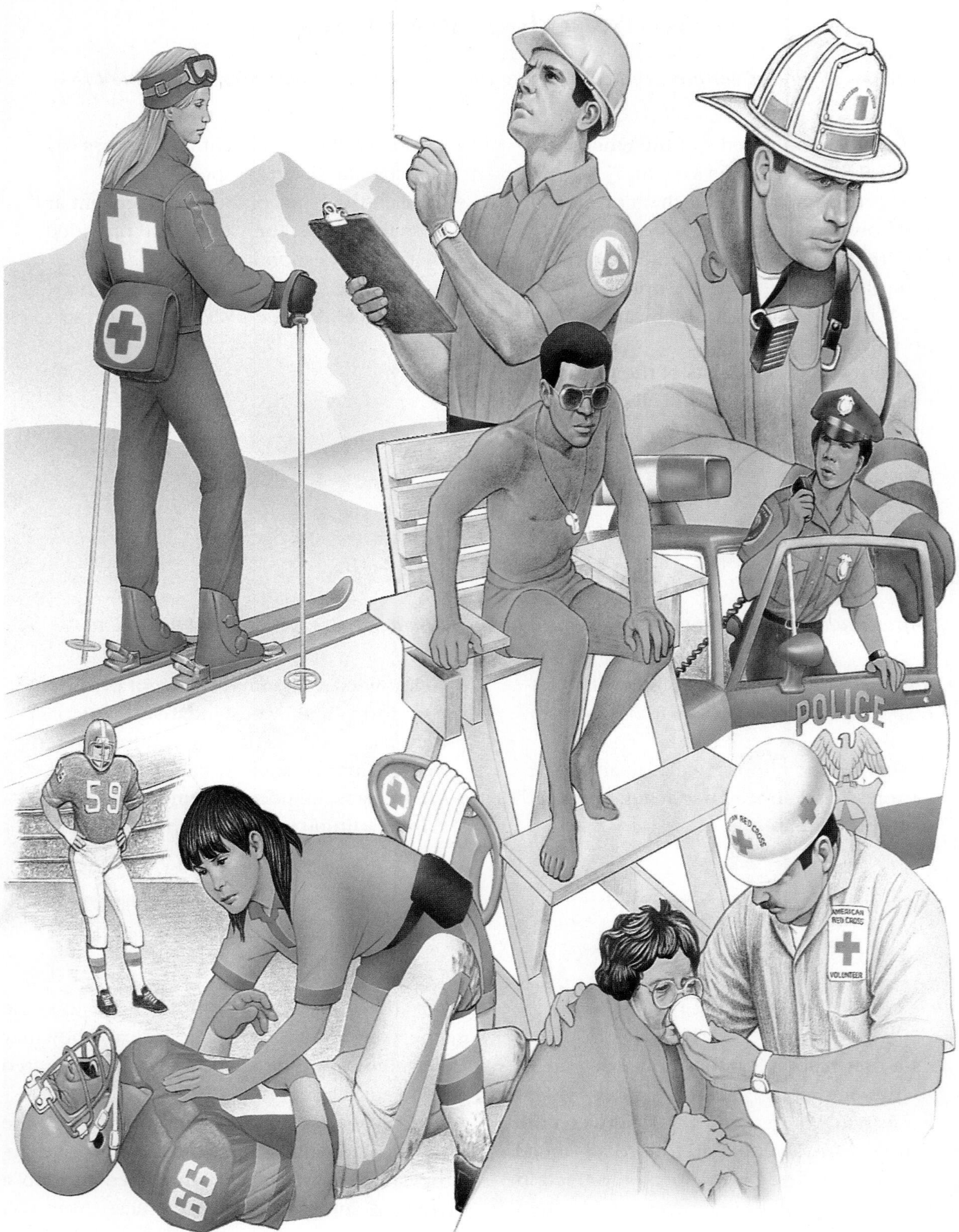

Figure 1-1 First responders are often summoned to provide care in an emergency.

emergencies. You will also learn how to minimize a victim's discomfort and prevent further complications until advanced medical personnel take over.

◆ THE EMERGENCY MEDICAL SERVICES (EMS) SYSTEM

The first responder is part of the ***emergency medical services (EMS) system,*** a network of community resources and medical personnel that provides emergency care to victims of injury or sudden illness. When bystanders at an emergency scene recognize an emergency and take action, they activate this system. The care provided by increasingly more highly trained professionals continues until an ill or injured person receives the level of care that he or she needs.

The development of this organized EMS network over the years has led to a higher quality of medical care in our society. As of 1966, the quality of emergency care outside the hospital was not regulated and standards of care were lower. Ambulance attendants had minimal training and rarely treated ill or injured people on the way to the hospital for emergency care. Ambulances were little more than fast transportation to the hospital.

In 1966, the National Academy of Sciences, in a landmark white paper entitled "Accidental Death and Disability: The Neglected Disease of Modern Society," brought to light the dismal quality of emergency care. The paper criticized both ambulance services and hospital emergency departments. As a result, in 1973, the United States Congress enacted the Emergency Medical Services Act. This act created a multi-tiered, nationwide system of emergency health care. From that beginning, the EMS system as we know it today evolved. The National Highway Traffic Safety Administration (NHTSA), a division of the U.S. Department of Transportation, has supported the development of training programs for the various levels of ***out-of-hospital care*** personnel. One of these programs is specifically titled "First Responder."

◆ COMPONENTS OF AN EMS SYSTEM

The goal of NHTSA of the U.S. Department of Transportation (DOT) is to reduce death and disabilities caused by motor vehicle crashes. NHTSA has created 10 components of an effective EMS system, and a method of assessing those areas. By measuring the progress of EMS systems against the standard set by NHTSA, states can ensure the EMS system is effective nationwide. The components developed by NHTSA are as follows: Regulation and Policy, Resource Management, Human Resources and Training, Transportation, Facilities, Communications, Public Information and Education, Medical Oversight, Trauma Systems, and Evaluation (Fig. 1-2).

◆ A CHAIN OF SURVIVAL

The EMS system functions as a series of events linked in a chain, a chain of survival (Fig. 1-3). The basic principle is to bring rapid medical care to the victim rather than the victim to medical care. From the onset of illness or injury until the victim receives hospital care, the survival and recovery of critically ill or injured persons depends on this chain of events. These events include—

1. Recognition of an emergency and initial care provided by citizen responders.
2. Early activation of the EMS system.
3. First responder care.
4. More advanced out-of-hospital emergency care.

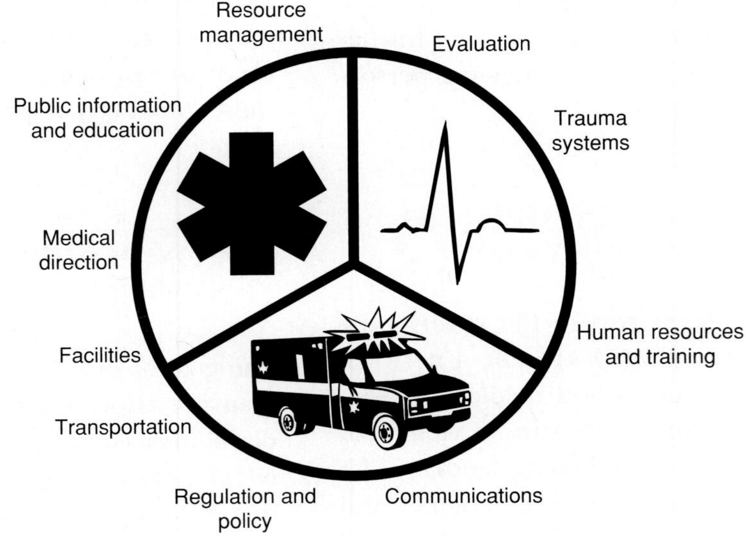

Figure 1-2 The National Highway Traffic Safety Administration's ten standards for EMS systems.

5. Hospital care.
6. Rehabilitation.

Citizen Responder

The first crucial link in the EMS system is the action of the ***citizen responder.*** This link depends on a responsible citizen who takes action when an injury or illness occurs. The person must first recognize that what has happened is an emergency. He or she must then activate the EMS system by dialing 9-1-1 or a local emergency number, or by notifying a nearby first responder, such as a police officer. In the Enhanced 9-1-1 (E-911) system, the call is recorded on a computer system that provides information about where the call originated. The public can be educated on how to access the EMS system through using public information campaigns, such as "Make the Right Call" or "Check, Call, Care."

While waiting for more highly trained personnel, the citizen responder can provide basic care to the ill or injured person. This initial care may be as simple as applying direct pressure on a bleeding wound or more complex, such as cardiopulmonary resuscitation (CPR). Often the care provided by citizen responders in these first few minutes is critical. However, their efforts may be futile without the immediate response of more highly trained emergency personnel.

Early Activation of the EMS System

The next link involves the EMS dispatcher who receives the call for help from either a citizen or a first responder already on the scene. The dispatcher quickly determines what help is needed and sends the appropriate professionals.

First Responder Care

The first person to arrive on the scene who is trained to provide a higher level of care than the citizen responder is often referred to as the first responder (Fig. 1-4). This person has the skills and training to better assess the victim's

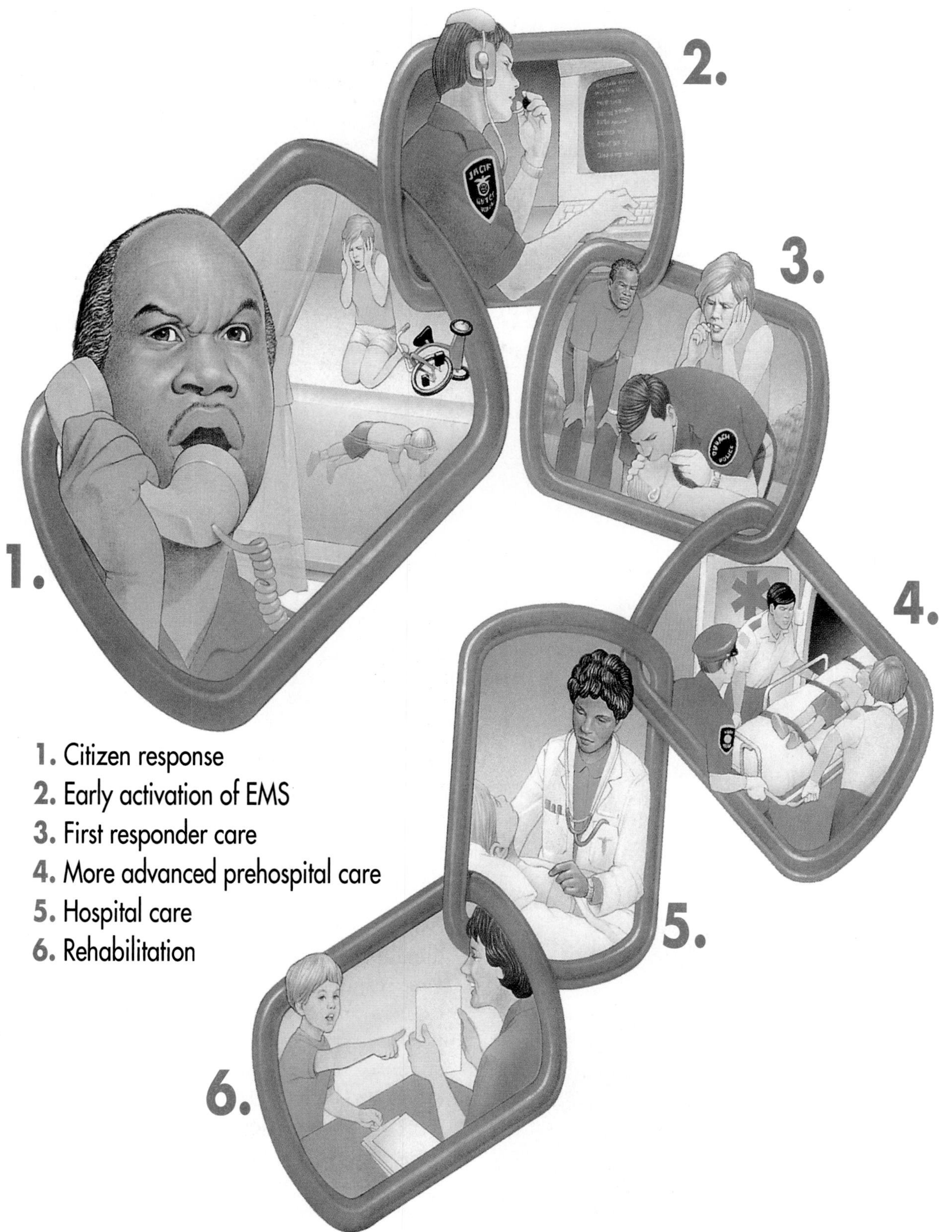

Figure 1-3 The Chain of Survival

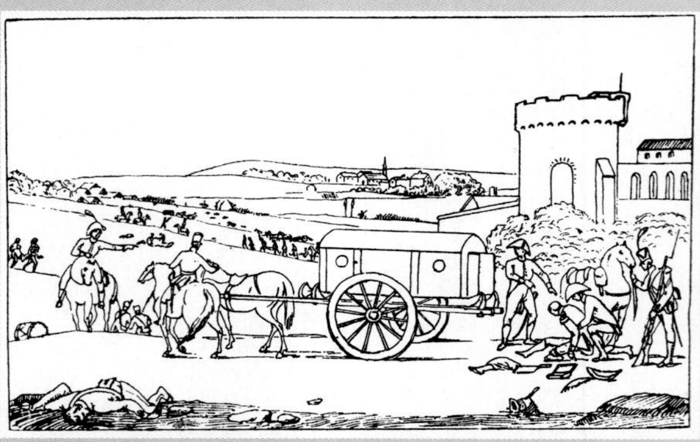

Yesterday's "Flying Ambulance." (Cabanes, Chirurgiens et Blessés à Travers l'Histoire, Paris, 1918.)

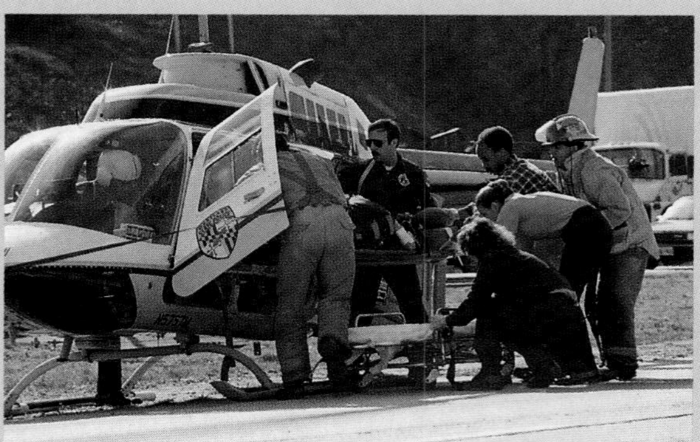

Craig C. Schleunes

Today's "Flying Ambulance"

From Horses to Helicopters: A History of Emergency Care

Emergency care originated during the French emperor Napoleon's campaigns in the late 1700s. The surgeon-in-chief for the Grand Army, Dominique Jean Larrey, became the first doctor to try to save the wounded during battles instead of waiting until the fighting was over.[1] Using horse-drawn litters, Larrey and his men dashed onto the battlefield in what became known as "flying ambulances."

By the 1860s, the wartime principles of emergency care were applied to everyday emergencies in some American cities. In 1878, a writer for *Harper's New Monthly Magazine* explained how accidents were reported to the police, who notified the nearest hospitals by a telegraph signal. He described an early hospital ambulance ride in New York City.

"A well-kept horse was quickly harnessed to the ambulance; and as the surgeon took his seat behind, having first put on a jaunty uniform cap with gold lettering, the driver sprang to the box and with a sharp crack of the whip we

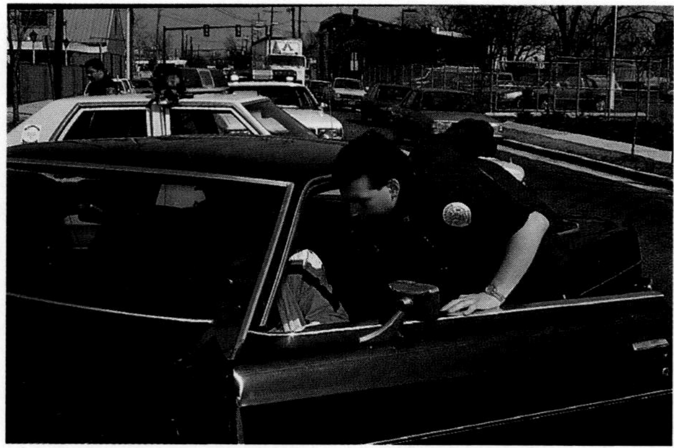

Figure 1-4 A first responder is often the first person trained to provide a higher level of care to arrive on the scene.

condition and take appropriate actions, which include caring for life-threatening conditions. First responders have traditionally been police officers and fire fighters. Besides these traditional first responders, others are routinely summoned to emergency situations. These responders include industrial response teams, athletic trainers, and people with similar responsibilities for the safety and well-being of others. Because of the nature of their jobs, first responders are often close to the scene and sometimes have appropriate supplies and equipment. First responder care often provides a critical transition between a citizen's initial

rolled off the smooth asphalt of the courtyard and into the street. . . . As we swept around corners and dashed over crossings, both doctor and driver kept up a sharp cry of warning to pedestrians."[2]

While booming industrial cities developed emergency transport systems, rural populations had only rudimentary services. In most small towns, the mortician had the only vehicle large enough to handle the litters, so emergency victims were just as likely to ride in a hearse to the hospital as in an ambulance.[3]

Cars gave Americans a faster system of transport, but over the next 50 years, car collisions also created the need for more emergency vehicles. In 1966, a major report questioned the quality of emergency services. Dismayed at the rising death toll on the nation's highways, Congress passed laws in 1966 and 1973 ordering the improved training of ambulance workers and emergency department staffs, an improved communications network, and the development of regional units with specialized care.

Today, the telegraph signal has been replaced in many areas by the 9-1-1 telephone code, which immediately connects a caller to a dispatcher who can send help. In some areas, a computer connected to the enhanced 9-1-1 system displays the caller's name, address, and phone number, even if the caller cannot speak. Ambulance workers have changed from coachmen to trained medical professionals who can provide lifesaving care at the scene. Horses have been replaced by ambulances and helicopters equipped to provide the most advanced out-of-hospital care available.

The EMS system has expanded in sheer numbers and in services. Today, New York City has 15 times as many hospitals as in the 1870s. Hospitals have also vastly improved their emergency care capabilities. If victims suffer from critical injuries, such as burns, spinal cord injuries, or other traumatic injuries, the EMS system now has developed regional trauma and burn centers where specialists are always available.

In two centuries, the EMS system has gone from horses to helicopters. As technology continues to advance, it is difficult to imagine what changes the next century will bring.

REFERENCES

1. Major R, M.D.: *A history of medicine,* Springfield, Ill, 1954, Charles C Thomas.
2. Rideing WH: Hospital life in New York, *Harper's New Monthly Magazine* 57:171, 1878.
3. Division of Medical Sciences, National Academy of Sciences–National Research Council: *Accidental death and disability: the neglected disease of modern society,* Washington, DC, September 1966.

actions and the care of more highly trained professionals.

More Advanced Out-of-Hospital Emergency Care

The arrival of ***emergency medical technicians (EMTs)*** represents the next link in the chain of survival. Depending on the level of training and certification (basic, intermediate, or paramedic), EMTs can provide more advanced care and life-support techniques. An EMT's training requires successful completion of a state-approved EMT training program, which provides experience in both out-of-hospital and hospital settings. In most parts of the United States, ambulance personnel must be certified at least at the basic EMT level.

Paramedics (EMT-P) are highly trained EMTs. In addition to performing basic EMT skills, paramedics can administer medications and intravenous fluids and deliver advanced care for breathing problems and abnormal heart rhythms. Paramedics usually provide the

Hundreds of Millions Served

The 9-1-1 service was created in the United States in 1968 as a nationwide telephone number for the public to use to report emergencies and request emergency assistance. It gives the public direct access to a Public Service Answering Point that is responsible for taking the appropriate action. The numbers 9-1-1 were chosen because they best fit the needs of the public and the telephone company. They are easy to remember and dial, and they have never been used as an office, area, or service code.[1]

When should you call 9-1-1? Call 9-1-1 whenever there is a threat to life or property, or the potential for injury. Fire and motor vehicle crashes are obvious emergencies that require calling 9-1-1. But you should also call 9-1-1 for other situations that threaten life or property or those that may cause injury, such as a dangerous animal running loose, a downed electrical line, a burglary, or an assault. If you are unsure whether you should call 9-1-1, make the call.

Hundreds of millions of people call 9-1-1 each year. The majority, approximately 80 percent of 9-1-1 calls, pertain to law enforcement. Fire and EMS comprise the rest. EMS professionals alone respond to more than 19 million 9-1-1 calls each year.

What advantages does 9-1-1 offer? It was designed to save time in a public safety agency's overall response (for example, fire, police, EMS) to a call for help. This includes the time it takes a citizen to telephone the correct agency or agencies for help. For example, imagine that a house is on fire in your neighborhood and your neighbor has been seriously burned. You run to call for help. Whom should you call first — the fire department to come and put out the fire so no one else is hurt, the ambulance so that EMTs can attend to your neighbor, or the police to help secure the area? Without 9-1-1 service, you may need to place separate calls to all three agencies.

With 9-1-1 service, regardless of your needs, you make only one call. When the call comes in, a 9-1-1 dispatcher answers the call, listens to the caller, gathers needed information, and dispatches help.

Perhaps one of the most exciting lifesaving advances in computer technology in the past few years has been the development of an Enhanced 9-1-1 system. This computer system automatically displays the telephone number, address, and name in which the phone is listed. So, even if the caller is unable to remain on the line or unable to speak or if the call is disconnected, the dispatcher has enough information to send help.

The latest advance in 9-1-1 system development is the use of Mobile Data Terminals (MDTs) in police cars, fire engines, and ambulances. By the time these personnel start their vehicles, the built-in MDT units provide them with the location information. These MDT units are also used to send messages, establishing a vital communication link among the caller, the dispatcher, and the field unit en route.

With all of its advantages and lifesaving capabilities, 9-1-1 service today covers approximately 75 percent of the U.S. population and 30 to 35 percent of the geographical area of the United States. Ninety to ninety-five percent of the coverage is via Enhanced 9-1-1. As more cities establish 9-1-1 systems, response times of emergency personnel will continue to improve, resulting in more lives being saved.

REFERENCES

1. National Emergency Number Association: *Nine one one 9-1-1 (what's it all about?).*
2. Stanton W, Executive Director, National Emergency Number Association: Interview, Feb 13, 1990.

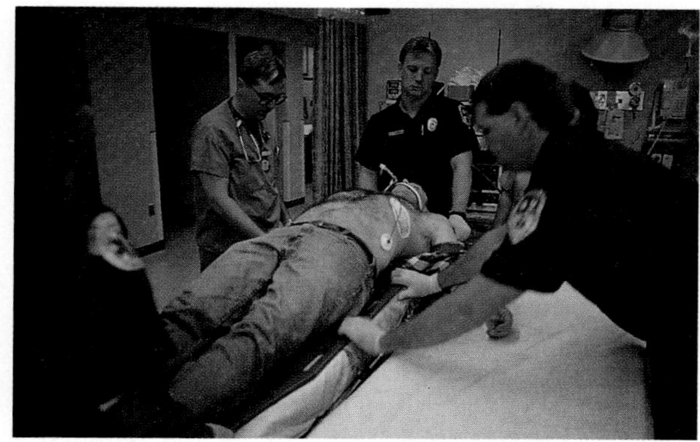

Figure 1-5 At the hospital, EMTs turn over care of the victim to the emergency department staff.

highest level of out-of-hospital care. They serve as the field extension of the emergency physician. Regardless of the level of training, the EMT's role is to reassess the victim's condition and to begin and continue appropriate care until the injured or ill person reaches the hospital.

Hospital Care

When the victim arrives at the hospital emergency department, the emergency department staff take over care (Fig. 1-5). Many personnel in this link become involved as needed, including nurses, physicians, and other health-care professionals.

Some areas may have facilities or centers for specific conditions. These specialty centers focus on **trauma,** burn, pediatric, or poisoning emergencies. The EMTs who care for and transport these victims may have to determine if a victim needs to be transported to one of these centers.

A nurse trained to assess the victim's condition is usually the first member of the emergency department staff involved. He or she quickly evaluates the victim's condition and identifies any immediate threats to the victim's life. Other specially trained emergency department nurses continue to provide needed care.

Most hospital emergency departments are staffed by emergency physicians trained to care for acutely ill or injured victims. They evaluate and provide care to stabilize critically ill or injured people. If other specialized care is required, the emergency physician involves the appropriate medical specialist, such as a **cardiologist, orthopedic surgeon, neurosurgeon,** or **trauma surgeon.**

In addition to nurses and physicians, many other allied health personnel may help provide care. These include respiratory therapists, radiologic (x-ray) technicians, and laboratory technicians.

Rehabilitation

The final link in the chain of survival is **rehabilitation.** The goal of rehabilitation is to return the injured or ill person to his or her previous state of health. This phase begins once the person has been moved from the emergency department. Other health-care professionals, including family physicians, consulting specialists, social workers, and physical therapists, work together to rehabilitate the victim.

◆ SUPPORTING THE EMS SYSTEM

The chain of survival depends on all people in the chain performing their roles correctly and promptly to make the EMS system work. Citizens must recognize emergencies and get help quickly by activating the system. They must learn what actions to take in the first critical minutes. They must also learn to prevent and prepare for emergencies. They need to support the EMS system in their community.

Professionals must respond quickly, effectively, and sensitively to emergencies when they are summoned. They must keep their training current and stay abreast of new issues in emergency response. When each link in the chain works effectively, the victim's chances for a full recovery are enhanced. Being a professional includes providing the highest-level

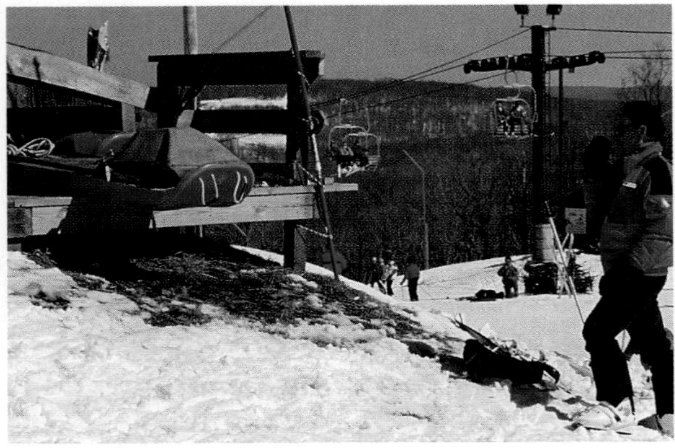

Figure 1-6 First responders may have ready access to emergency supplies and equipment.

standard of care to victims regardless of their age, gender, culture, position in society, or income level.

So what happens if one of these links in the chain of survival breaks? Since the victim's life may depend on each or all of these links, a broken link can cause serious consequences.

For instance, if a citizen responder does not recognize a life-threatening emergency, such as the early signals of a heart attack, and does not quickly call EMS personnel, the victim may not live. Poor information given to the EMS dispatcher may delay advanced care. Improper care of the ill or injured person before more advanced care arrives can result in the victim's condition worsening, possibly leading to permanent disability or death.

With a serious injury or illness, survival and recovery are not a matter of chance. Survival results from a carefully orchestrated chain of events in which all participants fulfill their roles. The EMS system can make the difference between life and death or a partial or full recovery. You as a first responder play a critical role in this system.

◆ THE FIRST RESPONDER

While on duty, first responders, unlike citizen responders, have a duty to respond to the scene of a medical emergency and to provide emergency care to the ill or injured person. They should have ready access to supplies and equipment for providing care until more advanced emergency medical care arrives (Fig. 1-6).

Some occupations, such as law enforcement and fire fighting, require personnel to respond to and assist at the scene of an emergency. These personnel are dispatched through an emergency number, such as 9-1-1, and often share common communication networks. When a person dials 9-1-1, he or she will contact police, fire, or ambulance personnel. These are typically considered **public safety personnel.** However, all first responders do not necessarily work for public safety agencies. People in many occupations other than public safety are called to help in the event of an injury or sudden illness, such as —

- Athletic trainers.
- Camp leaders.
- Emergency management personnel.
- First aid station members.
- Industrial response teams.
- Lifeguards.
- Ski patrol members.

In an emergency, these people are often required to provide the same minimum standard of care as traditional first responders. Their duty is to assess the victim's condition and provide necessary care, make sure that any necessary additional help has been summoned, assist other medical personnel at the scene, and document their actions.

Personal Characteristics and Roles

As an emergency care provider who deals with the public, you must be willing to take on responsibilities beyond giving care. These responsibilities require you to demonstrate certain characteristics that include —

- *Maintaining a caring and professional attitude.* Ill or injured people are sometimes difficult to work with. Be compassionate; try to understand their concerns and fears. Realize that any anger an injured or ill person may show often results from fear. A citizen who helps at the emergency may also be afraid. Try to be reassuring. Even though citizen responders may not have done everything perfectly, be sure to thank them for taking action. Recognition and praise help to affirm their willingness to act. Also, be careful about what you say. Do not volunteer distressing news about the emergency to the victim or to the victim's family or friends.

- *Controlling your fears.* Try not to reveal your anxieties to the victim or bystanders. The presence of blood, vomit, unpleasant odors, or torn or burned skin is disturbing to most people. You may need to compose yourself before acting. If you must, turn away for a moment and take a few deep breaths before providing care.
- *Presenting a professional appearance.* This helps ease a victim's fears and inspires confidence.
- *Keeping your skills and knowledge up-to-date.* Involve yourself in continuing education, professional reading, and refresher training.
- *Staying fit with daily exercise and a healthy diet.* Job stresses can adversely affect your health. Exercise and diet can help you manage physical, mental, and emotional stress.
- *Maintaining a safe and healthy lifestyle.* As a first responder, it is important to maintain a safe and healthy lifestyle both on and off the job. Completing the Healthy Lifestyles Awareness Inventory in Appendix B will help you identify the potential risks in your life so that you can take steps to reduce them.

Responsibilities

Since you will often be the first trained professional to arrive at many emergencies, your primary responsibilities center on safety and early emergency care. Your major responsibilities are to—

- *Ensure safety for yourself and any bystanders.* Your first responsibility is not to make the situation worse by getting hurt or letting bystanders get hurt. By making sure the scene is safe as you approach it, you can avoid unnecessary injuries.
- *Gain access to the victim.* Carefully approach the victim unless the scene is too dangerous for you to handle without help. Electrical or chemical hazards, unsafe structures, and other dangers may make it difficult to reach the victim. Recognize when a rescue requires specially trained emergency personnel.
- *Determine any threats to the victim's life.* Check first for immediate life-threatening conditions and care for any you find. Next, look for other conditions that could threaten the victim's life or health if not cared for.
- *Summon more advanced medical personnel as needed.* After you quickly assess the victim, notify more advanced medical personnel of the situation, if someone has not already done so.
- *Provide needed care for the victim.* Remain with the victim and provide whatever care you can until more advanced personnel take over.
- *Assist more advanced personnel.* Transfer your information about the victim and the emergency to any more advanced personnel (Fig. 1-7). Tell them what happened, how you found the victim, any problems you found, and any care you gave. Assist them as needed, and help with care for any other victims. When possible, try to anticipate the needs of those giving care.

In addition to these major responsibilities, you have secondary responsibilities that include—

- Summoning additional help when needed, such as special rescue teams.
- Controlling or directing bystanders or asking them for help.

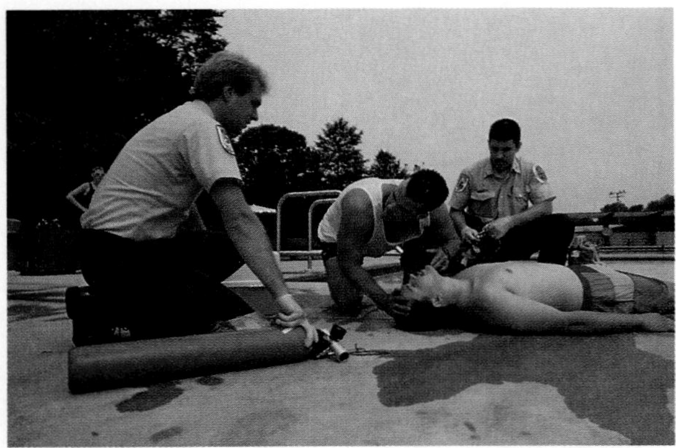

Figure 1-7 The first responder transfers information about the victim to more advanced medical personnel.

- Taking additional steps, if necessary, to protect bystanders from dangers, such as traffic or fire.
- Recording what you saw, heard, and did at the scene.
- Reassuring the victim's family or friends.

◆ MEDICAL OVERSIGHT

Medical oversight is the process by which a physician directs the care given by out-of-hospital providers to ill or injured victims. Usually this monitoring is done by a ***medical director,*** who assumes responsibility for the care given.

The physician also oversees training and the development of ***protocols*** (standardized procedures to be followed when providing care to victims of injury or illness). Since it is impossible for the medical director to be present at every incident that happens outside of the hospital, he or she can still direct care through ***standing orders.*** Standing orders allow EMTs to provide certain types of care or treatments without speaking to the physician. This kind of medical oversight is called ***indirect medical control.*** Indirect medical control includes education, protocol review, and quality improvement of emergency care providers. Other procedures that are not covered by standing orders require the EMTs to speak directly with the physician. This contact can be made via cellular phone, radio, or telephone. This kind of medical oversight is called ***direct medical control.***

◆ STATUTES AND REGULATIONS

Each state has very specific laws and rules that govern the practice of EMS in the out-of-hospital setting. First responders should become aware of these laws and regulations. Typical legal concerns and issues are addressed in Chapter 4.

◆ SUMMARY

The survival and recovery of a severely ill or injured person depend on all parts of the emergency medical services (EMS) system working together efficiently. Citizen response, rapid activation of EMS, first responder care, advanced out-of-hospital emergency care, hospital care, and extended care (rehabilitation) are the links in this chain of survival. You, as a first responder, are often the first trained person to arrive on the emergency scene and take over care of the victim from any citizen responders present.

After arriving on the scene, the first responder checks the scene for safety and then reaches the victim, gives care for any life-threatening conditions, and summons more advanced medical personnel if needed. The first responder should give arriving medical personnel any assistance they need.

Regardless of your profession, when you are called upon to help a victim of injury or sudden illness, you assume the role of an emergency care provider. When an emergency occurs, the people in your care, as well as assisting bystanders, will expect you to know what to do. Be prepared to think and act accordingly. What to do, however, often involves more than giving emergency care. Chapter 19 provides an overview of the first responder's role in assessing and managing emergency scenes. In addition to caring for victims, first responders have a responsibility to keep healthy and up-to-date in their knowledge and training.

As emergency care providers, many first responders work under the supervision of a medical director. By planning ahead and following protocols and standing orders, out-of-hospital providers are able to perform certain skills and procedures through direct or indirect medical control.

Use the activities in Unit 1 of your workbook to help you review the material in this chapter.

You Are the Responder

1. A terrified mother pulls her child from the bottom of a pool while a neighbor calls 9-1-1 for help. You are the first to arrive at the scene to see the neighbor trying to breathe air into the boy's limp body. The mother looks to you helplessly. How would you respond?

2. As a member of your company's emergency response team, you are radioed that a worker's arm is trapped in a piece of machinery. You arrive to find co-workers attempting to free the arm. How would you respond?

The Well-Being of the First Responder

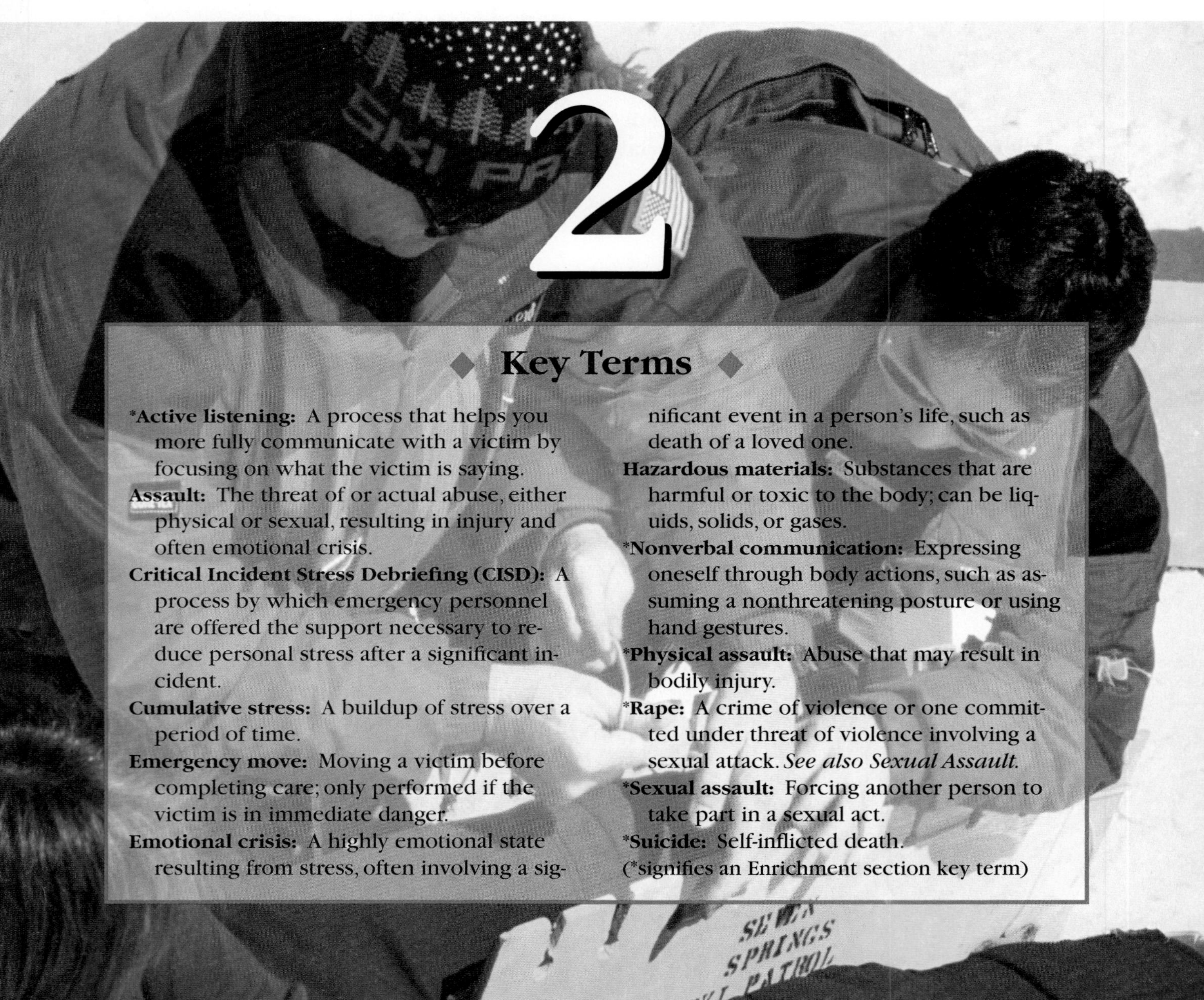

Key Terms

***Active listening:** A process that helps you more fully communicate with a victim by focusing on what the victim is saying.

Assault: The threat of or actual abuse, either physical or sexual, resulting in injury and often emotional crisis.

Critical Incident Stress Debriefing (CISD): A process by which emergency personnel are offered the support necessary to reduce personal stress after a significant incident.

Cumulative stress: A buildup of stress over a period of time.

Emergency move: Moving a victim before completing care; only performed if the victim is in immediate danger.

Emotional crisis: A highly emotional state resulting from stress, often involving a significant event in a person's life, such as death of a loved one.

Hazardous materials: Substances that are harmful or toxic to the body; can be liquids, solids, or gases.

***Nonverbal communication:** Expressing oneself through body actions, such as assuming a nonthreatening posture or using hand gestures.

***Physical assault:** Abuse that may result in bodily injury.

***Rape:** A crime of violence or one committed under threat of violence involving a sexual attack. *See also Sexual Assault.*

***Sexual assault:** Forcing another person to take part in a sexual act.

***Suicide:** Self-inflicted death.

(*signifies an Enrichment section key term)

◆ Knowledge Objectives ◆

After reading this chapter and completing the class activities, you should be able to—

- Identify the signs and symptoms of critical incident stress.
- Describe actions a first responder could take to reduce or alleviate stress.
- Describe the reactions a person might have when confronted with the dying or death of another person.
- List possible emotional reactions a first responder may experience when faced with trauma, illness, death, and dying.
- Explain the importance of understanding the response to death and dying and communicating effectively with the victim's family.
- Describe the steps a first responder might take when approaching the family of a dead or dying person.
- Explain the need to determine scene safety.
- Explain the importance of being an advocate for the use of appropriate protective equipment.
- List the personal protective equipment necessary for each of the following situations: hazardous materials, rescue operations, violent scenes, crime scenes, exposure to electricity, hazardous water and airborne pathogens.

◆ Attitude Objectives ◆

After reading this chapter and completing the class activities, you should be able to—

- Recognize possible reactions of the first responder's family to the responsibilities of a first responder.
- Communicate with empathy to victims and their family members and friends.

◆ INTRODUCTION

In one way or another, a serious injury, sudden illness, or death has an emotional impact on everyone involved: victims, family, friends, bystanders, first responders, and others. The degree of impact varies from person to person. For some, the impact is minimal. They accept situations involving injury or illness that results in hospitalization, disability, or even death, and handle them well. For others, however, even a minor injury can create an extreme ***emotional crisis,*** a highly emotional state resulting from stress. The way a person responds to an emergency largely depends on his or her emotional makeup and response patterns. Therefore the way one person responds to a stressful situation can differ substantially from the response of another person in a similar situation.

You may someday encounter a situation involving a victim who is experiencing an emotional crisis. Besides providing care for any specific injury or illness, you may need to provide emotional support. The emotional crisis may be more serious than any physical problem. In some instances, the victim will be so distraught that he or she will be entirely dependent on you and your directions. Being able to understand some of what the victim is feeling can help you cope with the situation.

As a first responder, you have a duty to respond to an emergency when summoned. Although you should immediately proceed to the scene of an emergency when notified, you must do so safely. When you arrive, carefully evaluate the entire scene. Emergency scenes are often dangerous. Never enter a dangerous emergency scene unless you have been trained to do so and have the necessary equipment. Follow your established operating procedures, including when and how to access the EMS system.

This chapter describes emotional aspects of emergency medical care and how to recognize and cope with stressful situations. It also discusses the responsibilities for preparing for an emergency response and for identifying and managing initial dangers at an emergency scene.

◆ EMOTIONAL ASPECTS OF EMERGENCY CARE

First responders encounter many stressful situations when providing emergency medical care to victims. Some of theses situations include terminal illness, death, major traumatic situations, and abuse.

Stressful Situations

While providing care, you may encounter angry, scared, and violent victims. You may encounter victims of serious illness and injury and their family members. You can be affected by personal feelings triggered by these situations. You will learn what to expect and how to assist the victims, their families, your family, yourself, and others in dealing with this stress. Although it is hard to predict which type of situation will trigger a stress response, probable situations include —

- Multiple casualty incidents.
- Trauma to infants or children.
- Injuries caused by trauma.
- Infant/child/elder/spouse abuse.
- Death/injury of co-worker or other public safety personnel.

Everyone involved in a serious injury, sudden illness, or death will face an emotional crisis. Their reactions to the crisis will depend on a number of factors and will differ from person to person. Often reactions will come during or immediately following the event, but the onset of the reaction may be delayed for hours, days, or even longer. This aspect is discussed later in this chapter.

More emotional crisis situations and crisis intervention techniques are presented in the Enrichment section of this chapter.

Death and Dying

You may be summoned to an emergency in which one or more victims have died or are dying. The cause could be natural, accidental, or intentional. Though your responses will vary according to the situation, you must recognize that death will have an emotional impact on you, as well as on others involved. Dying is part of the living process. Everyone is affected by death, and response is highly individualized. Be prepared to handle your feelings and the feelings of others. Remember that reactions to death and dying range from anxiety to acceptance. How well you and others handle the situation will depend on both personal feelings about death and the nature of the incident.

One of the most disturbing situations is sudden death. This situation could involve a person who suffers a sudden illness, becomes unconscious, and later dies. It could also involve a person in what appeared to be a minor motor vehicle collision, who is alert and talkative when you arrive, but who suddenly suffers a cardiac arrest. Especially disturbing to new parents is the sudden unexplained death of an infant in the first few weeks or months of life. In situations involving sudden death, there is no time to prepare for what has happened. Suddenly a man, woman, or child who had been alive only minutes earlier is now dead.

Sometimes you may be in a situation in which you think a victim has been dead for a while and you are unsure whether you should attempt to resuscitate the victim. The general rule is to always attempt to resuscitate a body that feels warm and a victim of extreme cold. Continue efforts to resuscitate until advanced medical personnel advise you to stop.

To determine that a person is dead, he or she is often placed on a heart monitor, and vital signs are assessed. When it is determined that the victim has no heart rhythm, no pulse, no respiration, and no blood pressure, the victim is declared dead. In some instances, this will be after prolonged resuscitation attempts. At other times, additional signs, such as decapitation, **rigor mortis, lividity,** and decomposition, will cause resuscitation attempts to be withheld.

Some victims may have advance directives or **Do Not Resuscitate (DNR)** orders, written legal documents saying that they do not wish to be resuscitated or kept alive by mechanical means. In most instances, you should honor the wishes of the victim expressed in writing. However, since state and local laws about these situations vary, you should summon more advanced medical personnel immediately to provide care. If you are in doubt about the validity of the advanced directives, attempt to resuscitate.

If you must confront a victim, family, friends, or bystanders during or following a situation in which death is probable, be cautious about what you say. Avoid making statements about the victim's condition. You can provide comfort with positive statements such as, "We are doing everything we can."

The Grieving Process

Everyone involved in a sudden, unexpected, and undesired event, such as life-threatening illness or injury or the death of a loved one, experiences grief. The grieving process involves an outpouring of emotions that often follows a common pattern with various stages. These stages are not separate entities and do not necessarily follow one after the other. Instead, they often blend together. These stages include—

Anxiety—A stage characterized by a feeling of worry, uncertainty, and fear. Signs and symptoms include rapid breathing and pulse, increased activity, rapid speech, loud talking or screaming, and agitation.

Denial/disbelief—A stage in which a person refuses to accept that the event, such as the death of a loved one or a debilitating injury, has occurred.

Anger—A stage that involves an expression of aggressive verbal or physical behavior. The anger is sometimes the result of the frustration of not being able to accept the event or a feeling that not enough was done or is being done to help.

Bargaining—A stage that involves an unspoken promise of something in exchange for an extension of life or return to the previous condition.

Guilt/depression—A stage that involves placing the blame for what happened on yourself, resulting in feelings of guilt or depression. A parent will often feel guilty for an event that involves a child. A family member may feel guilty for not being able to help another family member who committed suicide.

Acceptance—The final stage of grief in which the grieving process ends and the pain and discomfort are eased. The person accepts the event and the outcome. For some people, arriving at the stage of acceptance takes weeks, months, or even years after the event. For others, such as friends or family members who are aware that a victim's condition is terminal, this stage can occur much more rapidly.

Helping the Victim and the Family

Experiencing the dying process is difficult for most people. You can use the following measures to help the victim and family deal with the dying process:

- Recognize that the victim's needs include dignity, respect, sharing, communication, privacy, and control.
- Allow family members to express rage, anger, and despair.

- Listen empathetically.
- Do not falsely reassure.
- Use a gentle tone of voice.
- Let the victim know that everything that can be done to help will be done.
- Use a reassuring touch, if it is appropriate.
- Comfort the family.

Stress Management

Stress is the body's normal response to any situation that changes a person's existing mental, physical, or emotional balance. By learning how stress builds up, how to identify the signs and symptoms, and how to manage stress, you can enjoy the responsibilities of your work without an accumulation of feelings that could make you want to quit.

Warning Signs

Responding to an emergency can become overwhelming, even to the most experienced EMS personnel. Recognizing the warning signs of stress overload will help you to begin the process of dealing with the issues.

Managing Stress

Managing stress is not as difficult as people think it is. By developing healthy physical and mental habits, you can easily manage stress on a day-to-day basis without a lot of thought. Changing lifestyles can help prevent "job burnout." Reduce sugar, caffeine, and alcohol intake, and avoid foods that are high in fat. Exercise regularly, and practice relaxation techniques, meditation, and visual imagery. Balance work, recreation, family, and health.

If feelings and emotions caused by the stress of the responsibilities of being a first responder become too overwhelming, it is right and important to seek professional help. Mental health professionals, social workers, and clergy are examples of people who are well trained to help out in high-stress situations.

First responders sometimes do not recognize how much the stress of what they do can affect their family and friends. First responders sometimes complain that their loved ones show a lack of understanding for what they do. Frustration is caused by the first responder's unwillingness to share information and feelings about an incident. First responders do not always realize that family members and friends suffer fear of separation and are afraid of being ignored for something "more exciting." Many an EMS career has been cut short by the invisible dangers of unmanaged stress. By taking a serious look at your life and making necessary adjustments, you can ensure a healthy balance in all the things you choose to do.

Common Signs and Symptoms of Stress

Irritability towards co-workers, family, and friends

Inability to concentrate

Difficulty sleeping or nightmares

Anxiety

Indecisiveness

Guilt

Loss or increase in appetite

Loss of interest in sexual activities

Isolation

Loss of interest in work and family

◆ CRITICAL INCIDENT STRESS

Researchers have recognized for years that people who provide emergency care can experience high levels of stress. Incidents involving multiple casualties, rescues, children, failed resuscitation attempts, and death or serious injury to co-workers tend to cause more stress than other incidents. However, it has only been a few years since it was generally recognized that emergency personnel needed a support system to help relieve job-related stress.

From the time you begin to establish a rapport with the victim, you become involved in the victim's pain and stress. To some degree, you share the thoughts and emotions of the victim. As a result, the emotional impact of a situation may be too great for you to handle alone. For this reason, you may need counseling to deal with the stress. Signs and symptoms of stress include loss of appetite, anxiety, guilt, irritability, and loss of interest in work.

A critical incident is a specific situation that causes a first responder to have an unusually strong emotional reaction that interferes with his or her ability to function, either immediately or in the future. The emotional impact of the situation may be more than a first responder can handle without help from counseling. Such counseling is available through a process called ***Critical Incident Stress Debriefing (CISD).*** CISD is discussed later in this chapter. Critical incident stress can build up over a period of days, weeks, months, or even years. This kind of stress reaction is referred to as ***cumulative stress.***

Critical Incident Stress Management

As was stated earlier, stress is the body's normal response to any situation that changes a person's physical, mental, or emotional balance. Many agencies and organizations have a comprehensive plan to help first responders handle stress before a crisis stage is reached. Components of a comprehensive critical incident stress management plan are —

- Pre-incident stress education.
- On-scene peer support.
- One-on-one support.
- Disaster support services.
- Critical Incident Stress Debriefing (CISD).
- Follow-up services.
- Spouse/family support.
- Community outreach programs.
- Other health and welfare programs, such as wellness programs.

Techniques for Coping with Critical Incident Stress

Two techniques are commonly used to help deal with critical stress situations. These processes bring you together with peer counselors and mental health professionals who are trained in techniques to help accelerate the recovery process after a critical incident.

Critical Incident Stress Debriefing (CISD)

This type of meeting is usually held within 24 to 72 hours of a major incident. At this meeting, which is not an investigation or interrogation, participants are encouraged to have an open discussion of feelings, fears, and reactions triggered by the incident. All information shared at these meetings is confidential. CISD leaders and mental health professionals evaluate the information and offer suggestions on overcoming the stress.

CISD is not just used for those incidents involving death or major disasters. Any incident, such as a dramatic, lifesaving rescue, is a potential source of an emotional crisis. Even though the outcome of such an incident would be completely different from one involving death, the emotions and stress factors would still be present. It is important that the rescuer, rescue teams, and any others closely involved in an incident involving significant stress be debriefed. CISD can also benefit the layperson who performs CPR before you arrive, only to learn that the victim was pronounced dead soon after arriving at the hospital.

Critical Incident Stress Defusing

Defusings are much shorter than debriefings. They are less formal and less structured. Defusings are effective in the first few hours after the event and usually last 30 to 45 minutes. Advantages of defusings are that they allow for immediate, initial venting and may even eliminate the need for a formal debriefing. If the choice is made to have a formal debriefing meeting, discussions shared in the defusing may enhance the subsequent meeting. Defusings are often done on a one-on-one basis between the rescuer and a peer counselor.

When to Access CISD

Incidents that could lead to activation of the CISD team include—

- Line-of-duty death or serious injury.
- Multiple casualty incidents.
- Suicide of an emergency worker.
- Serious injury or death of children.
- Events with excessive media attention.
- Victims known to the emergency care personnel.
- Events that have unusual impact on the emergency care personnel.
- Any disaster.

Activation protocols of CISD teams vary from area to area. Your instructor should be able to supply you with information on how to access this service in your particular area.

Some people think that participating in CISD is an admission of weakness—quite the contrary. CISD should be, and in many areas is, a routine part of any overwhelming incident, such as an airline disaster. CISD can help in any situation, regardless of how minor you may think the event was. The most important thing you can do to minimize the effects of any emergency is to express your feelings and thoughts after the incident. Check with your local agency to see what resources are available to you.

Primary Responsibilities of the First Responder

1. Ensure safety for yourself and any bystanders.
2. Gain access to the victim.
3. Determine any threats to the victim's life.
4. Summon more advanced personnel as needed.
5. Provide needed care for the victim.
6. Assist medical personnel as needed.

◆ THE EMERGENCY SCENE

Almost every emergency response carries a certain risk to the safety of the first responder. Upon arrival at the emergency scene, safety should be the first priority of the first responder. Safety includes both personal safety and the safety of others.

Scene Safety

Scene safety requires the assessment of the scene and surroundings that provides valuable information about the emergency situation and helps ensure the well-being of the first responder.

Some emergency scenes are immediately dangerous. Others may become dangerous while you are providing care. Sometimes the dangers are obvious, such as fire or hostile victims or bystanders. Other dangers may be less obvious, such as the presence of a hazardous material or unstable structures.

Personal Safety

Of the primary responsibilities of the first responder discussed in Chapter 1, safety should always be foremost. You cannot overlook ensuring adequate safety for yourself. Often it requires only simple tasks to make an emergency scene safe.

Approach all emergency scenes cautiously until you can size up the situation. If you arrive at the scene by vehicle, park a safe distance away. If the scene appears safe, continue to evaluate the situation as you approach (Fig. 2-1).

Pay particular attention to the—

- Location of the emergency.
- Extent of the emergency.
- Apparent scene dangers.

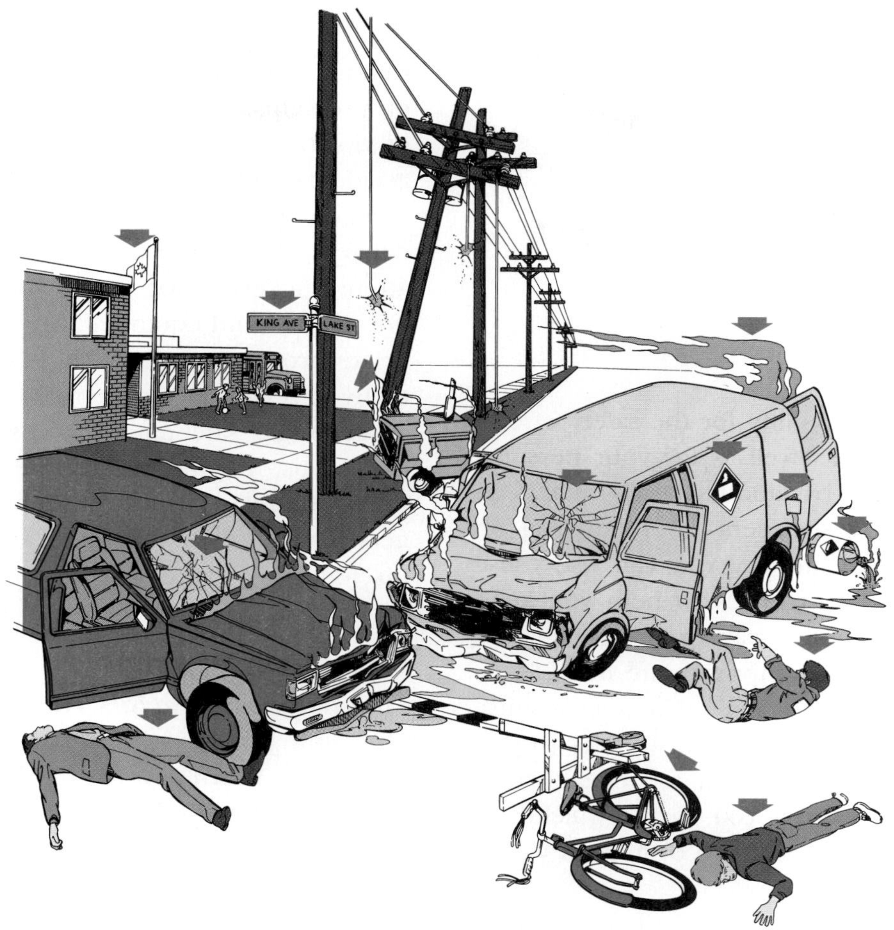

Figure 2-1 Note the location of the emergency, the dangers, the number of victims, and other important information while approaching an emergency scene.

- Apparent number of ill or injured people.
- Behavior of the victim(s) and bystanders.

If at any time the scene appears unsafe, retreat to a safe distance. Notify additional personnel and wait for their arrival. This principle cannot be overemphasized. *Never* enter a dangerous scene unless you have the training and equipment to do so safely. Well-meaning rescuers have been injured or killed because they forgot to watch for hazards. If your training has not prepared you for a specific emergency, such as a fire or an incident involving hazardous materials, notify appropriate personnel.

When arriving on an emergency scene, always follow these four guidelines to ensure your personal safety and that of the bystanders:

- Take time to evaluate the scene. Doing so will enable you to recognize existing and potential dangers.
- Wear appropriate personal protective equipment for the situation and be a constant advocate for the use of appropriate protective equipment at all times.
- *Do not attempt to do anything you are not trained to do.* Know what resources are available to help.
- Get the help you need. If you have not already done so, notify additional personnel. Be able to describe the scene and the type of additional help required.

Another important aspect of personal safety is protecting yourself from exposure to communicable diseases. This is especially important if providing care for a victim when body fluids may be present. Since it is impossible to know if a person may be infected or not, you should always take protective measures. These protective measures are known as body substance isolation (BSI) and are discussed in detail in Chapter 3.

Safety of Others

You have a responsibility for the safety of others at the scene, as well as for your personal safety. Discourage bystanders, family members, or unprepared responders from entering an area that appears unsafe. You can use these well-intentioned individuals to help you keep unauthorized people away from unsafe areas and to summon more appropriate help. Some dangers may require you to take special measures, such as placing physical barriers to prevent onlookers from getting too close. Other situations may require you to act quickly to free someone who is trapped or move a victim in immediate danger to safety.

Ideally, you should move victims only after you have assessed and properly cared for them. If, however, immediate dangers threaten a victim's life, you must decide whether to move him or her. If the situation is dangerous and you cannot move the victim, retreat to safety yourself. If you can move the victim, do so quickly and safely.

Situations that may require an **emergency move** include—

- The presence of explosives or other hazardous materials (such as a natural gas leak).
- Fire or the danger of fire.
- The inability to make the scene safe (such as a structure about to collapse).
- The need to get to other victims requiring lifesaving care.

Chapter 6 provides more detailed information on how to safely move injured or ill victims.

Specific Emergency Situations

Certain emergency scenes present a special set of problems. These situations include scenes of violence, scenes with dangers such as traffic accidents, and scenes with hazardous materials.

Since every emergency scene has potential dangers, always expect the unexpected. Never attempt a rescue for which you are not properly trained and equipped. Always wear appropriate protective gear, such as gloves and protective eyewear. Be aware that at any time even a seemingly safe emergency scene can turn dangerous. Always take the necessary precautions when you suspect or identify certain dangers. Several of the following situations are also discussed in Chapter 19.

Hazardous Materials

Hazardous materials (HAZMAT) are common and pose a special risk for responding personnel. When you approach an emergency scene, look for clues that indicate the presence of hazardous materials. These include—

- Signs (placards) on vehicles, storage facilities, or railroad cars identifying the presence of hazardous materials.
- Clouds of vapor.
- Spilled liquids or solids.
- Unusual odors.
- Leaking containers, bottles, or gas cylinders.
- Chemical transport tanks or containers.

Those who transport or store hazardous materials in specific quantities are required by the U.S. Department of Transportation to post placards identifying specific hazardous material, by name or number, and its dangers (Fig. 2-2).

Identification is important, and it is helpful to have binoculars on hand. Binoculars allow you to view the scene from a safe distance. If you do not see a placard but suspect a hazardous material is present, try to get information before you approach the scene. Do not approach a HAZMAT scene unless you are trained to do so and have appropriate personal

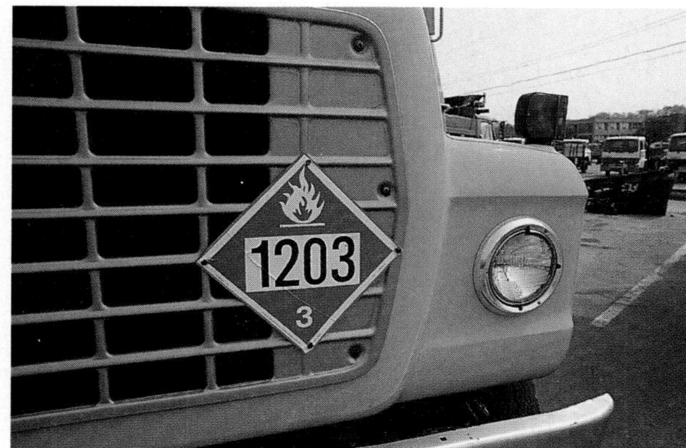

Figure 2-2 By law, specific types of placards must indicate the presence of hazardous materials.

protective equipment such as a self-contained breathing apparatus and chemical protective suit.

Motor Vehicle Crashes

The wreckage of automobiles, aircraft, or machinery may contain hazards, such as sharp pieces of metal or glass, fuel, and moving parts. Other potential threats to life are electricity, fire, explosion, hazardous materials, and traffic. The wreckage may be unstable. Do not try to rescue someone from wreckage unless you have the proper training and equipment, such as **turnout gear,** safety glasses, gloves, and a helmet. Specialized rescue teams can be called in for extensive or heavy rescue. Care for the victim is given only after the wreckage has been stabilized. Gather as much information as you can, and make sure advanced medical personnel have been called.

Violence

If you arrive at the scene of violence or a crime, do not try to reach any victim until you are sure the scene is safe. A victim of a shooting, stabbing, or other violence may have severe injuries, but until the scene is safe, there is nothing you can do to provide care. For the scene to be safe, law enforcement personnel must make it secure.

Police usually gather evidence at a crime scene, so do not touch anything except what you must to give care. Once you are approved to enter a crime scene to give care, make sure that law enforcement personnel are aware of your presence and actions and that you have appropriate equipment for protection against potentially infectious body substances (Table 2-1).

◆ SUMMARY

An emotional crisis often results from an unexpected, shocking, and undesired event, such as the sudden loss of a loved one. Although people react differently in different situations, everyone experiences some or all of the stages of grief. By considering the nature of the incident, you can begin to prepare yourself to deal with its emotional aspects.

Regardless of the nature of the event, however, the care you provide to victims of any emotional crisis is very similar. Your care involves both appropriate verbal and nonverbal communication. It also requires you to under-

Table 2-1 Responding to Specific Emergency Situations

Situation	Appropriate behavior
Hazardous materials	If you suspect hazardous materials, stay a safe distance away, upwind and uphill. *Do not* create sparks. Notify the fire department immediately.
Motor vehicle crashes	*Do not* attempt a rescue until wreckage has been stabilized.
Violence	*Do not* enter the scene until summoned by law enforcement personnel. *Do not* touch anything except what you must to give care.

stand that in some cases death is inevitable. In some situations, you may be overcome by emotion. Remember that self-help involves sharing your feelings with others.

Emergency scenes by their nature can be dangerous, so never approach a scene until you are sure it is safe. Your personal safety is always your first concern. Potential hazards at emergency scenes include traffic, fire, electricity, and hazardous materials. Other dangers include violence or crime scenes. If you have any doubt about the safety of a scene or if you are not trained and equipped to handle the situation, stay back and keep other untrained people out of the area. Be sure appropriate help has been called, and wait for properly trained and equipped personnel. Once you are sure the scene is safe, you will be expected to provide care to ill or injured victims.

Use the activities in Unit 2 of the workbook to help you review the material in this chapter.

You Are the Responder

1. You are summoned to a home where a 39-year-old father of three children has attempted suicide by carbon monoxide poisoning. He was found by his oldest child, age 14, in the car in the garage. You try to resuscitate the victim until more advanced medical personnel arrive and take over. As they begin to work on him, the victim's wife comes home. She immediately rushes screaming to her husband. You help restrain her so that the paramedics can continue to try to resuscitate him. You move her away, and the sobbing children run to her. Describe her emotions at this scene. How would you care for this woman and her children?
2. While trying to help a pedestrian who has been hit by a car, you are distracted because a noisy crowd has gathered. Should you move the victim? Why or why not? What should you do?

ENRICHMENT

◆ SPECIFIC EMOTIONAL CRISES

Many different situations can result in emotional crisis for the victim or bystanders. Examples commonly encountered by emergency personnel include attempted suicide, sexual or physical assault, the sudden death of a loved one, or a dying victim.

Suicide

You respond to a call for help from a distraught mother who states her 15-year-old son is having trouble breathing. She says he is in his bedroom crying uncontrollably. She also states that he has been depressed because of the recent death of a close friend and classmate.

When you arrive, you approach the bedroom and find the door closed and locked. You speak to the victim from outside the bedroom. He has stopped crying. You ask him to unlock the door. You can barely make out his shape in the darkened room as he opens the door. He appears to be breathing normally now. He requests that you and his mother leave him alone.

You suggest that he come out of the bedroom

to talk. He eventually complies and begins to talk about his problems dealing with the recent death of his girlfriend. He says no one understands how he feels. He also says he had thought once about killing himself.

Both you and the mother console him. Soon he appears better and states he is OK. You suggest to the mother, in the boy's absence, that she get psychological counseling for him immediately because of his suicide remark. You offer to call a counselor with a mental health agency. The mother says she has called her minister and he will arrive shortly. She also states that she will seek additional help later today after speaking with her husband who is out of town.

You leave the home, feeling as if you have averted an emotional crisis that could have had a serious consequence. You feel you did all you could and that the mother will get her son the professional help he needs. Unfortunately, you later find out that the boy went drinking several days later with friends and used a handgun to end his life.

In the time it took you to read this scenario, someone in the United States tried to end his or her life. More than 30,000 Americans kill themselves each year (Fig. 2-3). Many more make unsuccessful attempts. Males committing suicide outnumber females four to one. Suicide is the third leading cause of death among people ages 15 to 24. People commit suicide in a number of ways, but using a gun is the most common method, accounting for more than 50 percent of all suicide deaths. Many people who attempt suicide suffer some form of mental or emotional problem or illness. Substance misuse or abuse, primarily of alcohol and other drugs, plays a major role in attempted suicides.

What motivates a person to suddenly try to commit suicide? The motivation is often a combination of unbearable underlying tensions caused by a major event in a person's life, such as—

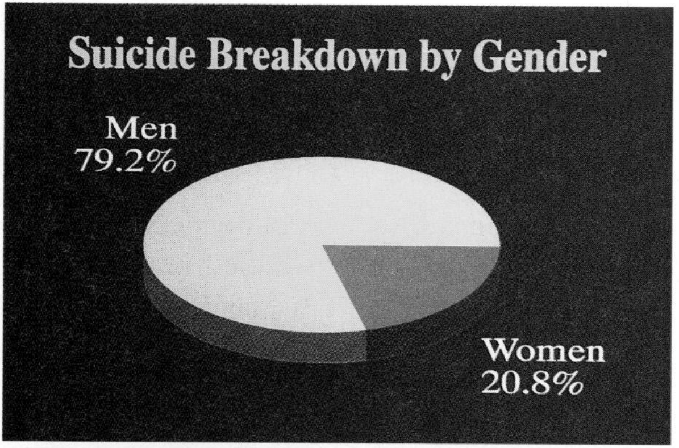

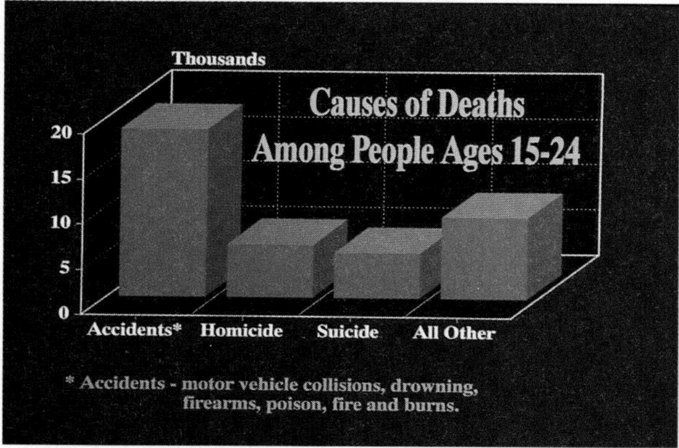

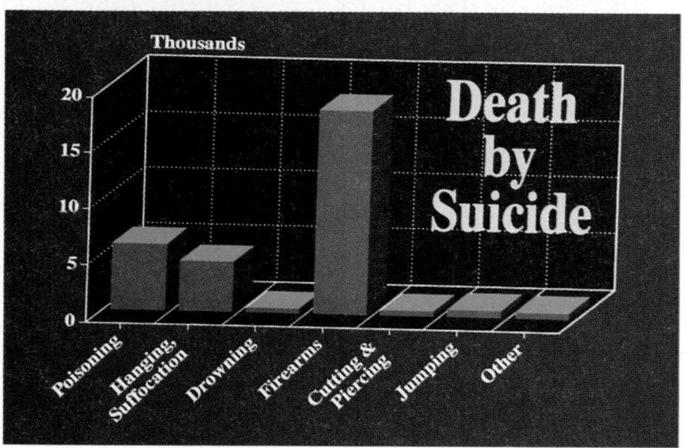

Figure 2-3 Suicide Statistics
(Data from National Safety Council, Accident Facts, 1991.)

- A failing or failed relationship with a spouse, family, or friend.
- Serious illness or death of a close family member or friend.
- Serious, prolonged, or chronic personal illness.
- A long period of failure at work or school.
- A long period of unemployment.

- Failure to achieve sufficient occupational, educational, or financial success.
- Dramatic change in the economy.

Assault

Assault is an all too common occurrence in our society. It can be threatened or actual, and physical, sexual, or both. It may result in injury and often emotional distress to the victim.

Sexual Assault

Sexual assault occurs when one person takes advantage of another by rape or forces a person to take part in any sexual act. ***Rape*** is a crime of violence, or one committed under threat of violence, that involves a sexual attack, either heterosexual or homosexual. Rape is a devastating experience for the victim. Victims often feel degraded, extremely frightened, and at further risk for attack. Victims of rape require significant emotional support.

Besides providing emotional support, you must care for any injuries the victim may have received. When caring for a victim of sexual assault, do the following:

- Cover the victim and protect him or her from unnecessary exposure.
- Clear the area of any bystanders except those friends or family able to help provide emotional support.
- Do not remove any clothing unless absolutely necessary to provide care for injuries.
- Care for any physical injuries.
- Discourage the victim from bathing, showering, or douching before a medical examination can be performed.
- Do not disrupt the crime scene by handling items unrelated to the victim's care.
- Do not question the victim about the specifics of the assault.
- Summon more advanced medical personnel and law enforcement personnel.

Physical Assault

Physical assault on a child, spouse, or the elderly occurs more frequently than reported. Unfortunately, when you are summoned, the assault has often resulted in more serious injuries. The emergency scene where a physical assault has occurred is not always safe. The attacker may still be present or nearby. If the scene involves domestic violence, it may not be clear what has happened. Substances, such as alcohol, may be involved. In such situations, remember that your first concern is always your personal safety. If you are not trained in law enforcement, do not approach the scene until it is determined to be safe. As with sexual assault, the scene is a crime scene. Therefore, do not handle items unrelated to the victim's care. Reassure and comfort the victim while providing care.

◆ CRISIS INTERVENTION

Regardless of the nature of the incident, caring for someone experiencing an emotional crisis involves offering emotional support, as well as caring for any specific injury. The most important initial step you can take is to communicate with the victim in an open manner. Communication can be both verbal and nonverbal.

Nonverbal communication refers to your actions. Sometimes your actions (body language) say more than you intend. You should always be aware of the messages you are sending with your body. General body posture is an important aspect of nonverbal communication. Begin by assuming a non-threatening posture. Doing so involves getting at eye level with the victim and looking at the victim as you talk. Avoid making physical contact. Also, avoid positions such as placing your arms across your chest, your hands on your hips, pointing at the victim, or leaning over and looking down at the victim.

As you begin to communicate verbally, remember that communication involves stimulating discussion and listening as much as talking. When you do talk, speak in a calm, reassuring manner. Ask the victim his or her name, and use it frequently in conversation. One technique used to help you more fully communicate is "active listening." The process of

active listening requires you to listen closely to what the person is saying. It involves four behaviors:

- Make every effort to understand fully what the victim is trying to say.
- Repeat back to the victim, in your own words, what he or she said.
- Avoid criticism, anger, or rejection of the victim's statements.
- Use open-ended questions such as, "What are you feeling?" or, "What problems are you having?" Generally, avoid questions that can be answered with "yes" or "no."

Victims of emotional crisis may be withdrawn or hysterical. Some may be entirely dependent on you to help. Avoid being judgmental. Do not place blame on the victim. The victim needs to be cared for gently and with respect. If care is needed for a minor injury, try to get the victim to help you (Fig. 2-4). By encouraging the victim to participate, you may help the victim regain a sense of control that he or she had lost.

Do not be fooled into thinking that you can manage a situation involving emotional crisis yourself. A suicidal person or a rape victim needs professional counseling. Summon more advanced personnel. They could include law enforcement, EMS, or local mental health or rape crisis center personnel. While waiting for others to arrive, continue to talk with the victim.

◆ DEALING WITH EMERGENCY SITUATIONS AT THE SCENE

In addition to the specific emergency situations discussed earlier that a first responder may encounter, other hazardous scenes require special consideration (Table 2-2). Remember to always expect the unexpected and make sure the scene is safe before entering. If it is not, then notify the necessary agencies to do what is necessary to provide you a safe working environment.

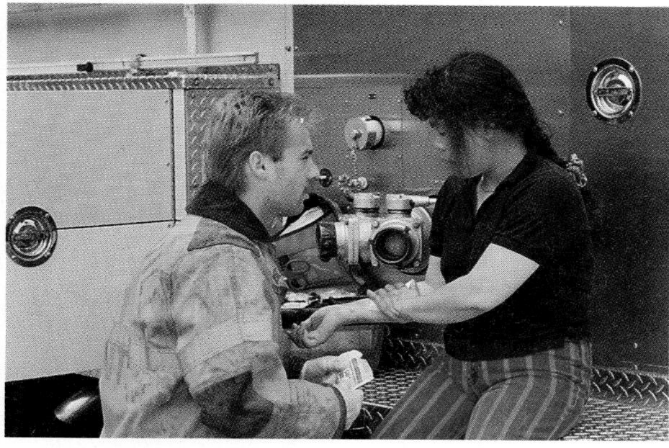

Figure 2-4 Have the victim help you when you give care.

Traffic

Traffic is often the most common danger you and other emergency personnel will encounter. If you drive to a collision scene, always try to park where your vehicle will not block other traffic, such as an ambulance that needs to reach the scene. The *only* time you should park in a roadway or block traffic is to —

- Protect an injured person.
- Protect any rescuers, including yourself.
- Warn oncoming traffic if the situation is not clearly visible.

Others can help you put reflectors, flares, or lights along the road. These items should be placed well back of the scene to enable oncoming motorists to stop or slow down in time.

Emergency personnel have been injured or killed by traffic at emergency scenes. If you are not a law enforcement officer, and dangerous traffic makes the scene unsafe, wait for more help to arrive before giving care.

Fire

Any fire can be dangerous. Make sure that the local fire department has been summoned. Only fire fighters, who are highly trained and use equipment that protects them against fire and smoke, should approach a fire. Do not let others approach. Gather information to help

Table 2-2 Additional Emergency Situations

Situation	Appropriate behavior
Traffic	Leave a path for arriving emergency vehicles. Put up reflectors, flares, or lights to direct dangerous traffic away from the scene.
Fire	Never approach a burning vehicle or enter a burning building without proper equipment and training. If in a burning building, *do not* open hot doors or use elevators, and stay close to the floor.
Electricity	Assume all downed wires are dangerous. *Do not* attempt to move them. *Do not* touch any metal fence, metal structure, or body of water in contact with a wire. Notify fire department and power company immediately.
Water and ice	Follow the rule of reach, throw, and row. Never enter water or go on ice unless you are trained to do so and have proper rescue equipment.
Unsafe structures	*Do not* enter structures that you suspect are unsafe. Call for trained and equipped personnel. Gather as much information as possible about the victim(s).
Natural disasters	Report to the person in charge. Follow the rescue plan. Avoid obvious hazards and be cautious when using equipment.
Multiple victims	Report to the person in charge. Care for victims with the most life-threatening conditions first.
Hostile situations	If the victim or bystanders threaten you, retreat to safety. Never try to restrain, argue with, or force your care on a victim. Summon law enforcement personnel.
Suicide	*Do not* enter until summoned by law enforcement personnel. *Do not* touch anything except what you must to give care.
Hostage situations	*Do not* enter until summoned by law enforcement personnel. Gather as much information as possible about the victims.

the responding fire and EMS units. Find out the possible number of people trapped, their location, the fire's cause, and whether any explosives or chemicals are present. Give this information to emergency personnel when they arrive. If you are not trained to fight fires or lack the necessary equipment, follow these basic guidelines:

- Do not approach a burning vehicle.
- Never enter a burning or smoke-filled building.
- If you are in a building that is on fire, always check doors before opening them (Fig. 2-5, *A*). If a door is hot to the touch, *do not* open it.
- Since smoke and fumes rise, stay close to the floor (Fig. 2-5, *B*).
- Never use an elevator in a building that may be burning.

Electricity

Downed electrical lines also present a major hazard to responders. Always look for downed wires at a scene, and always treat them as dan-

A 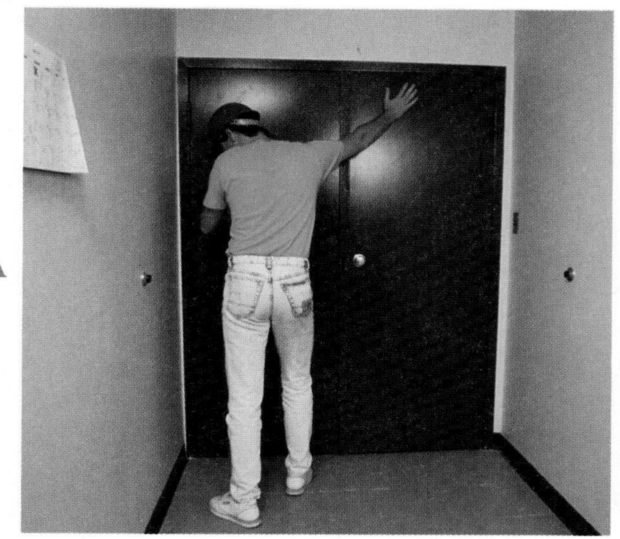 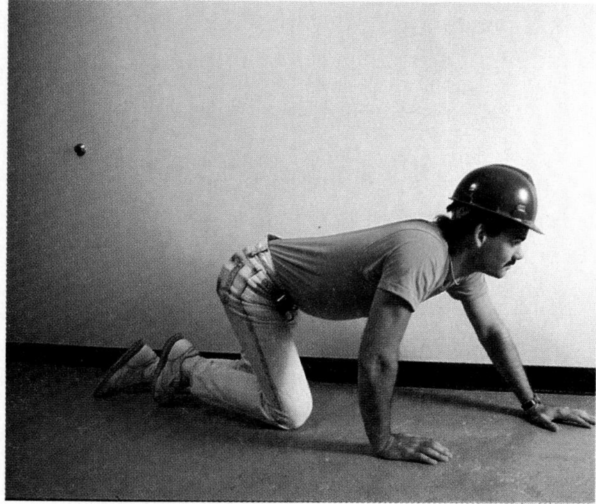 B

Figure 2-5 **A,** If a door in a burning building is hot to the touch, do not open it. **B,** Stay close to the floor to avoid rising smoke and fumes.

gerous. If you find downed wires, follow these guidelines:

- Move any crowd back from the danger zone. The safe area should be established at a point twice the length of the span (distance between the poles) of the wire.
- *Never attempt to move downed wires.*
- Notify the fire department and power company immediately. Always assume that the wires are energized, or live. Even if they are not energized at first, they may become energized later.
- *If downed wires contact a vehicle, do not touch the vehicle and do not let others touch it.* Tell anyone in the vehicle to stay still and stay inside the vehicle. Never attempt to remove people from a vehicle with downed wires across it, no matter how seriously injured they may seem.
- Do not touch any metal fence, metal structure, or body of water in contact with a downed wire. Wait for the power company to shut off the power source.

Water and Ice

Water and ice also can be serious hazards. To help a conscious person in the water, always follow the basic rule of "reach, throw, and row." You may reach out to someone in trouble with a branch, a pole, or even your hand, being careful not to be pulled into the water. When the person grasps the object, pull him or her to safety.

If you cannot reach the person, try to throw him or her something nearby that floats. If you have a rope available, attach a floatable object, such as a life jacket, plastic jug, ice chest, or empty gas can, to one end. *Never enter a body of water to rescue someone unless you have been trained in water rescue and then only as a last resort.*

Fast-moving water is extremely dangerous and often occurs with floods, hurricanes, and low head dams. Ice is also treacherous. It can break under your weight, and the cold water beneath can quickly overcome even the best swimmers. *Never enter fast-moving water or venture out on ice unless you are trained in this type of rescue.* Such rescues require careful planning and proper equipment. Wait until trained personnel arrive.

Unsafe Structures

Buildings and other structures, such as mines, wells, and unreinforced trenches, can become unsafe because of fire, explosions, natural disasters, deterioration, or other causes. An unsafe building or structure is one in which—

- The air may contain debris or hazardous gases.
- There is a possibility of being trapped or injured by collapsed walls, weakened floors, and other debris.

Try to establish the exact or probable location of anyone in the structure. Gather as much information as you can, call for appropriate help, and wait for the arrival of personnel who are properly trained and equipped.

Natural Disasters

Natural disasters include tornadoes, hurricanes, earthquakes, forest fires, and floods. Rescue efforts after a natural disaster are usually coordinated by local resources until they become overwhelmed. Then the rescue efforts are coordinated by a government agency such as the Federal Emergency Management Agency (FEMA) (Fig. 2-6). Typically, you would report to the person or people in charge at the scene, then work with the disaster response team and follow the rescue plan.

Natural disasters pose more risks than you might be aware of. More injuries and deaths result from electricity, hazardous materials, rising water, and other dangers than from the disaster itself. When responding to a natural disaster, be sure to carefully survey the scene, avoid obvious hazards, and use caution when operating rescue equipment. Never use gasoline-powered equipment, such as chain saws, generators, and pumps, in confined spaces.

Multiple Victims

Scenes that involve more than one victim are referred to as multiple casualty incidents (MCIs). Such scenes make your task more complex, since you must determine who needs immediate care and who can wait for more help to arrive. Multiple casualty incidents are covered in more detail in Chapter 19.

Hostile Situations

Environmental factors, such as hazardous materials, electricity, and unsafe structures, are not the only dangers you may encounter. You may sometimes encounter a hostile victim or family member. Any unusual or hostile behavior may be a result of the emergency. A victim's rage or hostility may be caused by the injury or illness or by fear. Many victims are afraid of losing control and may show this as anger. Hostile behavior may also result from the use of alcohol or other drugs, lack of oxygen, or an underlying medical condition.

If a person needing care is hostile toward you, try to calmly explain who you are and that you are there to help. Remember that you cannot give care without the person's consent. If the person accepts your offer to help, keep talking to him or her as you assess that person's condition. When the person realizes that you are not a threat, the hostility usually goes away.

If the person refuses your care or threatens you, withdraw from the scene. Never try to restrain, argue with, or force your care on a victim. If the victim does not let you provide care, wait for additional help. Sometimes a close friend or a family member will be able to reassure a hostile victim and convince that person to accept your care.

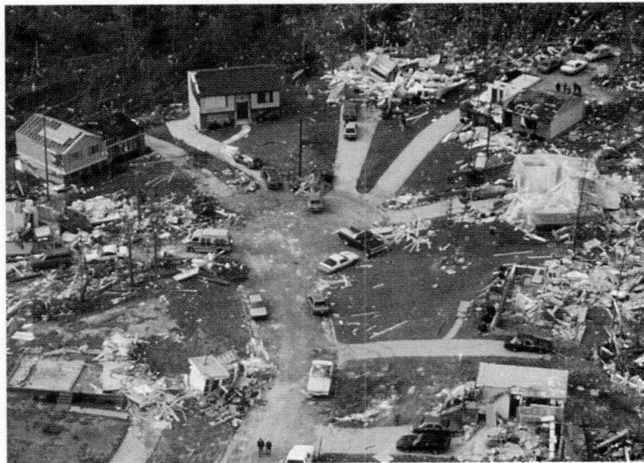

Figure 2-6 Rescue efforts after large natural disasters are often managed by the Federal Emergency Management Agency in coordination with local resources.

Family members or friends who are angry or hysterical, however, can make your job more difficult. Sometimes they may not allow you to provide care. At other times, they may try to move the victim before you have stabilized him or her. A terrified parent may cling to a child and refuse to let you help. When family members act this way, they often feel confused, guilty, and frightened. Be understanding and explain the care you are giving. By remaining calm and professional, you will help calm them.

Hostile crowds are a threat that can develop when you least expect it. As a rule, you cannot reason with a hostile crowd. If you decide the crowd at a scene is hostile, wait at a safe distance until law enforcement and EMS personnel arrive. Approach the scene only when police officers declare it safe and ask you to help. *Never approach a hostile crowd unless you are trained in crowd management and supported by other trained personnel.*

Suicide

Never enter a suicide scene unless police have made it secure. If the person is obviously dead, be careful not to touch anything at the scene such as a weapon, medicine bottle, suicide note, or other evidence. If the scene is safe and the person is still alive, give emergency care as needed. Concentrate on your care for the patient and leave the rest to law enforcement personnel.

Never approach an armed suicidal person unless you are a law enforcement officer trained in crisis intervention. Only approach if you have been summoned to provide care once the scene has been made secure.

If you happen to be on the scene when an unarmed person threatens suicide, try to reassure and calm the person. Make sure that appropriate personnel have been notified. You cannot physically restrain a suicidal person without medical or legal authorization. Listen to him or her, and try to keep the person talking until help arrives. Try to be understanding. Many suicide attempts are an attempt to get help. Do not dare the person to act or trivialize his or her feelings. *Unless your personal safety is threatened, never leave a suicidal person alone.*

Hostage Situations

If you encounter a hostage situation, your first priority is to not become a hostage yourself. Do not approach the scene unless you are specially trained to handle these situations. Assess the scene from a safe distance and call for law enforcement personnel. A police officer trained in hostage negotiations should take charge.

Try to get any information from bystanders that may help law enforcement personnel. Ask about the number of hostages, any weapons seen, and other possible hazards. Report any information to the first law enforcement official on the scene. Remain at a safe distance until law enforcement personnel summon you.

You Are the Responder

You are the first on the scene of a burning building. Smoke is pouring from the doors and windows. A young girl tells you her brother is still in the building. The fire department is en route, but it will be another 5 minutes before they arrive. You have no fire protection clothing or equipment and only minimal training. What should you do?

Preventing Disease Transmission

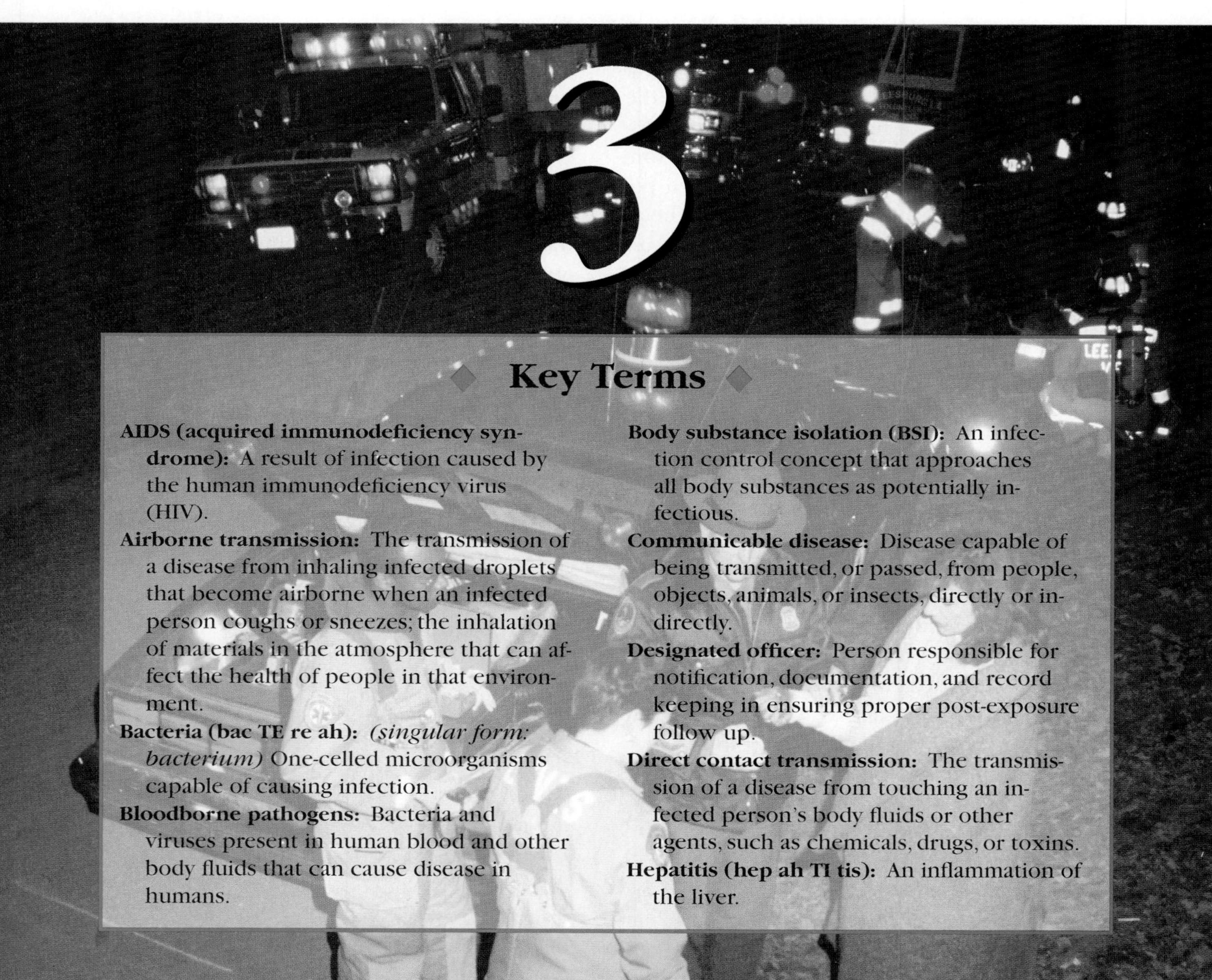

Key Terms

AIDS (acquired immunodeficiency syndrome): A result of infection caused by the human immunodeficiency virus (HIV).

Airborne transmission: The transmission of a disease from inhaling infected droplets that become airborne when an infected person coughs or sneezes; the inhalation of materials in the atmosphere that can affect the health of people in that environment.

Bacteria (bac TE re ah): *(singular form: bacterium)* One-celled microorganisms capable of causing infection.

Bloodborne pathogens: Bacteria and viruses present in human blood and other body fluids that can cause disease in humans.

Body substance isolation (BSI): An infection control concept that approaches all body substances as potentially infectious.

Communicable disease: Disease capable of being transmitted, or passed, from people, objects, animals, or insects, directly or indirectly.

Designated officer: Person responsible for notification, documentation, and record keeping in ensuring proper post-exposure follow up.

Direct contact transmission: The transmission of a disease from touching an infected person's body fluids or other agents, such as chemicals, drugs, or toxins.

Hepatitis (hep ah TI tis): An inflammation of the liver.

Herpes (HER pez) simplex: A viral infection that causes eruptions of the skin and mucous membranes.

HIV (human immunodeficiency virus): A virus that destroys the body's ability to fight infection. A result of HIV infection is referred to as AIDS.

Immune system: The body's group of responses for fighting disease.

Immunization (im u nĭ ZA shun): A specific substance containing weakened or killed pathogens introduced into the body to build resistance to specific infection.

Indirect contact transmission: The transmission of a disease from touching a contaminated object.

Infection: A condition caused by disease-producing microorganisms, called pathogens or germs, in the body.

Infectious disease: Disease caused by the invasion of the body by a pathogen, such as a bacterium, virus, fungus, or parasite.

Meningitis (men in JI tis): An inflammation of the brain or spinal cord caused by ral or bacterial infection.

Pathogen (PATH ah jen): A disease-causing agent; also called a microorganism or germ.

Standard precautions: Safety measures, such as body substance isolation, taken to prevent occupational-risk exposure to blood or other potentially infectious materials, such as body fluids containing visible blood.

Tuberculosis (tu ber ku LO sis) (TB): A disease, commonly respiratory, caused by a bacterium.

Vector transmission: The transmission of a disease by an animal or insect bite through exposure to blood or other body fluids.

Viruses (VI rusez): *(singular form: virus)* Disease-causing agents, or pathogens, that unlike bacteria, require another organism to live and reproduce.

◆ Knowledge Objectives ◆

After reading this chapter and completing the class activities, you should be able to—

- Describe how the immune system works.
- Identify ways in which diseases are transmitted and give an example of how each transmission can occur.
- Describe the conditions that must be present for disease transmission.
- Identify how each of the following communicable diseases is transmitted:
  Hepatitis A
  Hepatitis B (HBV)
  Hepatitis C
  Herpes
  Meningitis
  Tuberculosis
  Human immunodeficiency virus (HIV) infection
- Explain the importance of body substance isolation (BSI).
- Identify body substance isolation (BSI) techniques for protecting yourself against communicable disease.
- Describe the steps the first responder should take for personal protection from airborne and bloodborne pathogens.
- Describe the procedure a first responder would use to disinfect equipment, work surfaces, clothing, and leather items.

- Explain the importance of documenting an exposure to a communicable disease and post-exposure follow-up care.
- Explain how the OSHA guidelines for bloodborne and airborne pathogens influence your actions as a first responder.

◆ Attitude Objectives ◆

After reading this chapter and completing the class activities, you should be able to —

- Acknowledge the importance of knowing how various communicable diseases are transmitted.
- Appreciate the short- and long-term effects a person with an infectious disease may experience.
- Appreciate the importance of protecting yourself from disease transmission.
- Recognize the risks to the first responder from communicable diseases, and the importance of using proper body substance isolation (BSI).
- Appreciate the need for proper documentation and reporting should an exposure occur.

◆ Skill Objectives ◆

After reading this chapter and completing the class activities, you should be able to —

- Demonstrate the proper techniques for placing and removing personal protective equipment.
- Given a scenario in which potential communicable exposure takes place, the first responder will use appropriate personal protective equipment and will properly remove and discard the protective garments.

◆ INTRODUCTION

On December 6, 1991, the Occupational Safety and Health Administration (OSHA) issued final regulations on occupational exposure to bloodborne pathogens. These pathogens are bacteria and viruses that may be present in human blood and other potentially infectious materials (OPIM) and can cause disease in humans. These other potentially infectious materials include the following:

- Semen
- Vaginal secretions
- Cerebrospinal fluid (fluid that flows through the brain and spinal cord)
- Synovial fluid (fluid that lubricates many joints and tendons)

- Pleural fluid (fluid that lubricates the lungs)
- Pericardial fluid (fluid that lubricates the heart and the space it is in)
- Amniotic fluid (fluid that surrounds the fetus during pregnancy)
- Peritoneal fluid (fluid that lubricates the abdominal cavity)

OSHA has determined that employees are at risk when they are exposed on the job to blood and other materials that may cause infections. These materials may contain certain pathogens. These pathogens include hepatitis B virus (HBV), which causes hepatitis B, the hepatitis C virus (HCV), which also causes hepatitis, and human immunodeficiency virus (HIV), which causes AIDS. The agency further concludes that this hazard can be minimized or eliminated by using a combination of engineering and work practice controls, personal protective clothing and equipment, training, medical surveillance, hepatitis B vaccination, signs and labels, and other provisions.

The regulation defines the range of employees it covers. Any employee who has occupational exposure to blood or other potentially infectious materials is included within the scope of this standard. The hazard of exposure to infectious materials affects employees in many types of employment and is not restricted to the health care industry. Employees in the following jobs are automatically covered if they have occupational exposure:

- Employees in health-care facilities
- Employees in clinics in industrial, educational, and correctional facilities
- Employees whose job responsibilities are or include providing emergency first aid
- Employees who handle regulated (hazardous) waste
- Emergency medical technicians, paramedics, and other emergency medical services providers
- Fire fighters, law enforcement personnel, correctional officers, and employees in the private sector, the federal government, or a state or local government in a state that has an OSHA-approved state plan
- Linen service employees

The definition and the list of employees covered by the standard does not include any "Good Samaritan" acts that result in exposure to blood or other potentially infectious materials from assisting a fellow employee. However, OSHA requires employers to offer follow-up procedures in such cases.

As a first responder, you will be in situations in which disease transmission is a concern. For this reason, you need to understand how infections occur, how they are transmitted, and what you can do to protect yourself and others.

Infectious diseases that can be transmitted from people, objects, animals, or insects, directly or indirectly, are often called ***communicable diseases.*** Some diseases can be transmitted more easily than others. ***Infectious diseases*** are caused by invasion of the body by a pathogen such as a bacterium, virus, fungus, or parasite. A disease can be infectious but not communicable. This chapter presents basic concepts of **disease transmission.** You will learn how to recognize situations that have the potential for disease transmission and how to protect yourself and others from contracting disease.

◆ HOW INFECTIONS OCCUR

To better understand disease transmission, it helps to understand how diseases occur. This understanding will help you better identify the type of ***body substance isolation (BSI)*** techniques you should be using.

Disease-Causing Agents

The disease process begins when a ***pathogen*** invades the body. A pathogen is an extremely small disease-causing agent. It is also called a microorganism or germ. When pathogens enter the body, they can sometimes overpower the body's defense systems and cause illness. This condition is called an ***infection.*** Most infectious diseases are caused by one or another of the six types of pathogens identified in Table 3-1. The most common types of pathogens are viruses and bacteria.

Because they are the most common, viruses and bacteria are the pathogens of most concern to the first responder. ***Bacteria,*** one-celled microorganisms, are everywhere in our environment. Bacteria do not depend on other organisms for life and can live outside the human body. Most bacteria do not infect humans, but those that do may cause serious infections. Meningitis, scarlet fever, TB, and tetanus are examples of diseases caused by bacteria. It is difficult for the body to fight a bacterial infection. Physicians may prescribe medications called **antibiotics** that either kill the bacteria or weaken them enough for the body to eliminate them. Commonly prescribed antibiotics include penicillin, erythromycin, and tetracycline.

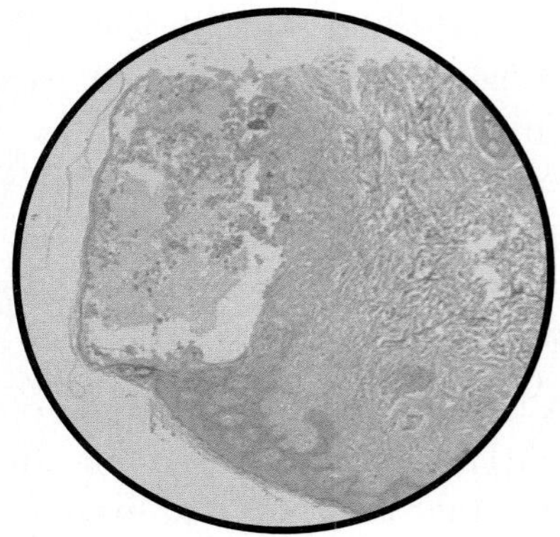

Figure 3-1 Herpes simplex virus type 2 is a microorganism that causes herpes simplex.

Table 3-1 Disease Causing Agents

Pathogen	Diseases they cause
Viruses	Hepatitis, measles, mumps, chicken pox, meningitis, rubella, influenza, colds, herpes, shingles, HIV infection including AIDS, genital warts
Bacteria	Tetanus, meningitis, scarlet fever, strep throat, tuberculosis, gonorrhea, syphilis, toxic shock syndrome, Legionnaires' disease, diphtheria, food poisoning
Fungi	Athlete's foot and ringworm
Protozoa	Malaria and dysentery
Rickettsia	Typhus, Rocky Mountain spotted fever

Unlike bacteria, ***viruses*** depend on other organisms to live and reproduce (Fig. 3-1). Viruses cause many diseases, including the common cold. Once they become established in the body, they are difficult to eliminate because very few medications effectively fight viral infections. Most antibiotics do not kill or weaken viruses. The body's immune system is the primary defense against viral infections.

The Body's Natural Defenses

The body's ***immune system*** is a highly effective, complex group of responses for fighting disease. The basic components are the white blood cells. Special white blood cells circulate in the bloodstream and identify invading pathogens. Once they detect a pathogen, these white blood cells gather around it and release infection-fighting proteins called **antibodies.**

These antibodies attack the pathogen and weaken or destroy it. Antibodies are usually effective at eliminating disease. However, once inside the body, certain pathogens can flourish and, under ideal conditions, overwhelm the immune system. Because the immune system may be overwhelmed, the body also depends on the skin as a protective mechanism to keep pathogens out.

This combination of limiting pathogens from entering the body and destroying them once they get inside is a constant process, essential to good health. Sometimes, despite its natural defenses, the body cannot fight off infection. When the infection is not destroyed, an invading pathogen can become established in the body, causing serious infection. Fever and a feeling of exhaustion often signal that the body is fighting an infection. Other common signs and symptoms include headache, nausea, and vomiting.

How Diseases Spread

For communicable diseases to be transmitted, all four of the following conditions must be met:

- A pathogen is present.
- The pathogen is in sufficient quantity to cause disease.
- A person is vulnerable to the specific pathogen.
- The pathogen is transmitted through the correct entry site.

Understanding these four conditions is the basis for understanding how communicable diseases occur. Think of these conditions as the pieces of a puzzle. All the pieces have to be in place for the picture to be complete (Fig. 3-2). If any one of these conditions is absent, a disease cannot spread.

Pathogens enter the body in four ways (Fig. 3-3):

- Direct contact
- Indirect contact
- Airborne
- Vector-borne

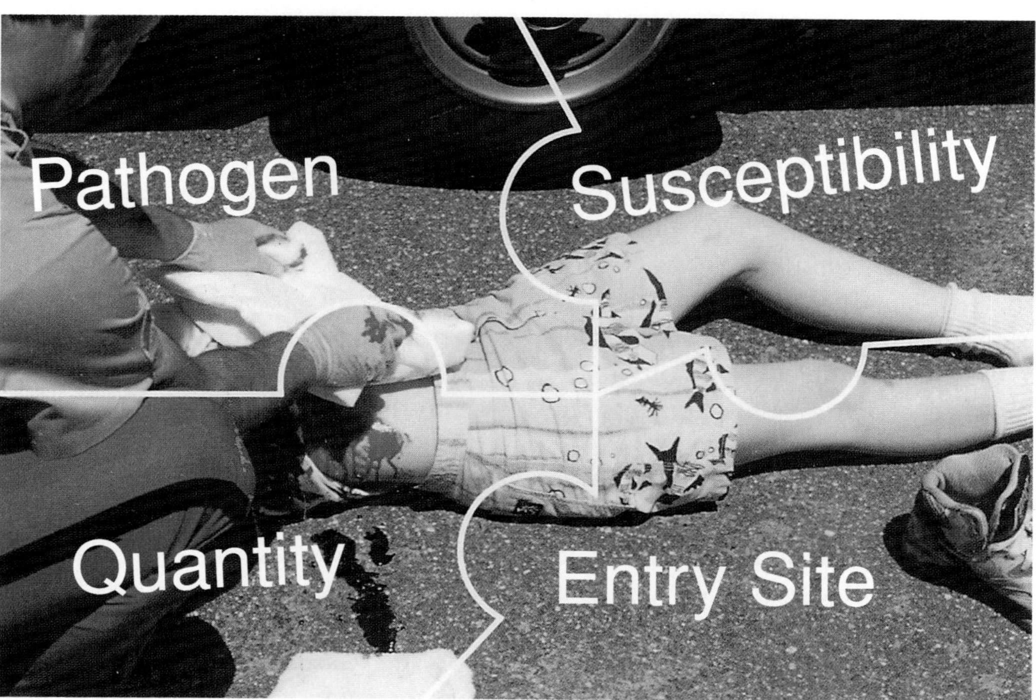

Figure 3-2 For an infection to occur, all four conditions must be present.

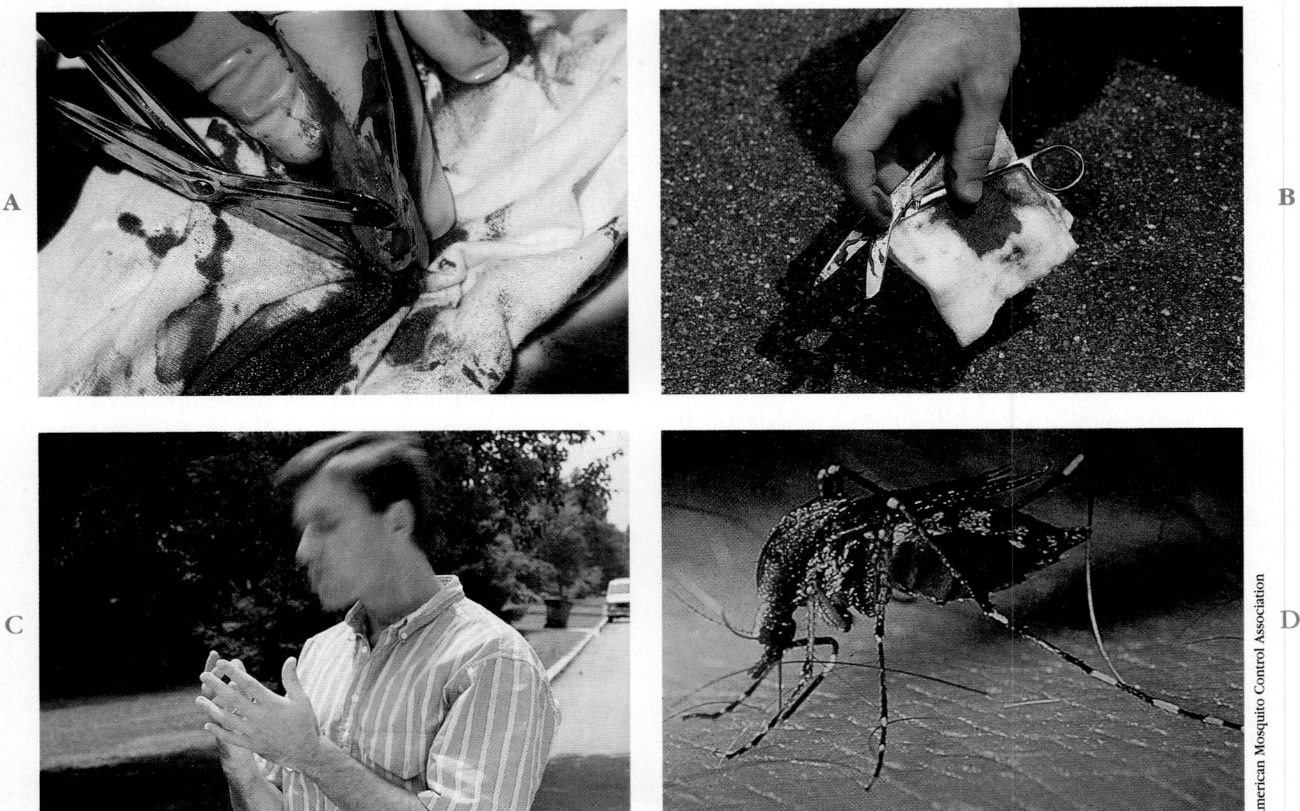

Figure 3-3 A, Direct contact transmission, **B,** Indirect contact transmission, **C,** Airborne transmission and, **D,** Vector transmission are the four ways pathogens can enter the body.

Not all pathogens can enter the body in all of these ways. For example, certain infections, such as Lyme disease and rabies, are vector-borne only.

Direct contact transmission occurs when a person touches an infected person's body fluids. This type of transmission presents the greatest risk for the first responder. ***Indirect contact transmission*** occurs when a person touches objects that have been contaminated by the blood or another body fluid of an infected person. These objects include dressings, equipment, and vehicle surfaces covered with blood or other potentially infectious material with which an infected person comes in contact. Contaminated sharp objects present a particular risk. Handled carelessly, they can pierce the skin and transmit infection.

Airborne transmission occurs when a person inhales infected droplets that have become airborne as an infected person coughs or sneezes. It can also occur from inhaling materials in the atmosphere that affect the health of people living in that environment. Airborne transmission from inhaling infected droplets is less likely than contact transmission for the first responder. If a person is coughing heavily, avoid face-to-face contact if possible.

Vector transmission occurs when an animal, such as a dog or raccoon, or an insect, such as a tick, transmits a pathogen into the body through a bite. The carrier is called a vector and passes the pathogens to another animal or person. Rabies and Lyme disease are transmitted in this manner. Lyme disease is discussed in Chapter 16. Those providing emergency care are not usually at risk for vector-borne transmission.

◆ DISEASES THAT CAUSE CONCERN

People transmit some diseases, such as the common cold, more easily than others. Although the common cold does cause minor discomfort for the sufferer, it is short-lived and rarely has serious consequences. Other diseases cause more severe problems. Hepatitis B, a liver infection, can last many months. The patient is often seriously ill and slow to recover. HIV infection, caused by the human immunodeficiency virus, destroys the body's ability to fight infection. Both infections can cause prolonged illness or death.

As an emergency care provider, you should be familiar with communicable diseases that can have severe consequences if transmitted. These include herpes, meningitis, tuberculosis, hepatitis, and HIV infection.

Herpes Simplex

Herpes simplex results from one of several viruses that cause infections of the skin and mucous membranes. It is highly contagious and transmitted by direct contact. For reasons that are not well understood, the herpes virus can lie dormant in sensory nerves until stimulated. The early stages of an acute infection may cause headache, sore throat, swelling of the lymph glands, and a general ill feeling. Sometimes swelling occurs around the lips and mouth where small, blisterlike sores may form (Fig. 3-4). These are commonly called cold sores.

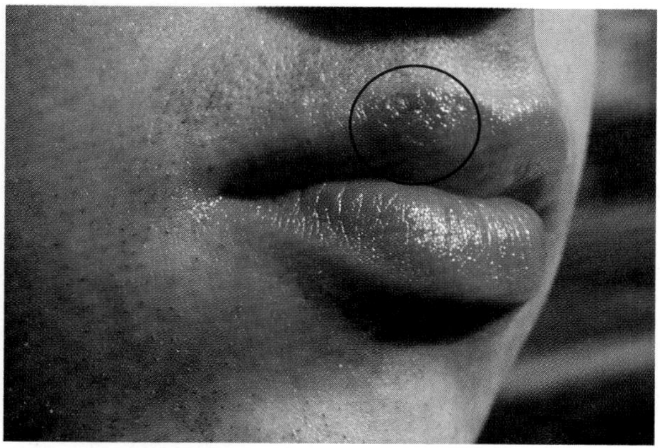

Figure 3-4 The herpes virus may cause blisterlike sores to erupt on or around the lips and mouth.

In a more serious form of herpes, sores form on the face, neck, and shoulders. Another form of herpes causes sores in the genital area. Since most antibiotics are not effective in combating viruses, the infection runs its course, becomes dormant for a while, then flares up again. Herpes is usually transmitted through an opening in the skin or through mucous membranes, such as those in the mouth or eyes, when a person makes direct contact with herpetic lesions. You should avoid unprotected contact with people who have active herpes.

Meningitis

Meningitis is a severe infection of the covering of the brain and spinal cord. It can be caused by either viruses or bacteria. It is transmitted easily by direct and airborne means. As a first responder, you are not normally at risk from the viral form of meningitis. Bacterial meningitis, however, can be transmitted through the mucous secretions of the nose and mouth. Transmission might occur if an infected person coughs near your face or if you directly contact the person's secretions. Unprotected rescue breathing and procedures like suctioning present a risk of contracting bacterial meningitis.

Although meningitis occurs more commonly

in infants and young children, adults are not immune. The first symptoms are often respiratory infections, sore throat, stiff neck, rash, nausea, and vomiting. An infected person may quickly become seriously ill. Advanced stages affect the person's level of consciousness. Meningitis, if treated early, is rarely fatal.

Tuberculosis (TB)

Tuberculosis (TB) is a communicable disease that most commonly affects the respiratory system. The bacteria that cause it can live in the lungs and other tissues. Transmission occurs primarily from inhaling infectious airborne droplets. The disease causes coughing, weight loss, night sweats, occasional fever, and a general feeling of fatigue. Because the signs and symptoms often develop gradually, early stages may go unnoticed. People with undiagnosed tuberculosis may even remain in relatively good health for a long time before they rapidly become ill.

Recently, a new strain of TB, multi-drug resistant TB (MDR.-TB), has been identified. This strain can result from an infected patient's failure to follow or complete prescribed treatment, resulting in an incomplete destruction of the TB bacteria. The remaining bacteria become resistant to the antibiotic and subsequently spread to the point that the patient suffers a relapse infection that no longer can be treated with the same medication. People who have been exposed to drug-resistant TB strains are also at risk, especially if they have damaged immune systems. Patients who have received ineffective treatment are at risk as well. Treatment for MDR.-TB is based upon timely diagnosis and appropriate administration of medications. Risk of exposure for resistant and nonresistant strains results from direct contact with respiratory secretions from coughing, spitting, speaking, or singing (Table 3-2).

Hepatitis

Hepatitis is a condition that results in inflammation of the liver. The liver makes, stores, and

Table 3-2 How Diseases are Transmitted

Disease	Signs and symptoms	Mode of transmission	Infective material
Herpes	Lesions, general ill feeling, sore throat	Direct contact	Broken skin, mucous membranes
Meningitis	Respiratory illness, sore throat, nausea, vomiting, headache, stiff neck	Airborne, direct and indirect contact	Food and water, mucus
Tuberculosis	Coughing, weight loss, night sweats, occasional fever, general ill feeling	Airborne	Saliva, airborne droplets
Hepatitis	Flulike, jaundice	Direct and indirect contact	Blood, saliva, semen, feces, food, water, other products
HIV Infection	Fever, night sweats, weight loss, chronic diarrhea, severe fatigue, shortness of breath, swollen lymph nodes, lesions	Direct and indirect contact	Blood, semen, vaginal fluid, breast milk

secretes bile; breaks down and stores fat; and renders some toxic chemicals harmless. The most common forms of hepatitis are caused by alcohol abuse, drugs, or other chemicals and cannot be transmitted. Viruses, however, also can cause hepatitis. The most common types of viral hepatitis are type A, type B, and type C.

Hepatitis A (HAV), also called infectious hepatitis, is common in young adults. Hepatitis A is often transmitted by contact with food or other products contaminated by the feces of an infected person. Parents may contract the disease from their children by changing diapers. Contaminated shellfish and water can also transmit hepatitis A.

People with hepatitis A initially feel as if they have flu. In later stages, their skin and eyes may become a yellowish color, a condition called **jaundice.** Jaundice occurs because the damaged liver cannot excrete bile, which then stays in the blood and colors the skin. Hepatitis A usually does not have serious consequences.

Hepatitis B (HBV), also called serum hepatitis, is a severe liver infection caused by the hepatitis B virus. Hepatitis B is transmitted by sexual contact and blood-to-blood contact from transfusions, needle sticks, cuts, scrapes, sores, and skin irritations. Hepatitis B is not transmitted by casual contact, such as shaking hands, or by indirect contact with a drinking fountain or telephone. Your risk while providing care most often occurs from unprotected direct or indirect contact with infected blood.

The signs of hepatitis B are similar to the flu-like signs of hepatitis A. Hepatitis B infections can be fatal. The disease may be in the body for up to 6 months before signs and symptoms develop. The person may then overlook the flu-like signs. Some people can even develop chronic hepatitis after recovering from the acute signs.

Hepatitis C (HCV) is a third form of hepatitis. It is transmitted in the same manner as hepatitis B. The signs and symptoms of hepatitis C are similar to those of hepatitis B. It is estimated that up to 85 percent of the people infected with the hepatitis C virus each year will develop chronic hepatitis. There are 3.9 million Americans chronically infected with HCV. First responders and other care providers who may come in contact with infected blood, instruments, or needles are at risk of acquiring hepatitis C. Currently, there is no vaccine available to immunize against the hepatitis C virus.

◆ HIV

AIDS (acquired immunodeficiency syndrome) is a result of HIV infection. It is caused by ***HIV (human immunodeficiency virus).*** This virus attacks white blood cells and destroys the body's ability to fight infection. The infections that strike people whose immune systems are weakened by HIV or other conditions are called **opportunistic infections.** Opportunistic infections common to HIV include severe pneumonia and fungal infections of the mouth and esophagus. HIV-infected people may also develop Kaposi's sarcoma, invasive cervical cancer, and other cancers (Fig. 3-5).

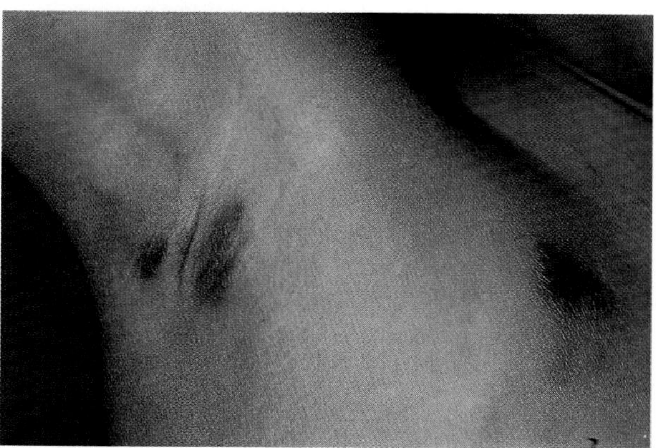

Figure 3-5 Kaposi's sarcoma is one of several opportunistic conditions that may strike the HIV-infected person.

People infected with HIV might look well, but they can still spread the virus to others. A person with HIV may have severe fatigue, fever, night sweats, unexplained weight loss, chronic diarrhea, shortness of breath, swollen lymph nodes, and skin lesions. However, people with other kinds of infections may also have these signs and symptoms. When the infected person shows certain signs of having a weakened immune system, he or she is diagnosed with having AIDS. Drugs for treating opportunistic infections and for attacking HIV itself are improving, and maximum survival after diagnosis with AIDS is not known. Most people with AIDS die because their bodies are so weak from repeated infections.

It is important to remember the following points about the transmission of HIV:

- HIV cannot be spread through casual contact.
- HIV is easily inactivated by alcohol, chlorine bleach, and other common germicides. It does not survive outside the body. You cannot reactivate a dead virus by adding water.
- HIV is transmitted through exposure to infected blood, semen, vaginal secretions, or through breast milk. This transmission can occur—
    - By having sex without a latex condom with an infected partner, male or female.
    - **Through blood-to-blood contact:**
    - Being exposed to blood through the use of contaminated equipment or supplies, needle stick injuries, or blood splashed on mucous membranes or broken skin. (Scientists estimate that the risk of HIV infection from a needle stick is less than 1%, based on several studies of health-care workers who received punctures from HIV-contaminated needles).
    - Sharing needles for street drug injection, steroids, ear-piercing, or tattooing.
- From an infected woman to her child during pregnancy, birth, or breast feeding.

Since 1985, all donated blood in the United States has been tested for signs of HIV. As a result, the risk of getting infected with HIV from blood transfusion is extremely low.

Childhood Diseases

Most people have been immunized against the common communicable childhood diseases, such as measles and mumps. An ***immunization*** is the introduction of a substance that contains specific weakened or killed pathogens into the body, which builds resistance to a specific infection.

You might not have been immunized against some childhood diseases. If you are not sure about which immunizations you have received or need, contact your doctor.

◆ PROTECTING YOURSELF FROM DISEASE TRANSMISSION

The best way to prevent disease transmission is to minimize your risk of exposure to possible infectious materials by protecting yourself and the environment you work in. Sometimes simply changing work habits will greatly reduce your chances of exposure.

Exposure Control Plan

Preventing communicable disease begins with preparation and planning. An Exposure Control Plan is an important step in eliminating or minimizing employee exposure to blood and other infectious materials. The Exposure Control Plan is the method by which an employer creates a system to protect its employees from infection and is, therefore, a key provision of the OSHA standard. This plan requires the employer to identify who will receive training, protective equipment, and vaccinations, and to provide post-exposure notification and treatment.

According to OSHA, an Exposure Control Plan should contain the following elements:

- Exposure determination
- A schedule and method for implementing other elements of the OSHA standard. These elements include—
  - Methods of compliance.
  - HIV and HBV research laboratories and production facilities.
  - Hepatitis B vaccination and post-exposure evaluation and follow-up communication of hazards to employees.
  - Recordkeeping.
  - Procedures for evaluating circumstances surrounding an exposure incident.

Exposure determination is one of the key elements of the Exposure Control Plan. It includes the identification and documentation of job classifications in which occupational exposure to blood or airborne pathogens can occur. The determination should be made without regard to using personal protective equipment. The Exposure Control Plan should be accessible to employees and must be updated annually or more often if changes in exposure occur.

Because of an increase in complaints about occupational exposure to TB, OSHA has begun to enforce policies and procedures for occupational exposure to tuberculosis in workplace settings where workers have a greater incidence of TB infection. These include—

- Health-care settings.
- Correctional institutions.
- Homeless shelters.
- Long-term care facilities for the elderly.
- Drug treatment centers.

Employers are required to provide employees with information and training regarding hazards of TB transmission, signs and symptoms, medical surveillance, and therapy and site-specific protocols, including the purpose and proper use of engineering and work practice controls. Although they are not part of the bloodborne pathogen standard, you should be aware of TB-related regulations that may affect your workplace.

Immunizations

For the individual, preventing communicable and other infectious diseases begins with maintaining good health and consistently practicing good personal hygiene, such as frequent hand washing (Fig. 3-6). Get immunizations for any childhood disease you have not had. The following immunizations are recommended:

- DPT (Diphtheria, pertussis, tetanus)
- Hepatitis B vaccine
- MMR (measles, mumps, rubella)
- Influenza
- Varicella (chicken pox)

Keep your immunizations up to date.

The OSHA standard requires that an employer inform employees about the hepatitis B vaccination and make it available to all employees who have occupational exposure. A post-exposure evaluation and follow-up should also be available to all employees who have an exposure incident (Table 3-3).

The employer shall ensure that all medical evaluations and procedures, including the hepatitis B vaccination series and post-exposure evaluation and follow-up, are—

- Made available at no cost to the employee.
- Made available to employees at a reasonable time and place.
- Provided by or under the supervision of a licensed physician or health-care professional. (Note: Persons receiving vaccinations should be monitored for at least 30 minutes after injection in case of adverse reaction to the vaccine.)
- Provided according to the current recommendations of the U.S. Public Health Service.

OSHA has also added special considerations

A

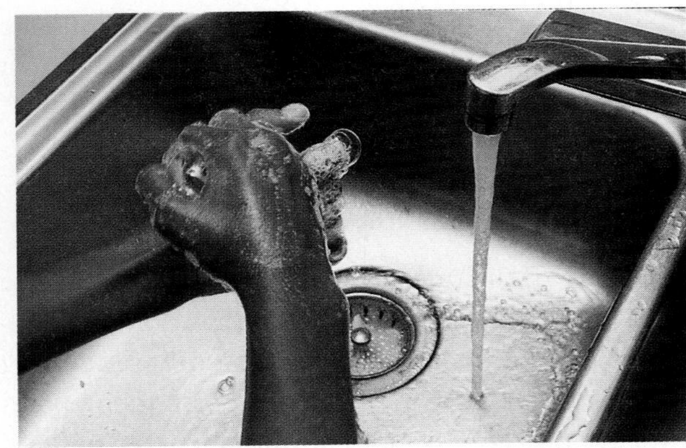

B

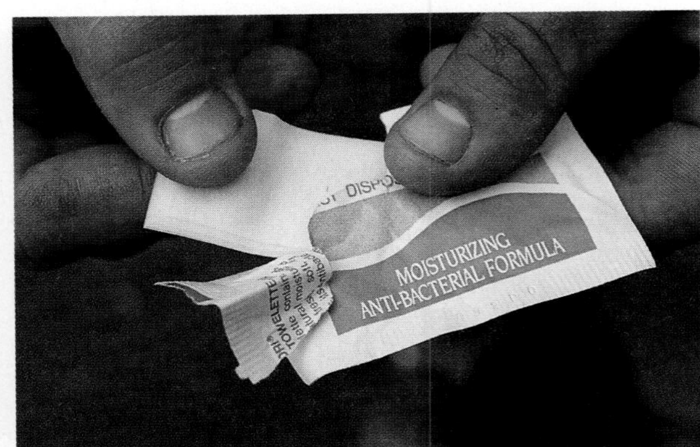

C

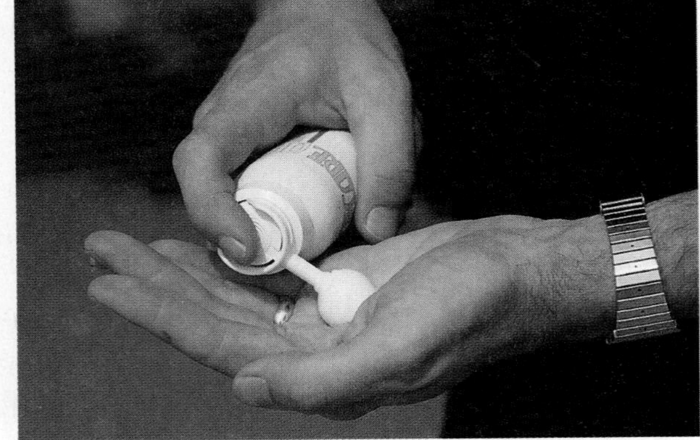

Figure 3-6 Thorough handwashing after giving care helps protect you against disease.

Table 3-3 Recommended Protective Equipment Against HIV and HBV. Transmission in Out-of-Hospital Settings

Task or activity	Disposable gloves	Gown	Mask	Protective eyewear
Bleeding control with spurting blood	Yes	Yes	Yes	Yes
Bleeding control with minimal bleeding	Yes	No	No	No
Emergency childbirth	Yes	Yes	Yes	Yes
Helping with an intravenous (IV) line	Yes	No	No	No
Oral/nasal suctioning, manually clearing airway	Yes	No	Yes	Yes
Handling and cleaning contaminated equipment and clothing	Yes	No, unless soiling is likely	No	No

Excerpt from Department of Health and Human Services, Public Health Services: *A curriculum guide for public-safety and emergency-response workers: prevention of transmission of human immunodeficiency virus and hepatitis B virus,* Atlanta, GA, February 1989, Dept Health and Human Services, Centers for Disease Control.

for employees whose routine work assignments do not include providing first aid for incidents occurring in the workplace. OSHA believes there is a low risk of exposure for these employees. The option of post-exposure prevention measures, including hepatitis B vaccination within 24 hours of exposure, is now available. OSHA believes that this option will minimize the risk to employees and lessen demands on limited supplies of the vaccine. The option does not apply to employees who provide first aid at a first aid station, clinic, or dispensary or to health care, emergency response, or public safety personnel expected to provide first aid in the course of their work.

OSHA considers the selection of this option a technical violation of the standard but does not impose any penalty on the employer. However, the following conditions must be met:

- The exposure control plan must include reporting procedures for first aid incidents involving exposure. The procedures must ensure that incidents are reported before the end of the shift in which they occur.
- Reports of first aid incidents must include the names of all first aiders involved and the details of the incident. The report must also include the date and time of the incident and if an exposure incident has occurred.
- Exposure reports must be included on lists of first aid incidents. They must be readily available to employees and provided to OSHA on request.
- First aid providers must be trained under the bloodborne pathogens standard that covers the reporting procedure specifics.

All first aiders who provide assistance in any incident involving blood or other potentially infectious materials, regardless of whether a specific exposure incident occurs, must be offered the full hepatitis B vaccination series. This immunization should be offered as soon as possible, but in no event later than 24 hours after exposure. If an exposure incident occurs, other post-exposure follow-up procedures must be initiated immediately.

Precautions

At times, we might consider varying the level of protection we use based on who our victims are, what they look like, or where they are located. However, the world of victim care is not that simple. Often you will not know the health status of the people you are called on to care for. The one time you let down your guard may be the very time that you become infected by someone who does not fit your preconceived notion of people who are likely to be infected.

Officials at the Centers for Disease Control and Prevention (CDC) have identified precautions to prevent occupational-risk exposure to blood and other potentially infectious material containing visible blood as ***standard precautions.*** Precautions taken to isolate or prevent the risk of exposure from any type of bodily substance are known as body substance isolation (BSI). Regardless of the type of exposure risk, you must follow basic precautions and safe practices each time you prepare to provide care (Fig. 3-7). These precautions and practices include the following four areas:

- Personal protective equipment
- Personal hygiene
- Engineering and work practice controls
- Equipment cleaning and disinfecting

Maintaining good personal hygiene habits, such as frequent hand washing, is an important secondary way to reduce the risk of disease transmission, regardless of any personal protective equipment you might use. Infection control products, such as waterless antiseptic hand cleansers, allow you to clean your hands when soap and water are not readily available. These simple methods of infection control can help prevent bacteria or other pathogens that may come in contact with the skin from transmitting an infectious disease.

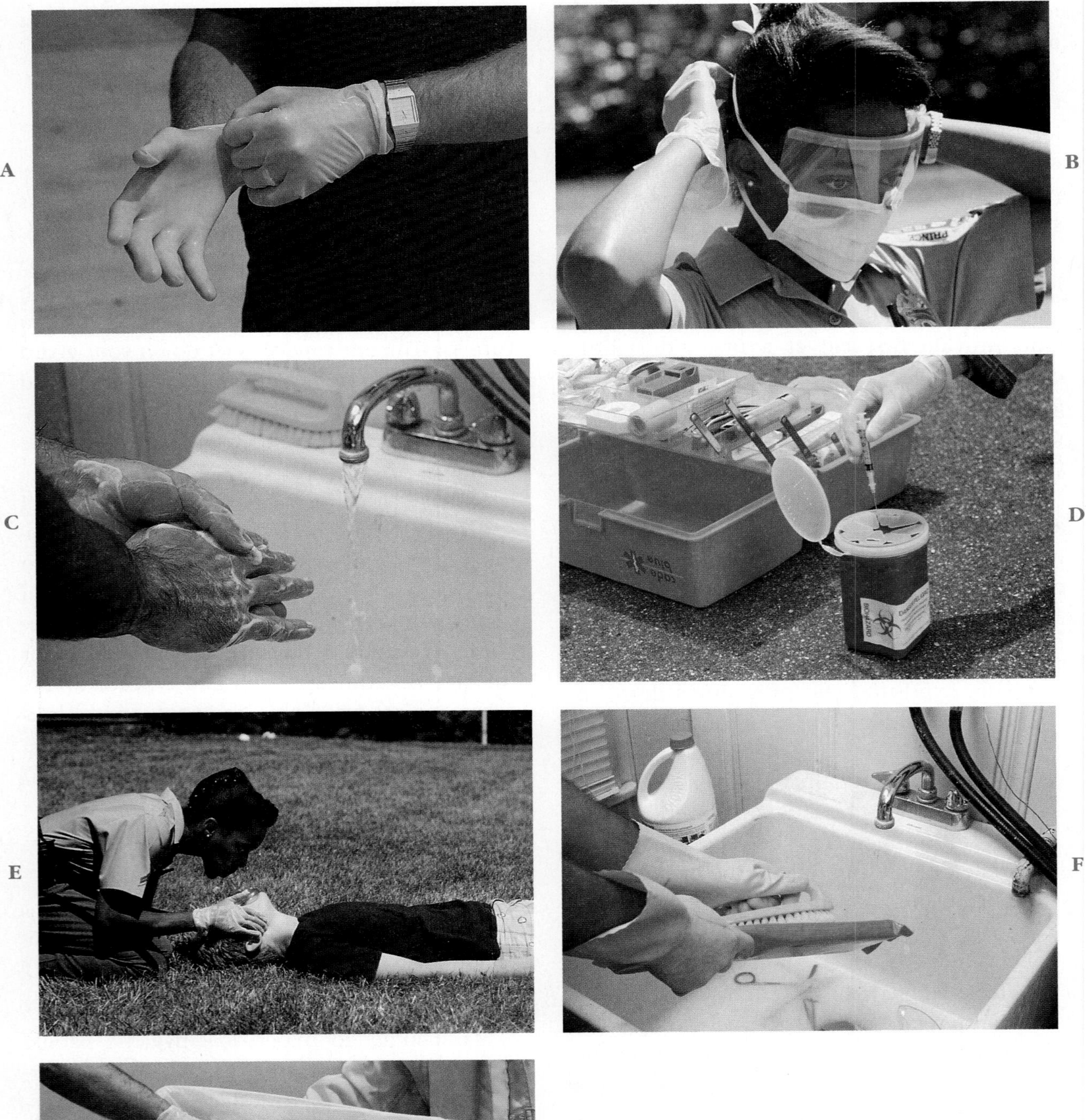

Figure 3-7 Following basic precautions decreases your risk of contracting or transmitting an infection.

Following good personal hygiene practices greatly reduces your chances of disease transmission.

Personal Protective Equipment

Personal protective equipment (PPE) includes all equipment and supplies that prevent you from making direct contact with infected materials. These supplies and equipment include disposable gloves, gowns, masks and shields, protective eyewear, and resuscitation devices. Following certain guidelines for the use of protective equipment can greatly decrease your risk of contracting or transmitting an infectious disease:

- Wear disposable (single-use) gloves, such as examination or surgical gloves, when there is a possibility you will contact blood or other potentially infectious material. Such contact may happen directly through contact with a victim or indirectly through contact with soiled clothing or other personal articles. Consider gloves contaminated as soon as you put them on. Use gloves made of latex or nitrile.
- Remove gloves by turning them inside out; beginning at the wrist, peel them off. When removing the second glove, do not touch the soiled surfaces with your bare, ungloved hand. Hook the *inside* of the glove at the wrist and peel the glove off.
- Discard discolored, torn, or punctured gloves.
- Do not clean or reuse disposable gloves.
- Avoid handling items such as pens, combs, steering wheels, or radios when wearing contaminated gloves.
- Change gloves when you give care to different persons.
- In addition to gloves, wear protective coverings, such as a mask, protective eyewear, and gown, whenever you are likely to contact blood or other body fluids that may splash.

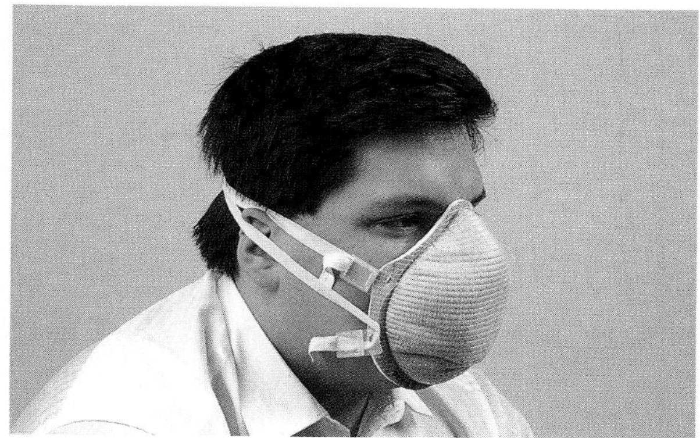

Figure 3-8 Use a NIOSH-approved high efficiency particulate air (HEPA) respirator if you are likely to be exposed to TB or other airborne pathogens.

- Cover any cuts, scrapes, or skin irritations before putting on protective body clothing.
- Use resuscitation aids, such as disposable resuscitation masks and airway devices. (Specific resuscitation aids are discussed in Chapter 9.)
- Use a NIOSH-approved respirator such as N95 if you are likely to be exposed to TB or other airborne pathogens (Fig. 3-8).

Personal Hygiene

Your personal hygiene habits are as important in preventing infection as any equipment you might use. These habits and practices serve as a second line of defense in preventing any materials that might have penetrated the protective equipment from remaining in contact with your body. Following certain guidelines for personal hygiene can greatly decrease your risk of contracting or transmitting a communicable disease:

- Wash your hands thoroughly with soap and water immediately after providing care. Use a utility or restroom sink, not one in a food preparation area.
- Avoid eating, drinking, smoking, applying cosmetics or lip balm, handling contact lenses,

and touching your mouth, nose, or eyes while providing care or before washing hands.

Engineering Controls

Engineering controls are safeguards intended to isolate or remove the hazard from the workplace. Engineering controls include puncture-resistant sharps containers and mechanical needle recapping devices. To ensure their effectiveness, engineering controls should be examined and maintained or replaced regularly. Once implemented, engineering controls are subject to periodic replacement and preventive maintenance.

Work practice controls reduce the likelihood of exposure by altering the manner in which a task is performed. Although they act on the source of the hazard, the protection provided by work practice controls is based on employer and employee behavior rather than installation of a physical device.

Engineering and work practice controls are used instead of other methods to ensure good industrial hygiene. Adhering to the following controls minimizes the risk of exposure in the workplace:

- Avoid needle stick injuries by *not* attempting to bend or recap any needles.
- Place sharp items (needles, scalpel blades, etc.) in puncture-resistant, leakproof, labeled containers (sharps containers).
- Perform all procedures so that splashing, spraying, splattering, and generation of droplets of blood or other potentially infectious materials are minimized.
- Clean and disinfect all equipment and work surfaces possibly contaminated by blood or other body fluids.
- Prohibit eating, drinking, smoking, applying cosmetics or lip balm, handling contact lenses, and touching the mouth, nose, or eyes in work areas where there is potential for occupational exposure.
- Remove blood-soiled protective clothing as soon as possible and place in properly marked plastic bags.
- Wash your hands and any other exposed skin area thoroughly after providing care.
- Make hand washing facilities readily accessible to employee's work areas.
- Provide antiseptic towelettes or hand cleanser where hand washing facilities are not available.
- Ensure all sharp instrument disposal containers are —
  - Puncture resistant.
  - Labeled or color-coded as **biohazard.**
  - Leakproof.
  - Able to prevent access to contents.

Equipment Cleaning and Disinfecting

It is important to clean and disinfect equipment to prevent transmission of communicable diseases. Handle all contaminated equipment, supplies, or other materials with the utmost care until they are properly cleaned and disinfected. Place all disposable items in labeled containers. Place all contaminated clothing in properly marked plastic bags for disposal or washing.

To disinfect equipment, such as stethoscopes, blood pressure cuffs, and splints, contaminated with blood or other potentially infectious materials, wash the equipment thoroughly with a solution of common household chlorine bleach and water. Approximately $\frac{1}{4}$ cup of bleach per gallon of water is all that is needed. Surfaces, such as floors, woodwork, ambulance and automobile seats, and countertops, should also be cleaned of any visible soil before a bleach solution is used.

Wash and dry protective clothing and work uniforms according to the manufacturer's instructions. Scrub contaminated boots, leather shoes, and other leather items, such as belts, with soap, a brush, and hot water. Do not wash contaminated clothing and uniforms with normal household laundry.

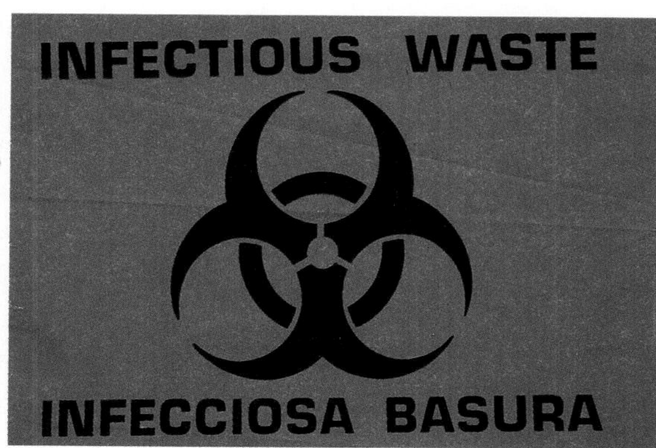

Figure 3-9 Biohazard warning label.

Biohazard warning labels are required on any container or equipment that has been or is potentially contaminated with infectious materials (Fig. 3-9). Signs should be posted at entrances of work areas where potentially infectious material may be present. Biohazard signs and labels should be entirely or predominately fluorescent orange or orange-red, with lettering or symbols in a contrasting color like black. Red bags or red containers may be substituted for labels.

In the event of an incident that creates disposable waste or contaminated laundry, the employer should provide properly labeled containers to store the materials until they are disposed of or laundered. The containers must have warning labels or signs to eliminate or minimize employee exposure. In addition to providing training, the employer must ensure that all employees understand and avoid the hazard.

The OSHA standard requires that the employer maintain the work site in a clean and sanitary condition. The employer is required to develop and implement a written schedule for cleaning and decontaminating at the work site. The schedule should be based on the location within the facility, the type of surface to be cleaned, the type of soil present, and the task or procedures being performed.

In addition, the employer must have a plan in place to deal with any spill of a potentially infectious substance that might occur. The plan should include a system for reporting the spill, the action to be taken to resolve the spill, a list of employees responsible for containment, instructions for cleanup, and the final disposition of the spill.

The first step in dealing with a spill is containment. Spill containment units designed for hazardous materials are available commercially and are very effective. However, any absorbent material, such as paper towels, can be used if the material is disposed of properly after use.

The steps for spill management are as follows:

- *Wear appropriate gloves and other personal protective equipment when cleaning spills.*
- Clean up spills immediately or as soon as possible after spills occur.
- If the spill is mixed with sharp objects, such as broken glass and needles, do not pick them up with your hands. Use tongs, broom and dustpan, or two pieces of cardboard.
- Use paper towels to absorb the spill, and dispose of the towels in a labeled biohazard container.
- Flood the area with bleach solution, and allow it to stand for at least 10 minutes.
- Use paper towels to absorb the solution, and discard towels in the biohazard container.

Following these precautions will usually remove at least one of the four conditions necessary for disease transmission. Remember, if only one condition is missing, infection will not occur.

◆ IF AN EXPOSURE OCCURS

If you suspect that you have been exposed to an infectious disease, wash any area of contact as quickly as possible and document the situation in which the exposure occurred. Exposures usually involve contact with potentially infectious blood or other potentially infectious materials through a needle stick, broken or scraped skin, or the mucous membranes of the eyes, nose, and mouth. Inhaling potentially infected airborne droplets may also constitute an exposure. Most employers have **protocols,** or standardized procedures, for reporting infectious disease exposure. These protocols should include the following elements:

- Types of exposure covered
- List of immediate actions to be taken by the exposed employee to reduce the chances of infection
- When or how quickly the exposure incident should be reported
- Where and to whom the exposure incident should be reported
- Which forms should be completed
- Directives for incident investigation
- Medical follow-up to be completed

If you think you have been exposed to a communicable disease, it is your responsibility to notify your superior and any necessary medical personnel immediately. The medical facility may test to determine if the victim has a communicable disease. If a disease is confirmed, you will be notified and given post-exposure care. Your superior or the hospital is responsible for notifying any other personnel who might have been exposed. If your system does not have a designated physician or nurse at a local hospital for follow-up care, see your personal physician. Usually, you will not know whether a person you are caring for has an infectious disease. If the hospital later diagnoses an infectious disease, you will be notified and given post-exposure care.

◆ OSHA REGULATIONS

The OSHA regulations on bloodborne and airborne pathogens have placed the following responsibilities on employers for protection of employees:

- Identifying positions or tasks covered by the standard
- Creating an Exposure Control Plan to minimize the possibility of exposure
- Using body substance isolation (BSI) to minimize the possibility of infection
- Creating a system for easy identification of contaminated material and its disposal
- Creating an annual training system for all covered employees
- Creating a system of record keeping that includes updates of protocols and Exposure Control Plans, employee training, employee medical records, and follow-up
- Hepatitis B vaccine program
- TB skin testing
- Compliance monitoring

◆ SUMMARY

Although the body's immune system defends well against disease, pathogens can still enter the body and sometimes cause infection. These pathogens can be transmitted in four ways: by direct contact with an infected person; by indirect contact with a contaminated object; by inhaling air exhaled by an infected person; and through a bite from an infected animal or insect.

Serious diseases include hepatitis, herpes, meningitis, tuberculosis, and HIV infection, including AIDS. You should know how the diseases are transmitted and take appropriate measures to protect yourself. Remember that all four conditions must be present for a disease to be transmitted.

The Occupational Safety and Health Administration (OSHA) has issued regulations on occupational exposure to bloodborne pathogens. The agency has determined that employees face a significant risk from occupational exposure to blood and other potentially infectious materials because they may contain bloodborne pathogens. OSHA concludes that this hazard can be minimized or eliminated using a combination of engineering and work practice controls, personal protective clothing and equipment, training, medical surveillance, hepatitis B vaccination, signs and labels, and other precautions. The OSHA regulation defines the range of employees covered by the standard, and it sets forth specific requirements that employers must meet to maintain work sites in a clean and sanitary condition.

Following OSHA guidelines, especially the standard precautions or BSI, greatly decreases your risk of contracting or transmitting an infectious disease. If you suspect you have been exposed to such a disease, always document it, or notify your superior or ***designated officer*** and other involved personnel. Seek medical help and participate in any follow-up procedures.

Keep these principles concerning infectious disease in mind as you read the following chapters about providing care in specific situations. Even when you must act quickly, as in restoring breathing or circulation, take these precautions to reduce the risk of infection.

Use the activities in Unit 3 of the workbook to help you review the materials in Chapter 3.

You Are the Responder

1. You are called to check on a woman having difficulty breathing. The woman is kneeling on the ground. She has a cough and looks very ill. What are your concerns regarding disease transmission?

2. You stop to assist a victim of an automobile crash. The victim has a large amount of blood on her head. She continues to bleed from a large cut on her face. What are your concerns regarding disease transmission? How would you protect yourself?

3. A man in the parking lot has collapsed next to an automobile. As the first trained person on the scene, you find the man bleeding from the mouth and face. Vomit and broken glass are around him. "His face hit the side-view mirror when he fell," a bystander says. He is not breathing. How would you respond? Do you have any concerns about contracting disease?

Legal and Ethical Issues

4

Key Terms

Abandonment: Ending the care of an ill or injured person without obtaining that person's consent or without ensuring that someone with equal or greater training will continue that care.

Competence: The victim's ability to understand the questions of the first responder and to understand the implications of decisions made.

Confidentiality: Protecting a victim's privacy by not revealing any personal information you learn about the victim except to law enforcement personnel or EMS personnel caring for the victim.

Consent: Permission to provide care, given by an ill or injured person to a rescuer.

Duty to act: A legal responsibility of some individuals to provide a reasonable standard of emergency care; a duty to act may be required by case law, statute, or job description.

Good Samaritan laws: Laws that protect people who willingly give emergency care without accepting anything in return.

Negligence: The failure to provide the level of care a person of similar training would provide, thereby causing injury or damage to another.

Refusal of care: The declining of care by a competent victim. A victim has the right to refuse the care of anyone who responds to an emergency scene.

Scope of practice: The range of duties and skills a first responder is allowed and expected to perform when necessary.

Standard of care: The criterion established for the extent and quality of a first responder's care.

◆ Knowledge Objectives ◆

After reading this chapter and completing the class activities, you should be able to—

- Define the first responder standard of care and scope of practice.
- Explain the importance and purpose of Do Not Resuscitate (DNR) orders, advance directives, and local or state provisions pertaining to EMS and how they affect the care a first responder provides.
- Define consent and describe the methods of obtaining consent.
- Differentiate between expressed consent and implied consent and explain the issues of consent when providing care to minors.
- Explain the implications for the first responder when a victim refuses transport.
- Explain abandonment, negligence, and battery and their implications for the first responder.
- State the conditions necessary for the first responder to have a duty to act.
- Explain the importance, necessity, and legality of maintaining confidentiality about the condition, circumstances, and care of the victim.
- List the actions that a first responder should take to help preserve a crime scene.
- Describe the situations that require a first responder to notify local law enforcement officials.
- Describe the fundamental components of documentation and related issues.
- *Explain the physiological changes that occur with age that a first responder should be aware of.
- *Identify reasons why a first responder might approach a child or infant victim differently than an adult victim.
- *Identify the special needs that a physically or mentally disabled victim might have and explain how a first responder might address those needs.

*Signifies an Enrichment section objective.

◆ Attitude Objectives ◆

After reading this chapter and completing the class activities, you should be able to—

- Recognize the need for compassion when caring for a victim's physical and mental needs.
- Communicate willingly and sensitively in the care of all victims.
- *Appreciate the specific needs of elderly victims.
- *Empathize with the daily challenges faced and overcome by victims with a visual, hearing, motor, or mental disability.

◆ LEGAL AND ETHICAL ISSUES

Many people are concerned about lawsuits. Lawsuits against those who give care at the scene of an emergency are not often successful. By becoming aware of some basic legal principles, you may be able to avoid the possibility of legal action (Fig. 4-1).

The following sections address in general terms some legal principles and a few ethical responsibilities that relate to emergency care. Because laws vary from state to state, your instructor will need to inform you on the laws in your state that apply to you or tell you where you can find such information.

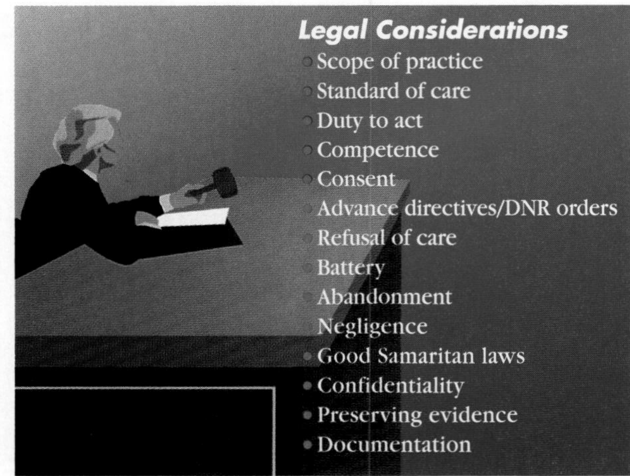

Legal Considerations
Scope of practice
Standard of care
Duty to act
Competence
Consent
Advance directives/DNR orders
Refusal of care
Battery
Abandonment
Negligence
Good Samaritan laws
Confidentiality
Preserving evidence
Documentation

Figure 4-1 First responders should be aware of these basic legal considerations.

Scope of Practice

The first responder's ***scope of practice*** is defined as the range of duties and skills a first responder is allowed and expected to perform when necessary. The first responder, like other out-of-hospital care providers, is governed by legal, ethical, and medical guidelines. These guidelines establish the scope and the limits of care the first responder provides. Since practice may differ from state to state or in regions of the same state, first responders must be aware of the variations existing for their level of training in their state or area.

Standard of Care

The public expects a certain ***standard of care*** from personnel summoned to provide emergency care. The standard of care is the criterion established for the extent and quality of first responder care. For instance, the standard of care for first responders is based on the training guidelines developed by the U.S. Department of Transportation and by the states and municipalities in which the first responders serve. When providing emergency care, first responders are expected to perform to at least the minimum standard set forth by their training. State laws and other authorities, such as national organizations, may govern the actions of other first responders. If your actions do not meet the set standards and harm another person, you may be successfully sued for negligence or malpractice.

Duty to Act

While on duty, the first responder has an obligation to respond to an emergency and provide care at the scene. This obligation is called a ***duty to act.*** This duty is governed either by **case law, statute,** or job description. This duty applies to public safety officers, certain government employees, licensed and certified professionals, and medical **paraprofessionals** while on duty. For instance, members of a volunteer fire department have a duty to act based on their agreement to participate in the fire department. An athletic trainer has a duty to give care to an injured athlete. Failure to adhere to these agreements could result in legal action.

If a first responder sees a motor-vehicle crash while driving to work, in most states, he or she has a moral obligation, as opposed to a legal obligation, to stop. However, once a first responder has begun care, he or she is legally obligated to continue until the victim is turned over to someone with equal or higher training.

Ethical Responsibilities

As a first responder, you have an ethical obligation to carry out your duties and responsibilities in a professional manner. This includes showing compassion when dealing with a victim's physical and mental needs, and communicating sensitively and willingly at all times. You must never become satisfied with meeting minimum training requirements but rather strive to professionally develop your skills to surpass the standards for your area. Doing so includes not only practicing and mastering the skills taught in this course but seeking out further training and information, such as through workshops, conferences, and supplemental or advanced educational programs. Your instructor may be able to provide ideas and information about opportunities in your area for increased education and professional development.

In addition to being the best you can be in providing care, be honest in reporting your actions and the events that occurred at a scene or when responding to an emergency. Make it a personal goal to be a person whom others trust and can depend on to give accurate reports and provide effective care.

The first responder should address responsibilities to the victim at each and every emergency. He or she must also periodically do a self-review of performance (victim care, communication, documentation, and so on) to help improve any areas of weakness.

Competence

Competence refers to the victim's ability to understand the questions of the first responder and to understand the implications of decisions made. First responders must obtain permission from competent victims before beginning any care. To receive consent or refusal of care, the first responder should determine competence. In certain cases, such as intoxication and drug abuse, the victim is not considered competent. In such cases, call advanced medical care and law enforcement personnel or send someone to call. If possible, the first responder should attempt to provide care but not endanger his or her safety. Always maintain a safe distance from potentially violent or hostile victims.

Consent

An individual has a basic right to decide what can and cannot be done to his or her body. Therefore to provide care for an ill or injured person, you must first obtain that person's ***consent.*** Usually, the person needs to tell you clearly that you have permission to provide care. To obtain consent, you must—

1. Identify yourself to the person.
2. Give your level of training.
3. Explain what you observe.
4. Explain what you plan to do.

Expressed Consent

After you have provided this information, the person can decide whether to give his or her **expressed (informed or actual) consent.** A person can withdraw consent for care at any time. If this should occur, step back and call for more advanced medical personnel. In some circumstances, you may be asked to explain why the person needs your care.

Implied Consent

A person who is unconscious or in your best judgment is confused, mentally impaired, or seriously ill or injured may not be able to give expressed consent. In these cases, the law assumes that the person would give consent for care if he or she were able to do so. This is termed **implied consent.** Implied consent also applies to minors who obviously need emergency assistance when a parent or guardian is not present.

Special Situations

Unless an illness or injury is life threatening, a parent or guardian who is present must give consent for **minors** before care can be given. If you encounter a parent or guardian who refuses to let you give care, try to explain to him or her the consequences of not giving the victim care. Use terms the parent or guardian will understand. A law enforcement officer can help obtain the necessary legal authority for care to be provided. If a law enforcement offi-

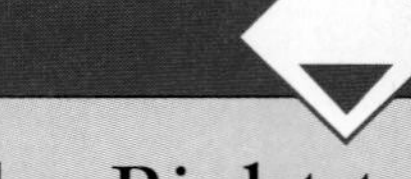

The Right to Choose

You respond to a call dispatched as a "heart attack." A woman has called saying that her husband was found unconscious and not breathing. Once on the scene, you ask how long he has been like this. The woman responds, "I don't know." You check a 60-year-old man for vital signs. No pulse! You are suddenly faced with the fact that the victim is clinically dead.

You've been trained to start CPR when there is no pulse, but the victim's wife tells you *not* to resuscitate him. She shows you papers that state he wishes not to receive medical care. Questions race through your mind. What are my moral and legal responsibilities? Is this document valid? Should I start CPR anyway? Should I call for advice? Should I follow my local protocols? Do my protocols cover this situation?

According to the 1992 Guidelines for CPR and Emergency Cardiac Care, "When a person suffers a cardiac arrest, prompt initiation of CPR is indicated. CPR should be provided by trained personnel unless generally accepted criteria for the determination of death are met or there is documentation or other reliable reasons to believe that CPR is not indicated, wanted, or in the victim's best interest."

Written instructions that describe a person's wishes about medical treatment are called *advance directives.* These instructions are used when the person can no longer make his or her own health care decisions.

Some examples of advance directives are *living wills* and *durable powers of attorney for health care.* The types of health care decisions covered by these documents vary depending on where you live. Talking with a legal professional can help determine which advance directive options are available in your state and what they do and do not cover.

Living wills generally allow a person to refuse only medical care that "merely prolongs the process of dying." A durable power of attorney for health care is a document authorizing someone to make medical decisions for an individual if that individual should become unable to make them for him or herself. This authorized person should support the needs and wishes of the victim, as outlined in the advance directive.

Another way to formalize preferences is by using *Do Not Resuscitate (DNR)* orders. A doctor could make DNR orders a part of an individual's medical record. Such orders would state that if

cer is not present, send someone to call or find one. If necessary, do so yourself. Do not argue with the parent or guardian. Doing so can create a potentially unsafe scene.

If the victim is an adult whom you know or learn is under a legal guardian's care, you must also get that guardian's consent to give care. Summon a law enforcement officer if necessary.

In certain situations, a person's cultural or religious beliefs may prevent that person from receiving care or being cared for by strangers or members of the opposite sex. In such a situation, you should respect the person's wishes and call for more advanced medical personnel.

Advance Directives and Do Not Resuscitate (DNR) Orders

Advance directives and **Do Not Resuscitate (DNR)** orders are written instructions from a physician that protect a victim's right to refuse efforts to resuscitate him or her. These orders are usually written for people who have a terminal illness. Advance directives and DNR orders may differ from state to state. You must be aware of your state and local legis-

the individual's heartbeat or breathing stops, he or she should not be resuscitated. The choice in deciding on DNR orders may be covered in a living will or in the durable power of attorney for health care.

Since these documents are sometimes still unclear about the exact level of care desired, a more recent approach has been to consider establishing *no-CPR* orders to avoid confusion. EMS personnel are encouraged to become familiar with the intent of the order and make provisions to identify persons who have *no-CPR* orders.

Interpreting advance directives in the out-of-hospital setting is fraught with difficulty; it requires the rescuer to interpret a legal document at the time of a medical emergency. So what is being done to make this decision easier?

EMS systems are developing protocols so that if confronted with an advance directive, the responder will know what to do. In some cases, first responders, EMTs, and paramedics initiate care but quickly notify their medical director of the situation. Since family members may be concerned that emergency medical personnel are not honoring the requests of the advance directive, personnel must sensitively and emphatically convey to the family emergency medical personnel's responsibility to initiate care while awaiting physician direction.

According to JAMA, "In certain cases, it may be difficult to determine if resuscitation should be started. For example, despite the presence of a no-CPR order, family members, surrogates, or the patient's physician may request that CPR be initiated. If there is reasonable doubt or substantive reason to believe the no-CPR order is invalid, CPR should be initiated. If evidence later indicates that resuscitation is inappropriate, CPR or other life support can be discontinued."

Advance directives are not limited to elderly people or people with a terminal illness. More people of all ages are choosing to make their wishes known through advance directives.

Prepare yourself for emergency situations by knowing how to handle advance directives. Check with your local EMS system. Inquire about how to deal with living wills, medical durable powers of attorney for health care, DNR orders, and no-CPR orders.

lation and protocols relative to these orders. Your state EMS office is a good source of this information.

Refusal of Care

Some ill or injured people may refuse care, even those who desperately need it. Even though the person may be seriously injured, you should honor his or her ***refusal of care.*** Try to convince the person of the need for care, but do not argue. Allow more advanced medical personnel to evaluate the situation. If possible, to make it clear that you did not abandon the person, have a witness hear and document the person's refusal. Many EMS systems have a "Refusal of Care" form that you can use in these situations.

Battery

Battery is the legal term used to describe the unlawful touching of a victim without the victim's consent. As mentioned, the first responder must obtain consent before giving care to a victim. Every person has a legal right to determine what happens to and who touches his or her body. If you try to give care or check a pulse on a patient who has refused your care, you could be charged with battery. The first responder must obtain consent (through the steps mentioned earlier) before even touching the victim.

Abandonment

Just as you must have the person's consent before beginning care, you must also continue to give care once you have begun. Once you have started emergency care, you are legally obligated to continue that care until a person with equal or higher training relieves you, you are physically unable to continue, or the victim refuses care. Usually, your obligation for care ends when more advanced medical professionals take over. If you stop your care before that point, you can be legally responsible for the ***abandonment*** of a person in need.

Negligence

Negligence is the failure to follow a reasonable standard of care, thereby causing or contributing to injury or damage to another. A person could be negligent either by acting wrongly or failing to act at all. The following scenario is an example of a case in which negligence may be suspected.

A car is traveling at a high rate of speed on an icy road. The driver loses control, and the car flips end over end. A passenger is ejected from the car and hurled 30 feet, landing on her back.

The arriving first responder notes the severity of the incident but fails to consider that the passenger may have a spinal injury. The first responder attempts to get the victim to stand up and move out of the road, even though there is no immediate threat of danger. This movement causes the victim to experience severe pain, and she suddenly loses feeling in her legs. In this case, the first responder may be negligent because he or she failed to follow a reasonable standard of care of a trained first responder.

Four components must be present for a lawsuit charging negligence to be successful:

- Duty
- Breach
- Cause
- Damage

As a first responder, you have a duty to respond in a professional manner, obeying traffic laws and following the protocols that govern your actions. If you fail to act within this duty, then you commit a breach of duty. If that breach is the cause of physical injury for which the person suffers damage, typically measured in financial terms, such as medical costs, lost wages, and future needs, then all the elements of a negligence claim are present.

Most states have enacted ***Good Samaritan laws,*** which protect people providing emergency care. These laws, which differ from state to state, may protect you from legal liability as a first responder as long as you act in good faith, are not negligent, and act within the scope of your training. Some Good Samaritan laws, however, do not provide coverage for individuals with a duty to respond. For this reason, it is important that you know the degree to which your state's Good Samaritan laws will help protect you while performing the duties of a first responder.

Confidentiality

While providing care, you may learn things about the victim that are generally considered private and confidential. Information such as previous medical problems, physical problems, and medications being taken, is personal to the victim. Respect the victim's privacy by maintaining ***confidentiality.*** Television and newspaper reporters may ask you questions. Attorneys may also approach you at the scene. Never discuss the victim or the care you gave with anyone except law enforcement personnel or other personnel caring for the victim. The only exceptions to this are in cases of suspected or known abuse or in injuries sustained in physical or sexual assault. Some state laws require the first responder to report such incidents to the applicable government agency or the proper EMS authority.

Potential Crime Scene / Evidence Preservation

Sometimes first responders may be called to give care to a victim of violence or crime.

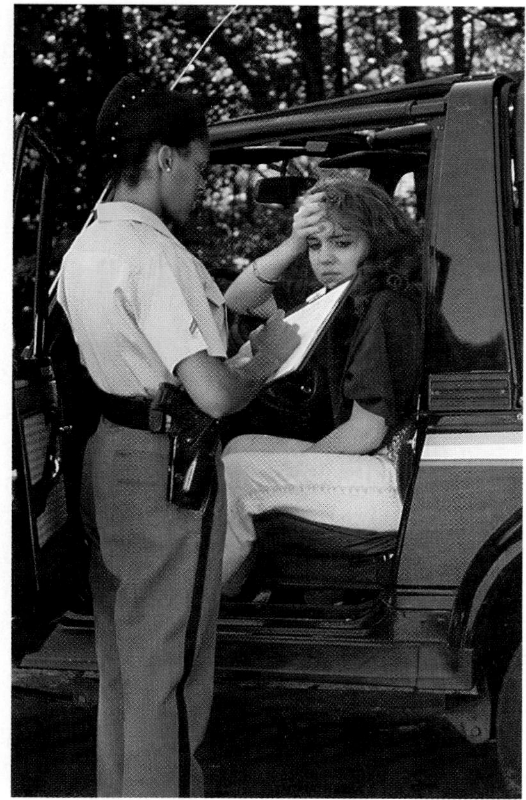

Figure 4-2 Record the conditions of the victim at the emergency scene as soon as possible.

Do not approach the scene if you believe it is unsafe. If you respond to this type of incident and law enforcement personnel are not present, they must be notified. An unsafe scene or situation is just cause for not providing or stoping care. Other responsibilities could include —

- Observing and documenting anything unusual at the scene.
- Preserving evidence.

Documentation

Documentation procedures are established by state regulations or laws or by local policy and may vary from state to state. Documenting your care is nearly as important as the care itself. Your record will help advanced health-care professionals assess the victim and continue care. Because a victim's condition may change before the victim arrives at the hospital, a record of the condition immediately after the emergency will provide useful information for EMTs and emergency department staff. They can compare the current condition to what you recorded earlier.

Your record is a legal document and is important if legal action occurs. Should you be called to court for any reason, your record will support what you saw, heard, and did at the scene of the emergency. It is important to write the record as soon as possible after the emergency while all the facts are fresh (Fig. 4-2). Many EMS systems have printed forms for first responders to use. Your instructor may be able to give you information about the report forms used in your system.

◆ SUMMARY

In your role as an emergency care provider, you are guided by certain legal parameters, such as the duty to act and professional standards of care. Victims of injury or illness have a right to expect competent initial care by a first responder. Part of a first responder's responsibility lies not only in giving competent care, but also in keeping up skills and knowledge through refresher programs and continuing education.

Regardless of your profession, when you are called to help a victim of injury or sudden illness, you assume the role of an emergency care provider. When an emergency occurs, the people in your care, as well as assisting bystanders, will expect you to know what to do. Be prepared to think and act accordingly. What to do, however, often involves more than giving emergency care. Chapter 1 includes an overview of the first responder's role in assessing and managing emergency scenes.

Keeping information that you learn about a victim confidential is very important. The information that you learn as you give care can directly affect the outcome of the victim's condition. Victims could lose trust in first responders who do not protect their confidentiality. Effective documentation is important in maintaining the standard of care for a victim and may provide legal protection for you and the organization you represent.

Use the activities in Unit 4 of your workbook to help you review the material in this chapter.

You Are the Responder

A 12-year-old basketball player was temporarily unconscious after hitting his head in a fall during a game. He is now awake but complaining of dizziness and nausea. You, the first responder, tell the player to go home and rest. At home, the player loses consciousness and his parents call for an ambulance. Later, at the hospital, the boy is diagnosed as having a severe head injury that could have been minimized if medical attention had been provided earlier. In your opinion, are there any grounds for legal action against you? State your reasons why or why not.

ENRICHMENT

◆ SPECIAL POPULATIONS

Some segments of the population may require special consideration when you are providing care. These groups include the elderly and people with disabilities.

The Elderly Victim

The elderly are generally considered those over 65 years of age. This segment of the population is quickly becoming the fastest growing group in the United States. A major reason for this occurrence is an increase in life expectancy because of advances in health care. Since 1900, there has been a 57 percent increase in life expectancy. For example, in 1900, the average life expectancy was 49 years. Today, the average life expectancy exceeds 75 years.

Many changes occur with age. Overall, there is a general decline in body function, with some changes beginning as early as age 30. One of the first body systems affected is the respiratory system. The capacity of the respiratory system begins to decrease around age 30. By the time we reach age 65, the respiratory system may be only half as effective as it was in our youth. The heart also suffers the effects of aging. The amount of blood pumped by the heart with each beat decreases and the heart rate slows. The blood vessels harden, causing increased work for the heart. The number of functioning brain cells also decreases with age. Hearing and vision usually decline, often causing some degree of sight and hearing loss. Reflexes become slower, and arthritis may affect joints, causing movement to become painful.

As a result of slower reflexes, failing eyesight and hearing, arthritis, and numbness (related to the blood vessels) the elderly are at increased risk of injury from falls. Falls frequently result in fractures because the bones become weaker and more brittle with age.

An elderly person is also at increased risk of serious head injuries. This is primarily because of the change in proportion between the brain and the skull. As we age, the size of the brain decreases, which results in increased space between the surface of the brain and the inside of the skull. This allows more movement of the brain within the skull, which can increase the likelihood of serious head injury. Occasionally, an elderly person may not develop the signs and symptoms of a head injury until days after a fall. Therefore, you should always suspect a head injury as a possible cause of unusual behavior in an elderly victim, especially if there is a history of a fall or blow to the head.

The elderly are also prone to nervous system disorders. The most common such disorder in the elderly is stroke, discussed in Chapter 15. In addition, the elderly are at increased risk of altered thinking patterns and confusion. Some deterioration in mental function caused by ag-

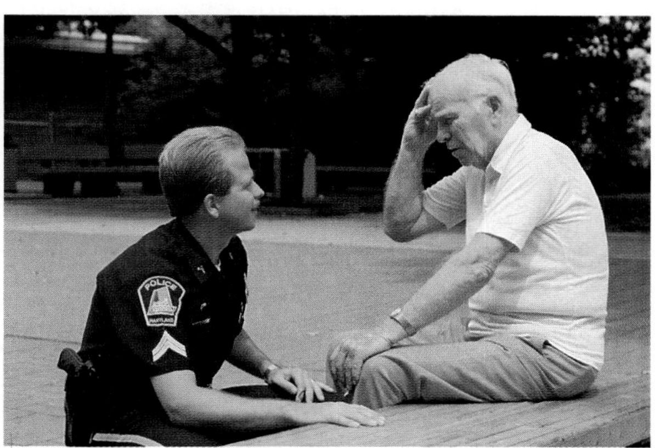

Figure 4-3 Speak to an elderly victim at eye level.

ing is normal. However, we have more recently learned that certain diseases occurring in some elderly persons also cause deterioration in mental function. The most common of these is **Alzheimer's disease,** a progressive, degenerative disease that affects the brain. It results in impaired memory, thinking, and behavior. Alzheimer's disease affects an estimated 2.5 million adults.

If you are providing care for a confused elderly person, try to determine whether the confusion is the result of injury or a preexisting condition. Get at the victim's eye level so he or she can see and hear you more clearly (Fig. 4-3). Sometimes confusion is actually the result of decreased vision or hearing.

Your care for the elderly victim requires you to keep in mind the special problems and concerns of the elderly and to communicate appropriately. Often, an elderly victim's problem will seem insignificant to him or her. However, he or she may not recognize the signs or symptoms of a serious condition. For example, an elderly person may complain of weakness. On further questioning, you may learn that she has been having fainting episodes with periods of numbness and tingling in one side of the body. Some elderly victims may purposely minimize their symptoms from fear of losing their independence or of being placed in a nursing home or similar institution. If the victim takes medications, you should gather them and see that they are with the victim if he or she is being taken to a medical facility.

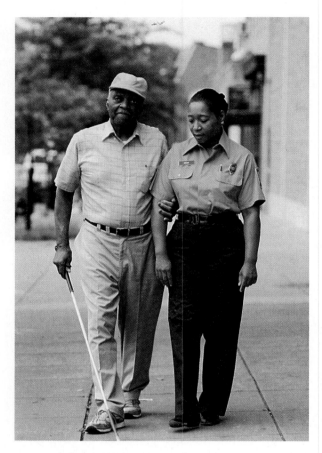

Figure 4-4 If a blind victim can walk, stand beside the victim and have him or her hold your arm.

The Victim with Physical or Mental Disabilities

Other special populations include people with physical or mental disabilities. The terms *physical* and *mental* disabilities mean different things to different people. What comes to mind when you hear these words? A person who uses a wheelchair? An amputee? Someone said to be mentally retarded?

A person who suffers a serious injury that results in the loss of a limb, or who is born without a limb, is often referred to as having a physical disability. So is someone who suffers the paralyzing effects of a stroke.

A **mentally disabled** person has an impairment of mental function that interferes with normal activity. Anyone at any age can find himself or herself disabled by a physical or mental impairment that interferes to some degree with normal activities. Some of the more common types of mental or physical disabilities that you will encounter include the people with visual impairments, hearing impairments, and physical and developmental disabilities.

Visually Impaired

People who are unable to see adequately or at all are often called blind or partially blind. These people are also said to be **visually impaired.** Blindness can occur from many causes. Some people are born blind. Others can see, then subsequently lose sight through injury or illness. Visual impairment is not necessarily a problem in the eyes. It can occur because of problems in the visual centers of the brain.

People who are visually impaired have usually adapted well to their condition and are not embarrassed by it. It should be no more difficult to communicate with this victim than with one who can see. It is not necessary to speak loudly or in overly simple terms. In fact, your assessment of the visually impaired victim should be little different from one of a victim who is not impaired. The victim may not be able to tell you certain things about how an injury occurred but can generally give you a good description based on his or her interpretation of sounds and touch.

If you are called to assist a person who is visually impaired, explain to him or her what is going on and what you are doing. This will help alleviate anxiety. It will also allow the victim to orient himself or herself to the environment and then provide you with information regarding his or her care. If you must move a visually impaired victim who can walk, stand beside the victim and have the victim hold on to your arm (Fig. 4-4). Walk at a normal pace and alert him or her to any hazards, such as stairs, during the move. If the victim has a seeing eye dog, try to keep them together. These dogs are usually not aggressive. If the victim has a cane, give it to the victim, or carry it yourself if the victim is unable to.

Hearing Impaired

People who are unable to hear or who suffer from any other type of hearing disability are termed **hearing impaired** and are often referred to as deaf or partially deaf. Deafness can occur as a result of injury or illness affecting the ear, the nerves leading from the ear to the brain, or the brain. As with blindness, deafness can be present at birth or can develop later as a result of injury or illness. Some rescuers become anxious when called to treat a hearing-impaired person. This anxiety is unnecessary. Hearing-impaired people should be cared for in basically the same manner as the hearing. You may only have to modify your assessment somewhat so that you can obtain necessary information.

You may not even be aware initially that a victim is deaf. Often, the victim will tell you. Others may point at their ear and shake their head, "No." A child may carry a card stating that he or she is deaf. You may see a hearing aid in a person's ear. The biggest obstacle you must overcome in caring for the hearing impaired is how to best communicate (Fig. 4-5). If you know how to use sign language, then you may communicate in this manner. Often the victim will be able to read lips. If the victim's illness or injury does not distract from the ability to read your lips, then communicate in this manner. Position yourself where the victim can see you. You must look at the victim when you speak and speak slowly. Do not modify the way you form words. If the victim cannot read lips and communication through sign language is impossible, you can write messages on paper and have the victim respond. This system is slow, but effective. Some hearing-impaired people have a machine called a Telecommunications Device for the Deaf (TDD), which is generally used for telephone communication. You can use this device to type messages and questions to the victim, and the victim can type replies to you.

Hearing-impaired persons are usually not embarrassed by their condition. They have adapted to it by learning to lip read, sign, or both. Most deaf people can also speak. One person's speech will be quite clear, whereas an-

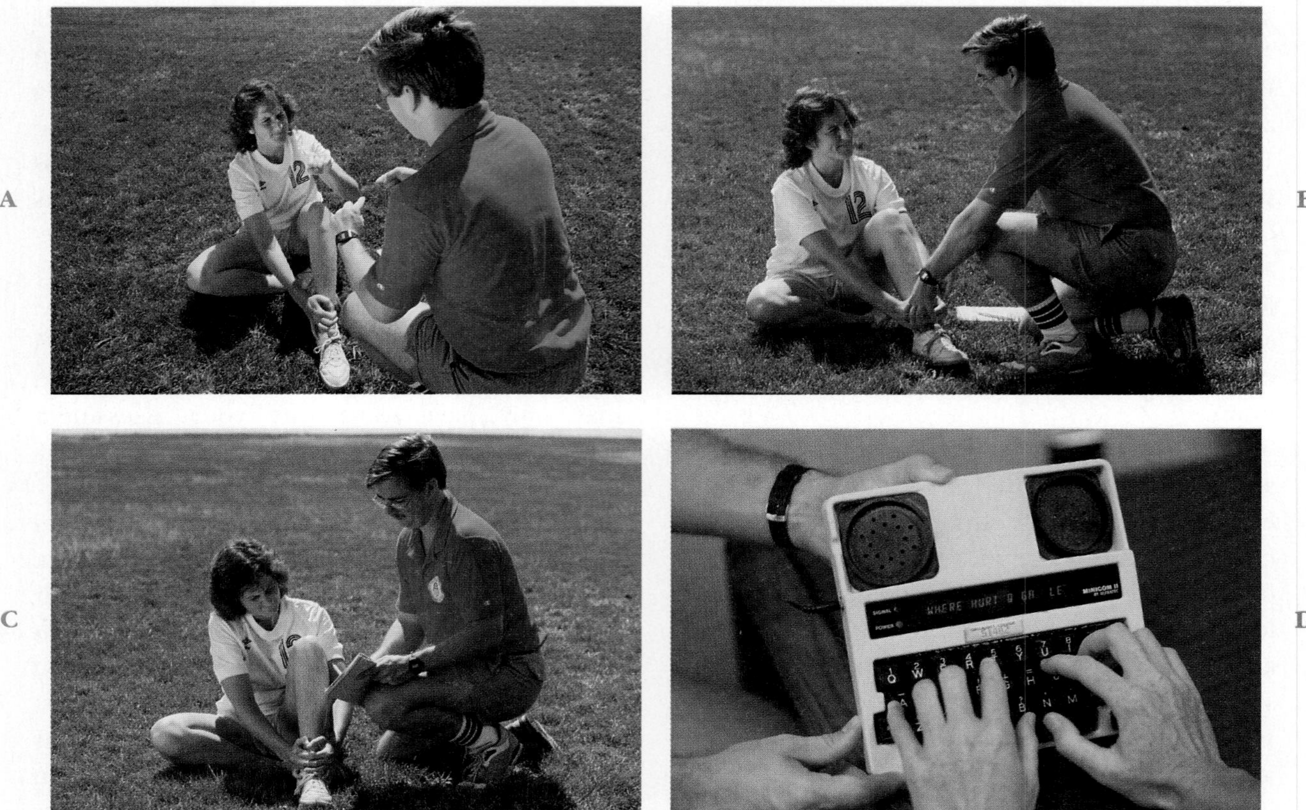

Figure 4-5 Communicate with a hearing-impaired victim in the best way possible: **A,** Signing; **B,** Lip Reading; **C,** Writing; **D,** TDD.

other's will be more difficult to understand. If you do not understand what the victim is saying, ask him or her to repeat. Do not pretend that you understand.

Physically Disabled

The term **physically disabled** refers to a person who is unable to move normally. The impairments causing a disability can be diverse. Physical disabilities generally result from problems with the muscles or bones or the nerves controlling them. Causes include stroke, cerebral palsy, multiple sclerosis, muscular dystrophy, polio, and brain and spinal cord injuries. Some physically disabled persons have adapted well to their situation and others have not. Care for the person who is physically disabled with respect and compassion. You will often need to be very patient. Many persons have adapted to life without assistance. Your presence may be perceived as a failure, and the person may refuse your assistance to prove that he or she does not need your help.

The physically disabled person who is injured poses unique problems because it may be difficult to determine which problems are new and which are preexisting conditions. If this situation occurs, and the person cannot respond to you, care for any detected problems as if they are new.

Developmentally Disabled

A person who has a mental disability is often described as being **developmentally dis-**

abled. As with physical impairments, mental impairments also can be diverse. Some types of mental impairment, such as Down syndrome, are genetic. Others result from injuries or infections that occur during pregnancy, after birth, or later in life. Some occur for reasons never determined.

Often you will be able to determine easily whether a person is developmentally disabled. However, in some situations, you will not be able to determine this. Always approach the victim as you would any other person in his or her age group. When you speak, try to determine the victim's level of understanding. If the person is confused, rephrase your statement or question in simpler terms. Listen carefully to what the victim is saying. People who are developmentally disabled often lead very orderly lives. A sudden illness or injury can interrupt the order in a person's life and cause a great deal of anxiety and fear. You should expect this concern and offer reassurance. Take time to explain to the victim who you are and what you are going to do. Try to gain the victim's trust. If a parent or guardian is present, ask him or her to assist you in providing care.

Human Body Systems

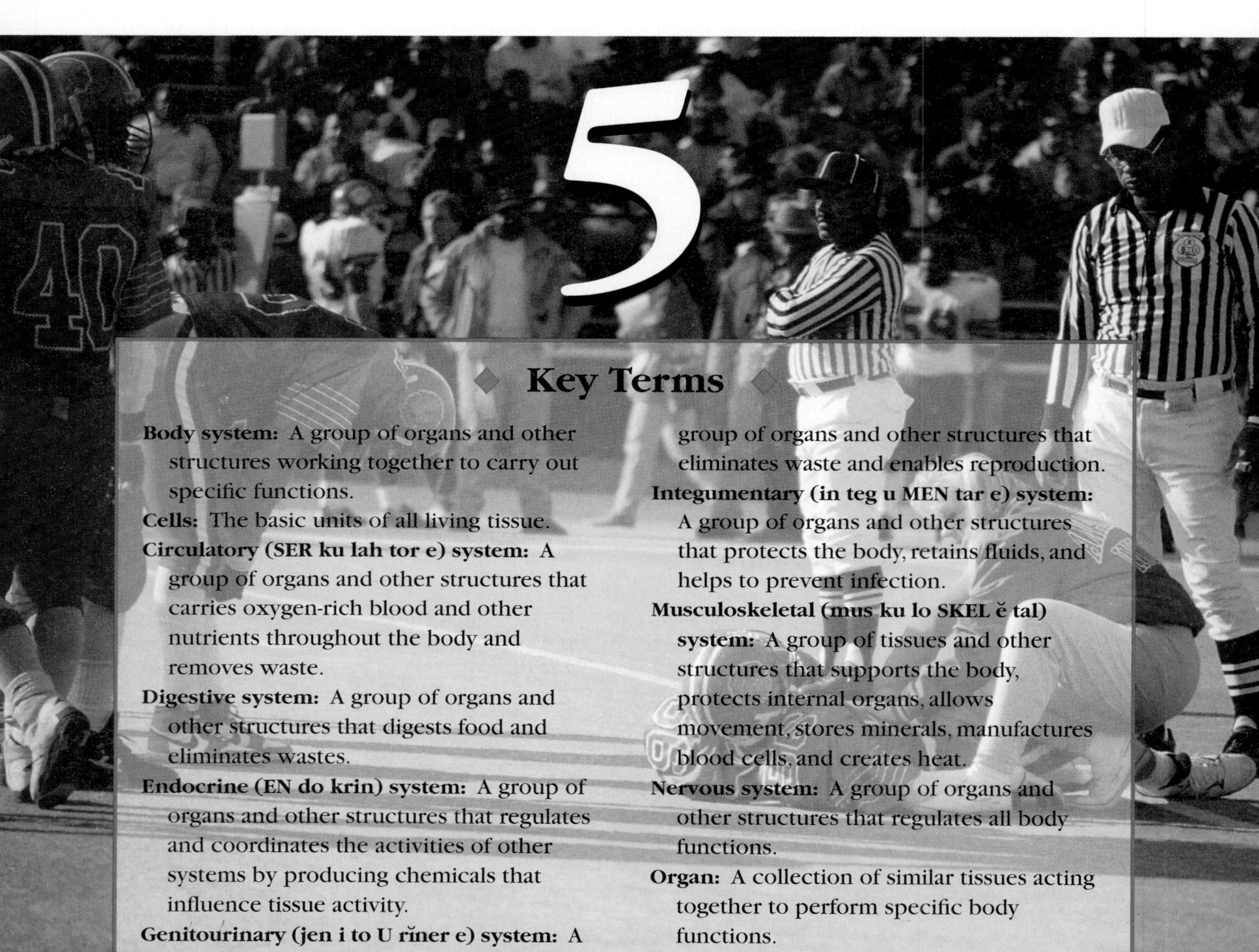

5

Key Terms

Body system: A group of organs and other structures working together to carry out specific functions.

Cells: The basic units of all living tissue.

Circulatory (SER ku lah tor e) system: A group of organs and other structures that carries oxygen-rich blood and other nutrients throughout the body and removes waste.

Digestive system: A group of organs and other structures that digests food and eliminates wastes.

Endocrine (EN do krin) system: A group of organs and other structures that regulates and coordinates the activities of other systems by producing chemicals that influence tissue activity.

Genitourinary (jen i to U rĭner e) system: A group of organs and other structures that eliminates waste and enables reproduction.

Integumentary (in teg u MEN tar e) system: A group of organs and other structures that protects the body, retains fluids, and helps to prevent infection.

Musculoskeletal (mus ku lo SKEL ĕ tal) system: A group of tissues and other structures that supports the body, protects internal organs, allows movement, stores minerals, manufactures blood cells, and creates heat.

Nervous system: A group of organs and other structures that regulates all body functions.

Organ: A collection of similar tissues acting together to perform specific body functions.

Respiratory (re SPI rah to re or **RES pah rah tor e) system:** A group of organs and other structures that brings air into the body and removes wastes through a process called breathing, or respiration.

Tissue: A collection of similar cells acting together to perform specific body functions.

Vital organs: Organs whose functions are essential to life, including the brain, heart, and lungs.

◆ Knowledge Objectives ◆

After reading this chapter and completing the class activities, you should be able to—

- *Describe the anatomical position.
- *Identify various anatomical terms commonly used to refer to the body.
- *Describe the various body cavities.
- *Identify the structure, function, and common problems of the digestive, endocrine, and genitourinary systems.
- Describe the structure and function of the respiratory, circulatory, musculoskeletal, nervous, and integumentary systems.
- *Provide examples of how body systems interrelate.
- *Describe what can happen to the body if a problem occurs in one or more of the body systems.

* Signifies an Enrichment section objective.

◆ Attitude Objectives ◆

After reading this chapter and completing the class activities, you should be able to—

- *Appreciate the interrelationships of the various body systems.

You see a car that has struck a tree. You stop and find the driver not wearing a seat belt and slumped in the front seat. The steering wheel is bent and the windshield is cracked. You see no signs of blood or other obvious injury. The person is breathing fast and does not respond when you speak to her. Which body systems may have been affected by the crash? What emergency care do you think she might need?

◆ INTRODUCTION

As a first responder, you need a basic understanding of normal human structure and function. Knowing the body's structures and how they work will help you more easily recognize and understand illnesses and injuries. Body systems do not function independently. Each system depends on other systems to function properly. When your body is healthy, your body systems are working well together. But an injury or illness in one body part or system will often cause problems in others. Knowing the location and function of the major organs and structures within each body system will help you to more accurately assess a victim's condition and provide the best care.

To remember the location of body structures, it helps to visualize the structures that lie beneath the skin. The structures you can see or feel are reference points for locating the internal structures you cannot see or feel. For example, to locate the pulse on either side of the neck, you can use the Adam's apple on the front of the neck as a reference point. Using reference points will help you describe the location of injuries and other problems you may find. This chapter provides you with an overview of important reference points, terminology, and the functions of specific body systems.

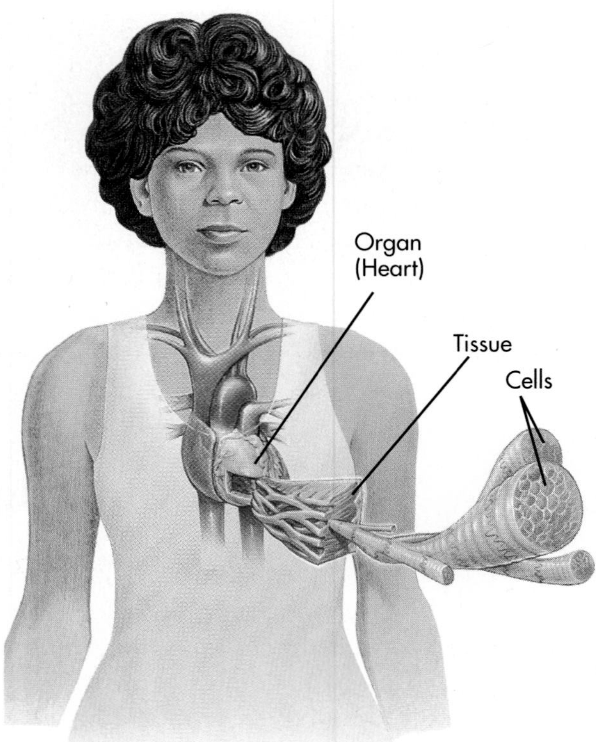

Figure 5-1 Cells and tissues make up organs.

◆ BODY SYSTEMS

The human body is a miraculous machine. It performs many complex functions, each of which helps us live. The body is made up of billions of microscopic ***cells,*** the basic unit of all living tissue. There are many different types of cells. Each type contributes in a specific way to keep the body functioning normally. Collections of similar cells form ***tissues,*** which form ***organs*** (Fig. 5-1).

Vital organs are organs whose functions are essential for life. They include the brain, heart, and lungs.

A ***body system*** is a group of organs and other structures that are especially adapted to perform specific body functions. They work together to carry out a function needed for life. For example, the heart, blood, and blood vessels make up the circulatory system. The ***circulatory system*** keeps all parts of the body supplied with oxygen-rich blood.

For the body to work properly, all of the following systems must work well together:

- Respiratory
- Circulatory
- Nervous
- Musculoskeletal
- Integumentary
- Endocrine
- Digestive
- Genitourinary

The Respiratory System

The ***respiratory system*** supplies the body with oxygen through breathing.

Structure and Function

The body must have a constant supply of oxygen to stay alive. When you **inhale,** air fills the lungs, and the **oxygen** in the air is transferred to the blood. The blood carries oxygen to all parts of the body. This same system removes carbon dioxide. Carbon dioxide is transferred from the blood to the lungs. When you **exhale,** air is forced from the lungs, expelling **carbon dioxide** and other waste gases. This breathing process is called **respiration.**

The respiratory system includes the airway and lungs. Figure 5-2 shows the parts of the respiratory system.

The **airway** is the passage through which air travels to the lungs. It begins at the nose and mouth, which form the upper airway. Air passes through the nose and mouth, through the **pharynx** (the throat), **larynx** (the voice box), and **trachea** (the windpipe) to reach the lungs (Fig. 5-3).

The **lungs** are a pair of organs in the chest that provides the mechanism for taking in oxygen and removing carbon dioxide during breathing. The trachea is also called the windpipe. Behind the trachea is the **esophagus,** which carries food and liquids from the mouth to the stomach. A small flap of tissue, the **epiglottis,** covers the larynx and the trachea when you swallow to keep food and liquids out of the trachea and the lungs.

Air reaches the lungs through two tubes called **bronchi.** The bronchi branch into increasingly smaller tubes (Fig. 5-4, *A*). These tubes eventually end in millions of tiny air sacs called **alveoli** (Fig. 5-4, *B*). Oxygen and carbon dioxide pass into and out of the blood through the thin cell walls of the alveoli and tiny blood vessels called capillaries.

Air enters the lungs when you inhale and leaves the lungs when you exhale. When you inhale, the chest muscles and the diaphragm contract. This contraction expands the chest and draws air into the lungs. When you exhale,

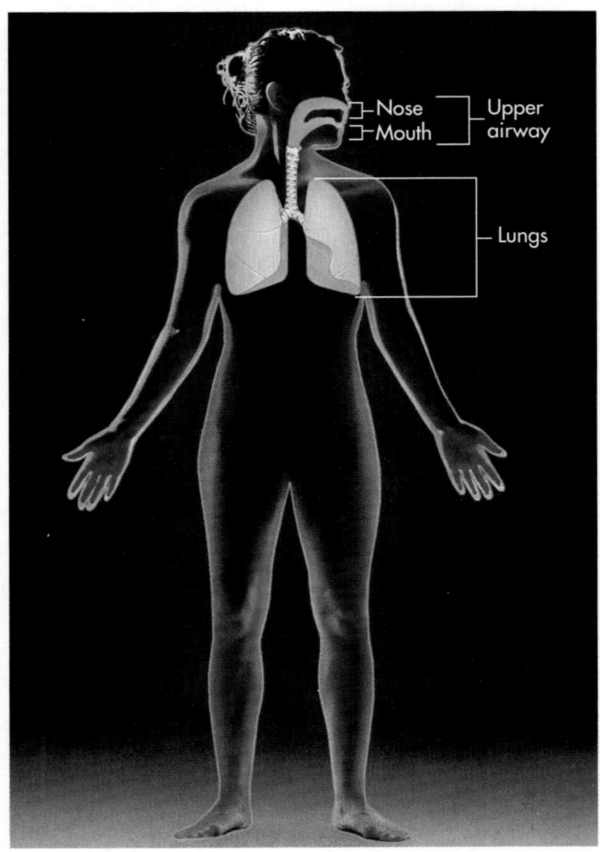

Figure 5-2 The Respiratory System

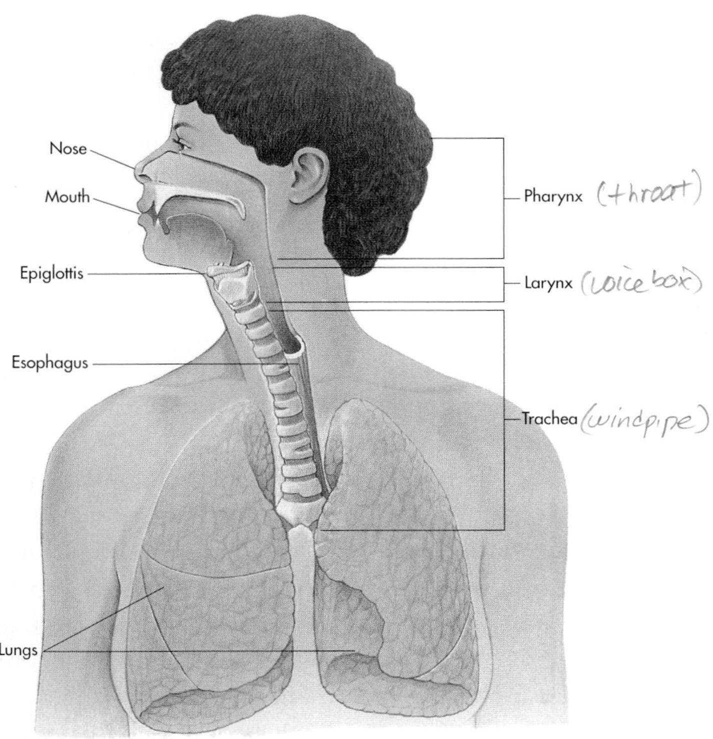

Figure 5-3 The respiratory system includes the pharynx, larynx, and trachea.

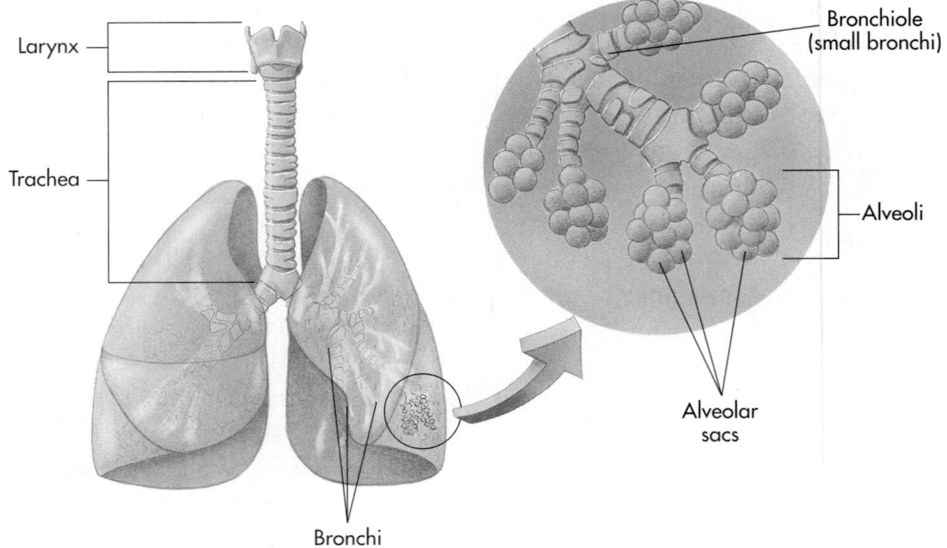

Figure 5-4 **A**, The bronchi branch into many small tubes. **B**, Oxygen and carbon dioxide pass into and out of blood through the walls of the alveoli and the capillaries.

the chest muscles and diaphragm relax, allowing air to exit from the lungs (Fig. 5-5).

The average adult breathes about 1 pint of air (500 ml) per breath and breathes about 10 to 20 times per minute. This ongoing breathing process is involuntary and is controlled by the brain.

Problems That Require Emergency Care

Because of the body's constant need for oxygen, it is important to recognize breathing difficulties and provide emergency care immediately. Some causes of breathing difficulties include asthma, allergies, and injuries to the chest. Breathing difficulty is referred to as **respiratory distress.**

If a person has breathing difficulties, you may hear or see noisy breathing or gasping. The victim may be conscious or unconscious. The conscious victim may be anxious or excited or may say that he or she feels short of breath. The victim's skin, particularly the lips and under the fingernails, may have a blue tint. This condition is called **cyanosis** and occurs when the tissues do not get enough oxygen.

If a person stops breathing, it is called **respiratory arrest.** Respiratory arrest is a life-threatening emergency. Without the oxygen obtained from breathing, other body systems fail to function.

Respiratory problems require immediate attention. Making sure the airway is open and clear is an important first step. You may have to breathe for a nonbreathing victim or give abdominal thrusts to someone who is choking. Breathing for a nonbreathing victim is called **rescue breathing.** These skills are discussed in detail in Chapter 8.

The Circulatory System

The circulatory system works with the respiratory system to carry oxygen to every cell in the body.

Structure and Function

The circulatory system, which includes the heart, blood, and blood vessels, also carries other nutrients throughout the body and removes waste. Figure 5-6 shows this system.

The **heart** is a muscular organ behind the

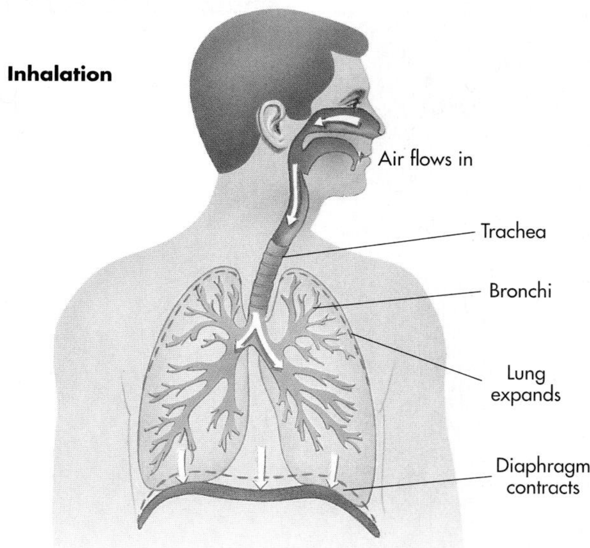

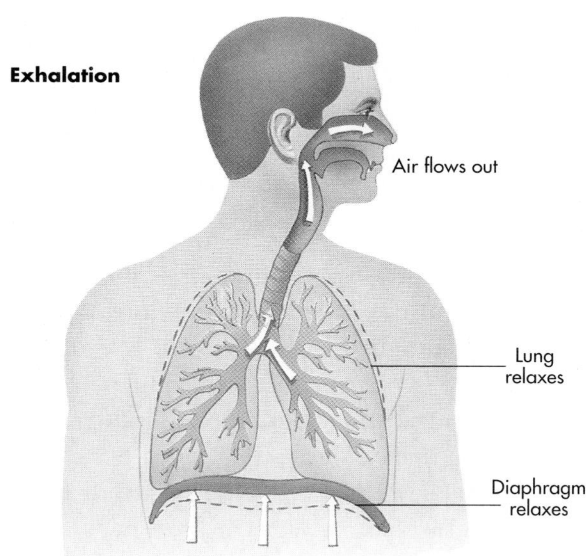

Figure 5-5 The chest muscles and the diaphragm contract as you inhale and relax as you exale.

sternum, or breastbone. The heart pumps blood throughout the body through veins and arteries. **Arteries** are large blood vessels that carry oxygen-rich blood from the heart to the rest of the body, except for the pulmonary arteries, which carry oxygen-poor blood from the heart to the lungs. The arteries subdivide into smaller blood vessels that become tiny capillaries. The **capillaries** transport blood to all the cells of the body and nourish them with oxygen.

After the oxygen in the blood is given to the cells, **veins** carry the oxygen-poor blood back to the heart, except for the pulmonary veins, which carry oxygen-rich blood back to the heart from the lungs. The heart pumps this oxygen-poor blood to the lungs to pick up more oxygen before pumping it to other parts of the body. This cycle is called the **circulatory cycle.** The cross section of the heart in Figure 5-7 shows how blood moves through the heart to complete the circulatory cycle.

The pumping action of the heart is called a **contraction.** Contractions are controlled by the heart's electrical system, which makes the heart beat regularly. You can feel the heart's contractions in the arteries that are close to the skin, for instance, at the neck or the wrist. The beat you feel with each contraction is called the **pulse.** The heart must beat continuously to deliver oxygen-rich blood to body cells to keep the body functioning properly.

Problems That Require Emergency Care

The following problems threaten the delivery of oxygen-rich blood to body cells:

- Blood loss caused by severe bleeding (e.g., a severed artery)
- Impaired circulation (e.g., a blood clot)
- Failure of the heart to pump adequately (e.g., a heart attack)

Body tissues that do not receive oxygen die. For example, when an artery supplying the brain with blood is blocked, brain tissue dies. When an artery supplying the heart with blood is blocked, heart muscle tissue dies. The death of heart muscle tissue can result in a life-threatening emergency, such as a heart attack.

When a person has a heart attack, the heart functions irregularly and may stop. If the heart stops, breathing will also stop. When the heart stops beating, it is called **cardiac arrest.** Victims of either heart attack or cardiac arrest need emergency care immediately. Cardiac ar-

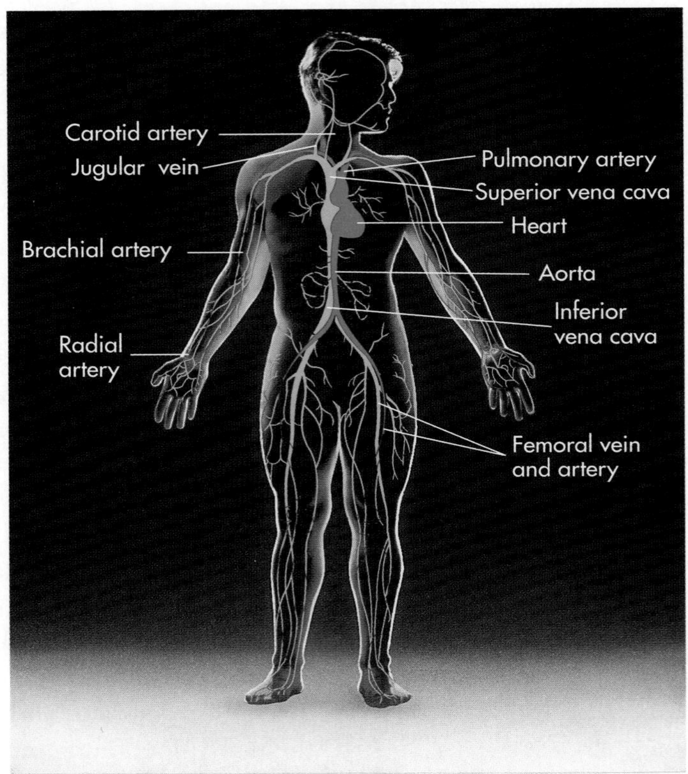

Figure 5-6 The Circulatory System

rest victims need to have their circulation maintained artificially by chest compressions and rescue breathing. This combination of compressions and breaths is called **cardiopulmonary resuscitation,** or **CPR.** You will learn more about the heart and how to perform CPR in Chapter 10.

The Nervous System

The ***nervous system*** is the most complex and delicate of all body systems. It relays information from the body to the brain and activates, coordinates, and controls the activity of all body systems.

Structure and Function

The **brain,** the center of the nervous system, is the master organ of the body. It regulates all body functions, including the respiratory and circulatory systems. The primary functions of the brain can be divided into three categories. These are the sensory functions, the motor functions, and the integrated functions of consciousness, memory, emotions, and use of language.

The brain transmits and receives information through a network of nerves. Figure 5-8 shows the nervous system. The **spinal cord,** a cylindrical structure consisting mainly of nerve cells covered by protective membranes, extends from the brain through a canal in the **spine,** or backbone. **Nerves** extend from the brain and spinal cord to every part of the body.

Nerves transmit information as electrical impulses from one area of the body to another. Some nerves conduct impulses from the body to the brain, allowing you to see, hear, smell, taste, and feel. These are the sensory functions. Other nerves conduct impulses from the brain to the muscles to control motor functions, or movement (Fig. 5-9).

The integrated functions of the brain are more complex. One of these functions is **con-**

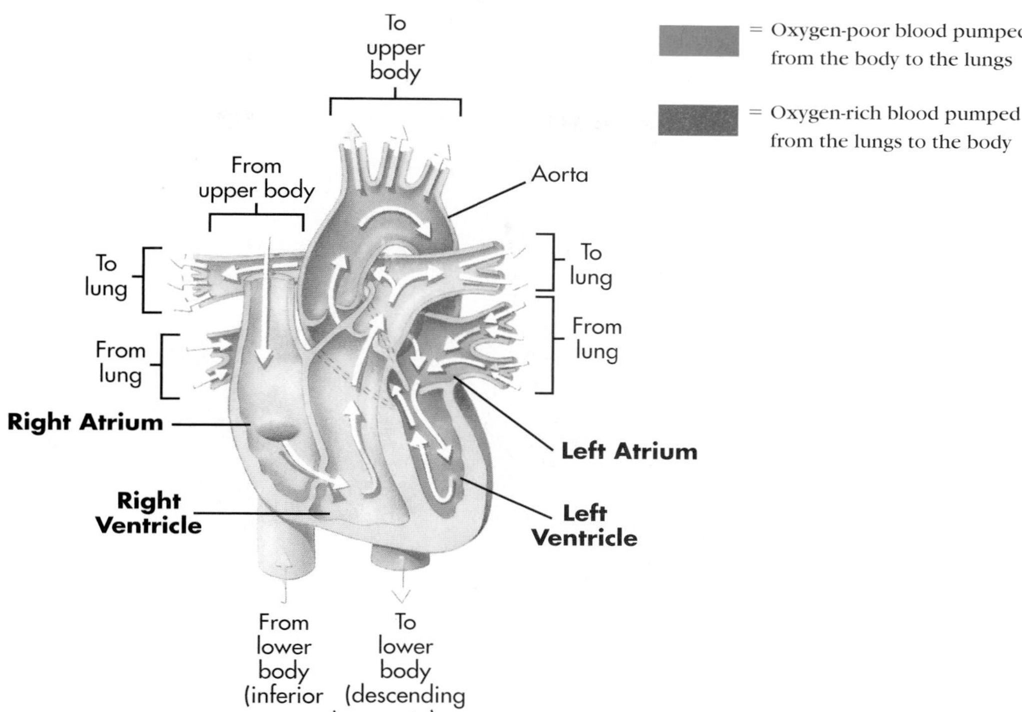

Figure 5-7 The heart is a two-sided pump made up of four chambers. A system of one-way valves keeps blood moving in the proper direction to complete the circulatory cycle.

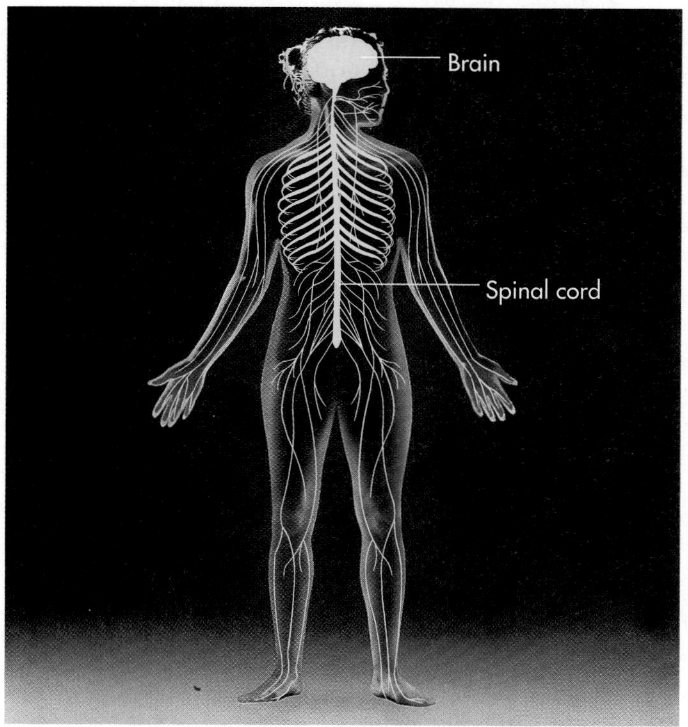

Figure 5-8 The Nervous System

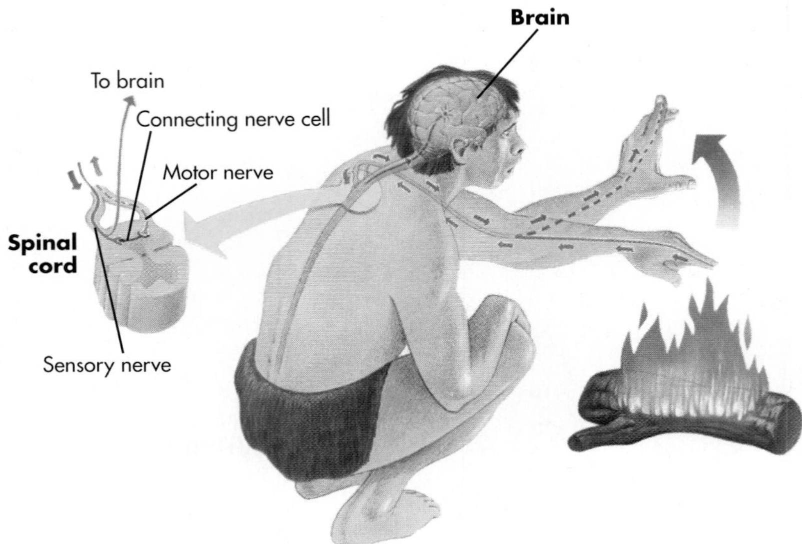

Figure 5-9 Messages are sent to and from the brain by way of the nerves.

sciousness. Normally, when you are awake, you are conscious. In most cases, being conscious means that you know who you are, where you are, the approximate date and time, and what is happening around you. There are various degrees of consciousness. Your level of consciousness can vary from being highly aware in certain situations to being less aware during periods of relaxation, sleep, illness, or injury.

Problems That Require Emergency Care

Brain cells, unlike other body cells, cannot regenerate, or grow back. Once brain cells die or are damaged, they are not replaced. Brain cells may die from disease or injury. When a particular part of the brain is diseased or injured, a person may lose forever the body functions controlled by that area of the brain. For example, if the part of the brain that regulates breathing is damaged, the person may stop breathing.

Illness or injury may change a person's level of consciousness. Consciousness may be heightened, in which case the victim may be intensely aware of what is going on. At other times, the victim's mind may seem to be dull or cloudy. Illness or injury affecting the brain can also alter memory, emotions, and the ability to use language.

A head injury can cause a temporary loss of consciousness. Any head injury causing a loss of consciousness can also cause brain injury and must be considered serious. These injuries require evaluation by medical professionals because injury to the brain can cause blood to form pools in the skull. Bleeding inside the skull puts pressure on the brain and limits the supply of oxygen to the brain cells.

Injury to the spinal cord or a nerve can result in a permanent loss of feeling and movement below the injury. This condition is called **paralysis.** For example, a lower back injury can result in paralyzed legs; a neck injury can result in paralysis of all four limbs. A broken bone or a deep wound can also cause nerve damage, resulting in a loss of sensation or movement. In Chapter 14, you will learn about techniques for caring for head, neck, and back injuries.

The Musculoskeletal System

The ***musculoskeletal system*** consists of the bones, muscles, ligaments, and tendons.

Structure and Function

The musculoskeletal system performs the following functions:

- Supporting the body
- Protecting internal organs
- Allowing movement
- Storing minerals and producing blood cells
- Producing heat

Muscles and Tendons

Muscles are made of special tissue that can lengthen and shorten, resulting in movement. Figure 5-10 shows the major muscles of the body. Muscles band together to form muscle groups. Muscle groups work together to produce movement (Fig. 5-11). Working muscles also produce heat. Muscles also protect underlying structures, such as bones, nerves, and blood vessels. **Tendons** are tissues that attach muscles to bones.

The nervous system controls muscle action. Nerves carry information from the muscles to the brain. The brain takes in this information and directs the muscles through the nerves (Fig. 5-12).

Muscle actions can be voluntary or involuntary. **Involuntary muscles,** such as the heart and intestines, are automatically controlled by the brain. You don't have to think about them to make them work. **Voluntary muscles,** such as leg and arm muscles, are most often under your conscious control. You are aware of telling them to move.

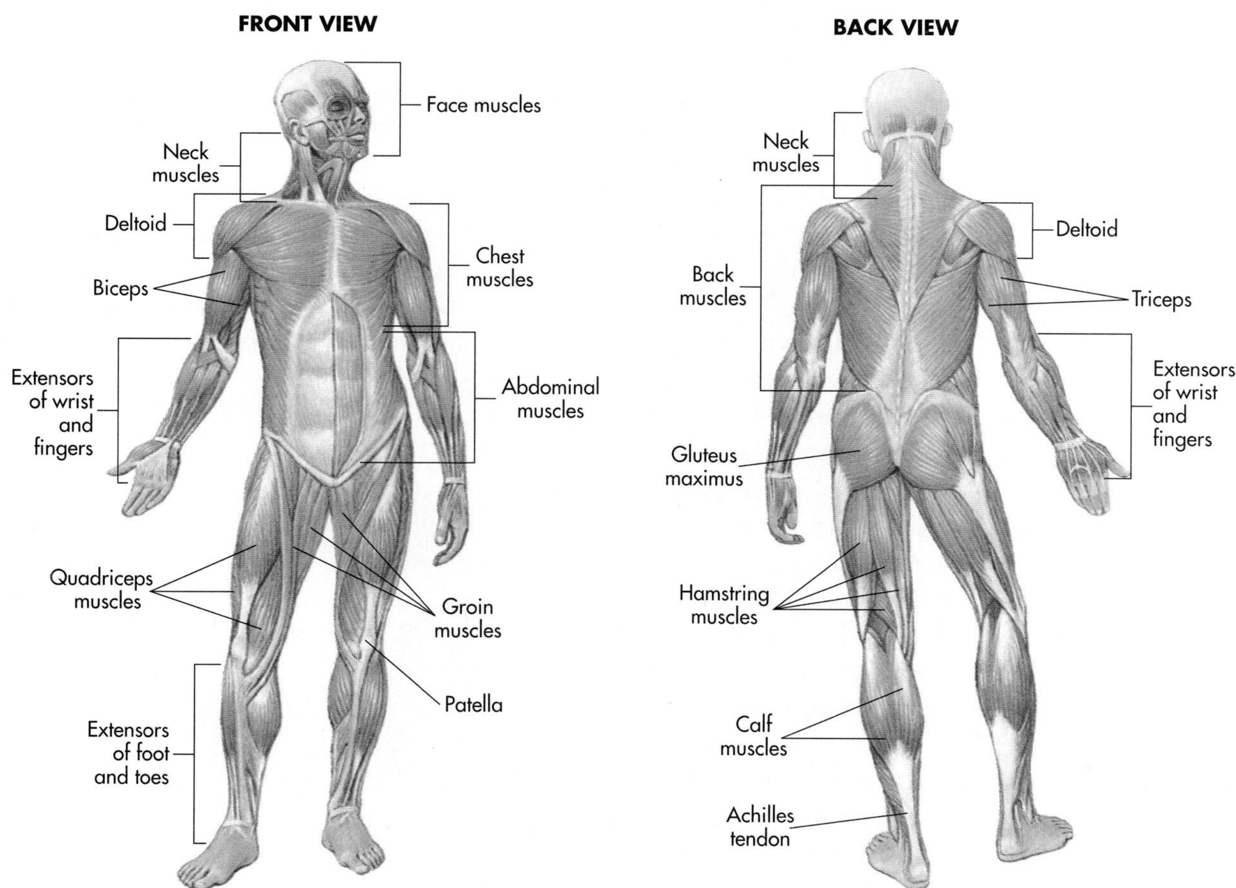

Figure 5-10 Major Muscles of the Body

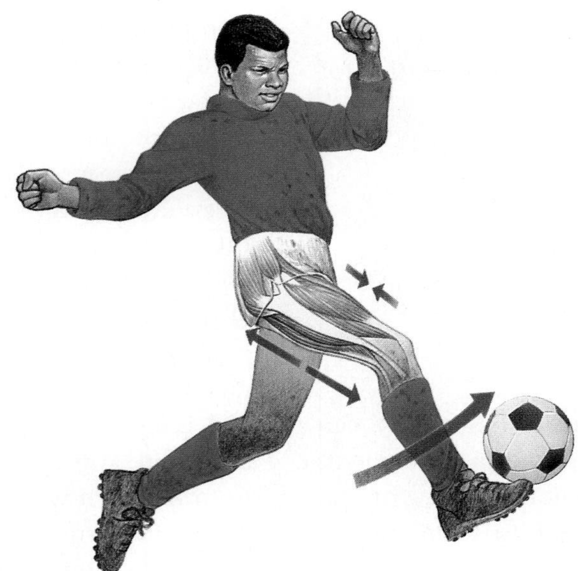

Figure 5-11 Muscle groups work together to produce movement.

Bones and Ligaments

Bone is hard, dense tissue that forms the skeleton. The 206 bones of the skeleton form the framework that supports the body (Fig. 5-13). Where two or more bones join, they form a **joint.** Figure 5-14 shows a typical joint. Bones are usually held together at joints by fibrous bands called **ligaments.** Bones vary in size and shape, allowing them to perform specific functions.

The bones of the skull protect the brain. The spine is made of bones called **vertebrae** that protect the spinal cord. The **ribs** are bones that attach to the spine and to the breastbone, forming a protective shell for vital organs, such as the heart and lungs.

In addition to supporting and protecting the body, bones aid movement. The bones of the arms and legs work like a system of levers and pulleys to position the hands and feet so that they can function. Bones of the wrist, hand, and fingers are progressively smaller to allow for fine movements like writing. The small bones of the feet enable you to walk smoothly. Together they work as shock absorbers when you walk, run, or jump. Bones also store minerals and produce certain blood cells.

Problems That Require Emergency Care

Injuries to bones and muscles include fractures, dislocations, strains, and sprains. A fracture is a broken bone. Dislocations occur when bones of a joint are moved out of place. Strains are injuries to muscles and tendons; sprains are injuries to ligaments. Although injuries to bones and muscles may not look serious, nearby nerves, blood vessels, and other organs may be damaged. Regardless of how they ap-

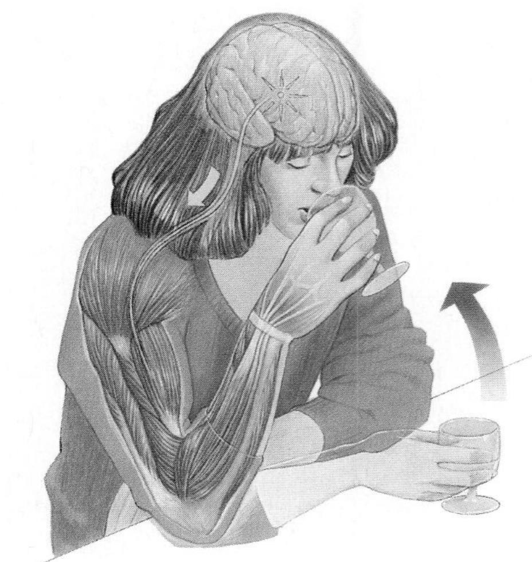

Figure 5-12 The brain controls muscle movement.

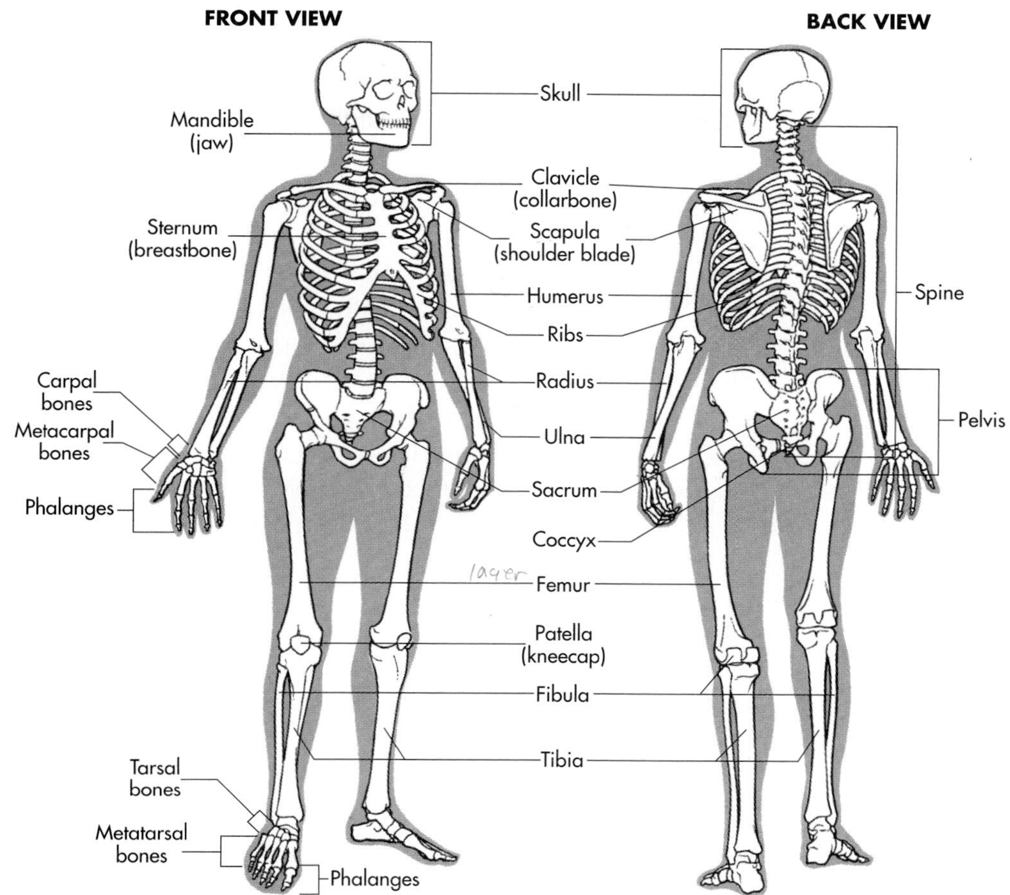

Figure 5-13 The Skeleton

pear, these injuries may cause lifelong disabilities or become life-threatening emergencies. For example, torn ligaments in the knee can limit activity, and broken ribs can puncture the lungs and threaten breathing.

When you give emergency care, remember that injuries to muscles and bones often result in additional injuries. You will learn more about musculoskeletal injuries and how to care for them in later chapters.

The Integumentary System

The ***integumentary system*** consists of the skin, hair, and nails (Fig. 5-15).

Structure and Function

Most important among these components is the skin because it protects the body. The skin helps keep fluids in. It prevents infection by keeping out disease-producing pathogens, or germs. The **skin** is made of tough, elastic fibers that stretch without easily tearing, protecting it from injury. The skin also helps make vitamin D and stores minerals.

The outer surface of the skin consists of dead cells that are continually rubbed away and replaced by new cells. The skin contains the hair roots, oil glands, and sweat glands. Oil glands help to keep the skin soft, supple, and waterproof. Sweat glands and pores help regulate body temperature by releasing sweat. The nervous system monitors blood temperature and causes you to sweat if blood temperature rises even slightly. Although you may not see or feel it, sweat is released to the skin's surface.

Blood supplies the skin with nutrients and helps provide its color. When blood vessels dilate (become wider), the blood circulates close to the skin's surface. This makes some people's

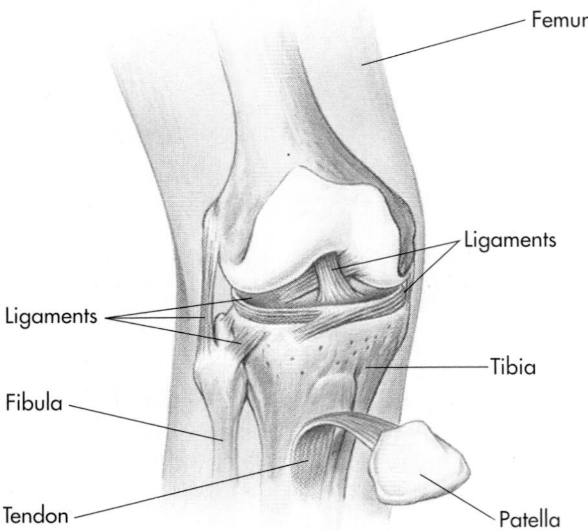

Figure 5-14 A typical joint consists of two or more bones held together by ligaments.

skin appear flushed or red and makes the skin feel warm. Reddening or flushing may not appear in darker skin. When blood vessels constrict (become narrower), not as much blood is close to the skin's surface, causing the skin to appear pale or ashen and feel cool. Nerves in the skin make it very sensitive to sensations such as touch, pain, and temperature. Therefore, the skin is also an important part of the body's communication network.

Problems That Require Emergency Care

Although the skin is tough, it can be injured. Sharp objects may puncture, cut, or tear the skin. Rough objects can scrape it, and extreme heat or cold may burn or freeze it. Burns and skin injuries that cause bleeding may result in the loss of vital fluids. Pathogens may enter the body through breaks in the skin, causing infection that can become a serious problem. In later chapters, you will learn how to care for skin injuries, such as burns and cuts.

◆ SUMMARY

The body includes a number of systems, all of which must work together for the body to function properly. The brain, the center of the nervous system, controls all body functions, including those of the other body systems. Knowing a few key structures, their functions, and their locations helps you to understand more about these body systems.

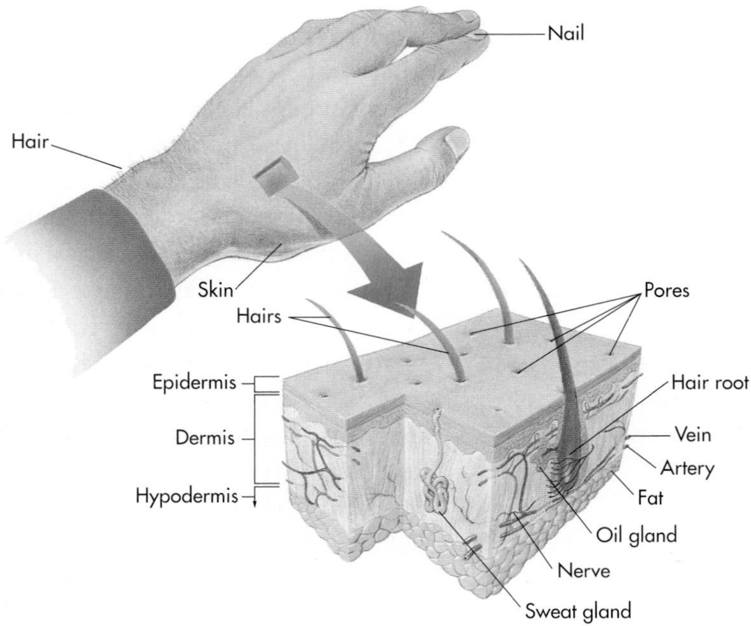

Figure 5-15 The skin, hair, and nails make up the integumentary system.

ENRICHMENT

Knowing certain anatomical terms, body cavities, and the structure and functions of other body systems will add to your ability to accurately communicate with other emergency care personnel about a victim's condition.

Anatomical Terms

To learn to use terms that refer to the body, you must first understand the "anatomical position." In this position, the body is standing, arms at the side, palms facing forward (Fig. 5-16, *A*). All medical terms that refer to the body are based on this position. A medical person you are speaking with may not be able to see the victim's actual position. You will make the situation clearer if you refer to parts of the body as if the body were in the anatomical position. Figure 5-16, *B* and *C*, shows the basic anatomical terms.

The simplest anatomical terms are based on an imaginary line. It runs down the middle of the body from the head to the ground, dividing the body into right and left halves. This line is called the **midline.** When you face a victim, you might tend to refer to that person in terms of what is your own right or left. However, in medical terms, right and left **always** refer to the victim's right and left.

Other terms related to the midline include lateral and medial. Anything away from the midline is called **lateral.** Anything toward the midline is called **medial.** For example, the inner side of the knee is the medial side because it is nearer to the midline. The outer side is the lateral side (Fig. 5-17).

Another reference line can be drawn through the side of the body, dividing it into front and back halves. Anything toward the front of the body is called **anterior;** anything toward the back is called **posterior.**

Other terms that refer to direction can also be useful. When comparing any two structures, such as two body parts, any part toward the patient's head is described as **superior.** Any part toward the patient's feet is described as **inferior.** For example, the abdomen is superior to the pelvis but is inferior to the chest. These terms can also be used to describe the location of an injury. For instance, bruising might be described as covering the superior portion of the chest.

Two other terms are generally used when referring to the arms and legs. These terms are proximal and distal. To understand these terms, you must think of the chest, abdomen, and pelvis as those areas that make up the **trunk** of the body. The arms and legs are the attachments to the trunk. Points on the body closer to the trunk are described as **proximal.** Points away from the trunk are described as **distal.** For example, the elbow is proximal to the hand because the elbow is closer to the trunk. The hand is distal to the elbow because it is farther from the trunk. Figure 5-18 shows other basic terms used for body regions and their specific parts.

These are all standard terms used by people who provide emergency care. Some terms will be familiar, whereas others may be new to you. Study these terms and learn to use them correctly when describing body parts.

Specific anatomical terms are used for the abdomen. The **abdomen** is the part of the trunk below the ribs and above the pelvis. By drawing two imaginary lines, one from the breastbone down through the navel to the lowest point in the pelvis and another line horizontally through the navel, you divide the abdomen into four areas called quadrants. These are the right upper quadrant, the left upper quadrant, the right lower quadrant, and the left lower quadrant. Figure 5-19 shows the abdomen divided into these four quadrants.

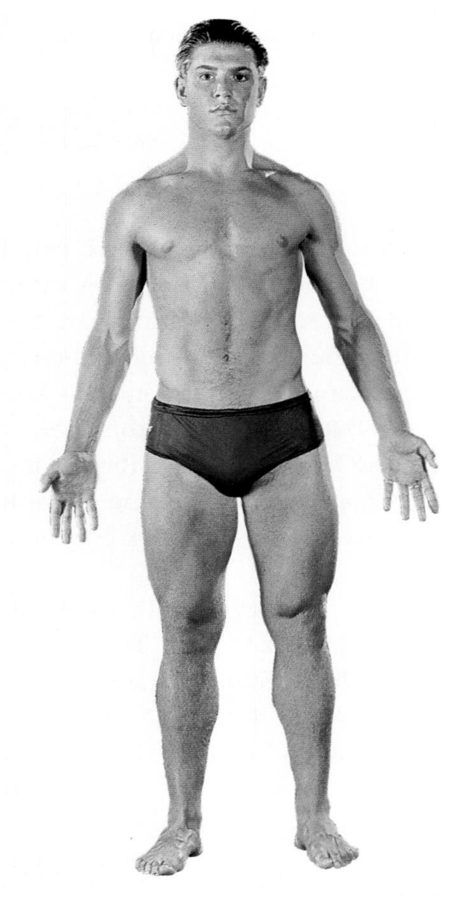

A

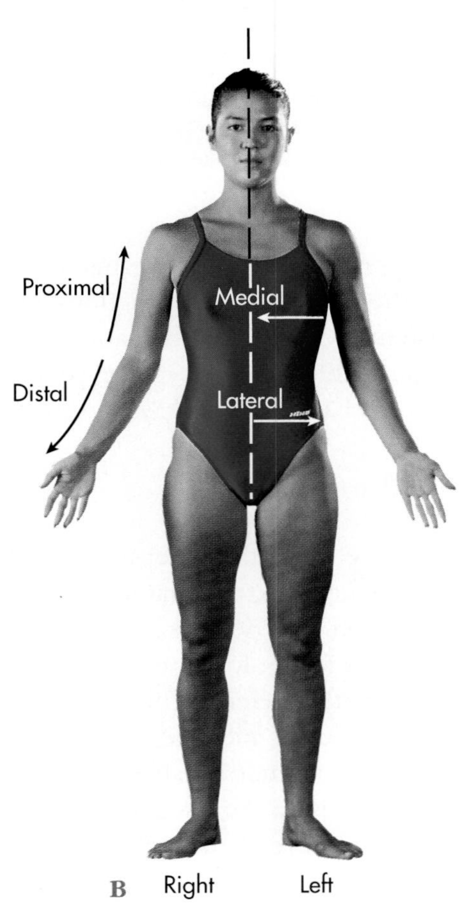

B

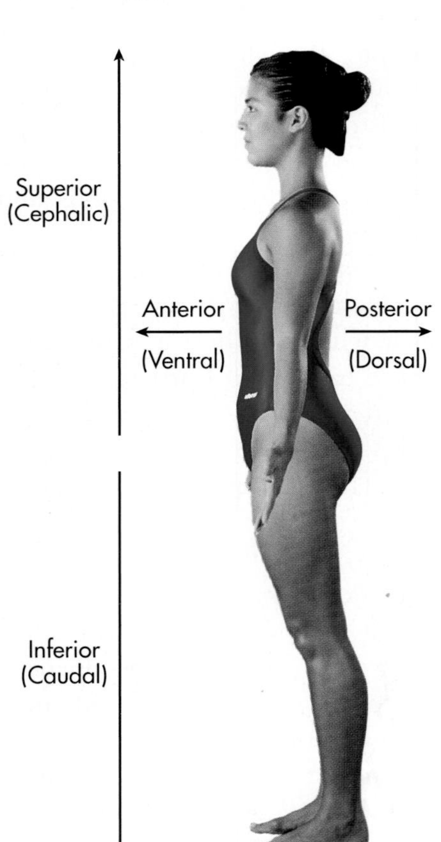

C

Figure 5-16 **A,** The Anatomical Position **B,** Medical use of the terms right and left refers to the victim's right and left. Medial refers to anything toward the midline; lateral refers to anything away from the midline. Proximal and distal are usually used to refer to extremities. **C,** Anterior refers to the front of the body; posterior refers to the back of the body. Superior refers to anything toward the head; inferior refers to anything toward the feet.

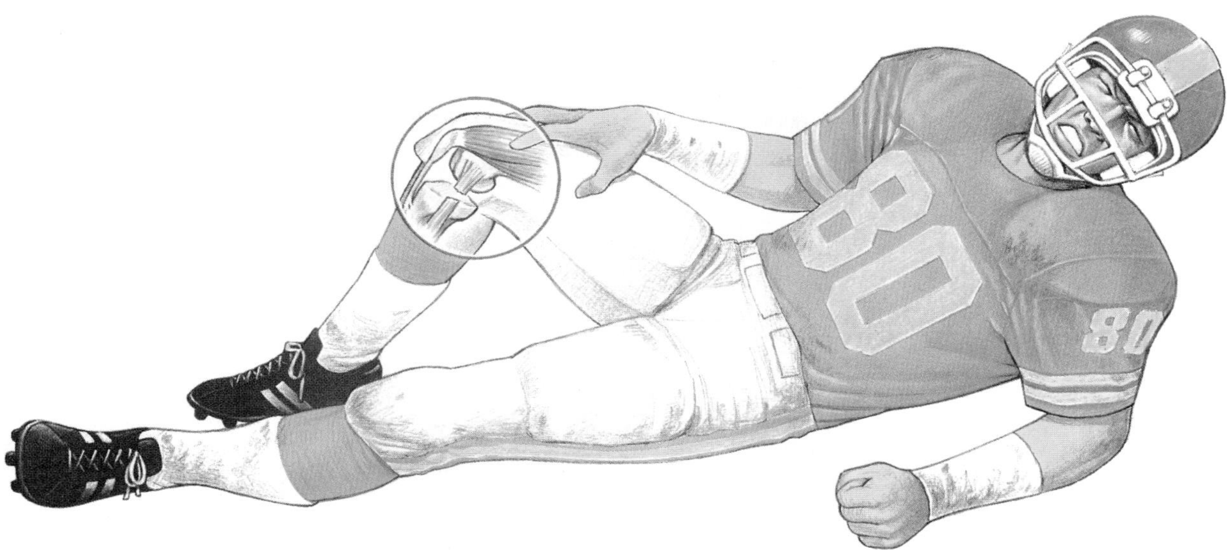

Figure 5-17 An injury to the medial side of the right knee.

These terms are important when describing injuries to the abdomen because different organs may be injured depending on the quadrant involved.

Of all these terms, it is most important to correctly use left and right, lateral and medial, and the basic terms that refer to body parts. Even though you may not use the other terms, you should know what they mean. You may need to understand what other emergency care personnel are saying when they use these terms to refer to injuries.

Body Cavities

A **body cavity** is a hollow place in the body that contains organs, such as the heart, lungs, and liver. The five major cavities, illustrated in Figure 5-20, are the—

- **Cranial cavity,** located in the head. It contains the brain and is protected by the skull.
- **Spinal cavity,** extending from the bottom of the skull to the lower back. It contains the spinal cord and is protected by the bones of the spine.
- **Thoracic cavity,** also called chest cavity, located in the trunk between the **diaphragm,** a dome-shaped muscle used in breathing, and the neck. It contains the heart, the lungs, and other important structures. The thoracic cavity is protected by the rib cage and the upper portion of the spine.
- **Abdominal cavity,** located in the trunk between the diaphragm and the pelvis. It contains many organs, including the liver, pancreas, intestines, stomach, kidneys, and spleen. Because the abdominal cavity is not protected by any bones, the organs in it are vulnerable to injury.
- **Pelvic cavity,** located in the pelvis, the lowest part of the trunk. It contains the bladder, the rectum, and the reproductive organs. It is protected by the pelvic bones and the lower portion of the spine.

Knowing the general location and relative

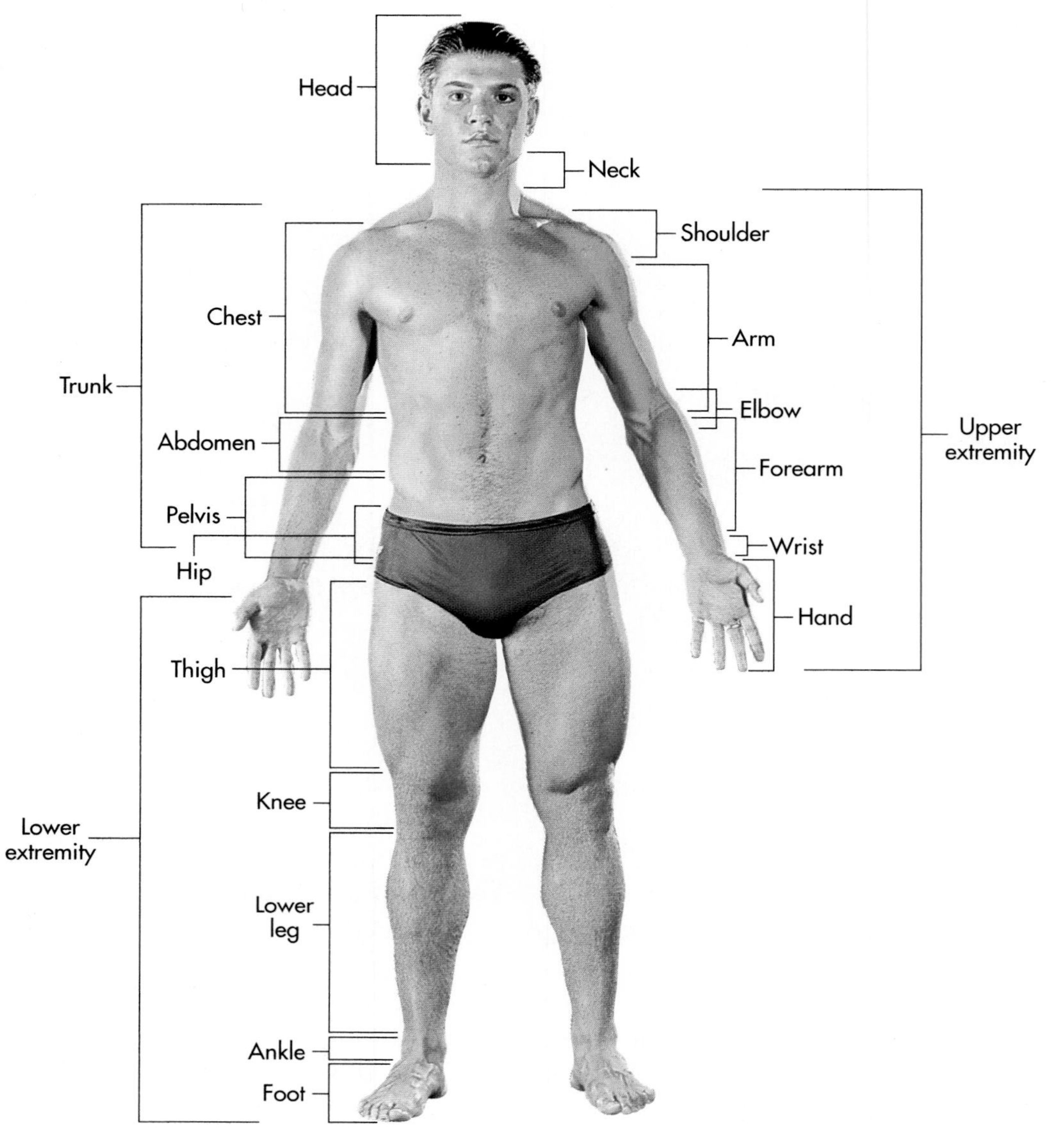

Figure 5-18 It is important to refer correctly to the parts of the body.

size of major organs in each cavity will help you assess a victim's injury or illness.

◆ MORE BODY SYSTEMS

Other body systems and their functions include—

The Digestive System

The ***digestive system,*** also called the gastrointestinal system, consists of organs that work together to break down food, absorb nutrients, and eliminate waste.

Structure and Function

Figure 5-21 shows the major organs of the digestive system. Food entering the system is broken down into a form the body can use. As food passes through the system, the body absorbs nutrients that can be converted for the cells to use. The unabsorbed portion continues through the system and is eliminated as waste.

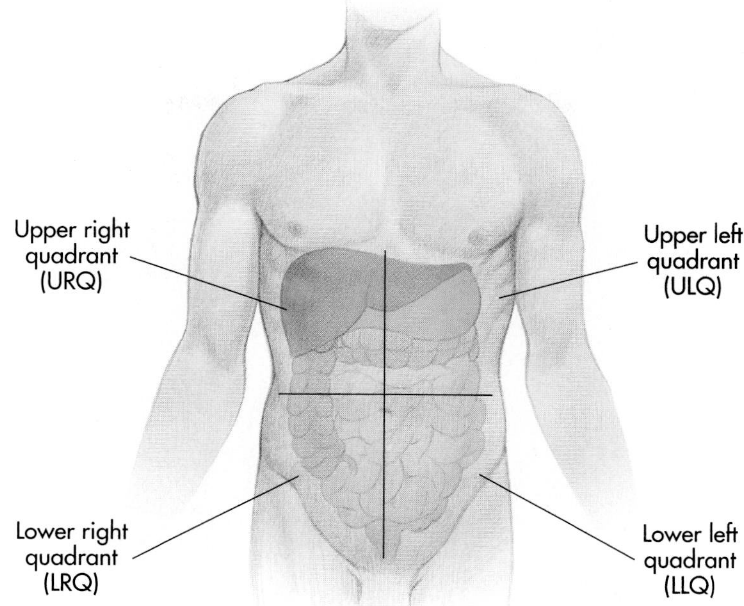

Figure 5-19 The Abdominal Quadrants

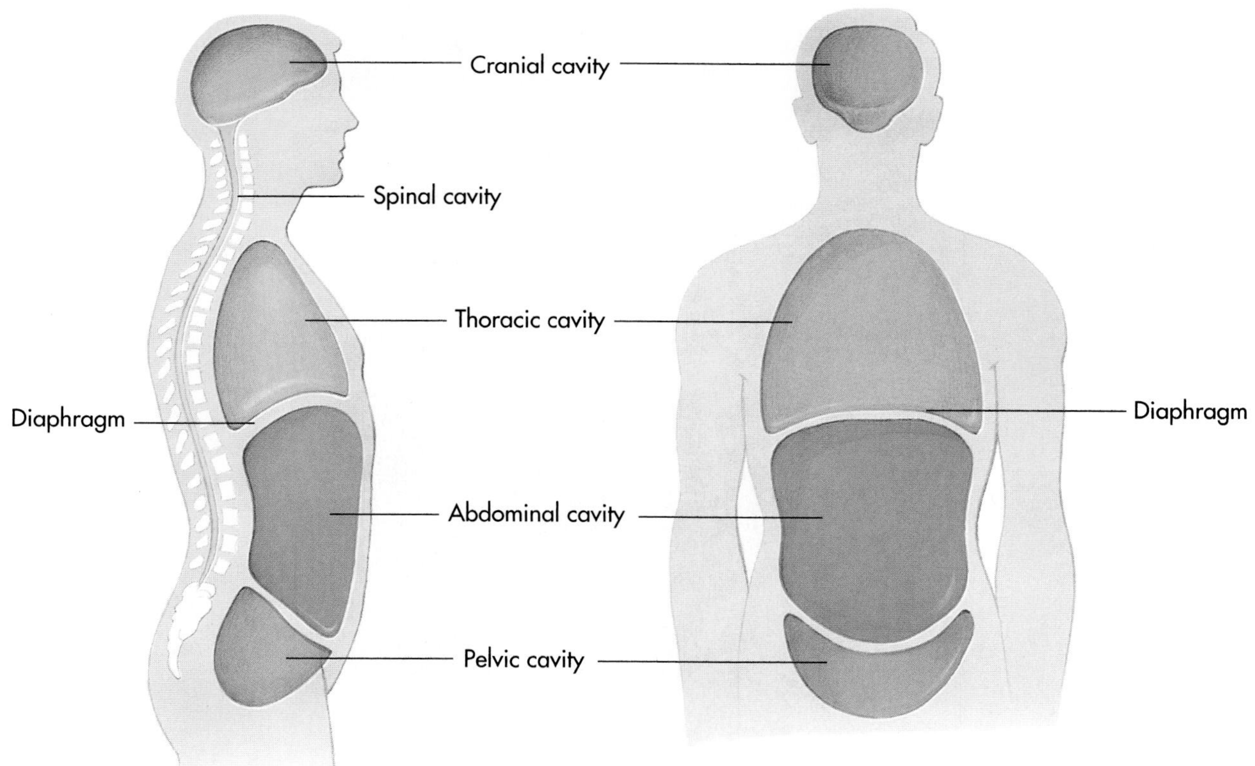

Figure 5-20 The Five Major Cavities of the Body

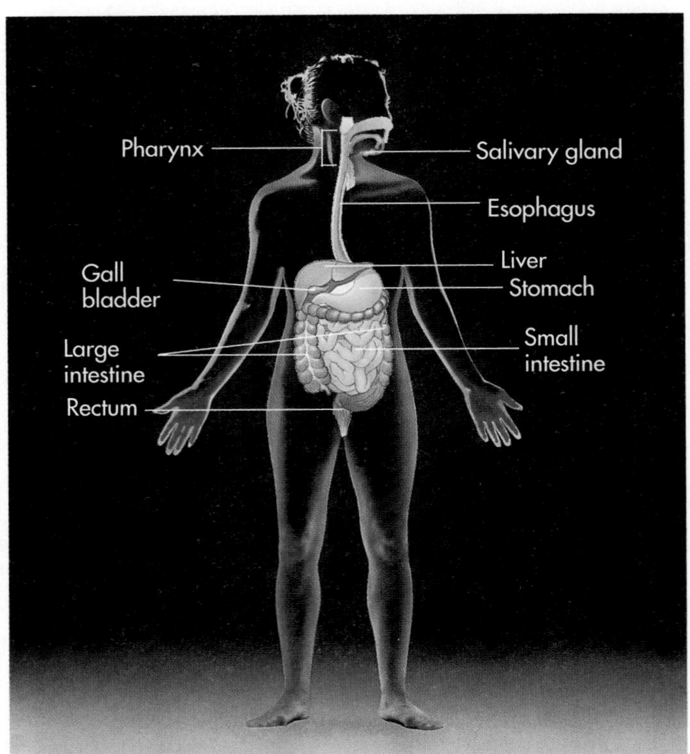

Figure 5-21 The Digestive System

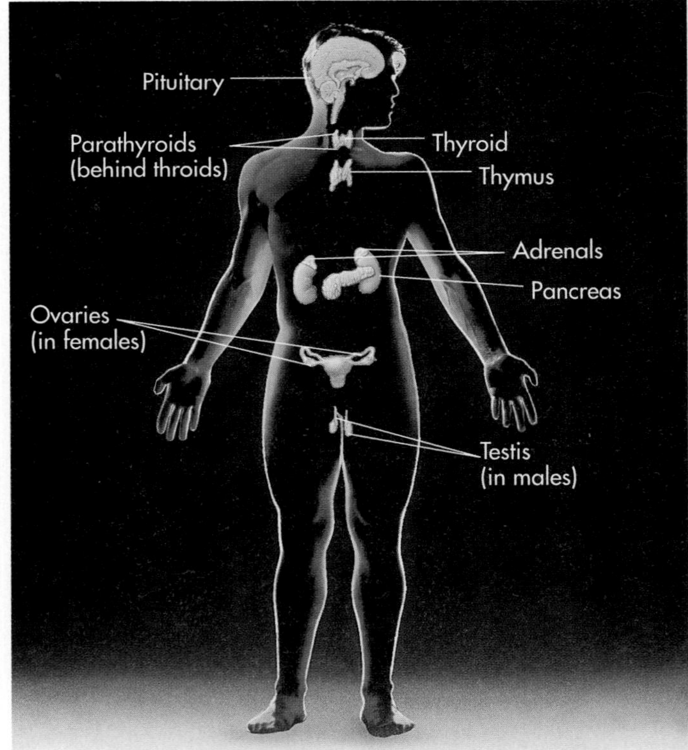

Figure 5-22 The Endocrine System

Problems That Require Emergency Care

Since most digestive system organs are in the unprotected abdominal cavity, they are very vulnerable to injury. Such an injury can occur, for example, if a person in a car strikes the steering wheel in a collision. These organs can also be damaged by a penetrating injury, such as a stab or gunshot wound. Damaged organs may bleed internally, causing severe loss of blood, or spill waste products into the abdominal cavity. This can result in severe infection. Chapter 12 discusses in more detail how to recognize and care for abdominal injuries.

The Endocrine System

The ***endocrine system*** is one of the two regulatory systems in the body.

Structure and Function

Together with the nervous system, the endocrine system coordinates the activities of other systems. The endocrine system consists of several glands (Fig. 5-22). **Glands** are organs that release fluid and other substances into the blood or onto the skin. Some produce **hormones,** chemical messengers that enter the bloodstream and influence tissue activity in parts of the body. For example, the thyroid gland makes a hormone that controls **metabolism,** the process by which all cells convert nutrients to energy. Other glands include the sweat and oil glands in the skin.

Problems That Require Emergency Care

A first responder does not need to know all the glands in the endocrine system or the hormones they produce. Problems in the endocrine system usually develop slowly and are seldom emergencies. Knowing how hormones work in general, however, helps you understand how some illnesses seem to develop suddenly.

For example, an emergency occurs when there is too much or too little of a hormone called insulin in the blood. Without insulin, cells cannot absorb the sugar they need from food. Too much insulin forces blood sugar rapidly into the cells, lowering blood sugar levels and depriving the brain of the blood sugar it needs to function normally. Blood sugar levels that rise or fall can make a person ill, sometimes severely so.

The Genitourinary System

The ***genitourinary system*** is made up of two organ systems: the urinary system and the reproductive system.

Structure and Function

The **urinary system** consists of organs that eliminate waste products filtered from the blood (Fig. 5-23). The primary organs are the kidneys and the bladder. The **kidneys** are located behind the abdominal cavity just beneath the chest, one on each side. They filter wastes from the circulating blood to form urine. Urine is then stored in the **bladder,** a small muscular sac. The bladder stretches as it fills and then shrinks back when the urine is released.

The male and female **reproductive systems** include the organs for sexual reproduction (Fig. 5-24). Because these reproductive organs are close to the urinary system, injuries to the abdominal or pelvic area can injure organs in either the reproductive system or the urinary system.

The female reproductive organs are smaller than many major organs and are protected by the pelvic bones. The soft tissue external structures are more susceptible to injury, although such injury is uncommon. The male reproductive organs are located outside of the pelvis and are more vulnerable to injury.

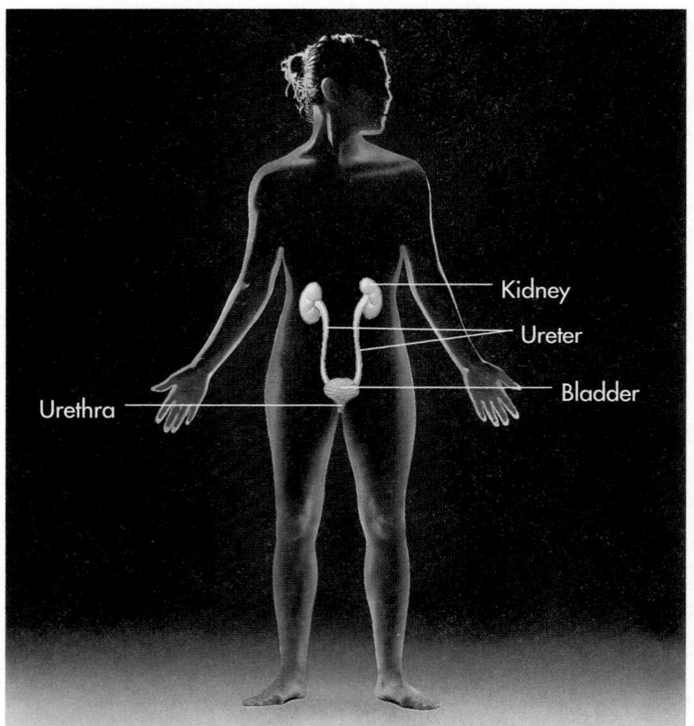

Figure 5-23 The Urinary System

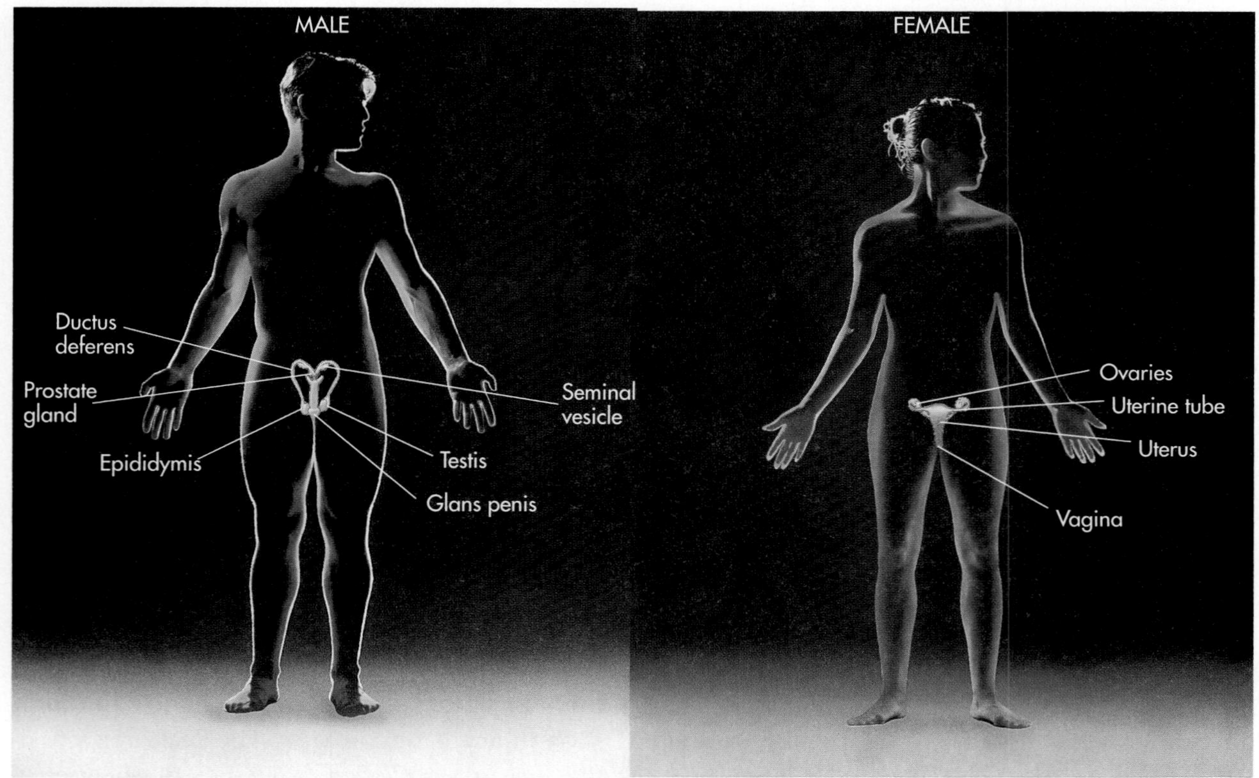

Figure 5-24 The Male and Female Reproductive Systems

Problems That Require Emergency Care

The frequency of injuries to the organs of the urinary system depends on their vulnerability. Unlike the abdominal organs, the kidneys are partially protected by the lower ribs, making them less vulnerable to injury. But the kidneys may be damaged by a significant blow to the back just below the rib cage or by a penetrating wound, such as a stab or gunshot wound. Anyone with an injury to the back below the rib cage may have injured one or both kidneys. Because of the kidney's rich blood supply, such an injury often causes severe bleeding.

The bladder is injured less frequently than the kidneys, but injuries to the abdomen can rupture the bladder, particularly when it is full. Bone fragments from a fracture of the pelvis can also pierce or rupture the bladder.

Injuries to urinary system organs may not be obvious but should be suspected if there are significant injuries to the back just below the rib cage or to the abdomen. Chapter 12 discusses signs and symptoms of urinary system injuries to watch for and how to provide care.

The external reproductive organs called **genitalia** have a rich supply of blood and nerves. Injuries to these organs may cause heavy bleeding that can be life threatening. Injuries to the genitalia are usually caused by a blow to the pelvic area but may be the result of sexual assault or rape. Such injuries almost always cause the victim extreme distress and a victim may refuse care.

◆ INTERRELATIONSHIPS OF BODY SYSTEMS

Each body system plays a vital role in survival. Body systems work together to help the body maintain a constant healthy state. When the environment changes, body systems adapt to the new conditions. For example, because your musculoskeletal system works harder when you exercise, your respiratory and circulatory systems must also work harder to meet your body's increased oxygen demands. Your body systems also react to the stresses caused by illness or injury.

Body systems do not work independently. The impact of an injury or a disease is rarely restricted to one body system. For example, a broken bone may result in nerve damage that will impair movement and feeling. Injuries to the ribs can make breathing difficult. If the heart stops beating for any reason, breathing will also stop.

In any significant illness or injury, body systems may be seriously affected. This may result in a progressive failure of body systems called **shock.** Shock results from the inability of the circulatory system to provide adequate oxygen to all parts of the body, especially the vital organs.

Generally, the more body systems involved in an emergency, the more serious the emergency. Body systems depend on each other for survival. In serious injury or illness, the body may not be able to keep functioning. In these cases, regardless of your best efforts, the victim may die.

Fortunately, basic care is usually all you need to give to support injured body systems until more advanced care is available. By learning the basic principles of care described in later chapters, you may be able to make the difference between life and death.

Lifting and Moving

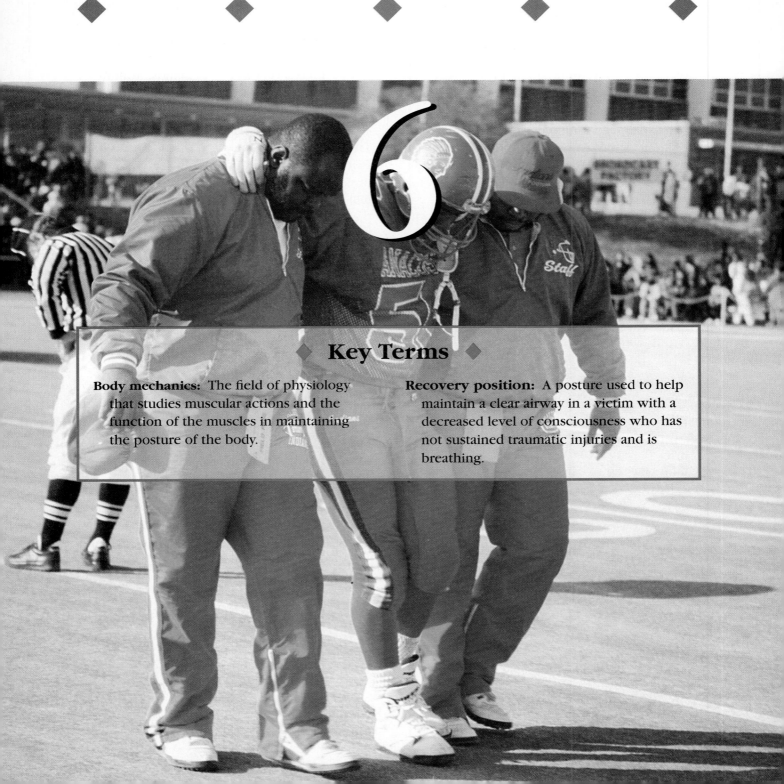

Key Terms

Body mechanics: The field of physiology that studies muscular actions and the function of the muscles in maintaining the posture of the body.

Recovery position: A posture used to help maintain a clear airway in a victim with a decreased level of consciousness who has not sustained traumatic injuries and is breathing.

◆ Knowledge Objectives ◆

After reading this chapter and completing the class activities, you should be able to—

- Define body mechanics.
- Explain the guidelines and safety precautions to follow when lifting a victim.
- Describe the conditions that require an emergency move.
- Describe the indications for assisting in non-emergency moves.
- Describe the various devices associated with moving a victim in the out-of-hospital setting.
- Explain the guidelines for lifting and moving victims.
- Explain the rationale for an emergency move.

◆ Skill Objectives ◆

After reading this chapter and completing the class activities, you should be able to—

- Demonstrate an emergency move.
- Demonstrate a non-emergency move.
- Demonstrate the ability to make appropriate decisions regarding the use of equipment for moving a victim in the out-of-hospital setting.

Your pager goes off just as you are preparing to leave work for the day. You are summoned to a recently remodeled adjacent building. As you proceed, you smell something burning. As you near the area, there is a sudden crackling sound followed by an explosion and screams.

You arrive to find smoke filling the area. Two people carry an employee through a doorway. Others stagger through and collapse to the ground. Smoke is blowing over them. Flames flicker inside the structure. You hear the sound of sirens, but they are still far off.

You quickly size up the scene and determine that for the next few minutes it is safe enough for you to rescue the victims who have collapsed. You recruit others and run to the collapsed victims. Two of them are unconscious. You recognize the immediate danger to the two unconscious victims and to the others who have escaped from the building. Time is critical. You need to get everyone to a safer place. With the help of others, you move victims away from the vicinity of the building. The fire fighters arrive.

◆ INTRODUCTION

You provide care for victims of injury and illness when it is safe to do so. Sometimes, you will not have easy access to the victim. At other times, the victim may be in a dangerous situation, but you can enter briefly and move the victim to safety. In this chapter, you learn how to quickly and safely move victims.

◆ ROLE OF THE FIRST RESPONDER

Usually when you provide care, you will not face hazards that require moving the victim immediately. In most cases, you can give care where you find the victim. Moving a victim needlessly can lead to further injury. For example, moving a victim who has a painful, swollen, deformed leg without taking the time to splint it could result in an open fracture if the end of the bone tears the skin. Soft tissue damage, damage to nerves, blood loss, and infection all could result unnecessarily. Needless movement of a victim with a head or spine injury could cause paralysis or even death.

Safety Precautions

Before you act, you must consider the factors affecting the situation. Consider the following factors:

- The distance the victim must be moved
- Dangerous conditions at the scene
- The size of the victim
- Your physical ability
- Whether others can help you
- The victim's condition
- Any aids to transport at the scene

You could be injured if you fail to consider these factors. If you become injured, you may be unable to move the victim and may risk making the situation worse. In this instance, you will have become part of the problem that arriving personnel with more advanced training will have to deal with. The situation will have become more complicated because now there is one more person to rescue.

Body Mechanics/Lifting Techniques

Body mechanics refers to the field of physiology that studies muscular actions and the function of the muscles in maintaining the posture of the body.

To protect yourself and the victim, follow these guidelines when moving someone:

- Only move a victim if the scene is too dangerous to remain or if you need to reach another victim to give care.
- Only attempt to move a person you are sure you can safely and comfortably handle.
- Know your physical limitations.
- Properly position your feet.
- Bend your body at the knees and hips.
- Lift with your legs, not your back.
- Lift without twisting.
- Keep the victim's weight as close to your body as possible.
- Walk carefully, using short steps.
- When possible, move forward rather than backward.
- Look where you are going.
- Support the victim's head and spine.
- Communicate clearly and frequently with your partner, the victim, and other EMS providers.
- Avoid bending or twisting a victim with possible head or spine injury.
- If the victim is conscious, explain what you are about to do. Tell the victim what is expected of him or her, such as not reaching out to grab anything.

◆ PRINCIPLES OF MOVING VICTIMS

Remember to protect yourself and the victim before making any emergency moves of victims. Is the move necessary? Can you do it safely?

General Considerations

Three general situations require you to perform an emergency move:

1. **Immediate danger**—Danger to you or the victim from fire, lack of oxygen, risk of drowning, possible explosion, collapsing structure, uncontrolled traffic hazards, or environmental conditions such as extreme cold.
2. **Gaining access to other victims**—A person with minor injuries may need to be moved quickly to reach other victims who may have life-threatening conditions.

3. **Providing proper care**—A victim with a medical emergency, such as cardiac arrest or heat stroke, may need to be moved to provide proper care. For example, someone in cardiac arrest needs CPR, which should be performed on a firm, flat surface with the victim on his or her back. If the person collapses on a bed or in a small bathroom, the surface or space may not be adequate to provide appropriate care. You may have to move the victim to give the proper care.

Moving Victims

There are many different ways to move a person to safety, *but no one way is best*. As long as you can move a person to safety without injuring yourself or causing further injury to the victim, the move is successful.

Moves used by first responders include assists, carries, and drags. The most common of these are the—

- Walking assist.
- Fire fighter's carry.
- Pack-strap carry.
- Two-person seat carry.
- Clothes drag.
- Blanket drag.
- Shoulder drag.
- Foot drag.
- Direct lift.
- Extremity lift.
- Direct carry.
- Draw sheet.

All of these moves can be done either by one or two people, and most of them do not require equipment. This is important because with most moves, equipment is not often immediately available and time is critical.

The greatest danger in moving a victim quickly is the possibility of aggravating a spinal injury. In an emergency, every effort should be made to pull the victim in the direction of the long axis of the body to provide as much protection to the spine as possible. It is impossible to remove a victim from a vehicle quickly and at the same time provide much protection to the spine.

Walking Assist

The most basic move is the **walking assist**. It is frequently used to help victims who simply need assistance to walk to safety. Either one or two rescuers can use this method with a conscious victim. To do a walking assist, place the victim's arm across your shoulders and hold it in place with one hand. Support the victim with your other hand around the victim's waist (Fig. 6-1). In this way, your body acts as a crutch, supporting the victim's weight while you both walk. A second rescuer, if present, can support the victim in the same way from the other side (Fig. 6-2).

If the victim is on the floor or ground, a first responder can use one of the following emergency moves to transport the victim.

Fire Fighter's Carry

The **fire fighter's carry** is useful for quickly moving a person from a dangerous situation.

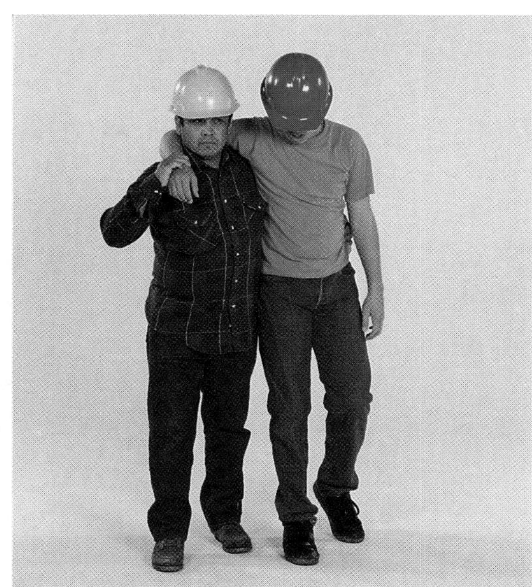

Figure 6-1 The most basic emergency move is the walking assist.

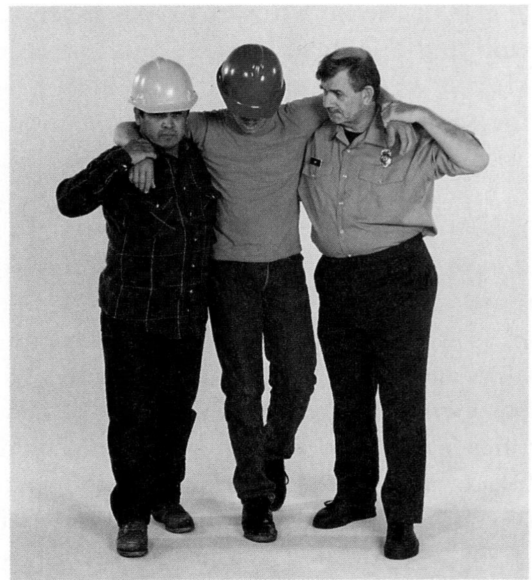

Figure 6-2 A second rescuer can support the victim from the other side.

The advantage of this carry is that it can be performed by one person and allows you to have one of your hands free while you carry the victim to safety. In addition, this method can be used with both conscious and unconscious victims. The disadvantages are that you may need help to position the victim across your shoulders. Also, the technique is not appropriate for victims with suspected head, spine, or abdominal injury, since the victim's body is twisted, the head is not supported, and the victim's abdomen bears the weight during movement. This carry works only if you are strong enough to carry a heavy weight on your shoulders. Practice this carry with someone lighter than you to get a feel for how heavy a person you can carry this way.

To perform a fire fighter's carry, kneel down and place the victim in a seated position facing you. Place one shoulder in the victim's abdomen and hoist the victim across your shoulders lengthwise, feet on one side, head on the other. Put one arm around the victim's legs and grasp one of the victim's arms with your other hand (Fig. 6-3, *A*). Keeping your back as straight as possible, stand up, using your legs (Fig. 6-3, *B*).

Pack-Strap Carry

The **pack-strap carry** can be used on both conscious and unconscious victims. To use it on an unconscious victim requires a second rescuer to help position the victim on your back. To perform the pack-strap carry, have the

A

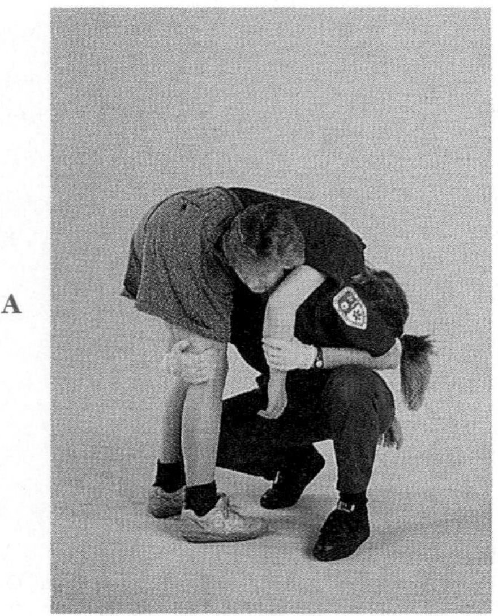

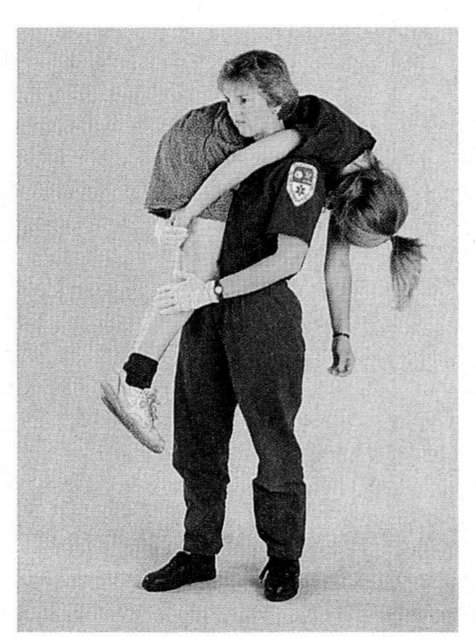

B

Figure 6-3 **A**, To perform a fire fighter's carry, hoist the victim across your shoulders lengthwise. Put one arm around the victim's legs and use your other hand to grasp one of the victim's arms. **B**, Stand up.

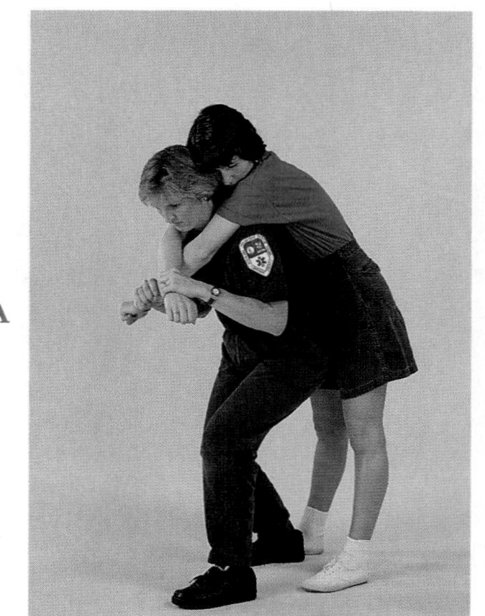

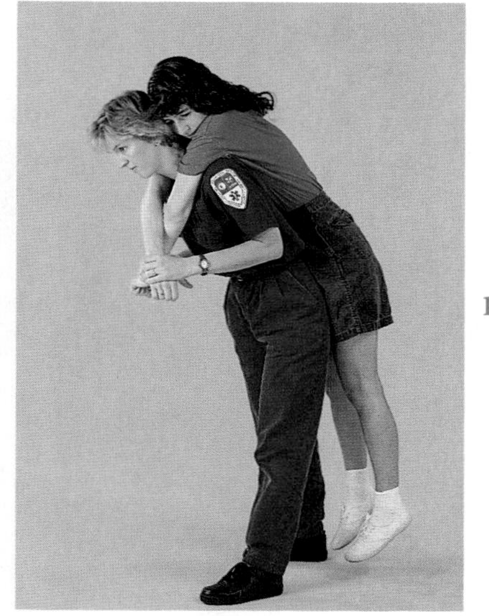

Figure 6-4 **A**, To perform the pack-strap carry, position yourself with your back to the victim. Cross the victim's arms in front of you and grasp the victim's wrists. **B**, Lean forward slightly and pull the victim onto your back.

victim stand or have a second rescuer help support the victim. Position yourself with your back to the victim, back straight, and knees bent so that your shoulders fit into the victim's armpits. Cross the victim's arms in front of you and grasp the victim's wrists (Fig. 6-4, *A*). Lean forward slightly and pull the victim up onto your back. Stand up and walk to safety (Fig. 6-4, *B*). Depending on the size of the victim, you may be able to hold both of the victim's wrists with one hand. This leaves your other hand free to help maintain balance, open doors, and remove obstructions.

Two-Person Seat Carry

The **two-person seat carry** is a method for moving a victim that requires a second rescuer. To perform the two-person seat carry, put one arm under the victim's thighs and the other across the victim's back. Interlock your arms with those of a second rescuer under the victim's legs and across the victim's back. The victim is then lifted in the "seat" formed by the rescuers' arms (Fig. 6-5, *A-C*). Keep your back straight and lift with your legs. The move should not be used for a victim suspected of having a serious head or spine injury.

Clothes Drag

The **clothes drag** is an appropriate emergency move for a person suspected of having a head or spine injury. This move helps keep the head and neck stabilized. To do a clothes drag, gather the victim's clothing behind the victim's neck. Using the clothing, pull the victim to safety. During the move, the victim's head is cradled by both the clothing and the rescuer's hands. Move carefully, since you will be moving backwards. Keep your back as straight as possible and bend your legs (Fig. 6-6). This type of emergency move is exhausting and may result in back strain for the rescuer, even when done properly.

Blanket Drag

The **blanket drag** is also a good way to move a victim in an emergency situation, when equipment is limited. Position a blanket (or tarp, drape, bedspread, or sheet) next to the victim. Keep the victim between you and the blanket. Gather half of the blanket and place it against the victim's side. Being careful to keep about 2 feet of blanket above the victim's head, roll the victim toward your knees and reach across and place the blanket so that it will be

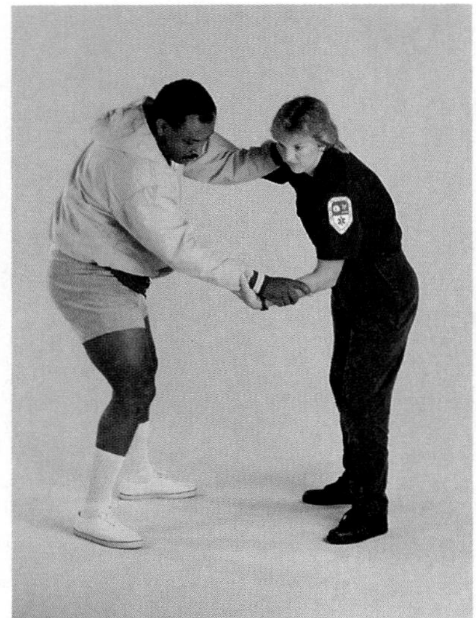
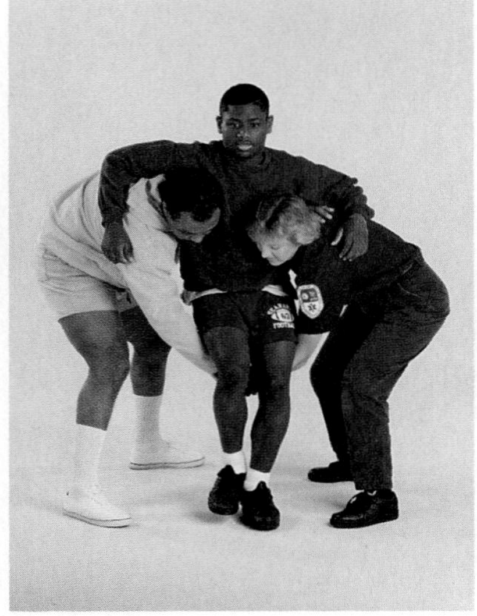
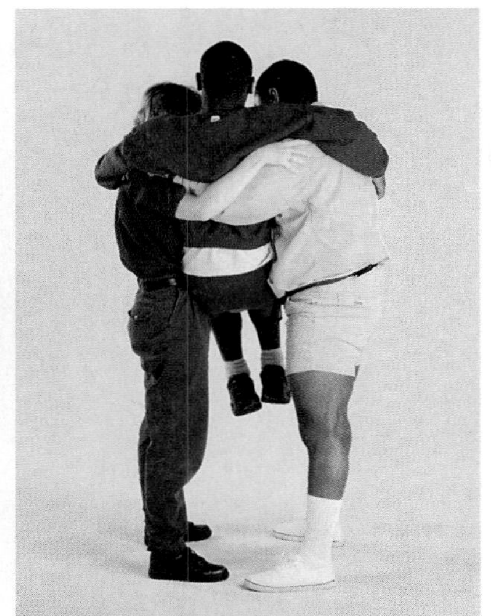

Figure 6-5 The Two-Person Seat Carry

positioned under him or her. Gently roll the patient onto the blanket. After smoothing out the blanket, wrap it around the victim, gather up the excess at the victim's head and drag, being sure to keep the victim's head as low as possible. Move carefully because you are moving backwards, and keep your back as straight as possible (Fig. 6-7).

Shoulder Drag

The shoulder drag is a variation of the clothes drag in which you reach under the victim's armpits (from the back), grasp the victim's forearms and drag the victim. Keep your back as straight as possible and do not twist. This move is exhausting and you should be careful because you are moving backwards. The move may result in back strain (Fig. 6-8).

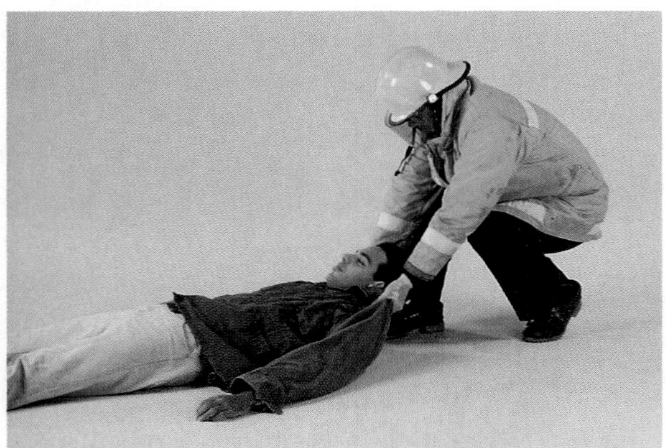

Figure 6-6 The clothes drag is most appropriate for moving a person suspected of having a head or spine injury.

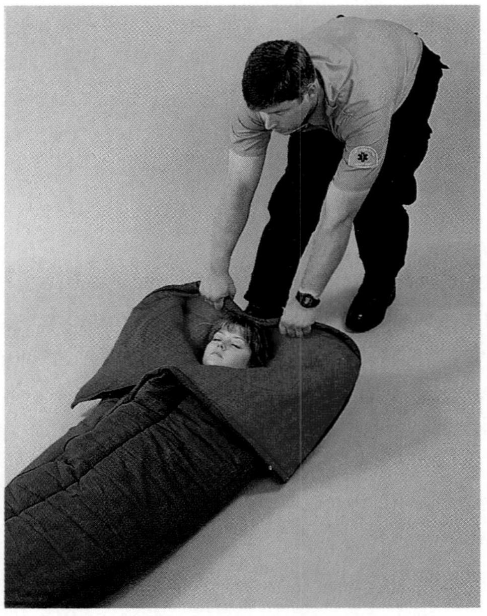

Figure 6-7 Blanket Drag

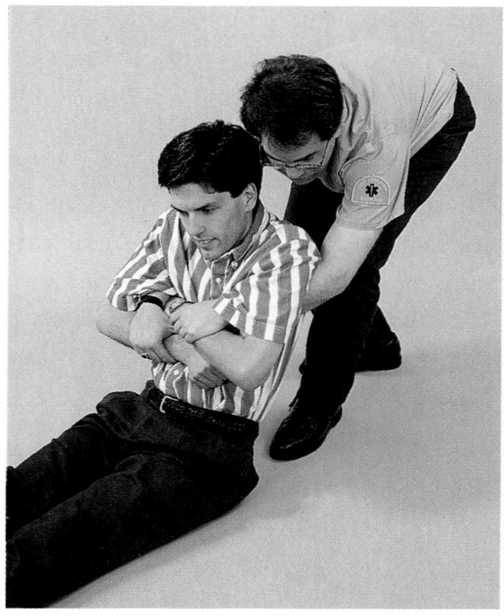

Figure 6-8 Shoulder Drag

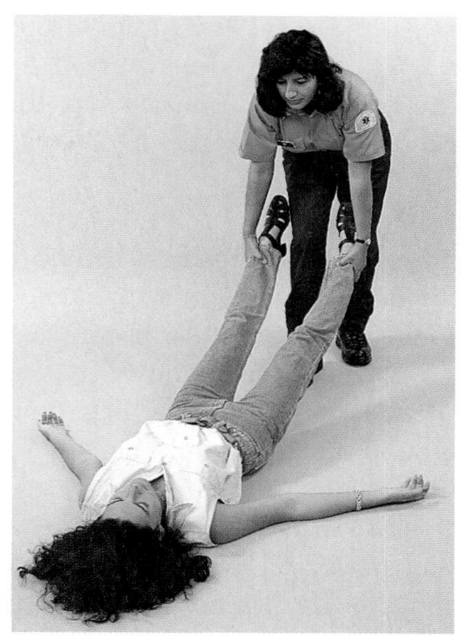

Figure 6-9 Foot Drag

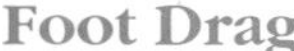

Foot Drag

In this move, you firmly grasp the victim's ankles and move backwards. Be careful to pull on the long axis of the body and not bump the victim's head. Keep your back as straight as possible and do not twist. Move carefully because you are moving backwards, which may result in back strain (Fig. 6-9).

Direct Lift

Three rescuers line up on one side of the victim and kneel close to the victim. The victim should cross his or her arms over the chest. The rescuer kneeling at the victim's head places one arm under the victim's shoulders, cradling the head and the other arm under the victim's upper back. The next rescuer places one arm under the victim's waist and the other under the buttocks. The third rescuer cradles the victim's hips and legs. On a signal from the rescuer at the victim's head, all three rescuers lift the victim to their knees and support the victim by rolling him or her against their chest (Fig. 6-10, *A-B*). On the next signal, all will rise

A

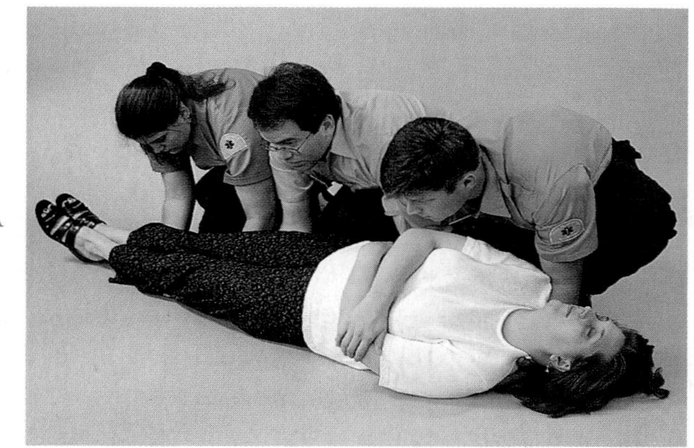

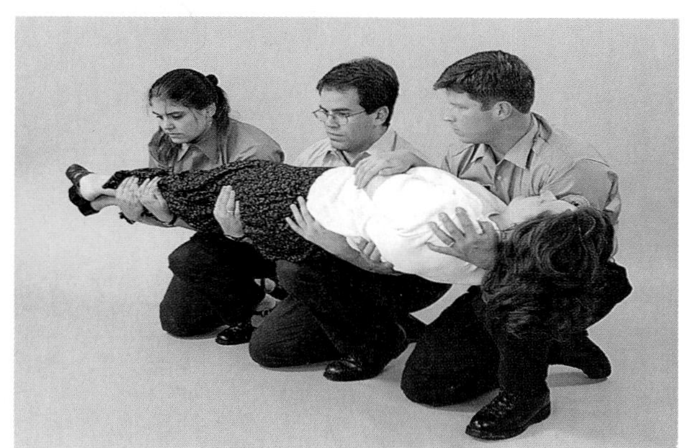

B

Figure 6-10 Direct lift: **A**, After the rescuers have properly placed their hands, the rescuer at the victim's head signals for all three rescuers to lift the victim to their knees. **B**, Next, the rescuers should support the victim by rolling him or her against their chest.

to their feet, and move the victim to the ambulance cot. These steps are reversed to lower the victim. Rescuers should keep the back straight and lift with the legs.

Extremity Lift

In this lift, one rescuer kneels behind the victim, keeping his or her back straight, and reaches under the victim's arms and grasps the victim's opposite wrist. The second rescuer kneels between the victim's legs and firmly grasps around the knees and thighs. On a signal from the rescuer at the victim's head, both rescuers move from a crouching position to a standing position. The rescuers then move the victim to the ambulance cot stretcher (Fig. 6-11).

The following two carries are designed to get a victim from a bed to an ambulance cot or vice versa.

Direct Carry

Position the stretcher at a right angle to the bed with the head of the stretcher at the foot of the bed. Two rescuers position themselves beside the bed at the same side as the cot. One rescuer slides his or her arms around the victim's shoulders and back while the second rescuer cradles the waist and hips. On a signal from the rescuer at the victim's head, the rescuers lift the victim simultaneously and curl the victim's body in toward their chests (Fig. 6-12, *A-B*). With a minimum of steps, the rescuers can then turn and place the victim on the cot. Rescuers should keep the back straight, lift with the legs and not twist the body.

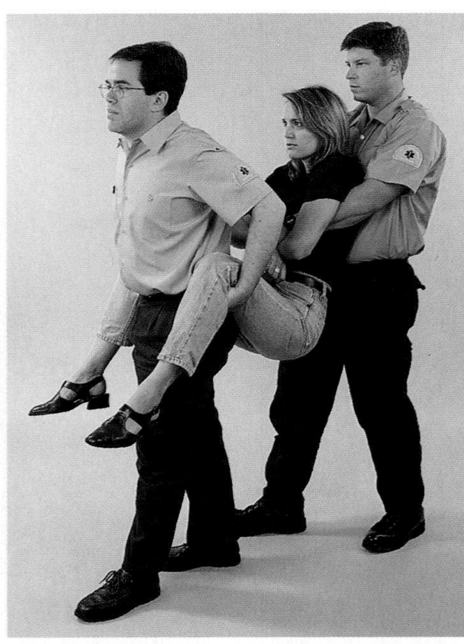

Figure 6-11 Extremity Lift

Draw Sheet

To transfer the victim from the stretcher to the bed, the rescuers loosen the bottom sheet on the stretcher. Position the stretcher along the side of the bed. Place rescuers beside the stretcher and on the other side of the bed. The rescuers on the bed side of the victim lean over the bed and grasp the sheet firmly at the victim's head and hips. The rescuers on the stretcher side grasp the sheets in the same place. The victim is then slid into the bed. If there are more rescuers available, they should be positioned to help support the victim's legs by grasping the sheet in the same manner as the initial rescuers (Fig. 6-13).

Victim Positioning

The victim's condition should guide the first responder's decision regarding patient positioning while awaiting transport. An unresponsive victim without trauma should be moved into the ***recovery position*** by rolling the victim onto his or her side (preferably the left). Bend the top leg and move it forward; hold the victim in that position. Support the head so that it is angled toward the ground. A victim with trauma should not be moved until additional EMS resources can evaluate and stabilize the victim. A victim experiencing pain or discomfort or difficulty breathing should be allowed to assume a position of comfort. A victim who is nauseated or vomiting should be allowed to remain in a position of comfort; however, the first responder should be positioned appropriately to manage the airway (Fig. 6-14).

A 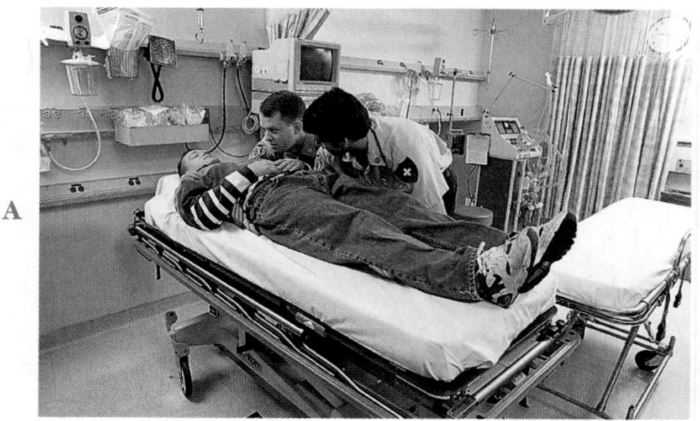

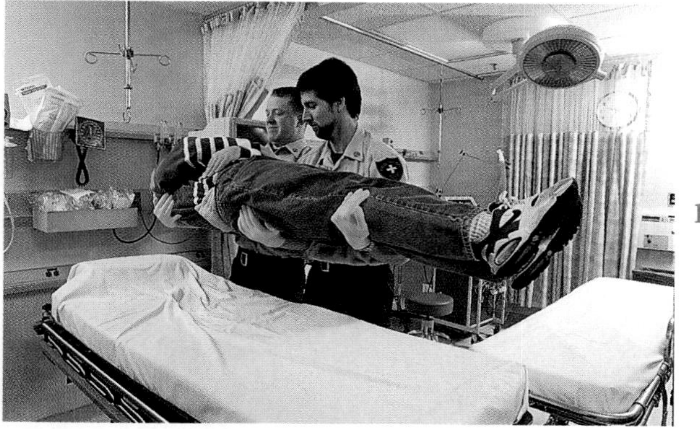 B

From McSwain N: *The Basic EMT: Comprehensive Prehospital Patient Care*, St. Louis, 1997, *Mosby Lifeline*.

Figure 6-12 Direct carry: **A**, With the stretcher positioned at a right angle to the bed with the head of the stretcher at the foot of the bed the rescuers position their hands. **B**, Once the rescuers are in position, one supporting the victim's head and shoulders and one cradling the waist and hips, the rescuer at the victim's head gives a signal to lift the victim and curl the victim's body toward their chests.

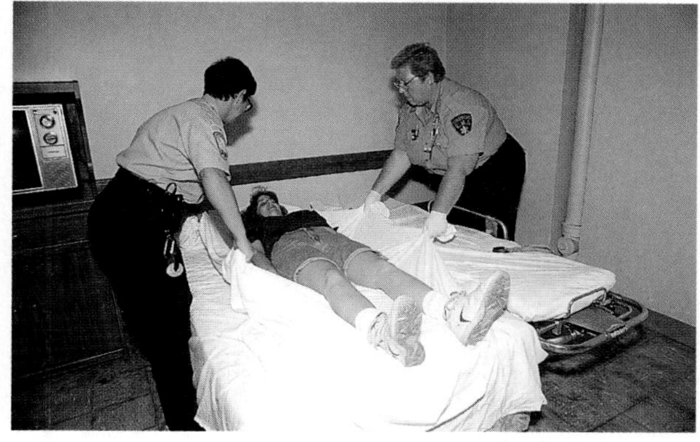

From McSwain N: *The Basic EMT: Comprehensive Prehospital Patient Care*, St. Louis, 1997, *Mosby Lifeline*.

Figure 6-13 Draw Sheet Method

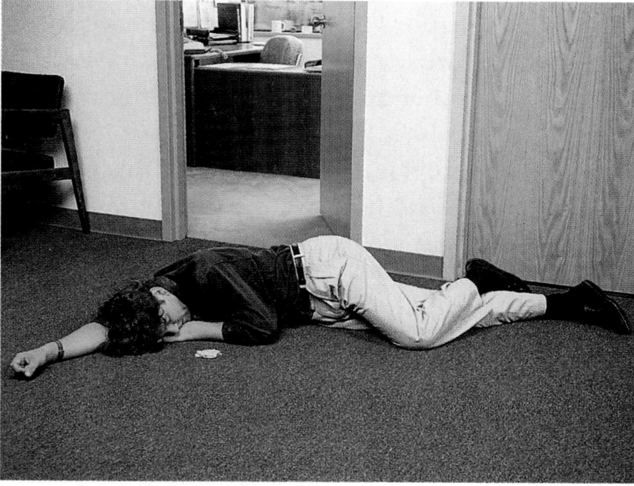

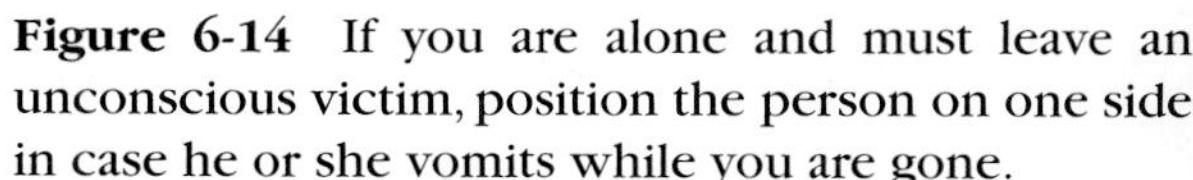

Figure 6-14 If you are alone and must leave an unconscious victim, position the person on one side in case he or she vomits while you are gone.

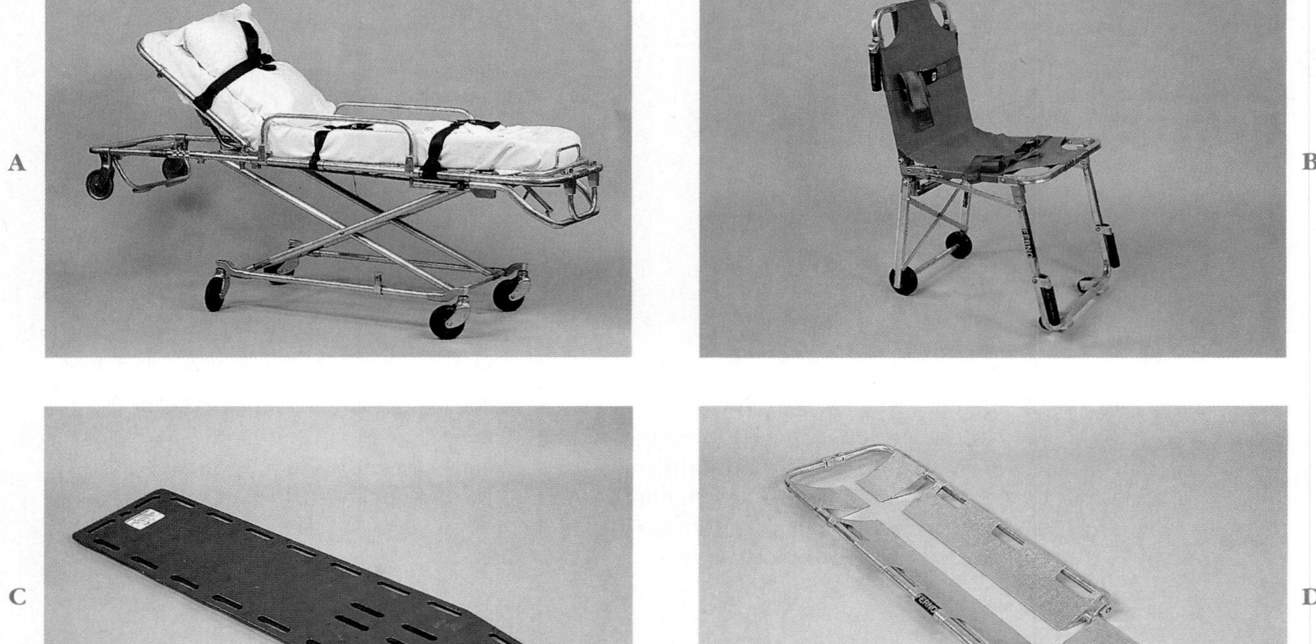

Figure 6-15 A, Ambulance Cot; B, Stair Chair; C, Backboard; D, Scoop or Orthopedic Stretcher.

◆ EQUIPMENT FAMILIARITY

As a first responder, you may not find yourself working in situations in which you will have to move and secure victims to different kinds of stretchers or other transport devices. Because you will be handing over the care of the victim to other EMS providers, it is important that you become familiar with some of the equipment. At times, you may be asked to help move, lift, or secure your victim before transport. Some of the commonly used transport devices that you will see include—

- Ambulance cots (6-15, *A*).
- Stair chair (6-15, *B*).
- Long backboard (6-15, *C*).
- Scoop or orthopedic stretchers (6-15, *D*).

Whenever using any of these devices, you should follow the manufacturer's direction for use, maintenance, and cleaning. If you have access to any of this equipment, take the opportunity to practice with it.

◆ SUMMARY

Take the time to survey the scene and determine if moving the victim is absolutely necessary before attempting to do so. Remember that your safety, and the safety of your partner, always comes first. This is especially true in incidents involving hazardous materials.

Avoid the common mistake of forcibly moving an ill or injured person unnecessarily. If you recognize a potentially life-threatening situation that requires the victim be moved immediately, use one of the techniques described in this chapter. Use the safest and easiest method to rapidly move the victim without causing injury to either yourself or the victim.

It is important for you to familiarize yourself with some of the typical equipment used in the local EMS systems. You should practice using the different types of stretchers and backboards, as you could be called on to assist the EMS providers in your area.

Use the activities in Unit 6 of the workbook to help you review the material in this chapter.

You Are The Responder

You are inspecting the work being done at a construction site. Suddenly you hear the crash of metal scaffolding on which you saw two men standing. As you and others rush back to the scene, you notice that one of the workers is conscious but is in obvious pain and is holding his leg. The other worker, lying a few feet away, is unconscious. There is a possibility that more of the scaffolding close by will fall. Should these victims be moved? If you decide to move them, how would you do so?

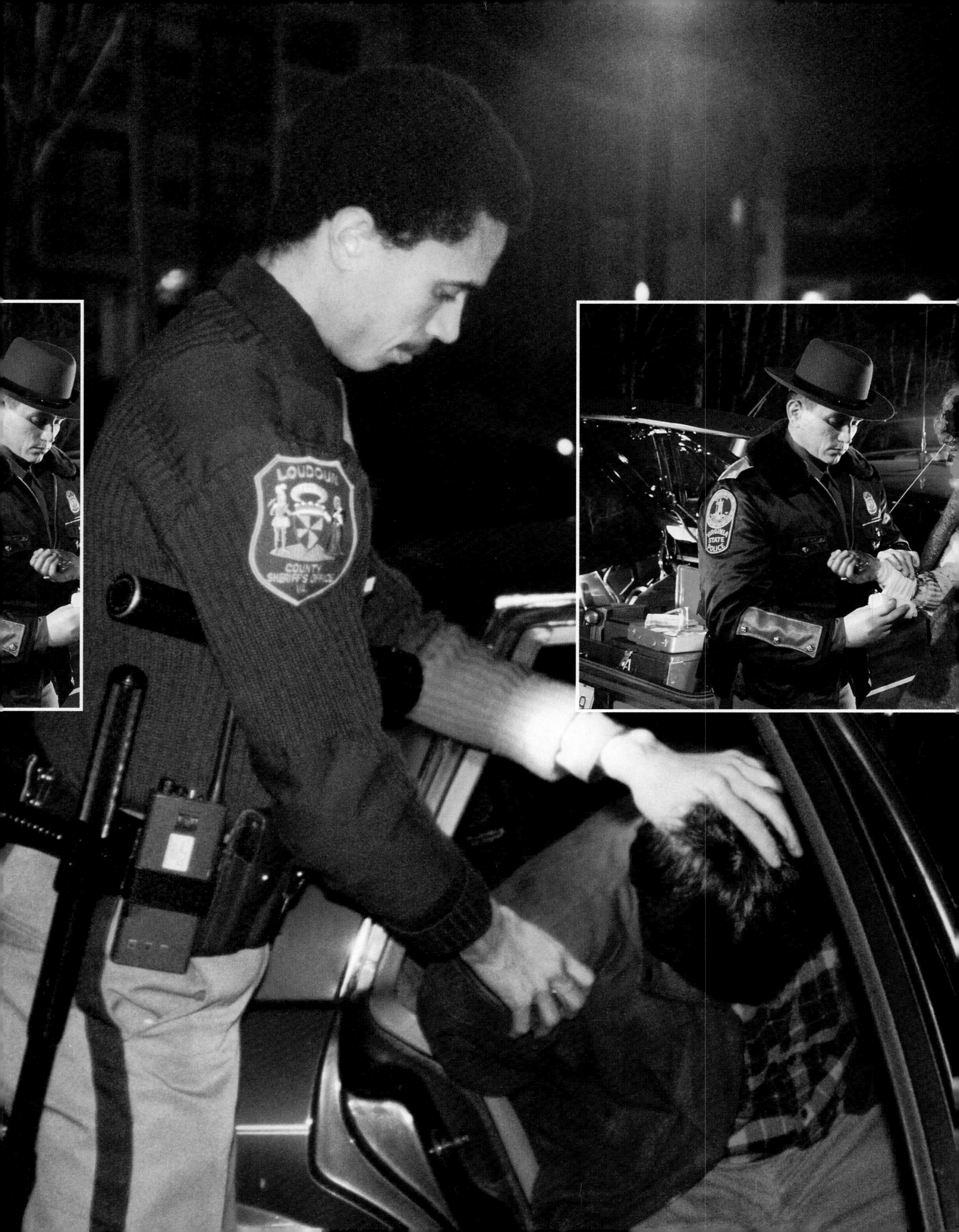
LOUDOUN
COUNTY
SHERIFF'S OFFICE
VIRGINIA
STATE
POLICE

Module Two

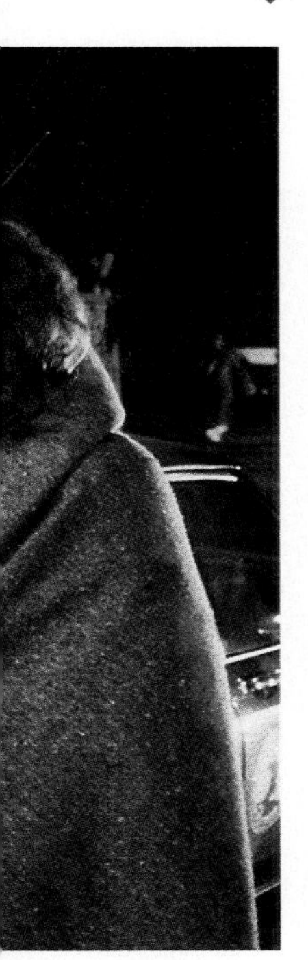

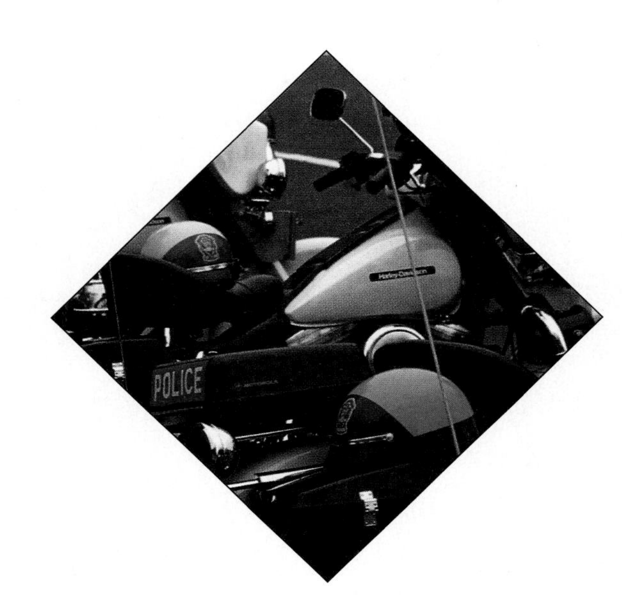

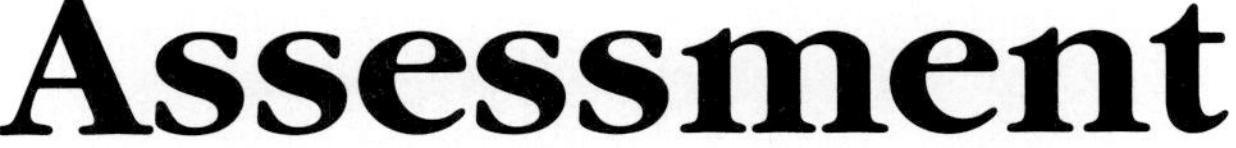

Assessment

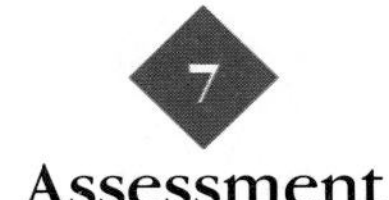

7

Assessment

Assessment

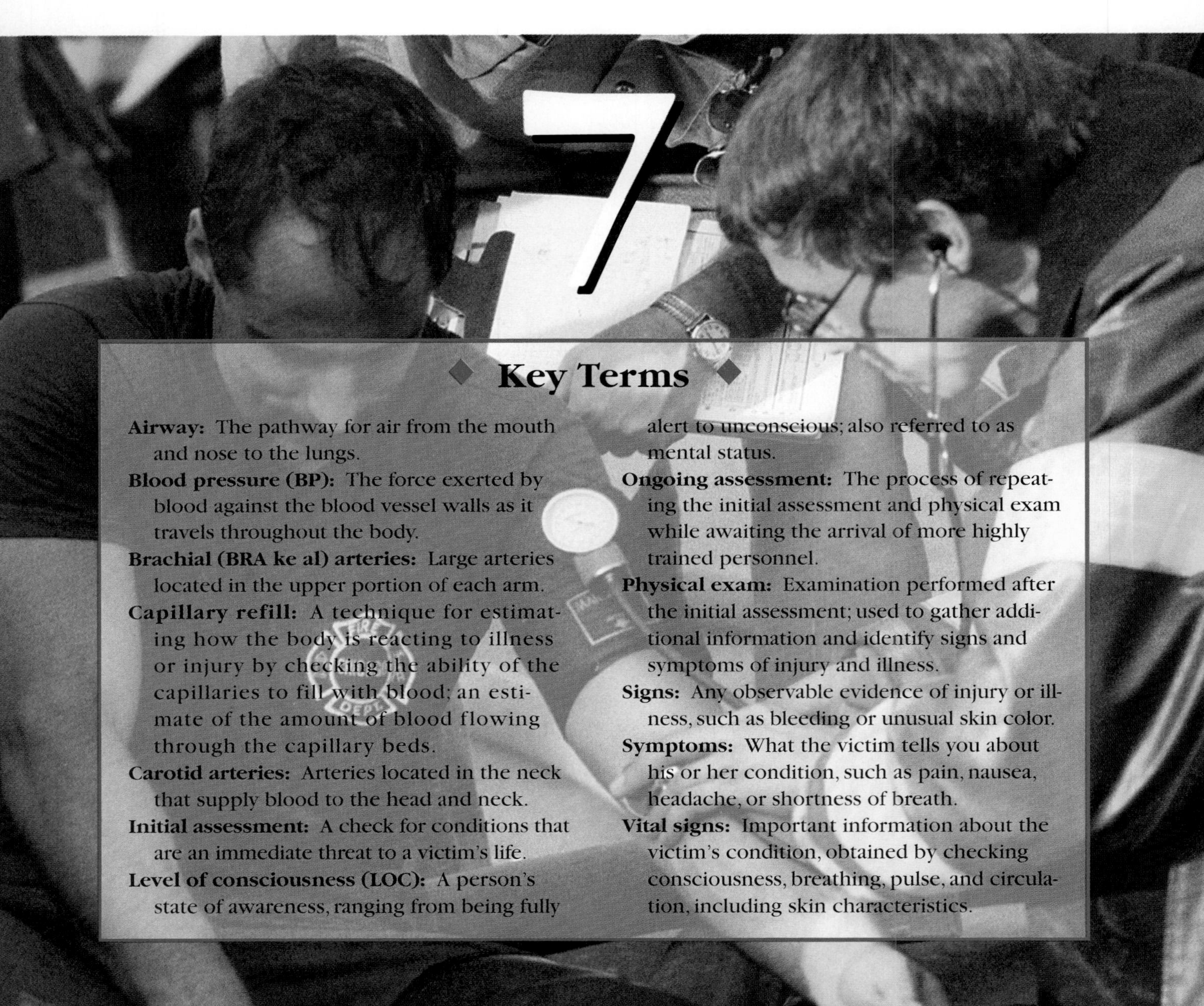

Key Terms

Airway: The pathway for air from the mouth and nose to the lungs.

Blood pressure (BP): The force exerted by blood against the blood vessel walls as it travels throughout the body.

Brachial (BRA ke al) arteries: Large arteries located in the upper portion of each arm.

Capillary refill: A technique for estimating how the body is reacting to illness or injury by checking the ability of the capillaries to fill with blood; an estimate of the amount of blood flowing through the capillary beds.

Carotid arteries: Arteries located in the neck that supply blood to the head and neck.

Initial assessment: A check for conditions that are an immediate threat to a victim's life.

Level of consciousness (LOC): A person's state of awareness, ranging from being fully alert to unconscious; also referred to as mental status.

Ongoing assessment: The process of repeating the initial assessment and physical exam while awaiting the arrival of more highly trained personnel.

Physical exam: Examination performed after the initial assessment; used to gather additional information and identify signs and symptoms of injury and illness.

Signs: Any observable evidence of injury or illness, such as bleeding or unusual skin color.

Symptoms: What the victim tells you about his or her condition, such as pain, nausea, headache, or shortness of breath.

Vital signs: Important information about the victim's condition, obtained by checking consciousness, breathing, pulse, and circulation, including skin characteristics.

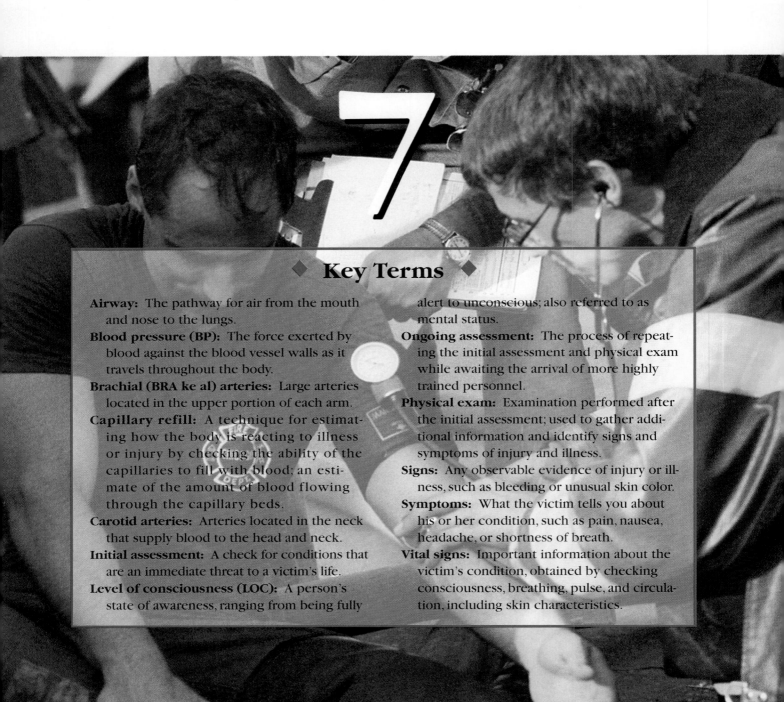

◆ Knowledge Objectives ◆

After reading this chapter and completing the class activities, you should be able to —

- Identify the components of a scene size-up.
- Describe common hazards found at the scene of a trauma or a medical emergency.
- Explain why first responders should evaluate scene safety before entering.
- Explain how to determine if a scene is safe to enter.
- Describe common mechanisms of injury and nature of illness.
- Summarize the reasons for forming a general impression of the victim.
- Explain the reasons for identifying the need for additional help.
- Explain the purpose of the initial assessment.
- Describe methods for assessing level of consciousness (mental status).
- Explain the differences in assessing the level of consciousness (mental status) of an adult, child, and infant.
- Describe methods of assessing whether a victim is breathing.
- Distinguish a victim with adequate breathing from a victim with inadequate breathing.
- Describe the methods used to assess circulation.
- Explain the differences in obtaining a pulse in an adult, child, and infant.
- Explain the need to assess a victim for external bleeding.
- Describe how to assess pulse rate and quality, breathing rate and quality, and skin appearance.
- Explain the importance of properly assessing a victim's vital signs.
- Explain the components of a physical exam.
- State the areas of the body that are evaluated during the physical exam.
- Identify further questions that may be asked during the physical exam.
- Explain the components of the SAMPLE history.
- Identify the components of the ongoing assessment.
- * Explain the importance of properly assessing a victim's blood pressure.
- * Describe the techniques used to measure blood pressure.

*signifies an Enrichment objective

◆ Attitude Objectives ◆

After reading this chapter and completing the class activities, you should be able to —

- Serve as a positive role model for others when —
  - Evaluating scene safety.
  - Evaluating the mechanism of injury or nature of illness.
  - Assessing a victim of injury or illness.
- Empathize with the feelings that victims may experience during assessment.
- Value the need for a caring attitude when performing victim assessment.

◆ Skills Objectives ◆

After reading this chapter and completing the class activities, you should be able to—

- Demonstrate how to assess mental status.
- Demonstrate how to assess airway, breathing, and circulation.
- Demonstrate how to assess for severe external bleeding.
- Demonstrate how to assess skin color, temperature, and moisture and capillary refill (infants and children).
- Demonstrate how to use the "SAMPLE" format to question a victim.
- Demonstrate how to perform a physical exam and an ongoing assessment.
- * Demonstrate how to measure blood pressure by auscultation and palpation.

◆ INTRODUCTION

In previous chapters, you learned how to prepare for an emergency, the precautions to take when approaching the scene, and how to recognize a dangerous situation. You also learned about your roles and responsibilities as a first responder. You learned that you can make a difference in an emergency—you may even save a life. But to make a difference, you must learn how to provide care for an ill or injured person. More important, you need to learn how to set priorities for the care you provide.

In this chapter, you will learn a plan of action to guide you through any emergency. When an emergency occurs, you may at first feel confused. But you can train yourself to remain calm and to think before you act. By following a standardized plan of action for any emergency, you can easily recall what to do and how to provide effective care.

◆ ESTABLISHING A PLAN OF ACTION

From the time you arrive at the scene until the time the victim is turned over to more advanced personnel, your plan involves five steps:

1. Scene size-up
2. Performing an initial assessment
3. Performing a physical exam
4. Gathering pertinent history
5. Performing an ongoing assessment

Summon more advanced medical personnel any time you discover a problem that requires greater care than you are able to provide (Table 7-1). In some cases, the need for greater care will be immediately obvious when you arrive at the scene. At other times, you may not determine the need for advanced care until later in your assessment. These five steps can ensure your safety and that of the victim and bystanders. They will also increase the victim's chance of survival if he or she has a serious illness or injury.

Step One: Scene Size-up

Once you recognize that an emergency has occurred and decide to act, you must size up, or survey, the scene. There are four main components to consider during a scene size-up:

1. Scene safety
2. The mechanism of injury/ nature of illness
3. The number of victims
4. The resources needed

Table 7-1 When to Summon More Advanced Medical Personnel

Condition	Signs and symptoms
Unconscious or not easily aroused	Victim does not respond to tapping, loud voices, or other attempts to arouse
Difficulty breathing	Noisy breathing, such as wheezing or gasping
Victim feels short of breath	Skin has a flushed, pale, ashen, or bluish appearance
No breathing	You cannot see the victim's chest rise and fall
	You cannot hear and feel air escaping from the nose and mouth
No pulse	You cannot feel the carotid pulse in the neck or the radial and brachial pulses in the arms
Severe bleeding	Victim has bleeding that spurts or gushes from the wound
Persistent pain in the chest or abdomen	Victim has persistent pain or pressure in the chest or abdomen that is not relieved by resting or changing positions
Vomiting blood or passing blood	You can see blood in vomit, urine, or feces
Poisoning	Victim shows evidence of swallowed, inhaled, or injected poison, such as presence of drugs, medications, or cleaning agents
	Mouth, nose, or lips may be burned
Sudden illness requiring assistance	Victim has seizures, severe headaches, changes in level of consciousness, unusually high or low blood pressure, or a known diabetic problem
Head, neck, or back injuries	How the injury happened; for example, a fall, severe blow, or collision suggests a head, neck, or back injury
Victim complains of severe headaches, neck or back pain	
Victim is unconscious	
Bleeding, clear fluid, or deformity of the scalp, face, or neck	
Possible broken bones	How the injury happened; for example, a fall, severe blow, or collision suggests a fracture
Evidence of damage to blood vessels or nerves, for example, slow capillary refill in a child or infant, no pulse below the injury, loss of sensation in the affected part	
Inability to move body part without pain or discomfort	
Painful, swollen, deformed area	

Always begin by making sure the emergency scene is safe for you, other rescuers, the victim(s), and any bystanders. Before approaching the victim, look for anything that may threaten your safety and that of others. Examples of dangers that may be present were previously discussed in Chapter 2. They include—

- Crash or rescue scenes requiring extrication or traffic control.

- The presence of hazardous materials.
- The potential for violence at crime scenes.

Other dangers include—

- Unstable surfaces or structures.
- Environmental conditions, such as water, ice, fire, or lightning.
- Downed power lines.

Take the necessary precautions when in a dangerous environment. If you are not properly trained and do not have the necessary equipment, do not approach the victim. Summon the necessary personnel. Nothing is gained by risking your safety. An emergency that begins with one victim could end up with two if you are hurt. If you suspect the scene is unsafe, wait and watch until the necessary personnel and equipment arrive. If conditions change, you may then be able to approach the victim.

As you approach the victim, consider the **mechanism of injury** or **nature of illness**. Doing so involves trying to find out what happened. Look around the scene for clues to what caused the emergency and the extent of the damage. Consider the force that may have been involved in creating an injury. This consideration will cause you to think about the possible type and extent of the victim's injuries. Take in the whole picture. How a motor vehicle is crushed or nearby objects, such as shattered glass, a fallen ladder, or a spilled medicine container, may suggest what happened (Fig. 7-1). If the victim is unconscious, considering the mechanism of injury or nature of illness may be the only way you can determine what happened.

When you size up the scene, look carefully for more than one victim. You may not see everyone at first. For example, in a vehicle collision, an open door may be a clue that a victim has left the car or was thrown from it. If one victim is bleeding or screaming loudly, you may overlook another victim who is unconscious. It is also easy in any emergency situation to overlook an infant or small child if he or she is not crying. Ask anyone present how many people may be involved. If you find more than one victim, ask bystanders to help you provide care.

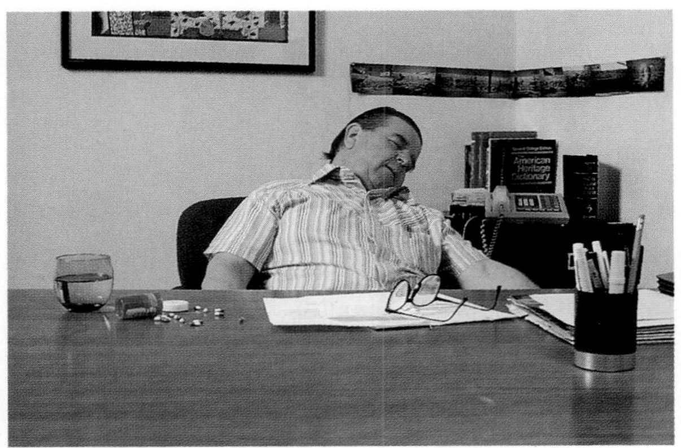

Figure 7-1 If the victim is unconscious, nearby objects may be your only clue to what has happened.

Look for bystanders who are in potential danger and tell them to move to safety. If the scene is safe and you need help, look for bystanders who may be able to assist you. Bystanders may be able to tell you what happened or help in other ways. A bystander who knows the victim may know whether he or she has any medical conditions or allergies. Bystanders can meet and direct the ambulance to your location, help keep the area free of unnecessary traffic, and help you provide care.

Once you reach the victim, quickly survey the scene again to see if it is still safe. At this point, you may see other dangers, clues to what happened, or victims or bystanders that you did not notice before. For example, you might respond to an automobile crash where a car has veered off the road and landed in a ditch. After surveying the scene and deciding it is safe to approach, you move to the car. As you come closer, you see a woman lying motionless on the ground near the car. But you also smell gasoline. What should you do? Is there a danger? Should you move her away from the car or try to care for her there?

As a rule, you should not move a victim unless there is an immediate danger, such as a fire, poisonous fumes, or an unstable structure. The odor of gasoline by itself is not sufficient cause to move the victim. If the area is dangerous and

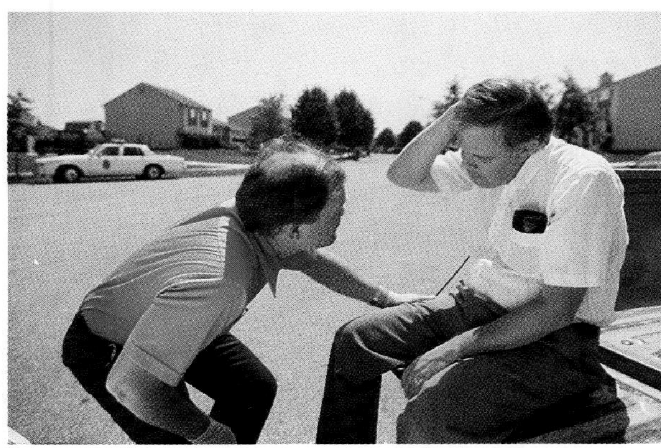

Figure 7-2 When talking to the victim, position yourself close to the victim's eye level and speak in a calm and positive manner.

the victim does not seem to be seriously injured, ask the victim to move to safety where you can help him or her. If the area is dangerous and the victim cannot move, you may try to move the victim as quickly as possible without making his or her condition worse. Emergency moves are discussed in Chapter 6. If there is no immediate danger, tell the victim not to move.

When you reach the victim, use appropriate BSI (body substance isolation) precautions. Try to position yourself close to the victim's eye level (Fig. 7-2). Speak in a calm and positive manner. If the victim is conscious, identify yourself and ask if you can help. Doing so lets a conscious victim know that a caring and skilled person is willing to help.

Step Two: Performing an Initial Assessment

In every emergency situation, you will perform an ***initial assessment.*** This is a check for conditions that are an immediate threat to a victim's life. The initial assessment has several components:

- Forming a general impression
- Assessing the victim's level of consciousness (LOC), or mental status
- Assessing the victim's airway, breathing, and circulation

Once you reach the victim and begin your assessment, you will be able to form a general impression of the victim's condition. This includes—

- Determining the victim's chief complaint or problem.
- Determining if the victim is injured or ill.
- Determining the victim's gender and approximate age.

This general impression may alert you that the victim has a serious problem that requires additional resources or only a minor problem that you can easily care for. You will discover these problems by looking for any signs and symptoms that the victim may have. ***Signs*** are evidence of injury or illness that you can observe, such as bleeding or unusual skin appearance. ***Symptoms*** are what the victim tells you he or she is experiencing, such as pain, nausea, headache, or shortness of breath.

As you perform the initial assessment, check to see if the victim—

- Is conscious.
- Has an open airway.
- Is breathing.
- Has a pulse.
- Is not bleeding severely.

Checking takes only seconds to perform and can tell you how the body is responding to injury or illness. Look for changes over time that may indicate a positive or negative change in the victim's condition. Recheck about every 5 minutes for a victim with a serious problem (unstable) and about every 15 minutes for a victim with a lesser problem (stable).

Level of Consciousness (Mental Status)

One of the most important indicators of a person's condition is his or her ***level of consciousness (LOC)***, or mental status. A person's level of consciousness can range from being fully alert to being unconscious. In describing a person's LOC, a four-level scale is used. The letters *A, V, P*, and *U* each refer to a stage of awareness (Table 7-2).

Table 7-2 Levels of Consciousness

Level	Characteristic behavior
Alert	Able to respond appropriately to questions
Verbal	Responds appropriately to verbal stimuli
Painful	Only responds to painful stimuli
Unresponsive	Does not respond

A - Alert: This implies that the person is aware of his or her surroundings and is able to respond appropriately to your questions, such as—

- What happened?
- What is your name?
- Where are you?
- What day of the week is it?

A person who is able to answer these questions is responsive and considered to be alert and oriented. Someone who is unable to answer these questions correctly or who may be unusually slow to respond is said to be disoriented.

V - Verbal: Sometimes a person only reacts to sounds, such as your voice. This person may appear to be lapsing into unconsciousness. A person who has to be stimulated by sound is described as responding to verbal stimuli.

P - Painful: If a person only responds when someone inflicts pain, then he or she is described as responding to painful stimuli. Pinching the earlobe or the skin above the collarbone are examples of painful stimuli used to try to get a response (Fig. 7-3).

U - Unresponsive: A person who does not respond to any stimuli is described as unconscious, or unresponsive to stimuli.

If you arrive and find a victim lying motionless, appearing to be asleep, gently tap him or her and ask "Are you okay?" (Fig. 7-4). The victim may just be resting with his or her eyes closed. Do not jostle or move the victim. A victim who can respond to you by speaking or crying is conscious, breathing, and has a pulse.

If the victim is unable to respond, he or she may be unresponsive (unconscious), which can indicate a life-threatening condition. When a person is unconscious, the tongue relaxes and may fall to the back of the throat, blocking the airway. This can cause breathing to stop. Soon after, the heart will stop beating.

You should be aware that infants and young children may not be able to respond to methods used to assess level of consciousness in adults. For example, they may not be able to respond to your questions because of an inability to speak or understand your questions, fear of a stranger, or because they are crying.

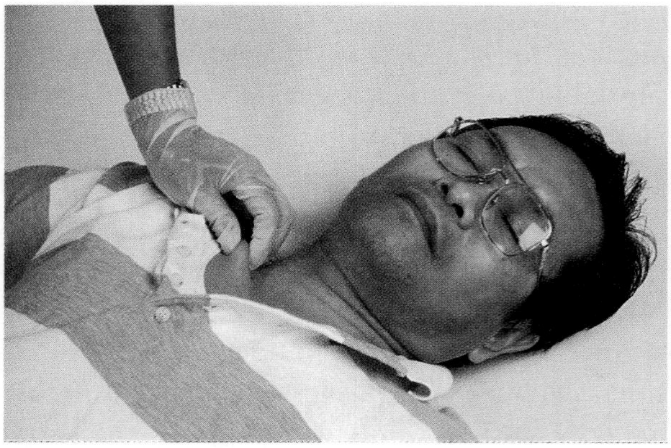

Figure 7-3 Pinching the skin above the collarbone is an example of a painful stimulus used to get a response.

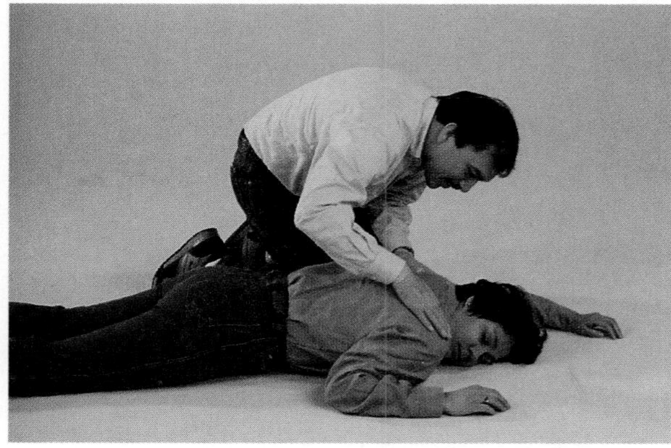

Figure 7-4 Determine if the person is conscious by gently tapping and asking, "Are you okay?"

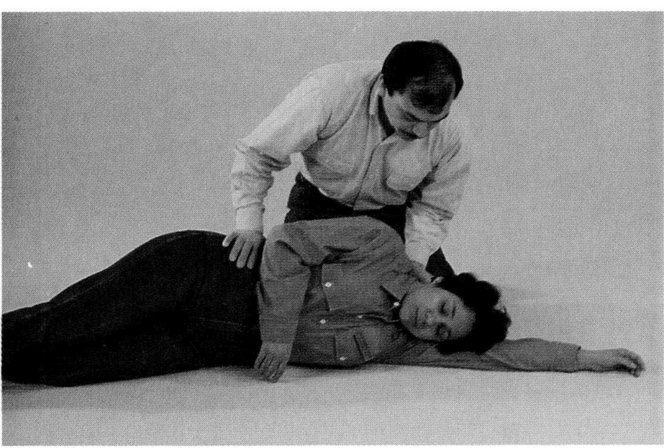

Figure 7-5 If the victim's position prevents you from checking the ABCs, roll the victim gently onto his or her back.

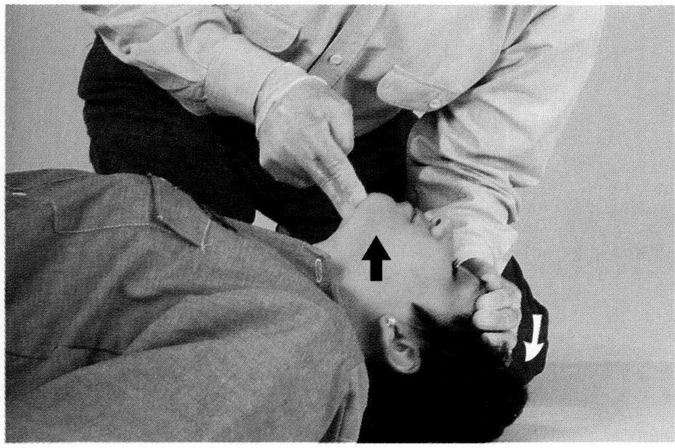

Figure 7-6 Tilt the head and lift the chin to open the airway.

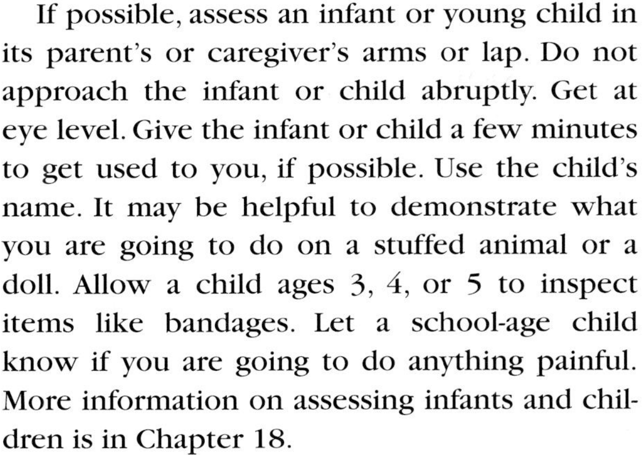

If possible, assess an infant or young child in its parent's or caregiver's arms or lap. Do not approach the infant or child abruptly. Get at eye level. Give the infant or child a few minutes to get used to you, if possible. Use the child's name. It may be helpful to demonstrate what you are going to do on a stuffed animal or a doll. Allow a child ages 3, 4, or 5 to inspect items like bandages. Let a school-age child know if you are going to do anything painful. More information on assessing infants and children is in Chapter 18.

Once you have assessed the victim's LOC, the next thing you must do is to check the victim's airway, breathing, and circulation. Remembering these steps is easy. The three steps are commonly referred to as the ABCs.

A = Airway

B = Breathing

C = Circulation (pulse, severe bleeding, skin characteristics)

If you can, try to check the ABCs in whatever position you find the victim, especially if you suspect the victim has a head, neck, or back injury. Sometimes, however, the victim's position, such as being facedown, prevents you from effectively checking the ABCs. In this case, you may roll the victim gently onto his or her back, keeping the head, neck, and back in as straight a line as possible (Fig. 7-5).

Checking the Airway

The pathway for air from the mouth and nose to the lungs is commonly called the ***airway***. Without an open airway, the victim cannot breathe. Remember, a victim who can speak or cry is conscious, has an open airway, is breathing, and has a pulse.

It is more difficult to tell if an unconscious victim has an open airway. To open an unconscious victim's airway, consider whether the victim has suffered an illness or injury. If the victim has not suffered an injury to the head, neck, or back, you should open the airway by tilting the head back and lifting the chin (Fig. 7-6). *If there is any possibility of head or spine trauma, open the airway by using the jaw thrust without head tilt* (Fig. 7-7). Both of these techniques move the tongue away from the back of the throat, allowing air to enter the lungs. After opening the airway, check for breathing.

Sometimes, opening the airway does not result in a free passage of air. Air does not pass freely when a victim's airway is blocked by liquid, food, or other objects. In this case, you will need to remove the obstruction. Chapter 8 describes how to care for an obstructed airway.

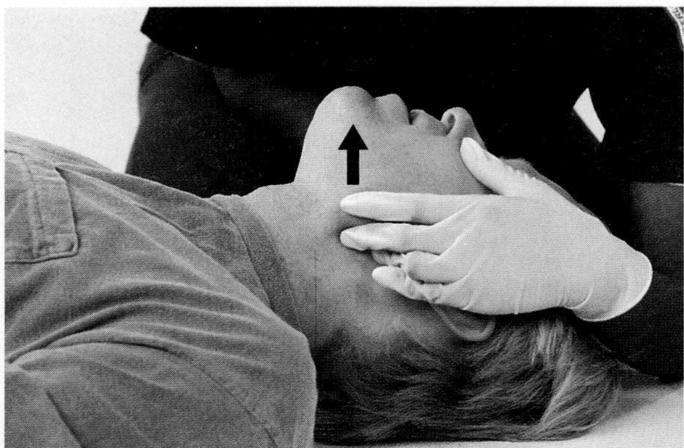

Figure 7-7 Use a two-handed jaw thrust when a chin-lift fails to open the airway of a victim with a suspected head or spine injury.

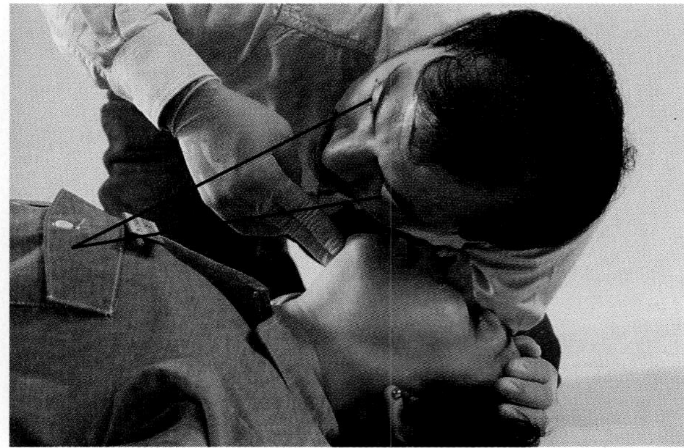

Figure 7-8 To check breathing, look, listen, and feel for breathing for about 5 seconds.

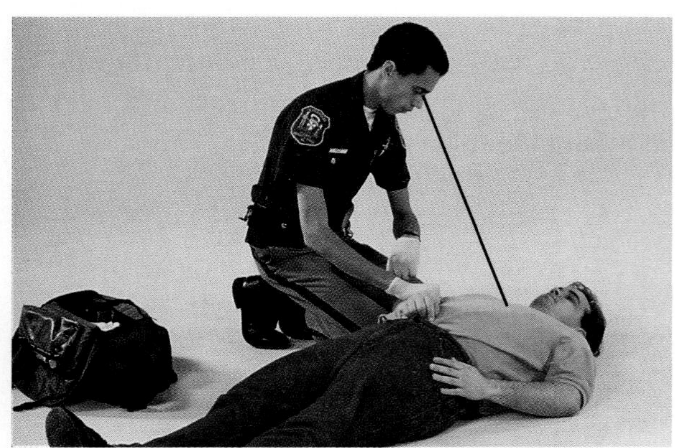

Figure 7-9 Look, listen, and feel for breathing to determine the rate and quality of breathing.

Checking Breathing

If the victim is breathing, the chest will rise and fall. However, chest movement by itself does not mean air is reaching the lungs. You must also listen and feel for signs of breathing. Position yourself so that you can hear and feel air as it escapes from the victim's nose and mouth. At the same time, watch the chest rise and fall. Take the time to look, listen, and feel for breathing for about 5 seconds (Fig. 7-8).

If the victim is breathing, assess the rate and quality of the breathing effort. A healthy person breathes regularly, quietly, and effortlessly. The normal breathing rate for an adult is between 12 and 20 breaths per minute. However, some people breathe slightly slower or faster. Excitement, fear, or exercise will cause breathing to increase and become deeper. Certain injuries or illnesses can also cause both the breathing rate and quality to change.

To determine the breathing rate, listen for the sounds as the person inhales and exhales. Count the number of times a person breathes (inhales and exhales) in 30 seconds and multiply that number by 2 (Fig. 7-9). The number you get is the number of breaths per minute.

Abnormal breathing may indicate a potential problem. The signs and symptoms of abnormal breathing include —

- Gasping for air.
- Noisy breathing, including whistling sounds, crowing, gurgling, or snoring.
- Excessively fast or slow breathing.
- Painful breathing.

Try to check for the rate and quality of breathing without the victim's awareness. If a victim realizes that you are checking his or her breathing, he or she may attempt to change his or her breathing pattern without being aware of doing so. In later chapters, you will learn more about what changes in breathing may mean and what specific care to provide.

If the victim is not breathing, you must breathe for him or her. Begin by giving 2 slow breaths. Each breath should be given until the chest gently rises. The breaths will get air into the victim's lungs. The longer a victim goes without oxygen, the more likely he or she is to suffer brain damage or die. This process of breathing for the victim is called **rescue breathing**. You will learn how to give rescue breathing in Chapter 8.

Checking Circulation

Once you have assessed the victim's airway and breathing, you should assess blood circulation. If the heart has stopped, blood will not circulate throughout the body. If blood does not circulate, the victim will suffer severe brain damage or die because the brain will not get any oxygen.

Pulse

The most commonly used method of checking for adequate circulation is to check for a pulse. With every heartbeat, a wave of blood moves through the blood vessels. This creates a beat called the **pulse**. You can feel it with your fingertips in arteries near the skin.

When the heart is healthy, it beats with a steady rhythm. This beat creates a regular pulse. A normal pulse for an adult is between 60 and 100 beats per minute. A well-conditioned athlete may have a pulse of 50 beats per minute or lower. An infant can have a normal pulse of greater than 100 beats per minute. If the heartbeat changes, so does the pulse. An abnormal pulse may be a sign of a potential problem.

Signs of an abnormal pulse include—

- Irregular pulse.
- Weak and hard-to-find pulse.
- Excessively fast or slow pulse.

When someone is ill or severely injured, the heart may beat unevenly, producing an irregular pulse. The rate at which the heart beats can also change. The pulse speeds up when a person is excited, anxious, in pain, losing blood, or under stress. It slows down when a person is relaxed. Some heart conditions or medications can also speed up or slow down the pulse rate. Sometimes changes may be very subtle and difficult for you to detect. The most important change to note is a pulse that changes from being present to no pulse at all.

Checking a pulse is a simple procedure. It involves placing two fingers on top of a major artery where it is located close to the skin's surface. Pulse sites that are easy to locate are the carotid arteries in the neck, the radial artery in the wrist, and the brachial artery in the upper arm (Fig. 7-10). There are also other pulse sites you may use (Fig. 7-11). To check the pulse rate, count the number of beats in 30 seconds and multiply that number by 2. The number you get is the number of heartbeats per minute.

An ill or injured victim's pulse may be hard to find. If you have trouble finding a pulse, keep checking for one periodically. Take your time. Remember, if a victim is breathing, his or her heart is also beating. However, there may be a loss in circulation to the injured area, causing a loss of pulse. If you cannot find the pulse in one place, check it in another major artery, such as in the other wrist. In later chapters, you will learn more about what any changes in pulse may mean and what care to provide.

If the victim is conscious and breathing, check the victim's pulse to determine the rate and quality of the pulse. For adults and children, you usually check the **radial pulse** on the thumb side of the victim's wrist. For infants, you should check the ***brachial artery*** located on the inside of the upper arm, midway between the shoulder and elbow (Fig. 7-12).

If the victim is unconscious, you must find out whether he or she is breathing and whether his or her heart is beating at all. If the victim is not breathing, you are not concerned with the rate and quality of the pulse, only whether it is present or absent. Check the pulse for an adult or child at either of the ***carotid arteries*** located in the neck. Check the brachial pulse of an infant in the middle of the upper arm (Fig. 7-13).

To find the carotid pulse, feel for the Adam's apple at the front of the neck, then slide your fingers into the groove at the side of the neck. Sometimes the pulse may be difficult to find,

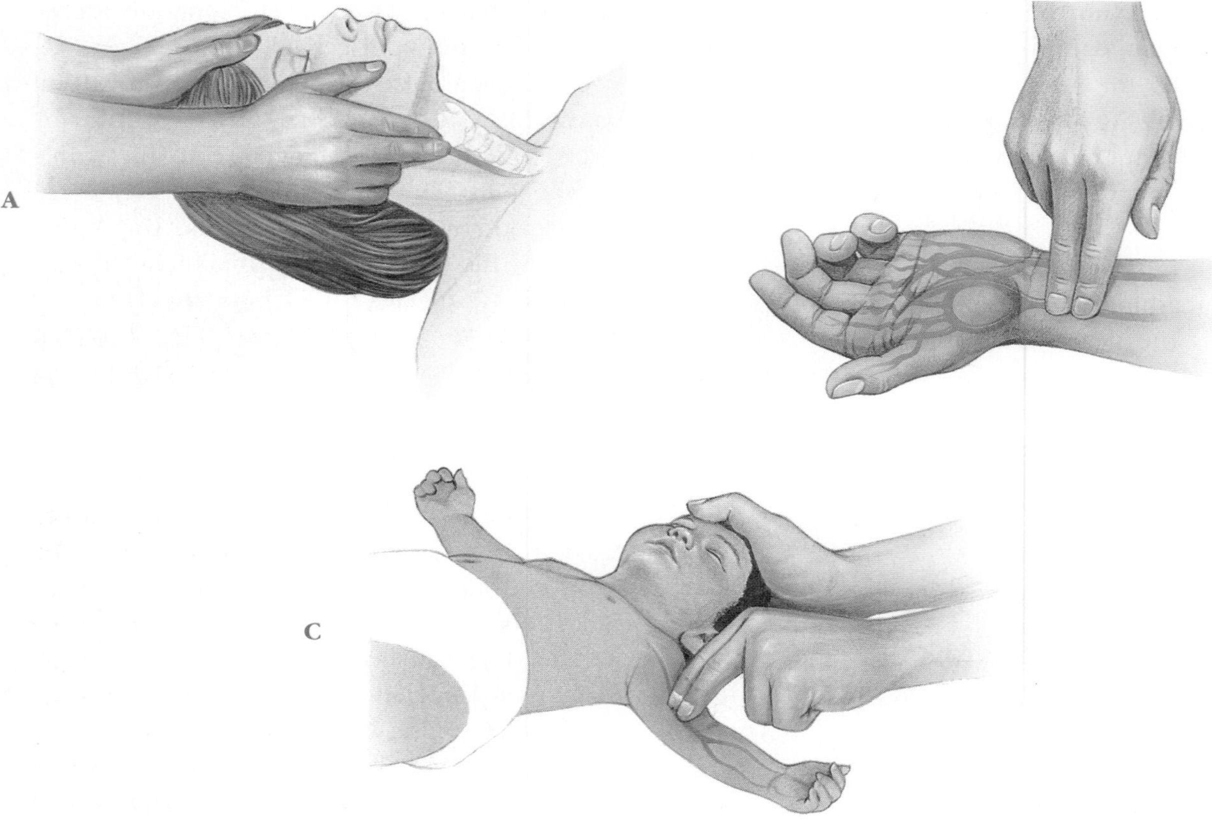

Figure 7-10 A pulse can be checked in arteries that circulate close to the surface, such as the carotid artery, the radial artery, and for infants, the brachial artery.

since it may be slow or weak. If at first you do not find a pulse, relocate the Adam's apple and again slide your fingers into place. When you think you are in the right spot, take 5 to 10 seconds to feel for the pulse.

If the victim does not have a pulse, you need to keep oxygen-rich blood circulating. This involves doing rescue breathing to get oxygen into the victim's lungs and chest compressions to circulate the oxygen to the brain. This procedure is called cardiopulmonary resuscitation (CPR) and is described in Chapter 10.

Severe bleeding

Checking circulation also means looking for severe bleeding. Bleeding is severe when blood spurts from the wound or cannot be controlled. Severe bleeding is life threatening. Check for it by looking from head to toe for signs of external bleeding (Fig. 7-14). Severe bleeding must be controlled before you provide any further care. Techniques for controlling severe bleeding are described in Chapter 11.

Skin characteristics

The appearance of the skin and its temperature can also indicate something about the victim's circulation. Checking the skin characteristics requires you to look at and feel the skin. The skin conditions to note are —

- Color — pale, ashen, or flushed.
- Temperature — hot or cold.
- Moisture — moist or dry.
- Capillary refill — normal or slow.

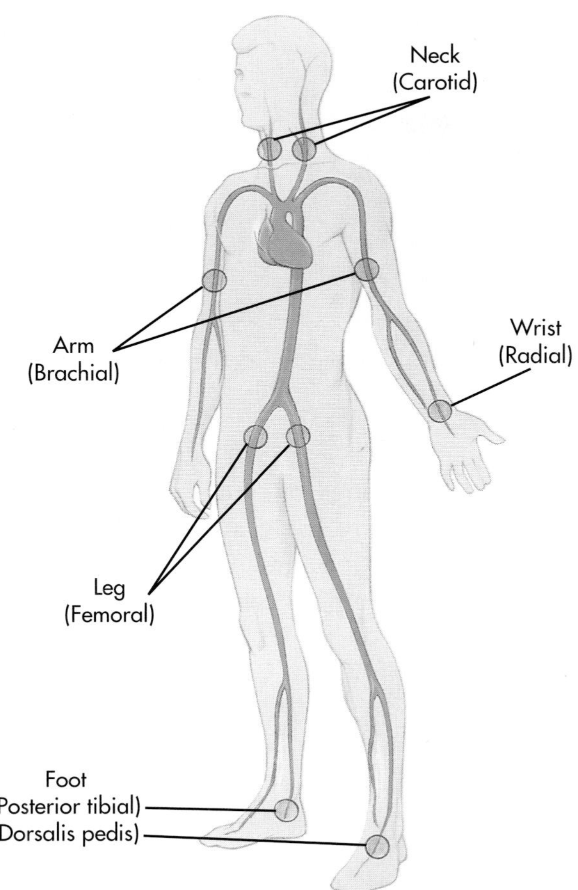

Figure 7-11 Easily Located Pulse Sites

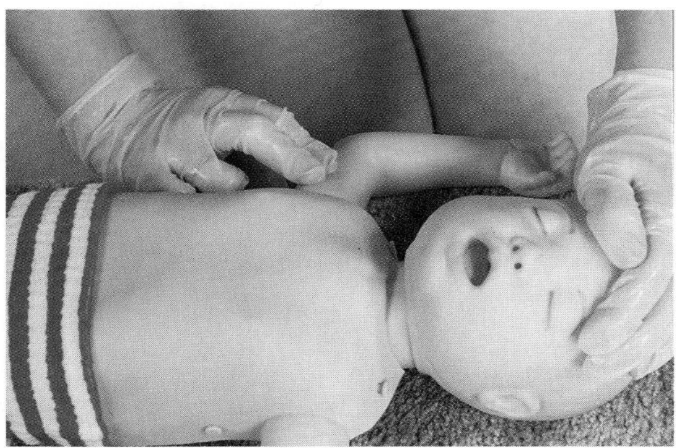

Figure 7-12 To find an infant's pulse, feel for the brachial artery in the upper arm.

In some people, the skin looks red when the body is forced to work harder. The heart pumps faster to get more blood to the tissues. This increased blood flow causes reddened skin and makes the skin feel warm. In contrast, the skin may look pale or bluish and feel cool and moist if the blood flow is inadequate. When a person with darker skin becomes pale, the skin turns **ashen**, a grayish color. Any of these skin conditions may indicate a problem.

One technique for estimating how the body is reacting to illness or injury is to check the ability of the capillaries to refill with blood. This technique, known as capillary refill, is used on children and infants. ***Capillary refill*** is an estimate of the amount of blood flowing through the capillary beds, such as those in the fingertips. The capillary beds in the fingertips are normally rich with blood, which causes the pink color under the fingernails. When a serious illness or injury occurs, the body attempts to conserve blood in the vital organs. As a

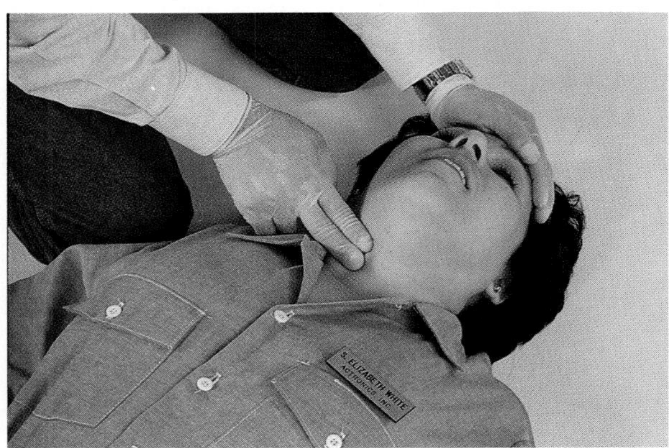

Figure 7-13 Determine if the heart is beating by feeling for a carotid pulse at either side of the neck.

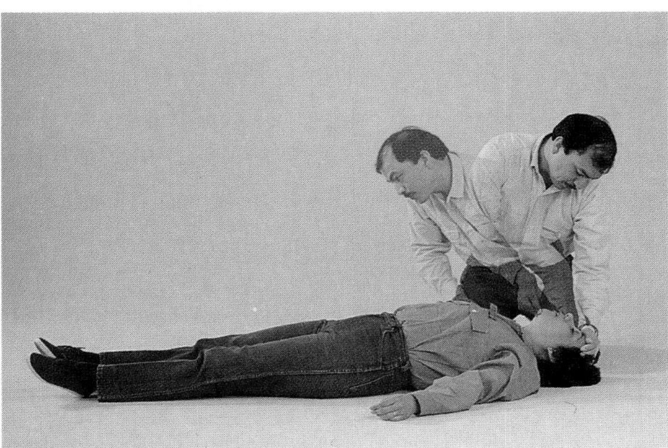

Figure 7-14 Visually check for signs of severe bleeding by looking from head to toe.

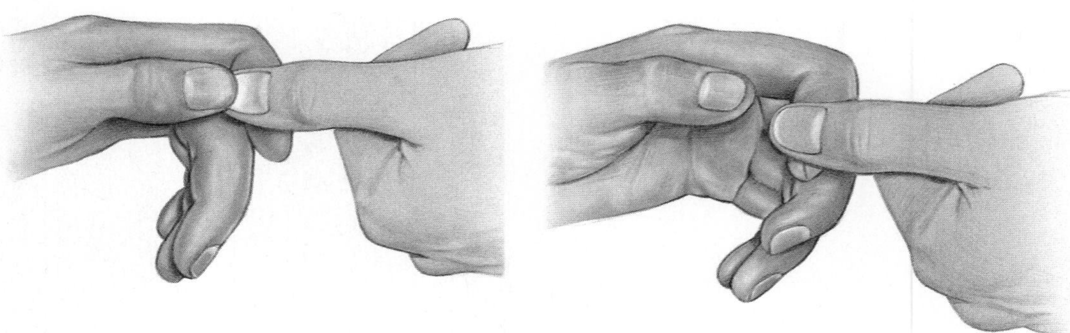

Figure 7-15 Checking capillary fill is a technique sometimes used to estimate whether blood is circulating properly in the extremities.

result, capillaries in the fingertips are among the first blood vessels to constrict, thereby limiting their blood supply.

To check capillary refill, squeeze the victim's fingernail for about 2 seconds and then release. In a healthy person, the normal response is for the area beneath the fingernail to turn pale as you press it and immediately turn pink again as you release and it refills with blood (Fig. 7-15). If the area does not return to pink within 2 seconds (the time it takes to say "capillary refill"), this indicates insufficient circulation and a potentially serious illness or injury. Be aware, however, that environmental temperature can play a role in the effectiveness of this technique. If the victim is exposed to cold temperature, the capillary refill will normally be slow. Refill slows because blood is directed away from the peripheral areas of the body, like the fingertips, in an effort to maintain core body temperature.

Consciousness, breathing, and circulation, including pulse and skin characteristics, are called ***vital signs***. Check the vital signs often as you monitor a victim while you wait for more advanced medical personnel to arrive.

Step Three: Performing a Physical Exam

Once you are certain that the victim has no life-threatening conditions that require your care, you can begin the physical exam. If you find life-threatening conditions, such as unconsciousness, no breathing, no pulse, or severe bleeding during the initial assessment, do not waste time with a physical exam. Instead, focus your attention on providing care for the life-threatening conditions.

The ***physical exam*** is a systematic "head-to-toe" examination that helps you gather additional information about injuries or medical conditions that may need care. These injuries or conditions are not immediately life threatening but could become so if not cared for. For example, you might find minor bleeding or possible broken bones as you conduct the exam. Begin the physical exam by telling the victim what you are going to do and asking the victim for consent.

Note the information you find during the physical exam. Sometimes you may need to have someone else write down the information or help you remember it. You can give this information to more advanced medical personnel when they arrive. This information may help determine what type of medical care the victim will receive later.

As you perform the physical exam, try not to move the victim. Most injured people will find the most comfortable position for themselves. For example, a person with a chest injury who is having difficulty breathing may be sitting up and supporting the injured area. Let the victim continue to do this. Do not ask him or her to change positions.

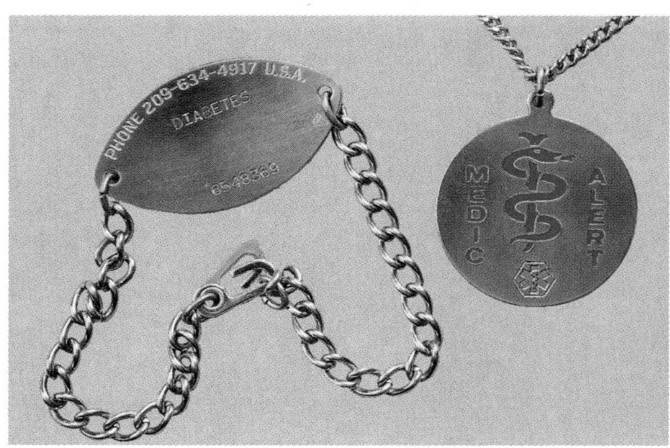

Figure 7-16 Medical alert tags can provide important medical information about the victim.

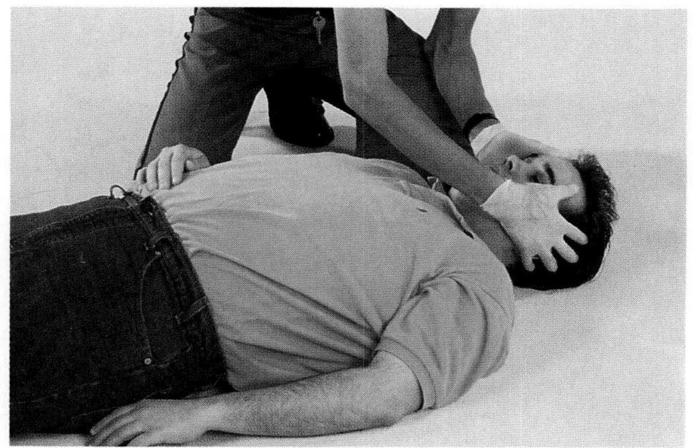

Figure 7-17 During the head-to-toe examination, inspect the entire body, starting with the head.

When you perform the physical exam, use your senses — sight, sound, smell, and touch — to detect anything abnormal. For example, you may smell an unusual odor that could indicate a victim has swallowed poison. You may see a bruise or feel a deformed body part. As you inspect (look) and palpate (feel) the victim's body, use the mnemonic DOTS to help you remember what you are trying to find. DOTS stands for —

- *D*eformity.
- *O*pen injuries.
- *T*enderness.
- *S*welling.

Ask the victim to remain still. Though a victim may be moving around in pain, he or she usually will not move a body part that is injured. Ask the victim to tell you if any areas hurt. *Avoid touching any painful areas or having the victim move any area in which there is discomfort.* Watch facial expressions; listen for a tone of voice that may reveal pain. Look for a medical alert tag on a necklace or bracelet (Fig. 7-16). This tag may help you determine what is wrong, whom to call for help, and what care to give.

As you conduct the physical exam, think about how the body normally looks and feels. Be alert for any sign of injuries — anything that looks or feels unusual. If you are uncertain whether your finding is unusual, check the other side of the body. Inspect the entire body, starting with the head. You might see abnormal skin color from bruising, a body fluid, such as blood, or a body part in an unusual position. You may see and feel odd bumps or depressions. The victim may seem groggy or faint. In most situations, you will not need to examine the entire body. For example, an isolated injury to the hand from a power saw accident does not require you to check other areas of the victim's body. In other situations, such as a pedestrian struck by a motor vehicle, a complete body exam is necessary.

Begin the physical exam by checking the head (Fig. 7-17). Look for blood or clear fluid in or around the ears, nose, and mouth. Blood or clear fluid can indicate a serious skull or spine injury.

Next, look and feel for any abnormalities in the neck (Fig. 7-18). If the victim has not suffered an injury involving the head or trunk and does not have any pain or discomfort in the head, neck, or back, then there is little likelihood of spinal injury. You should proceed to check other body parts. If you suspect a possible head, neck, or back injury because of the nature of the incident, such as a motor vehicle collision or a fall from a height, minimize movement to the victim's head and spine. If you suspect head, neck, or back injuries, take care of

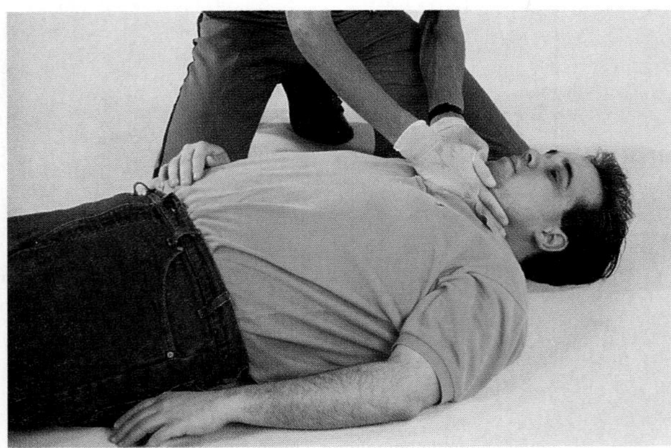

Figure 7-18 To check the neck, look and feel for any abnormalities. If there are no abnormalities, the victim has not suffered any injury involving the head or trunk, and the victim has no pain, have the victim turn his head gently from side to side.

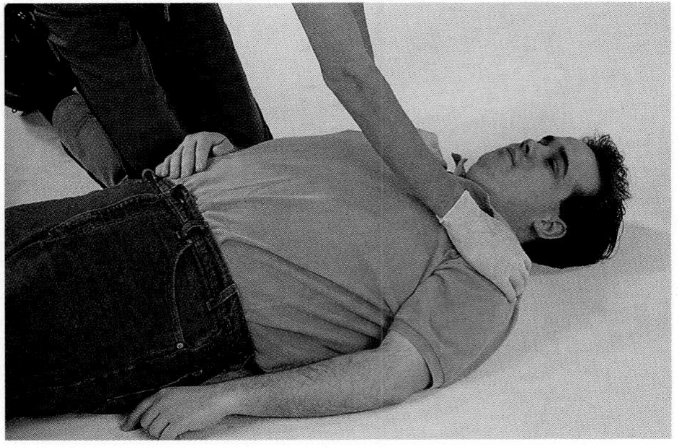

Figure 7-19 Check the shoulders by looking and feeling for deformity. Ask the victim to shrug his shoulders.

them first. Do not be concerned about finishing the physical exam. You will learn techniques for stabilizing and immobilizing the head, neck, and back in Chapter 16.

Continue your exam by checking the collarbones and shoulders by looking and feeling for deformity (Fig. 7-19). If the victim does not have any pain or possible head, neck, or back injury, ask the victim to shrug his or her shoulders. Check the chest by asking the victim to take a deep breath and then blow the air out. Look and listen for signs of difficulty breathing. Feel the ribs for deformity (Fig. 7-20). Ask the victim if he or she is experiencing any pain during breathing.

Next, ask if the person has any pain in the abdomen. If not, apply slight pressure to each side of the abdomen, high and low (Fig. 7-21). The abdomen should be soft. If it is rigid, this indicates a problem. Check the pelvis, asking the person if he or she has any pain. If the victim does not have any pain, place your hands on both sides of the pelvis and push down and inwards to check for fractures (Fig. 7-22).

Next, determine if the victim has any pain in the extremities. Start with the arms and hands. Inspect the arms for any deformity (Fig. 7-23).

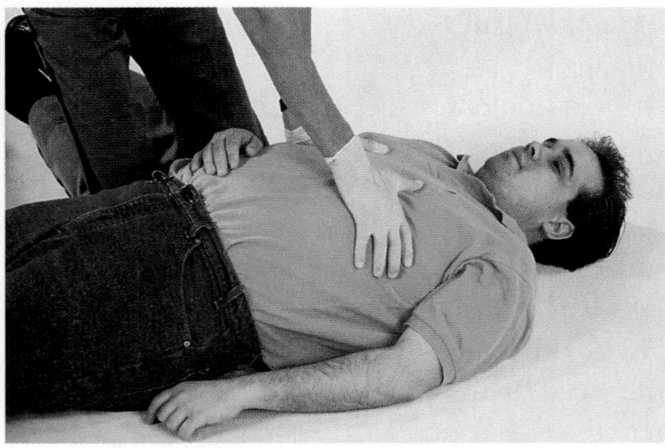

Figure 7-20 Check the chest by feeling the ribs for deformity. Ask the victim to take a deep breath and exhale.

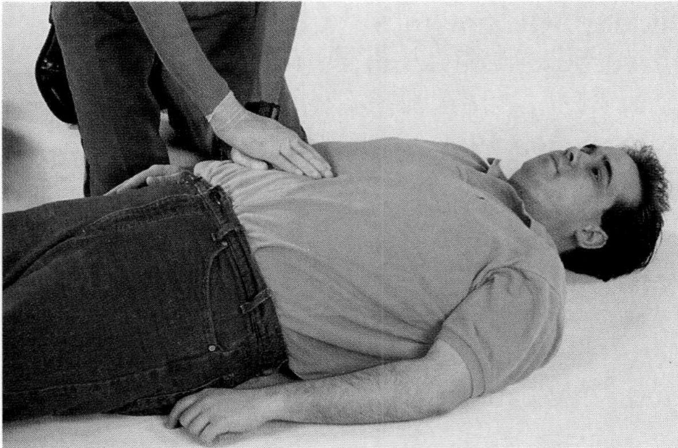

Figure 7-21 Apply slight pressure to the abdomen to see if it is soft or rigid.

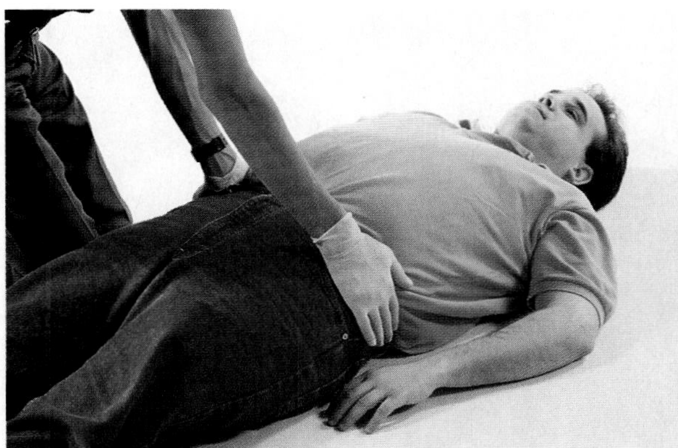

Figure 7-22 To check the pelvis, place your hands on both sides of the pelvis and push down and in, asking the victim if he feels any pain.

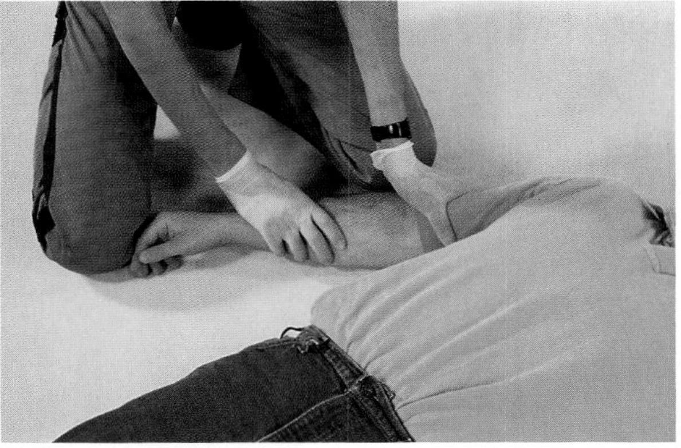

Figure 7-23 Check the arms by feeling for any deformity. If there is no apparent sign of injury, ask the victim to bend the arms and move the hands and fingers.

It is best to check only one extremity at a time. If there is no apparent sign of injury, ask the person if he or she can move the fingers, hand, and arm. Repeat this procedure with the other arm. Look and feel each leg as you did the arms (Fig. 7-24). Ask the victim to move his or her toes, foot, and leg. Finally, check the back by gently reaching under the victim (Fig. 7-25). If the victim is found lying facedown or on his or her side and needs to be rolled over, you could quickly check the back before any other part of the body and then roll the victim over if you do not suspect spinal injury.

If the victim is unable to move a body part or is experiencing pain or dizziness, recheck the ABCs. Provide care for any conditions you find. Help the victim rest in the most comfortable position, and maintain normal body temperature by keeping the victim from getting chilled or overheated. Reassure the victim and summon more advanced medical personnel.

As you perform this examination, keep watching the victim's level of consciousness, breathing, pulse, and skin color. *If any life-threatening problems develop, stop whatever you are doing and provide care immediately.*

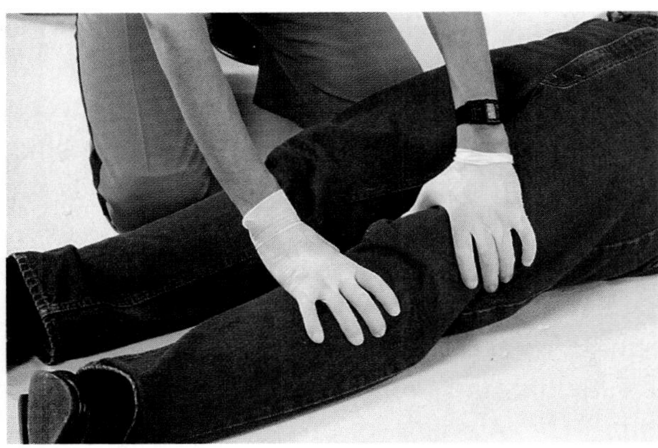

Figure 7-24 Check the legs by feeling for any deformity. If there is no apparent sign of injury, ask the victim to bend the legs and move the feet and toes.

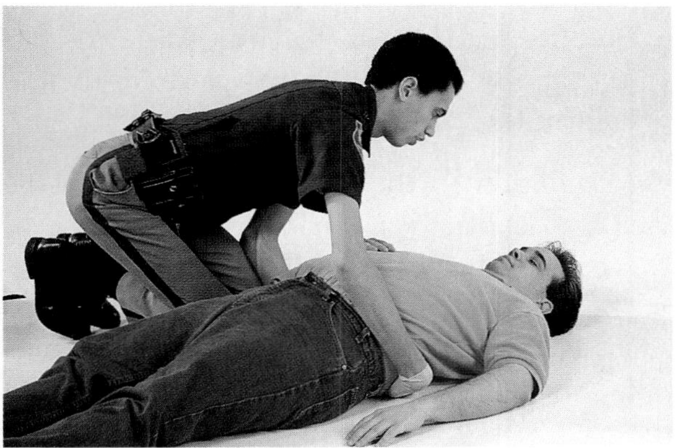

Figure 7-25 Gently reach under the victim to check the back.

Step Four: Obtaining a SAMPLE History

Asking the victim about the incident and any existing conditions is commonly called obtaining a "history." Obtaining a history should not take much time and may be done before or during the physical exam. Ask the victim's name. Using his or her name will make the victim more comfortable.

Using the mnemonic SAMPLE, determine the following six items for the history:

1. ***S*igns and *S*ymptoms**—Signs include seeing bleeding, hearing breathing distress, and feeling cool, moist skin. Symptoms include pain, nausea, headache, and difficulty breathing.
2. ***A*llergies**—Determine if the victim is allergic to any medications, food, or environmental elements, such as pollen or bees.
3. ***M*edications**—Determine if the victim is presently using any medications, prescription or non-prescription.
4. ***P*ertinent past history**—Determine if the victim is under a physician's care for any condition or if the victim has had a similar problem in the past or been recently hospitalized.
5. ***L*ast oral intake**—This intake includes solids or liquids and can include food, fluid, and medication.
6. ***E*vents leading up to the incident**—Determine what the victim was doing before and at the time of the incident.

In addition to the SAMPLE history, ask the victim to explain what happened. Ask if he or she has any pain. If so, ask him or her to describe it. You can expect to get descriptions such as burning, throbbing, aching, or sharp pain. Ask when the pain started. Ask how bad the pain is.

Sometimes the victim will be unable to give you the information. This is often the case with a child or with an adult who momentarily lost consciousness and may not be able to recall what happened or is disoriented. These victims may be frightened. Be calm and patient. Speak normally and in simple terms. Offer reassurance. Ask family members, friends, or bystanders what happened (Fig. 7-26). They may be able to give you helpful information, such as telling you if a victim has a medical condition you should be aware of. They may also be able to help calm the victim if necessary.

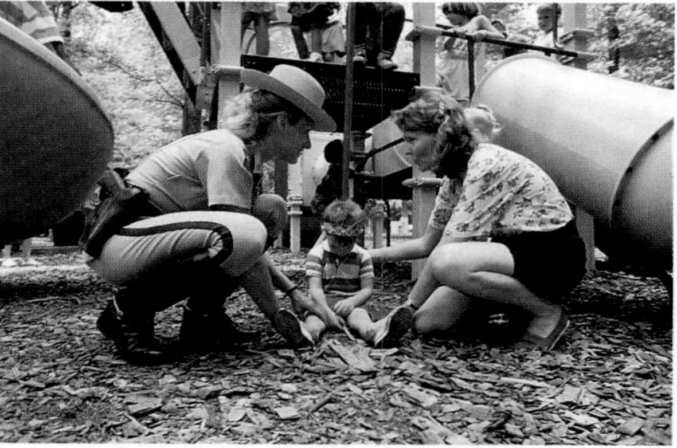

Figure 7-26 Parents or other adults may be able to provide information about a child who is sick or injured.

Step Five: Performing an Ongoing Assessment

Completing the initial assessment, physical exam, and SAMPLE history does not mean that your care for the victim is over. Instead, provide care for what you found, summon more advanced medical personnel whenever necessary, and perform an ongoing assessment. As its name implies, the ***ongoing assessment*** is the process of repeating the initial assessment while awaiting the arrival of more highly trained personnel. The initial assessment should be repeated every 5 minutes for unstable victims and every 15 minutes for stable victims. The physical exam and history do not need to be repeated unless there is a need. Record additional findings and turn this information over to more advanced medical personnel when they arrive.

◆ THE NEED FOR MORE ADVANCED MEDICAL PERSONNEL

As you may recall from Chapter 1, one of your major responsibilities, besides providing care for the victim, is to summon advanced medical personnel as needed. Your standard procedures will tell you when and whom to call. If you are not part of the EMS system, summoning other personnel will involve contacting EMS by calling 9-1-1 or the local emergency number. The EMS system works more effectively if you can provide information about the victim's condition as soon as possible. The information you provide will help to ensure that the victim receives proper medical care as quickly as possible.

If your communication network is not directly linked to the EMS system, you will need to use a telephone to call for more advanced medical personnel. If possible, ask another first responder or a bystander to call the emergency number for you. Sending someone else to make the call will enable you to stay with the victim to provide care. If you do send another person to make the call, tell that person to report back to you after the call is made.

Whether placing the call yourself or sending someone to call, follow these steps:

1. Dial the local emergency number. This number is 9-1-1 in many communities. Dial "O" (the operator) only if you do not know the emergency number for the area. Sometimes the emergency number is listed on the inside front cover of telephone directories and on pay phones.
2. Provide the dispatcher with the necessary information:
   a. *Where the emergency is located.* Give the exact address or location and the name of the city or town. It is helpful to give the names of nearby intersecting streets (cross streets), landmarks, the name of the building, the floor, and the room number.
   b. *Telephone number from which the call is being made.*
   c. *Caller's name.*
   d. *What happened*—for example, a motor vehicle collision, fall, or fire.
   e. *The number of people involved.*
   f. *Condition of the victim(s)*—for example, chest pain, difficulty breathing, no pulse, bleeding.
   g. *Care being given.*
3. Do not hang up until the dispatcher has finished gathering information. It is important to make sure the dispatcher has all the information needed to send the appropriate help immediately.

With your training, you can do two important things that can make a difference in the outcome of a seriously ill or injured person: (1) give care for life-threatening conditions, and (2) summon more advanced medical personnel as quickly as possible.

At times, you may be unsure if more advanced medical personnel are needed. For example, the victim may say not to call an ambulance because he or she is embarrassed about creating a scene. Sometimes you may be unsure if the victim's condition is severe enough to require more advanced care. Your training as a first responder will help you make the decision. As a general rule, summon more advanced medical personnel for any of the following conditions:

- Unconsciousness or altered level of consciousness
- Breathing problems (difficulty breathing or no breathing)
- Persistent chest or abdominal pain or pressure
- No pulse
- Severe bleeding
- Vomiting or passing blood
- Suspected poisoning
- Seizures, severe headache, or slurred speech
- Suspected or obvious injuries to head or spine
- Painful, swollen, deformed areas

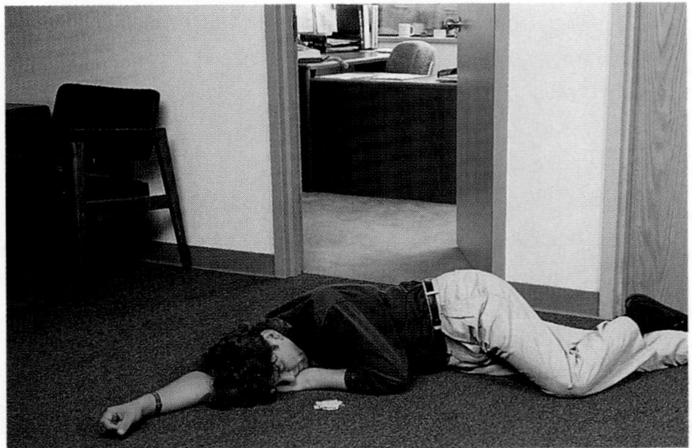

Figure 7-27 Place an unconscious victim in the recovery position if you must leave him alone.

These conditions are by no means a complete list. It is impossible to provide a definitive list, since there are always exceptions. Trust your instincts. If you think there is an emergency, there probably is. It is better to have more advanced personnel respond to a nonemergency than arrive at an emergency too late to help.

If you must leave the victim for any reason, such as to call 9-1-1 or the local emergency number, and the victim is unconscious, place him or her in the **recovery position** to help keep the airway open (Fig. 7-27). Place the victim on one side, bend the top leg, and move it forward to hold the victim in that position. Support the head so that it is angled toward the ground. In this position, if the victim vomits, the airway will stay clear.

To provide general care for the victim until more advanced medical personnel arrive, follow these steps:

1. Do no further harm.
2. Help the victim rest in the most comfortable position.
3. Keep the victim from getting chilled or overheated.
4. Reassure the victim.
5. Repeat the initial assessment and physical exam as needed (as part of your ongoing assessment).
6. Provide any specific care needed. (This care is discussed in following chapters.)

◆ SUMMARY

When you respond to an emergency, guide your actions by following a standardized plan. This plan reminds you of what to do and when to do it. It helps ensure your safety and the safety of others. It also helps ensure that necessary or urgent care is provided for life-threatening emergencies.

First, size up the scene. Make sure there are no dangers to you, the victim, and bystanders. Consider the mechanism of injury or nature of illness.

Second, perform an initial assessment. Check consciousness, airway, breathing, and circulation. Determine if there are any immediate threats to life, such as the absence of breathing or pulse or the presence of severe external bleeding.

Third, perform a physical exam to find and care for any other problems that are not an immediate threat to life but might become serious if you do not recognize them and provide care. This "head-to-toe" physical exam involves looking and feeling the body for abnormalities. Use the mnemonic DOTS as you perform the physical exam.

Fourth, obtain pertinent history from the victim. This is especially important if the victim is suffering from an illness that has already been diagnosed and is being cared for by a physician. Whether you obtain the history before, after, or during the physical exam does not matter. Use the mnemonic SAMPLE to gather all of the necessary information.

Fifth, perform an ongoing assessment until more advanced personnel arrive and take over. Repeat the initial assessment every 5 minutes for unstable victims and every 15 minutes for stable ones. Repeat the physical exam and history as needed.

Although this plan of action can help you decide what care to give in any emergency, providing care is not an exact science. Because each emergency and each victim is unique, an emergency may not occur exactly as it did in a classroom setting. Even within a single emer-

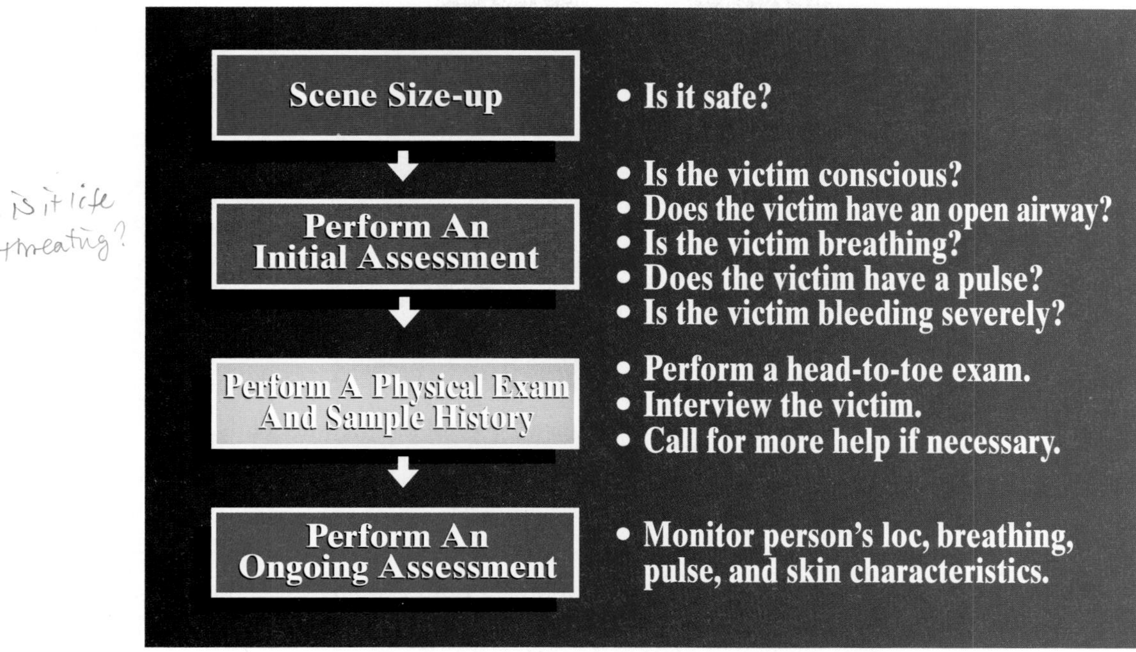

gency, the care needed may change from one moment to the next. For example, the initial assessment may indicate the victim is conscious, breathing, has a pulse, and has no severe bleeding. However, during your physical exam, you may notice that the victim begins to experience difficulty breathing. At this point, there is a need to summon more advanced medical personnel, if this has not already been done, and provide appropriate care. Provide necessary information about the victim's condition once these personnel arrive.

Scene Size-up
• Is it safe?
Perform An Initial Assessment
• Is the victim conscious?
• Does the victim have an open airway?
• Is the victim breathing?
• Does the victim have a pulse?
• Is the victim bleeding severely?
Perform A Physical Exam And Sample History
• Perform a head-to-toe exam.
• Interview the victim.
• Call for more help if necessary.
Perform An Ongoing Assessment
• Monitor person's loc, breathing, pulse, and skin characteristics.

Many variables exist when dealing with emergencies. You do not need to "diagnose" what is wrong with the victim to provide appropriate care. Use this plan of action as a guideline to help you assess any victim's condition.

As you read the remaining chapters, remember the steps of this plan. They form the basis for providing care in any emergency (Fig. 7-28). **Use the activities in Unit 7 of the workbook to help you review the material in this chapter.**

You Are the Responder

During a basketball game, two players collide while diving for a loose ball. Both players fall to the floor. One player is holding her knee, screaming in pain. The second player is lying motionless. Which player are you inclined to check first and why? What would you do for both players?

ENRICHMENT

◆ BLOOD PRESSURE

Another vital sign that helps to indicate a person's condition is blood pressure. ***Blood pressure (BP)*** is the force exerted by the blood against the blood vessel walls as it travels throughout the body. Blood pressure is a good indicator of how the circulatory system is functioning. If a person's circulatory system is working normally, blood pressure remains constant and within a normal range. If the circulatory system is failing, blood pressure reflects this failure by dropping. Blood pressure is necessary to move the oxygen and nutrients in the blood to the body's organs and muscles. It is also necessary to move waste products, such as carbon dioxide, to various parts of the body for removal.

Blood pressure is created by the pumping action of the heart. The pumping action involves two phases: the working (contracting) phase and the resting (refilling) phase. During the working phase, the **ventricles** (lower chambers) of the heart contract. This contraction causes blood to be pumped through the arteries to all parts of the body. During the resting phase, the ventricles relax and refill with blood before the next contraction.

Because a person's blood pressure can vary greatly, blood pressure is only one of several factors that give you an overall picture of a person's condition. Stress, excitement, illness, or injury often affect blood pressure. When a person is ill or injured, a single blood pressure measurement is often of little value. A more accurate picture of a person's condition immediately after an injury or the onset of an illness is whether his or her blood pressure changes over time while you provide care. For example, a person's initial blood pressure reading could be uncommonly high as a result of the stress of the emergency. Providing care, however, usually relieves some of the fear, and blood pressure may return to within a normal range. At other times, blood pressure will remain unusually high or low. For example, an injury resulting in a severe loss of blood may cause blood pressure to remain unusually low. You should be concerned about unusually high or low blood pressure or a large change in blood pressure whenever signs and symptoms of injury or illness are present.

To accurately assess a person's blood pressure, you need a **blood pressure** cuff. The cuff is a strip of fabric that is wrapped around the arm. Cuffs come in sizes for small, average, and large arms (Fig. 7-29). Inside the cuff is a rubber bladder, similar to an inner tube, that can be inflated. A pressure gauge, inflation bulb, and regulating valve are connected to the bladder by rubber tubing. Figure 7-30, *A* shows the parts of a blood pressure cuff.

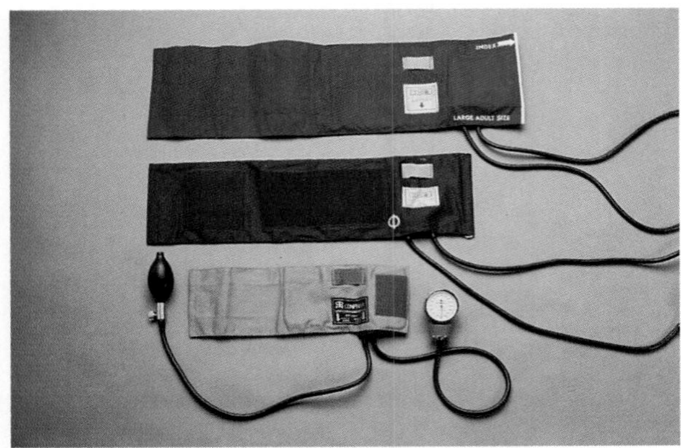

Figure 7-29 Blood pressure cuffs come in sizes for small, average, and large arms.

Blood pressure is measured in units called millimeters of mercury (mm Hg). These units, written on the blood pressure gauge, range from 20 to 300 mm Hg. In measuring blood pressure, two different numbers are usually recorded. The first number reflects the pressure in the arteries when the heart is working, or contracting. This pressure is called the **systolic blood pressure**. The second number reflects the pressure in the arteries when the heart is at rest and refilling. This is called the **diastolic blood pressure**. Both the systolic and diastolic blood pressures are normally measured in even numbers.

You report blood pressure by giving the systolic number first, then the diastolic (S/D). Average adult systolic blood pressure is approximately 120 mm Hg. Average adult diastolic blood pressure is approximately 80 mm Hg. When you express this blood pressure in writing, it looks like this: BP 120/80. When reporting 120/80, you would say "one twenty over eighty."

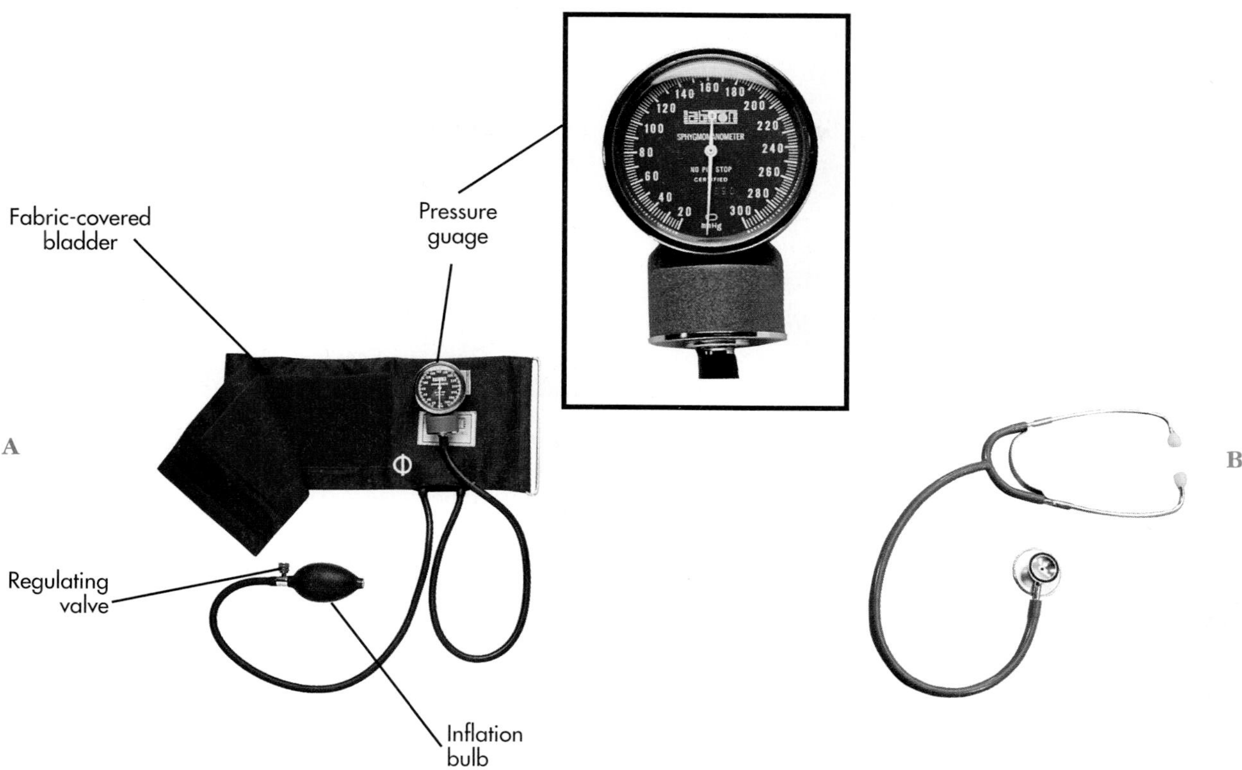

Figure 7-30 Equipment needed to measure blood pressure includes, **A**, a blood pressure cuff, and **B**, a stethoscope.

To determine both the systolic and diastolic pressure, you need a **stethoscope** (Fig. 7-30, *B*). The stethoscope enables you to hear the pulsating sounds of blood moving through the arteries with each contraction of the heart. Sometimes, however, you may not have a stethoscope or, because of noise, are unable to use one. You can still determine the systolic blood pressure through a method known as palpation. **Palpation** requires you to feel (palpate) the radial artery as you inflate the blood pressure cuff (Fig. 7-31).

To determine blood pressure by palpation, begin by having the person sit or lie down. Wrap the blood pressure cuff around the person's arm so that the lower edge is about 1 inch above the crease at the elbow. The center of the cuff should be over the major artery of the arm, the brachial artery on the inside of the upper arm (Fig. 7-32). Next, locate the radial pulse. Close the regulating valve by turning the valve clockwise and begin to inflate the cuff. Inflate the cuff until you can no longer feel the radial pulse. Note the number on the gauge.

Continue to inflate the cuff for another 20

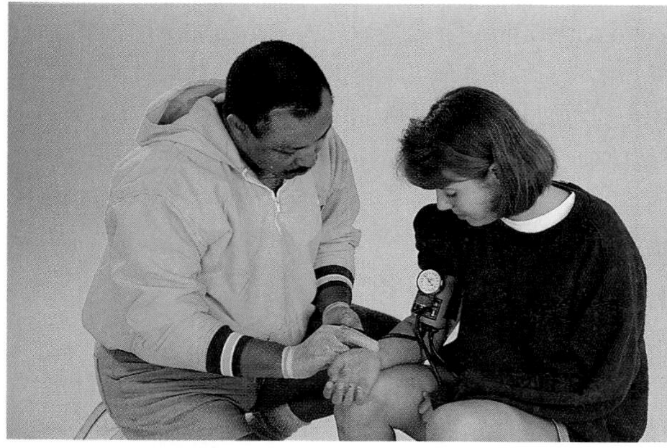

Figure 7-31 Estimating a systolic blood pressure requires you to feel for the radial pulse.

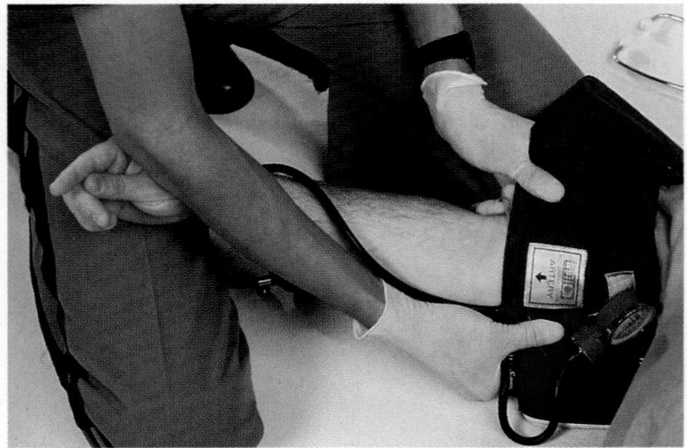

Figure 7-32 To obtain an accurate blood pressure reading, center the cuff over the brachial artery, about 1 inch above the crease of the elbow.

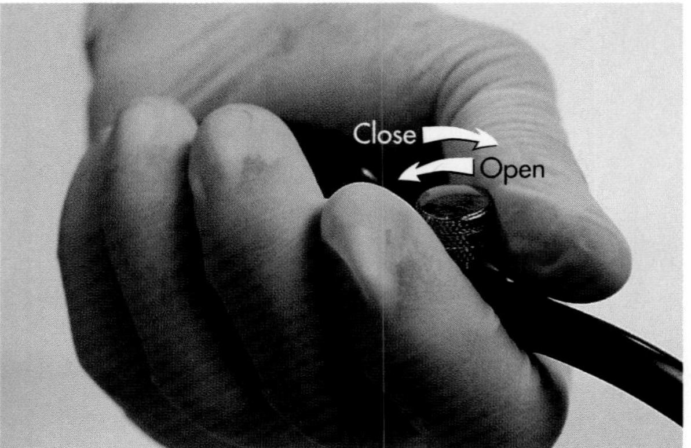

Figure 7-33 To close the regulating valve, turn the valve clockwise. To open the regulating valve, turn it counterclockwise.

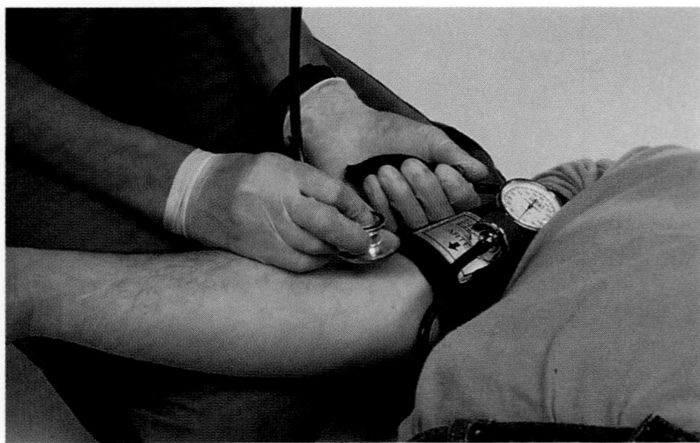

Figure 7-34 To auscultate blood pressure, position the cuff, find the brachial pulse, and position the stethoscope over it.

mm Hg beyond this point. Slowly release the pressure in the cuff by turning the regulating valve counterclockwise (Fig. 7-33). Allow the cuff to deflate at a rate of about 2 mm Hg per second. Continue to feel for the radial pulse as the cuff deflates. The point at which the pulse returns is the approximate systolic blood pressure by palpation. This blood pressure reading is expressed as one even number only, such as 130/P. The systolic pressure is 130, and P refers to palpation. Once you know the approximate systolic pressure, quickly deflate the cuff. Record the systolic pressure and whether the person was sitting or lying down when the blood pressure was taken.

The process of using a blood pressure cuff and stethoscope to listen for characteristic sounds is called **auscultation**. To auscultate means to listen. This method allows you to get accurate systolic and diastolic pressures. To auscultate blood pressure, begin by determining the systolic pressure using the palpation method. Next, locate the brachial pulse. Place the earpieces of the stethoscope in your ears and the other end, the diaphragm, over the spot where you found the brachial pulse (Fig. 7-34). Close the valve and begin to inflate the cuff. Inflate the cuff to 20 mm Hg above the approximate systolic blood pressure.

Slowly deflate the cuff at a rate of about 2 mm Hg per second. As you deflate the cuff, listen carefully for the pulse. In some instances, it may sound like a tapping sound. The point at which the pulse is first heard is the systolic pressure.

As the cuff deflates, the pulse sound will fade. The point at which the sound disappears is the diastolic pressure. Release the remaining air quickly. Record the blood pressure as two numbers, such as 130/80. Also record whether the person was sitting or lying down.

Initial Assessment

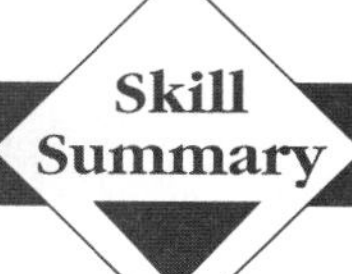

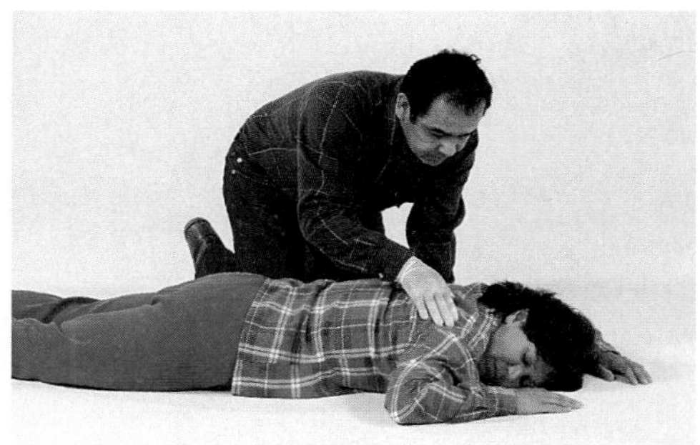

1. Check for consciousness.

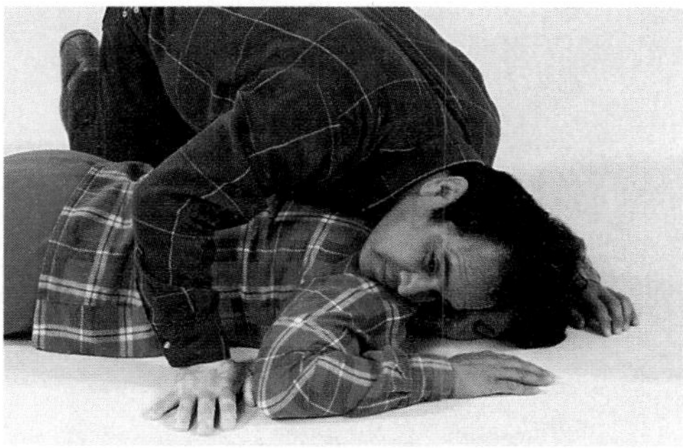

2. Check for breathing. If breathing, determine rate and quality.

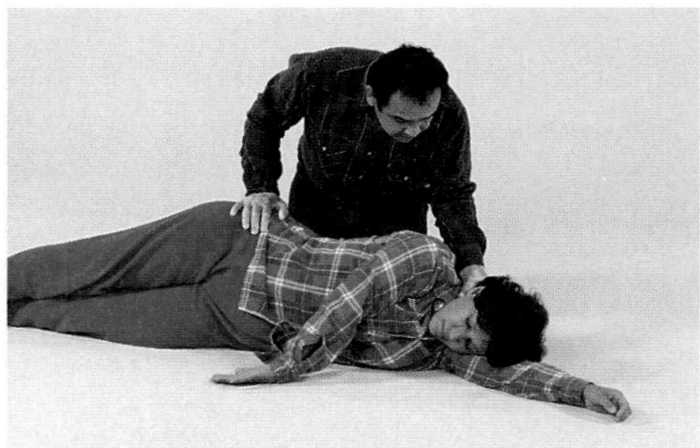

3. If uncertain whether victim is breathing, roll victim onto back, supporting head and back.

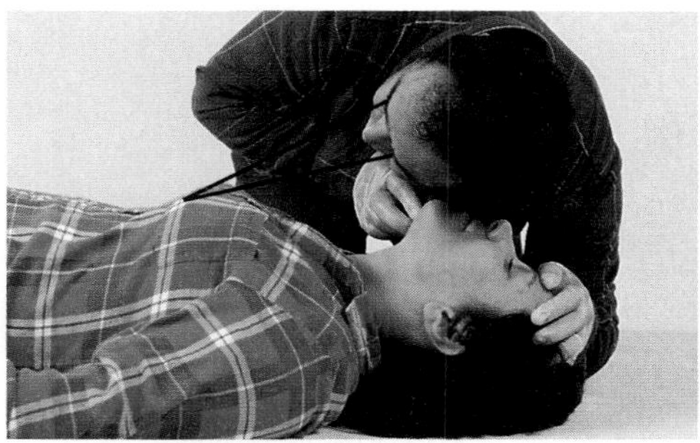

4. Open airway and recheck breathing. Use head-tilt/chin lift for victims without trauma. For trauma victims, use jaw thrust without head tilt.

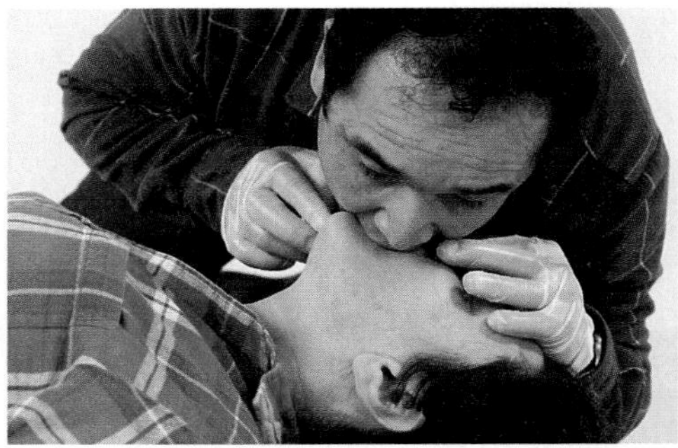

5. If not breathing, give 2 slow breaths. Use a barrier device whenever available.

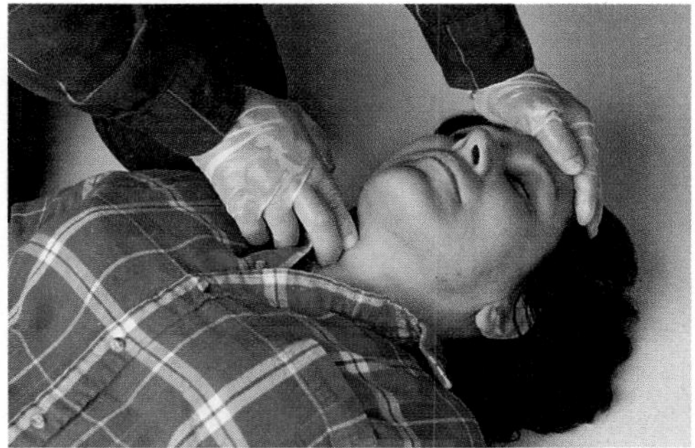

6. Check for a pulse. If the victim is breathing, determine pulse rate and quality. If not breathing, only determine absence/presence of pulse.

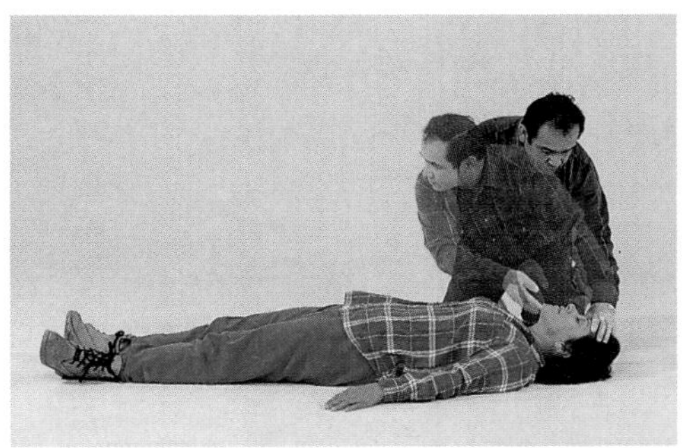

7. Check for severe bleeding and skin characteristics.

Physical Exam and History

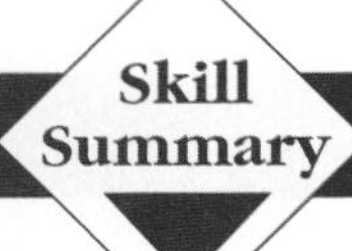

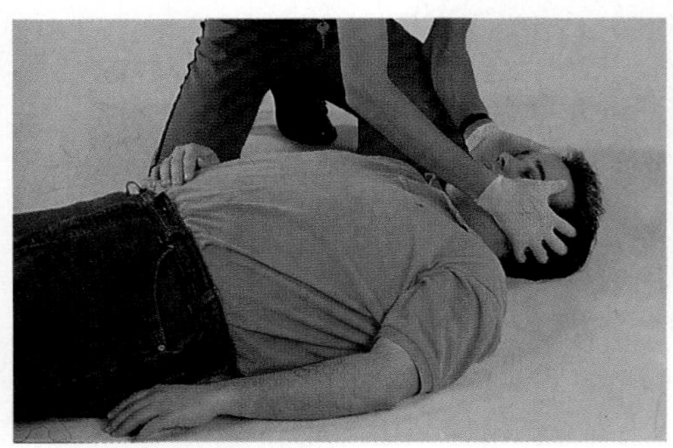

1. Perform physical exam beginning with the head and neck.

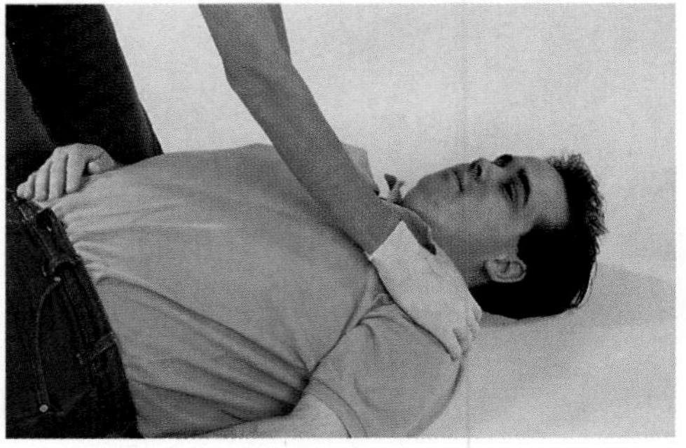

2. Check shoulders.

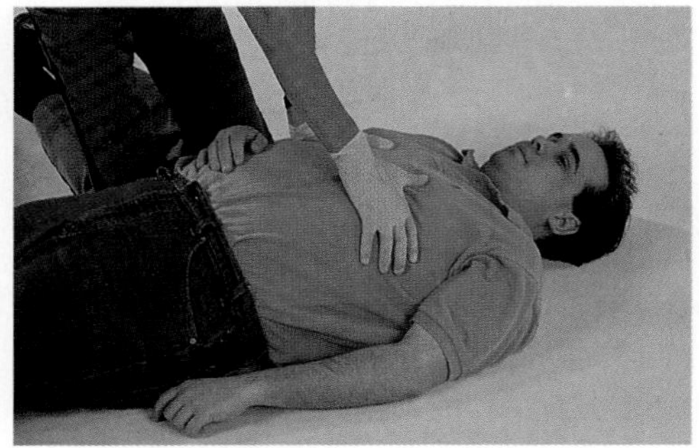

3. Check chest.

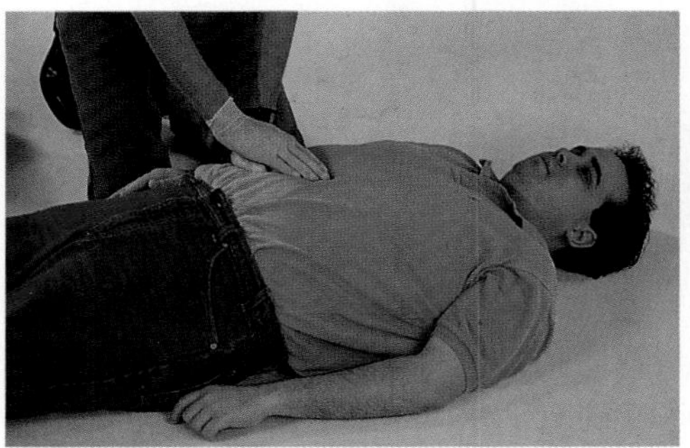

4. Check abdomen.

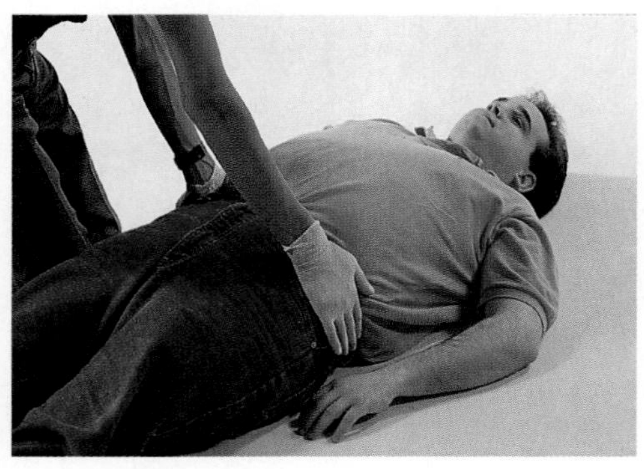

5. Check pelvis.

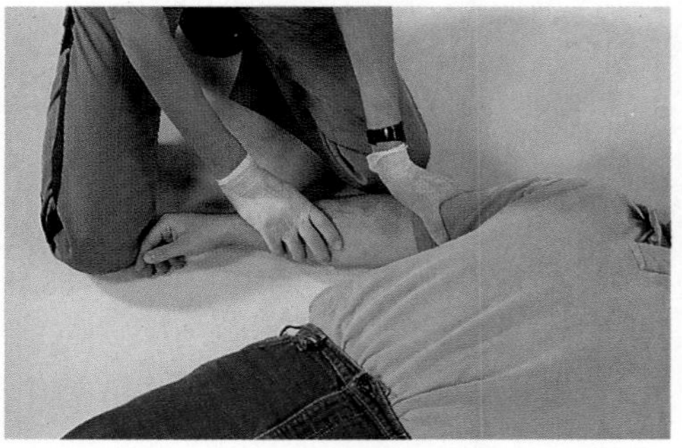

6. Check arms and hands.

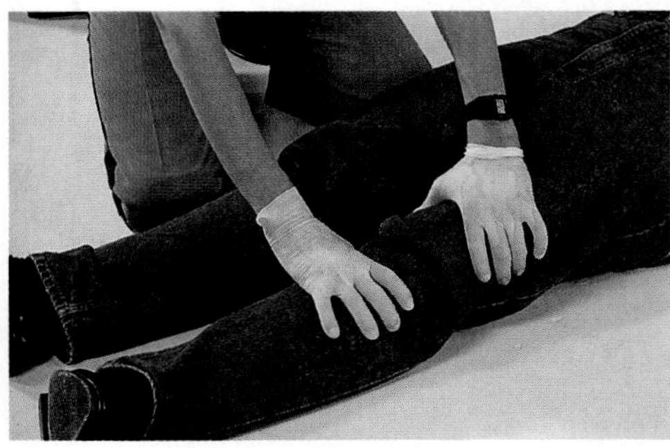

7. Check legs and feet.

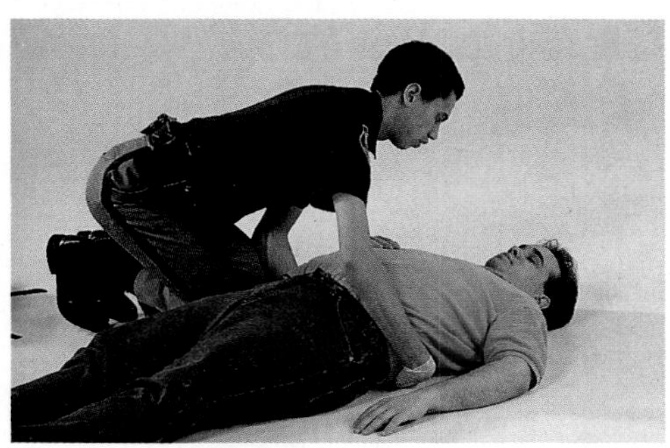

8. Check victim's back.

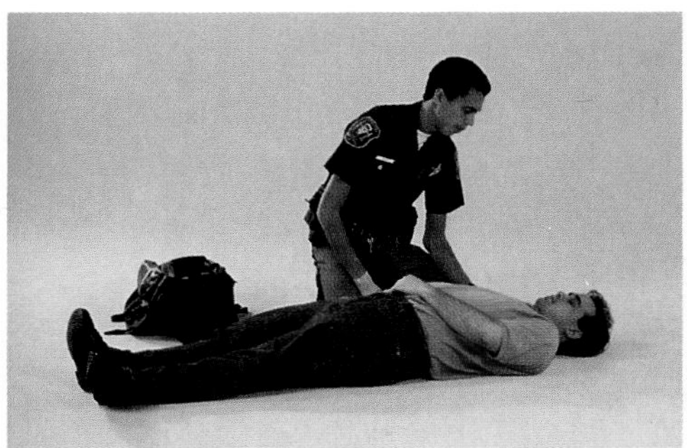

9. Interview the victim to obtain **SAMPLE** history.

Measuring Blood Pressure (Palpation)

Skill Summary

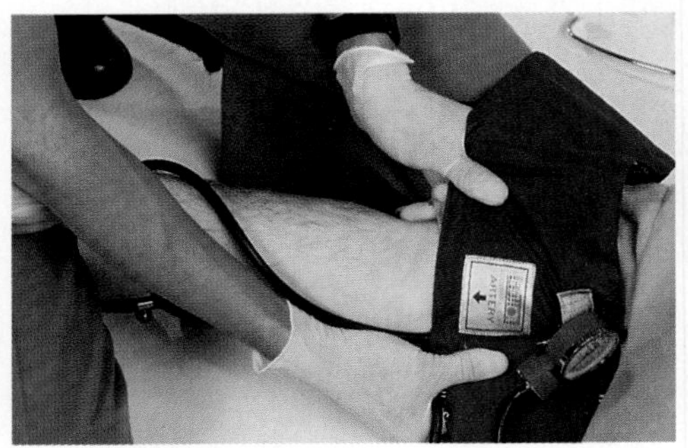

1. Position cuff.

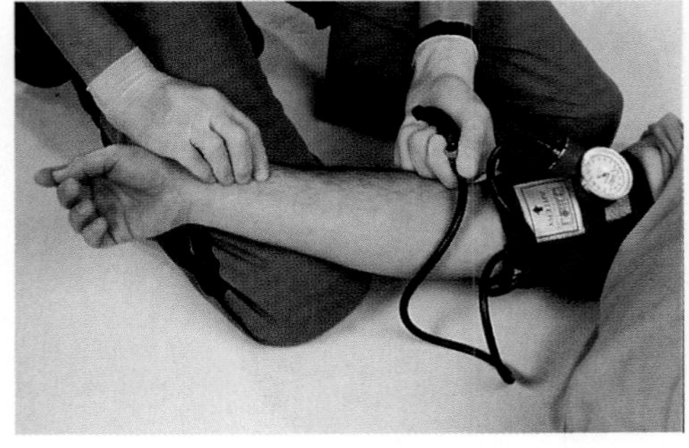

2. Locate radial pulse.

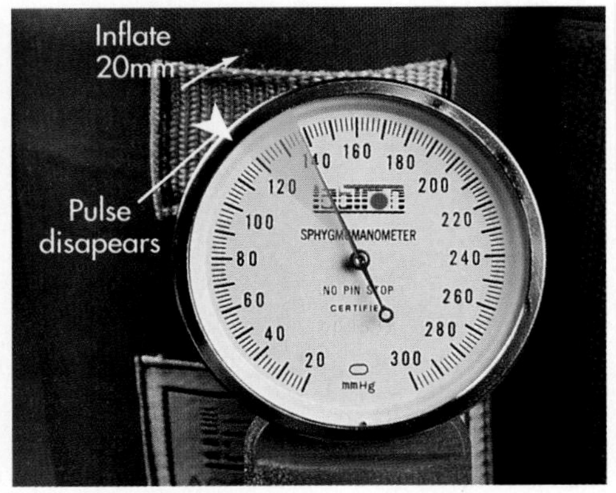

3. Inflate cuff—beyond point where pulse disappears.

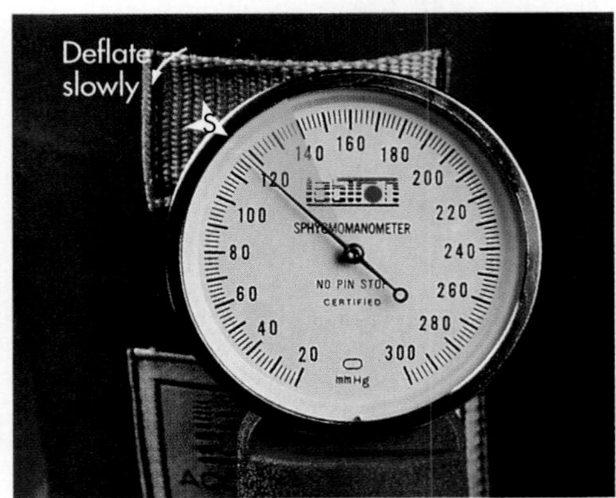

4. Deflate cuff slowly until pulse returns. This is the approximate systolic blood pressure.

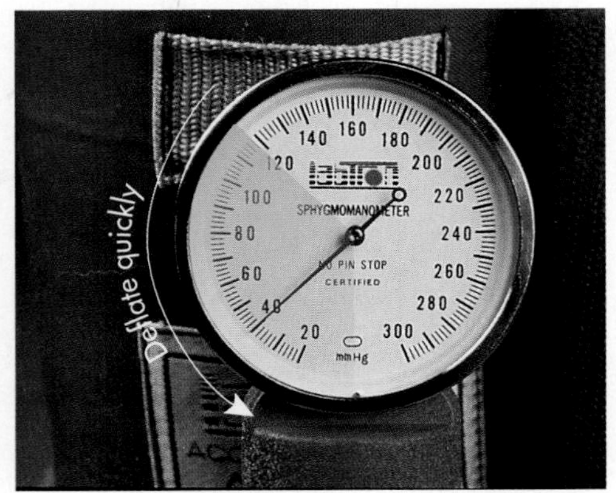

5. Quickly deflate cuff by opening valve.

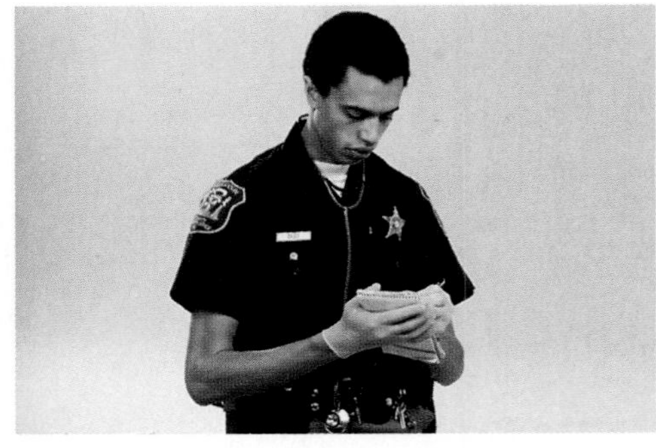

6. Record approximate systolic blood pressure.

Measuring Blood Pressure (Auscultation)

Skill Summary

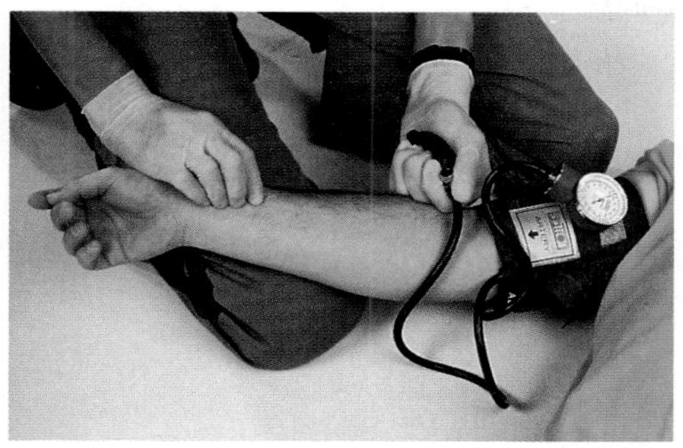

1. Approximate systolic blood pressure.

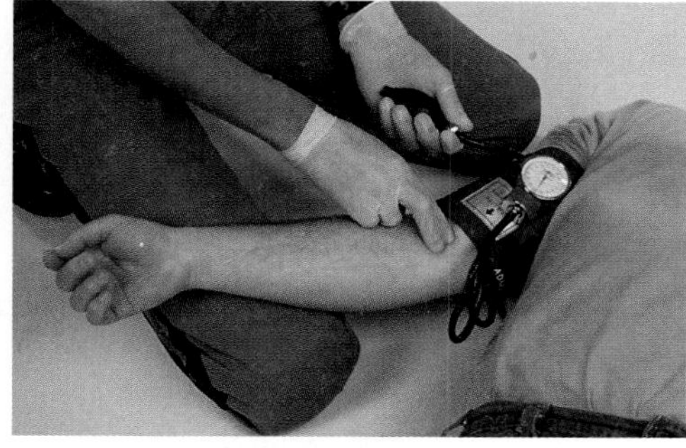

2. Locate brachial pulse.

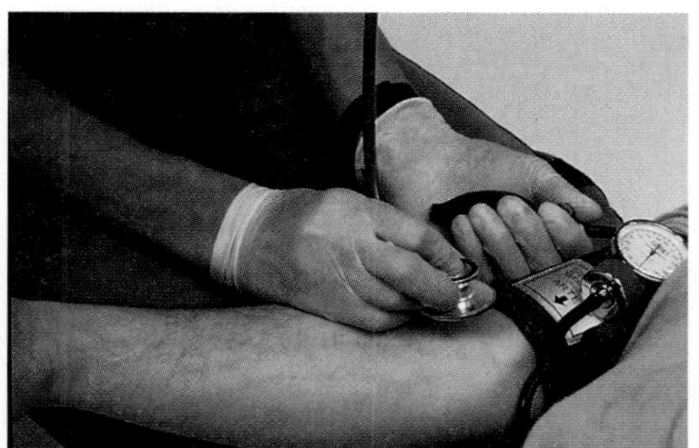

3. Position stethoscope.

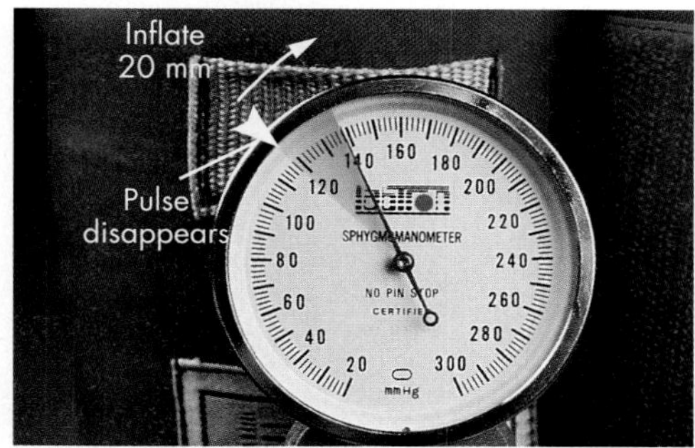

4. Inflate cuff — 20 mm Hg beyond approximate systolic blood pressure.

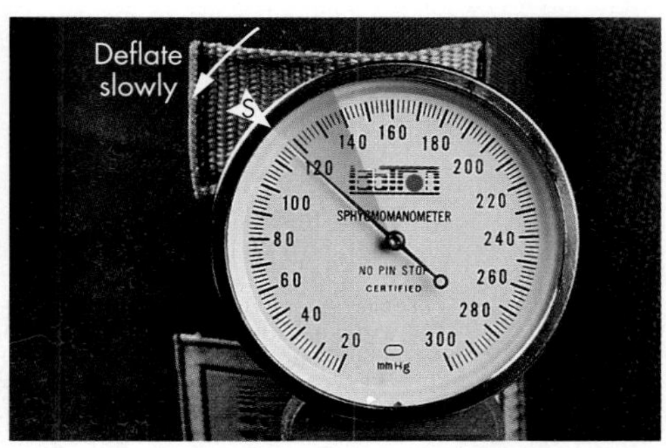

5. Deflate cuff slowly until pulse is heard (systolic).

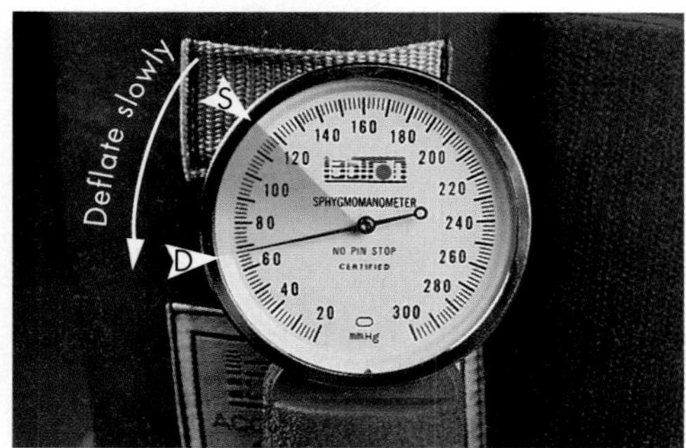

6. Continue deflating cuff until pulse disappears (diastolic).

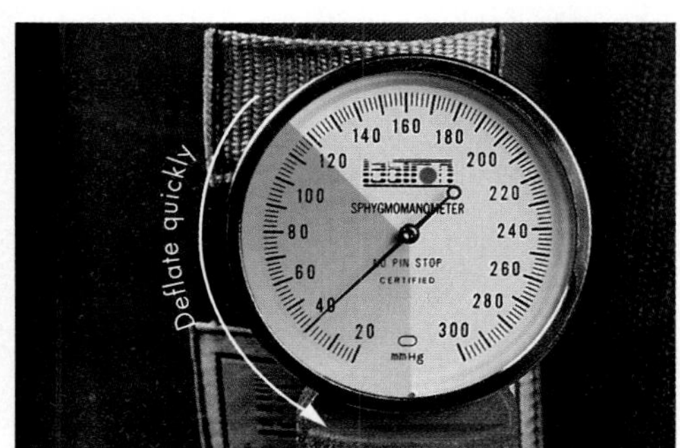

7. Quickly deflate cuff.

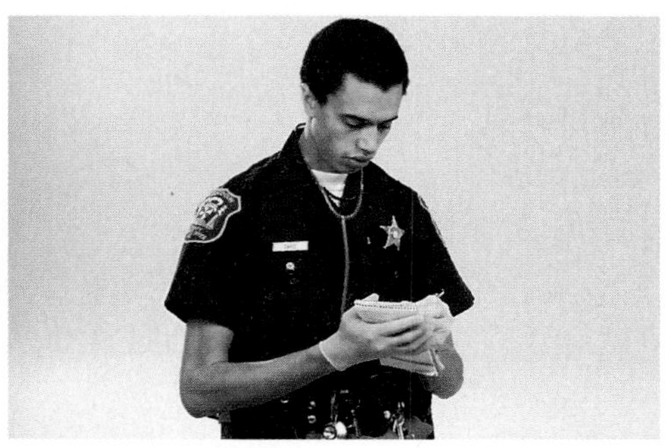

8. Record blood pressure (S/D).

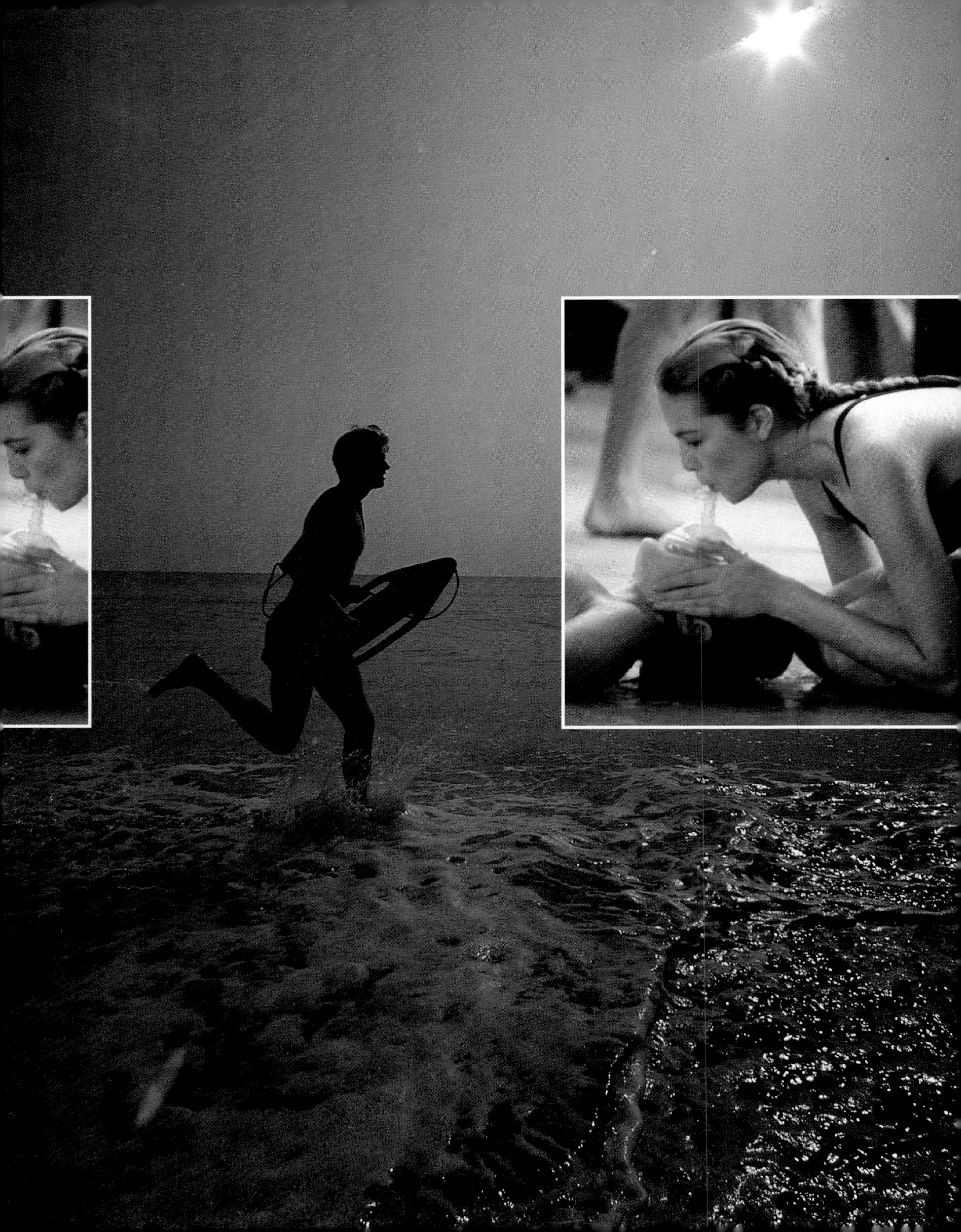

Module Three

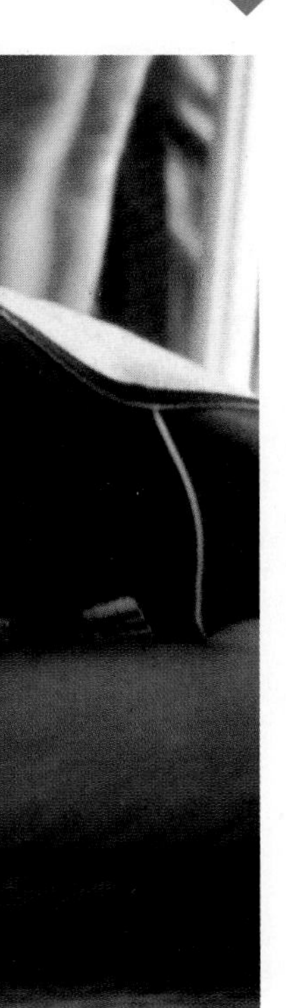

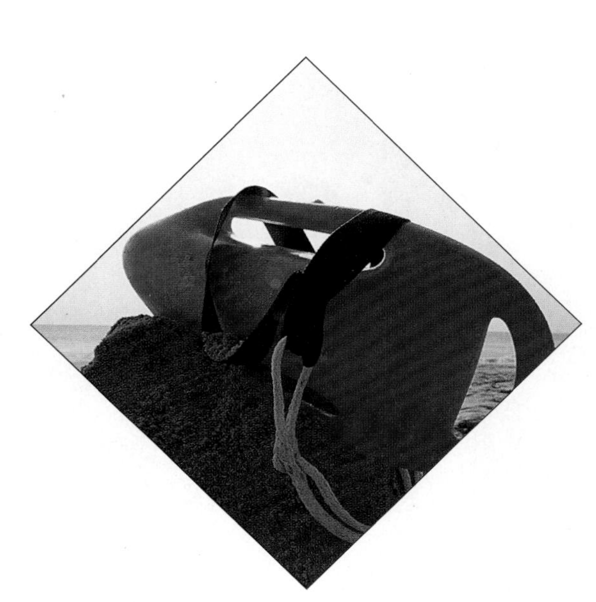

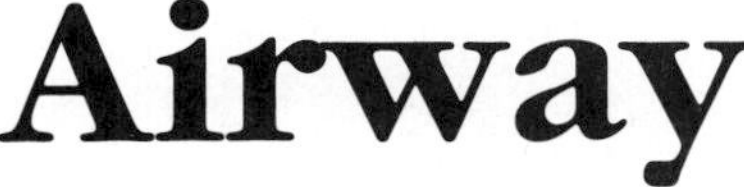

Airway

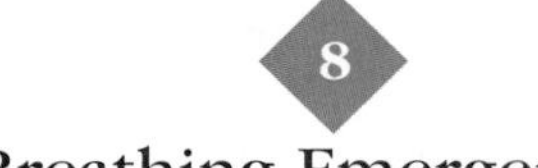

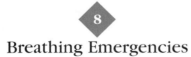

Breathing Emergencies

8

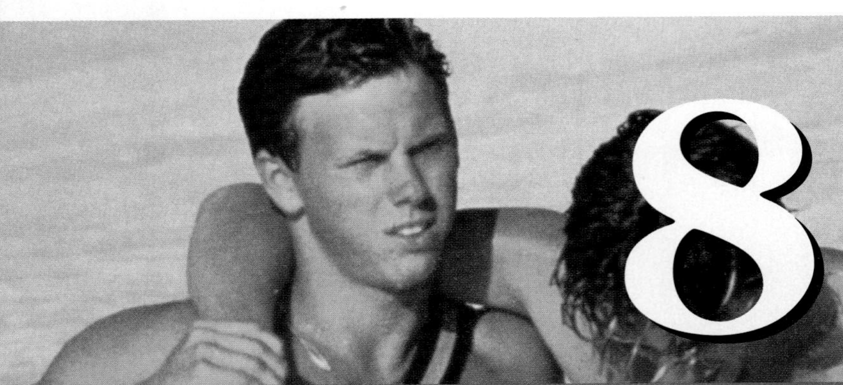

Key Terms

Airway obstruction: A blockage of the airway that prevents air from reaching a person's lungs.

Aspiration (as pĭ RA shun): Taking blood, vomit, saliva, or other foreign material into the lungs.

Breathing emergency: An emergency in which breathing is so impaired that life can be threatened; also called a respiratory emergency.

Cyanosis: A condition in which the victim's skin or the nail beds of the fingers or toes appear blue.

Finger sweep: A technique used to remove foreign material from a victim's airway.

Head–tilt/chin–lift: A technique for opening the airway.

Jaw thrust: A technique for opening the airway that avoids moving the head.

Rescue breathing: A technique of breathing for a nonbreathing victim.

Respiratory arrest: A condition in which breathing has stopped.

Respiratory distress: A condition in which breathing is difficult.

◆ Knowledge Objectives ◆

After reading this chapter and completing the class activities, you should be able to—

- Describe the structure and function of the respiratory system.
- List the signs of inadequate breathing.
- Describe how to care for a victim experiencing respiratory distress.
- Describe how to open the airway using the head-tilt/chin-lift technique.
- Describe how to open the airway using the jaw thrust technique.
- Relate the technique used to open the airway to the mechanism of injury.
- Explain why basic airway management and rescue breathing skills take priority over most other basic life-support skills.
- Distinguish the differences in the steps used to give rescue breathing to an adult, child, and infant.
- Describe how to perform mouth-to-mouth, mouth-to-nose, and mouth-to-stoma rescue breathing.
- Describe how to clear an airway obstruction in a conscious and unconscious adult, child, and infant.

◆ Skill Objectives ◆

After reading this chapter and completing the class activities, you should be able to—

- Demonstrate how to open the airway using the head-tilt/chin-lift and jaw-thrust technique.
- Demonstrate how to give rescue breathing to an adult, child, and infant.
- Demonstrate how to clear an airway obstruction in a conscious and unconscious adult, child, and infant.

You arrive at a scene to find a distraught mother who says, "I can't wake my baby up." You determine that the infant is unconscious, is not breathing, but has a pulse. What do you do?

◆ INTRODUCTION

In Chapter 5, you learned the parts of the airway and how the respiratory system functions. In Chapter 7, you learned that once you are sure the scene is safe, you begin an initial assessment of the victim. The initial assessment detects any life-threatening conditions. First, check to see if the victim is conscious. Then check the ABCs.

A - Airway
B - Breathing
C - Circulation

In this chapter, you will learn how to care for breathing emergencies. Because oxygen is vital to life, you must always ensure that the victim has an open airway and is breathing. You will often detect a breathing emergency during the initial assessment. In a ***breathing emergency,*** a person's breathing is so impaired that life is threatened. This kind of emergency can occur in two ways—breathing becomes difficult or breathing stops. A person who is having difficulty breathing is in ***respiratory distress***. A person who has stopped breathing is in ***respiratory arrest.***

◆ THE BREATHING PROCESS

Air enters the respiratory system through the nose and mouth and passes through the pharynx (Fig. 8-1). The pharynx divides into two passageways: one for food, the esophagus, and one for air, the trachea. The epiglottis protects the opening of the trachea when a person swallows so that food and liquid do not enter the lungs.

The body requires a constant supply of oxygen for survival. When a person breathes oxygen into the lungs, the oxygen is transferred to the blood. The blood transports the oxygen to the brain, organs, muscles, and other parts of the body where it is used to provide energy. This energy allows the body to perform its many functions, such as breathing, walking, talking, digesting food, and maintaining body temperature. Different functions require different levels of energy and therefore different amounts of oxygen. For example, sitting in a chair requires less energy and less oxygen than jogging around the block. A body fighting off an illness, even the common cold, uses more energy and oxygen than a body in its normal healthy state. With illness, the body must carry out all normal functions while also fighting the illness. Some tissues, such as brain tissue, are very sensitive to oxygen starvation. Without oxygen, brain cells begin to die in as few as 4 to 6 minutes (Fig. 8-2). Other vital organs will also be affected unless oxygen supplies are restored.

The brain is the control center for breathing. It adjusts the rate and depth of breaths according to the oxygen and carbon dioxide levels in the body. Breathing requires the respiratory, circulatory, nervous, and musculoskeletal systems to work together. As you read in Chapter 5, injuries or illnesses that affect any of these systems may cause breathing emergencies. For example, if the heart stops beating, the victim will stop breathing. Injury or disease in areas of the brain that control breathing may impair breathing or stop it entirely. Damage to muscles or bones of the chest and back can make breathing difficult or painful.

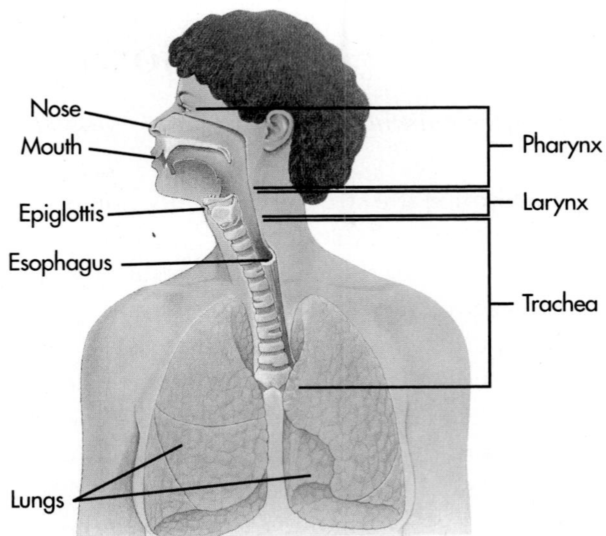

Figure 8-1 The respiratory system includes the pharynx, larynx, and trachea.

Breathing emergencies can be caused by the following:

- An obstructed airway (choking)
- Illness, such as pneumonia
- Respiratory conditions, such as emphysema and asthma
- Electrocution
- Shock
- Drowning
- Heart attack or heart disease
- Injury to the chest or lungs
- Allergic reactions, such as to food or to insect stings
- Drugs
- Poisoning, such as inhaling or ingesting toxic substances
- Hyperventilation

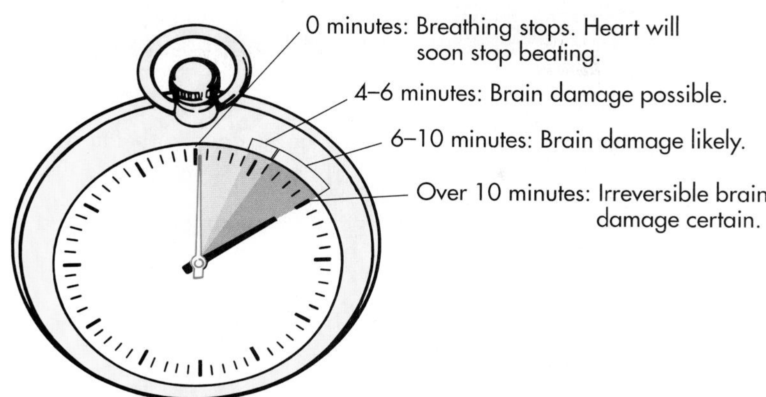
0 minutes: Breathing stops. Heart will soon stop beating.
4–6 minutes: Brain damage possible.
6–10 minutes: Brain damage likely.
Over 10 minutes: Irreversible brain damage certain.

Figure 8-2 Time is critical in starting lifesaving measures. If the brain is without oxygen for 6 minutes, brain damage is likely to occur.

The causes of breathing emergencies not discussed in this chapter are discussed in those chapters that cover conditions such as shock, injury to the chest, and so on.

◆ RESPIRATORY DISTRESS

Respiratory distress is the most common type of breathing emergency. It is not always caused by injuries or illnesses. It may also result from excitement or anxiety. Learn to recognize the signs and symptoms of respiratory distress.

Signs and Symptoms of Respiratory Distress

The signs and symptoms of respiratory distress are usually obvious. Victims may look as if they cannot catch their breath or they may gasp for air. They may make grunting sounds. Their breaths may be unusually fast, slow, deep, or shallow. Slow respirations are often less than 8 per minute for adults and less than 10 per minute for children and infants. Victims may make unusual noises, such as wheezing or gurgling or high-pitched, shrill sounds.

The victim's skin may also signal respiratory distress. At first, the skin may be unusually moist and appear flushed. Later, it may appear pale, ashen, or bluish as the oxygen level in the blood falls. When the victim's skin or the nail beds of the fingers or toes appear blue, the condition is called ***cyanosis***.

Victims may say they feel dizzy or lightheaded. Sometimes breathing may be painful. Victims may feel pain in the chest and tingling in the lips, hands, or feet. They may be apprehensive or fearful. They often display an increased effort to breathe. Any of these signs and/or symptoms is a clue that the victim may be in respiratory distress. Table 8-1 lists the signs and symptoms of respiratory distress.

Specific Types of Respiratory Distress

Although respiratory distress is often caused by injury, several other conditions also may cause it. These include asthma, emphysema, hyperventilation, and anaphylaxis (severe allergic reaction).

Asthma

Asthma is a condition that narrows the air passages and makes breathing difficult. During an asthma attack, the air passages become constricted, or narrowed, by a spasm of the muscles lining the bronchi, red mucus secretions, or by swelling of the bronchi themselves. Victims may become anxious or frightened because breathing is difficult.

Asthma is most commonly found in children and young adults. It may be triggered by an al-

Table 8-1 Signs and Symptoms of Respiratory Distress

Conditions	Signs and symptoms
Abnormal breathing	Breathing is unusually slow, rapid, deep, or shallow
	Victim is gasping for breath
	Victim is wheezing, gurgling, or making high-pitched shrill noises
Abnormal skin appearance	Skin is unusually moist
	Skin has a flushed, pale or ashen, or bluish appearance
How the victim feels	Short of breath
	Dizzy or lightheaded
	Pain in the chest or tingling in hands and feet

lergic reaction to food, pollen, a drug, or an insect sting. Emotional stress may also trigger it. For some people, physical activity induces asthma. Normally, someone with asthma controls attacks with medication. These medications help to reverse the muscle spasm, opening the airway and making breathing easier.

A characteristic sign of asthma is wheezing when exhaling, which occurs because the airway is constricted. Air trapped in the lungs may also make the victim's chest appear larger than normal, particularly in small children.

Emphysema

Emphysema is a disease in which the lungs lose their ability to exchange carbon dioxide and oxygen effectively. Emphysema is often caused by smoking and usually develops over many years.

Victims suffer from shortness of breath. Exhaling is extremely difficult. They may cough and may have cyanosis or fever. Victims with advanced cases may be restless, confused, and weak and can go into respiratory or cardiac arrest. People with chronic (long-lasting or frequently recurring) emphysema will get worse over time.

Hyperventilation

Hyperventilation occurs when someone breathes faster than normal. This rapid breathing upsets the body's balance of oxygen and carbon dioxide. Hyperventilation often results from fear or anxiety and is more likely to occur in people who are tense and nervous. It is also caused by injuries, such as head injuries, severe bleeding, or conditions such as high fever, heart failure, lung disease, or diabetic emergencies. It can be triggered by asthma or exercise.

A characteristic sign of hyperventilation is shallow, rapid breathing. Despite their breathing efforts, victims say that they cannot get enough air or that they are suffocating. Therefore they are often fearful and apprehensive or may appear confused. They may say they feel dizzy or that their lips, fingers, and toes feel numb or tingly.

Anaphylaxis (Severe allergic reaction)

While at a company picnic, a co-worker is stung by a hornet. You provide care for the sting and she returns to her activity. A few minutes later, she develops a rash and begins to feel tightness in her chest and throat. She is having difficulty breathing. She states that she feels her neck, face, and tongue are beginning to swell. She is a victim of a life-threatening condition known as anaphylaxis.

Anaphylaxis is a severe allergic reaction. The air passages may swell and restrict the victim's breathing. Anaphylaxis may be caused by insect stings, food, or medications such as penicillin. Some people know that they have a severe allergic reaction to certain substances.

They may therefore have learned to avoid these substances and may carry medication to reverse an allergic reaction. Medication may be carried in an **anaphylaxis kit**. People who know they are allergic may also wear a medical alert necklace or bracelet.

The signs and symptoms of anaphylaxis can include a rash, a feeling of tightness in the chest and throat, and swelling of the face, neck, and tongue. The person may also feel dizzy or confused. Anaphylaxis is a life-threatening emergency requiring advanced medical care.

Care for Respiratory Distress

Recognizing the signs and symptoms of respiratory distress and providing emergency care are often the keys to preventing other emergencies. Respiratory distress may signal the beginning of a life-threatening condition. For example, it can be the first signal of a more serious breathing emergency or even a heart attack. Respiratory distress can lead to respiratory arrest, which, if not cared for, will result in death.

Many of the signs and symptoms of different kinds of respiratory distress are similar. You do not need to know the specific cause to provide care. If the victim is breathing, you know the heart is beating. Make sure the victim is not bleeding severely. Help him or her rest in a comfortable position. Usually, sitting is more comfortable than lying down because breathing is easier. If the victim is in a hot, stuffy room, consider opening a window to reduce the heat or add moisture. Reassure and comfort the victim. Have bystanders move back. Make sure that more advanced medical personnel have been summoned.

The victim who is experiencing difficulty breathing may have trouble talking. Talk to any bystanders who may know about the victim's problem. The victim can confirm answers or answer yes-or-no questions by nodding. If possible, try to help reduce any anxiety; it may contribute to the victim's difficulty breathing. Help the victim take any medication prescribed by his or her physician for the condition, if it is available and you are trained or authorized to do so. This medication may be oxygen or an **inhalant** (bronchial dilator). Continue to look and listen for any changes in the victim's vital signs. Calm and reassure the victim. Keep the victim from getting chilled or overheated.

If the victim's breathing is rapid and there are signs of an injury or an underlying illness or condition, call for more advanced help immediately. If the victim's breathing is rapid and you suspect that it is caused by emotion, such as excitement, try to calm the victim to slow his or her breathing. Reassurance is often enough to correct hyperventilation. But you can also ask the victim to try to breathe with you. Breathe at a normal rate, emphasizing inhaling and exhaling.

If the condition does not improve, the victim may become unconscious. Summon more advanced medical personnel, if this has not already been done. Keep the victim's airway open and monitor breathing. In many cases, hyperventilation caused by emotion will correct itself after the victim becomes unconscious.

Care for Respiratory Distress

- Complete an initial assessment.
- Contact more advanced personnel.
- Help the victim rest comfortably.
- Do a physical exam.
- Obtain a SAMPLE history.
- Reassure the victim.
- Assist with medication if you are authorized to do so.
- Keep the victim from getting chilled or overheated.
- Monitor vital signs.

◆ RESPIRATORY ARREST

Respiratory arrest is the condition in which breathing stops. It may be caused by illness, in-

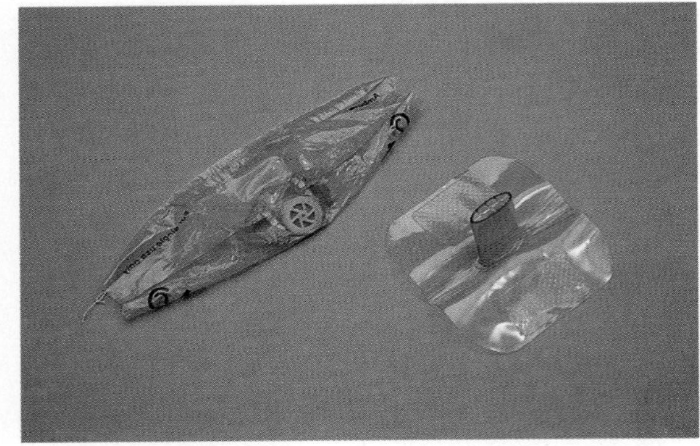
A

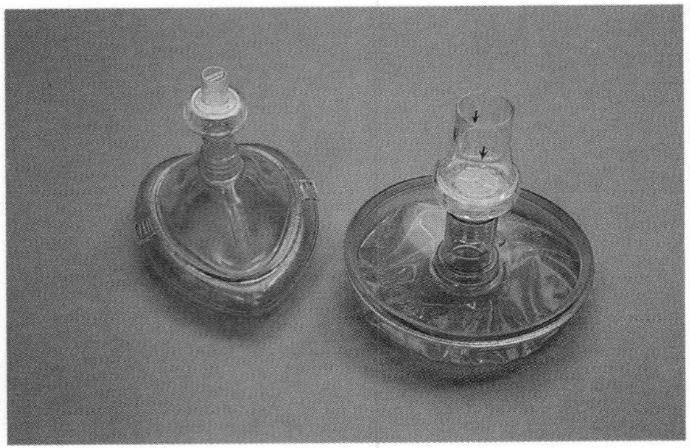
B

Figure 8-3 **A**, A face shield or, **B**, a mask, when placed between your mouth and nose and the victim's, can help prevent you from contacting a person's saliva or other body fluids.

jury, or an obstructed airway. The causes of respiratory distress can also lead to respiratory arrest. In respiratory arrest, the person gets no oxygen. The body can function for only a few minutes without oxygen before body systems begin to fail. Without oxygen, the heart stops functioning. This causes the circulatory system to fail. When the heart stops, other body systems will also start to fail. However, you can keep the person's respiratory system functioning artificially with rescue breathing.

Rescue Breathing

Rescue breathing is a technique of breathing air into a person to supply him or her with the oxygen needed to survive. Rescue breathing is given to victims who are not breathing but still have a pulse.

Rescue breathing works because the air you breathe into the victim contains more than enough oxygen to keep that person alive. The air you take in with every breath contains about 21 percent oxygen, but your body uses only a small part of that. The air you breathe out of your lungs and into the lungs of the victim contains about 16 percent oxygen, enough to keep someone alive.

A first responder should follow BSI (body substance isolation) precautions during rescue breathing. This includes the use of a barrier shield or resuscitation mask whenever giving rescue breaths (Fig. 8-3, *A-B*). Before you can use these devices, you need to learn how to perform rescue breathing. You also should be able to perform rescue breathing in the event a device is not readily available. In this chapter, you will learn the basics of performing rescue breathing. You will learn how to use a resuscitation mask in Chapter 9.

You will determine if you need to give rescue breathing after you open the victim's airway and check for breathing. If you cannot see, hear, or feel signs of breathing, position the head and give 2 slow breaths immediately to get air into the victim's lungs. Then check circulation by feeling for the pulse and looking for severe bleeding. Summon advanced medical personnel if you have not already done so.

If the victim is not breathing, begin rescue breathing. To give breaths, keep the airway open with the head-tilt/chin-lift (Fig. 8-4, *A*). The ***head-tilt/chin-lift*** technique not only opens the airway by moving the tongue away from the back of the throat, but also moves the epiglottis from the opening of the trachea. Gently pinch the victim's nose shut with the thumb and index finger of your hand that is on the victim's forehead. Next, make a tight seal around the victim's mouth with your mouth. Breathe slowly into the victim until you see the victim's chest gently rise (Fig. 8-4, *B*). Each

A 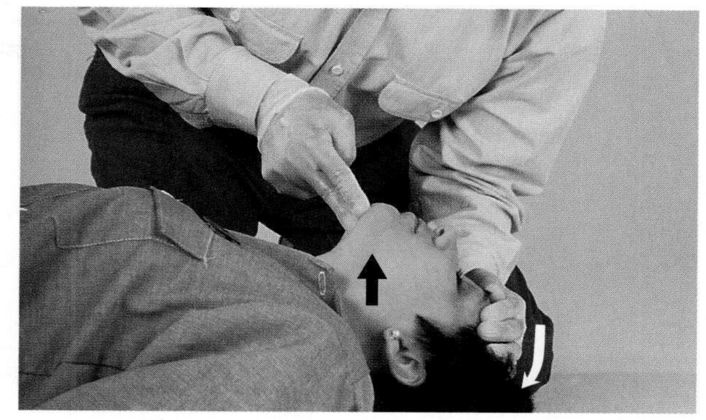

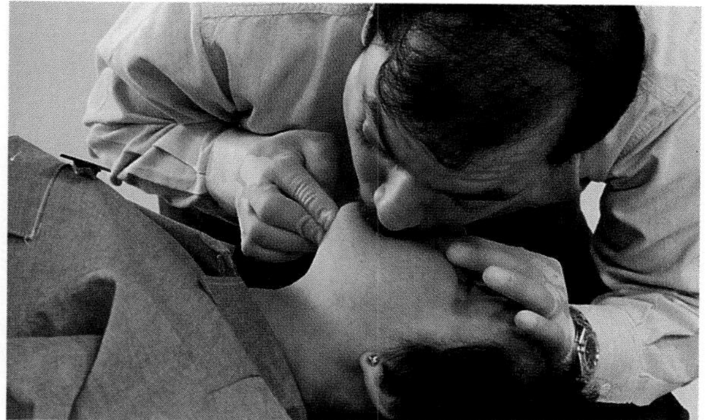 B

Figure 8-4 **A**, The head-tilt/chin-lift opens the victim's airway. **B**, To breathe for a nonbreathing victim, seal your mouth around the person's mouth and breathe slowly into the person.

breath should last about 1½ to 2 seconds, with a pause between breaths to let the air flow back out. Watch the victim's chest rise each time you breathe to make sure that your breaths are actually going in.

If you do not see the victim's chest rise *and fall* as you give breaths, you may not have the head tilted back far enough to open the airway adequately. Retilt the victim's head and try again to give breaths. If your breaths still do not go in, assume the victim's airway is obstructed. You must give the care for an obstructed airway that is described later in this chapter.

Check for a pulse after giving 2 breaths. If the victim has a pulse but is not breathing, continue rescue breathing by giving 1 breath every 5 seconds (for an adult). A good way to time the breaths is to count, "one one-thousand, two one-thousand, three one-thousand." Then take a breath on "four one-thousand" and breathe into the victim on "five one-thousand." Counting this way ensures that you give 1 breath about every 5 seconds. Remember, breathe slowly into the victim. Each breath should last about 1½ seconds.

After 1 minute of rescue breathing (about 12 breaths), recheck the pulse to make sure the heart is still beating. If the victim still has a pulse but is not breathing, continue rescue breathing. Check the pulse every minute. Do not stop rescue breathing unless one of the following occurs:

- The victim begins to breathe on his or her own.
- The victim has no pulse. Begin CPR (see Chapter 10).
- Another rescuer with training equal to yours or greater takes over.
- You are too exhausted to continue.
- The scene becomes unsafe.

Special Considerations for Rescue Breathing

There are several considerations that you should be aware of when you provide rescue breathing. These include—

- Air in the stomach.
- Vomiting.
- Mouth-to-nose breathing.
- Mouth-to-stoma breathing.
- Victims with dentures.
- Suspected injury to the spine.

Air in the Stomach

When you perform rescue breathing, air normally enters the victim's lungs. Sometimes, air may enter the victim's stomach. This may

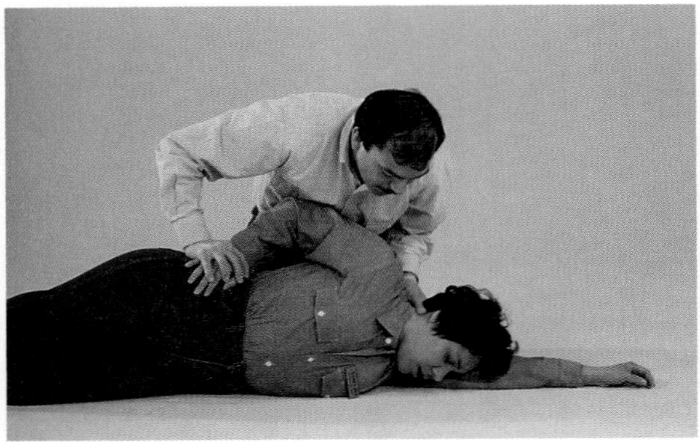

Figure 8-5 If vomiting occurs, turn the victim on his or her side, and clear the mouth of any matter.

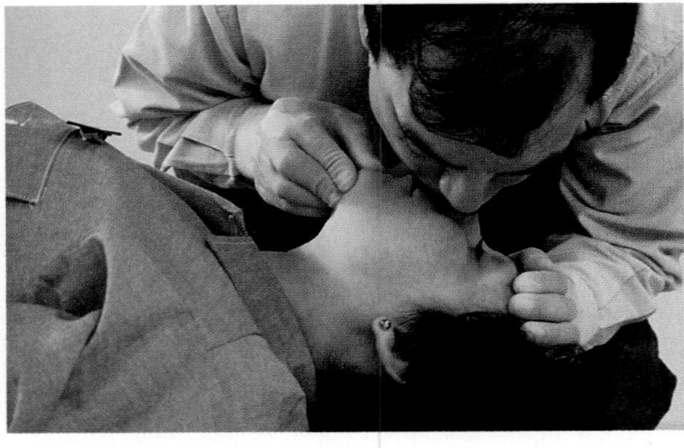

Figure 8-6 For mouth-to-nose breathing, close the victim's mouth and seal your mouth around the victim's nose. Breathe full breaths, watching the chest to see if the air goes in.

occur for several reasons. One, breathing into the victim longer than 2 seconds may cause extra air to fill the stomach. To avoid putting air in the stomach, do not overinflate the victim's lungs. Stop the breath when the chest rises. Two, if the victim's head is not tilted back far enough, the airway will not open completely. As a result, the chest may only rise slightly. If the chest only rises a little, you will probably breathe more forcefully, causing air to enter the stomach. Three, breaths given too quickly create more pressure in the airway, causing air to enter the stomach. Long, slow breaths minimize pressure in the air passages.

Excess air in the stomach is called **gastric distention**. Gastric distention can be a serious problem because it can make the victim vomit. When an unconscious victim vomits, stomach contents may get into the lungs, obstructing breathing. Taking such foreign material into the lungs is called ***aspiration***. Because aspiration can hamper rescue breathing, it may eventually be fatal.

To avoid forcing air into the stomach, be sure to keep the victim's head tilted back far enough. Breathe slowly into the victim, just enough to make the chest rise. Pause between breaths long enough for the victim's lungs to empty and for you to take another breath.

Vomiting

When you give rescue breathing, the victim may vomit whether there is gastric distention. If the victim vomits, turn the victim's head and body together as a unit to the side (Fig. 8-5). This position helps prevent vomit from entering the lungs. Quickly wipe the victim's mouth clean, carefully reposition the victim on his or her back, and continue with rescue breathing.

Mouth-to-Nose Breathing

Sometimes you may not be able to make an adequate seal over a victim's mouth to perform rescue breathing. For example, the person's jaw or mouth may be injured or shut too tightly to open, or your mouth may be too small to cover the victim's. If so, provide mouth-to-nose rescue breathing as follows:

- Maintain the head-tilt position with one hand on the forehead. Use your other hand to close the victim's mouth, making sure to push on the chin, not on the throat.
- Open your mouth wide, take a deep breath, seal your mouth tightly around the victim's nose, and breathe full breaths into the victim's nose (Fig. 8-6). Open the victim's mouth between breaths, if possible, to let air escape.

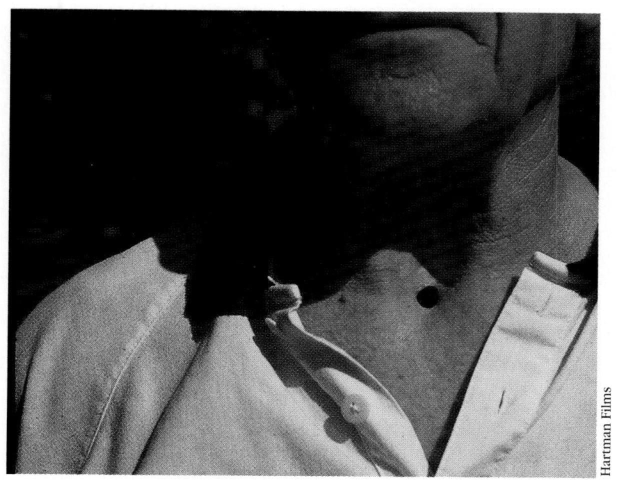

Figure 8-7 You may need to perform rescue breathing on a victim with a stoma.

Mouth-to-Stoma Breathing

Some people have had an operation that removed all or part of the **larynx**, the upper end of the windpipe. They breathe through an opening called a **stoma** in the front of the neck (Fig. 8-7). Air passes directly into the trachea through the stoma instead of through the mouth and nose.

Most people with a stoma wear a medical alert bracelet or necklace or carry a card identifying this condition. You may not see the stoma immediately. You will probably notice the opening in the neck as you tilt the head back to check for breathing.

To give rescue breathing to someone with a stoma, you must give breaths through the stoma instead of the mouth or nose. Follow the same basic steps as in mouth-to-mouth breathing, except—

1. Look, listen, and feel for breathing with your ear over the stoma (Fig. 8-8, *A*).
2. Give breaths into the stoma, breathing at the same rate as for mouth-to-mouth breathing (Fig. 8-8, *B*).
3. Remove your mouth from the stoma between breaths to let air flow back out.

If the chest does not rise when you give rescue breaths, suspect that the victim may have had only part of the larynx removed. That means that some air continues to flow through the larynx to the lungs during normal breathing. When giving mouth-to-stoma breathing, air may leak through the nose and mouth, diminishing the amount of your rescue breaths that reach the lungs. If air leaks, you need to seal the nose and mouth with your hand to prevent air from escaping during rescue breathing (Fig. 8-9).

A

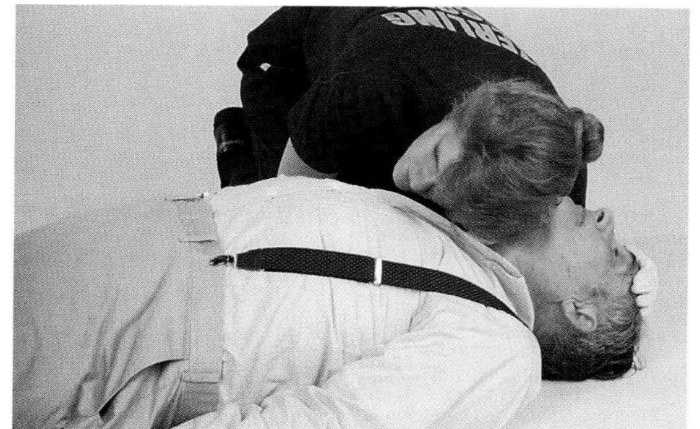

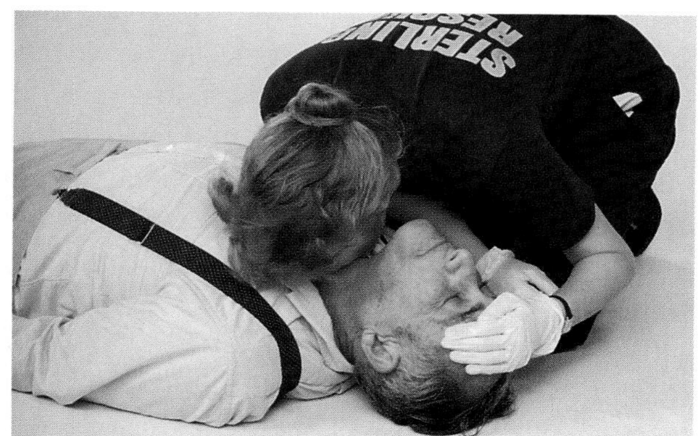

B

Figure 8-8 **A**, Look, listen, and feel for breathing with your ear over the stoma. **B**, Seal your mouth around the stoma and breathe into the victim. You may need to tilt the head back to get the chin out of the way.

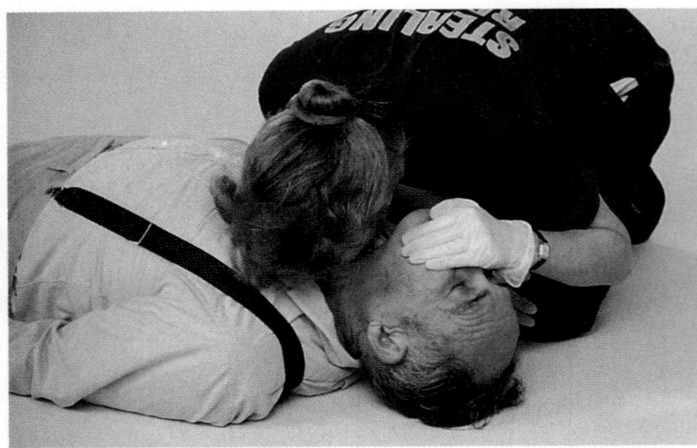

Figure 8-9 When performing rescue breathing on a person with a stoma, you may need to seal the victim's nose and mouth to prevent air from escaping.

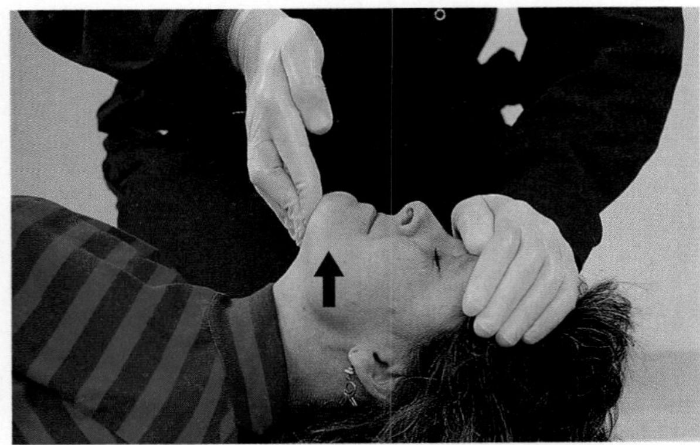

Figure 8-10 If you suspect head or spine injuries, try to open the airway by lifting the chin without tilting the head.

Victims with Dentures

If you know or see the victim is wearing **dentures**, do not automatically remove them. Dentures help rescue breathing by supporting the victim's mouth and cheeks during mouth-to-mouth breathing. If the dentures are loose, the head-tilt/chin-lift technique may help keep them in place. Remove the dentures *only* if they become so loose that they block the airway or make it difficult for you to give breaths.

Suspected Head, Neck, or Back Injuries

You should suspect head, neck, or back injuries in victims who have suffered a violent force, such as that caused by a motor vehicle crash, a fall, or a diving or other sports-related incident. If you suspect the victim may have an injury to the head, neck, or back, you should try to minimize movement of the head and neck when opening the airway. Minimizing movement requires you to change the way you open the airway.

Try to open the victim's airway by lifting the chin *without* tilting the head back (Fig. 8-10). In most cases, doing so will allow air to pass into the lungs. Since it is sometimes difficult to keep the jaw lifted with one hand, you can perform a two-handed ***jaw thrust*** (Fig. 8-11, *A*). Open the airway by placing your fingers under the angles of the jaw and lifting. Place your mouth over the victim's, using your cheek to close the nose, and breathe (Fig. 8-11, *B*). These techniques allow you to open the airway and provide rescue breathing without moving the head.

Infants and Children

The airway structures of an infant or child are different from those of an adult. These structures are smaller and more easily obstructed than an adult's. In addition, a child's tongue takes up proportionally more space in the mouth than an adult's. Also, the trachea is more flexible and fragile, making it more susceptible to injury.

Uncorrected breathing emergencies in children and infants are the primary cause of cardiac arrest. For this reason, rescue breathing is extremely crucial to the survival of a child or infant who has stopped breathing. Rescue breathing for infants and children follows the same general procedure as that for adults. The minor differences take into account the infant's or child's undeveloped physique and moderately faster heartbeat and breathing rate. Rescue breathing for infants and children uses less air in each breath, and breaths are delivered at a slightly faster rate.

A 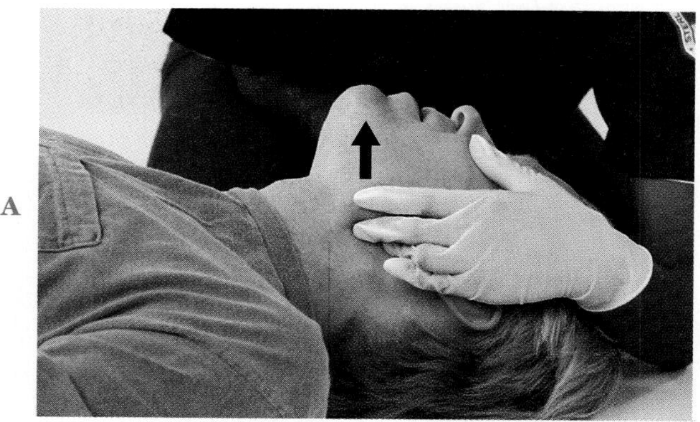

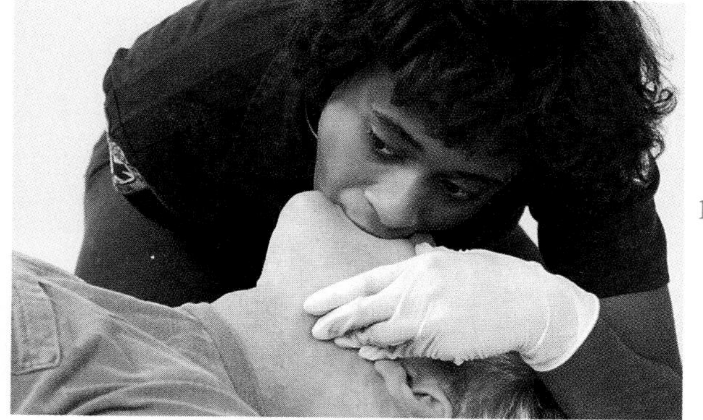 B

Figure 8-11 **A**, Use a two-handed jaw thrust when a chin-lift fails to open the airway of a victim with a suspected head or spine injury. **B**, Seal the nose with your cheek, and breathe into the victim.

You do not need to tilt a child's or infant's head as far back as an adult's to open the airway. Tilt the head back only far enough to allow your breaths to go in. Tilting an infant's or child's head back too far may cause injury that will obstruct the airway. Give 1 slow breath every 3 seconds for both a child and an infant. Figure 8-12 shows the distance the head normally needs to be tilted back during rescue breathing for an adult, a child, and an infant.

It is easier to cover both the mouth and nose of an infant with your mouth when giving breaths. Remember to breathe slowly into the victim. Each breath should last about 1½ seconds. Be careful not to overinflate a child's or infant's lungs. Breathe only until you see the chest rise. After 1 minute of rescue breathing (about 20 breaths in a child or in an infant), recheck the pulse.

◆ AIRWAY OBSTRUCTION

Airway obstructions are the most common cause of respiratory emergencies. The two types of airway obstruction are anatomical and mechanical.

An **anatomical obstruction** occurs when the airway is blocked by an anatomical structure like the tongue or swollen tissues of the mouth and throat. This type of obstruction may result from injury to the neck or a medical emergency, such as anaphylactic shock. The most common obstruction in an unconscious person is the tongue, which drops to the back of the throat and blocks the airway. The tongue drops back because muscles, including those in the tongue, relax when deprived of oxygen.

A **mechanical obstruction** occurs when the airway is blocked by a foreign object, such as a piece of food, a small toy, or fluids such as vomit, blood, mucus, or saliva. Someone with a mechanical obstruction may be choking.

Common causes of choking include—

- Trying to swallow large pieces of poorly chewed food.
- Drinking alcohol before or during meals. Alcohol dulls the nerves that aid swallowing, making choking on food more likely.
- Wearing dentures. Dentures make it difficult for you to sense whether food is fully chewed before you swallow it.
- Eating while talking excitedly or laughing or eating too fast.
- Walking, playing, or running with food or objects in the mouth.

A person whose airway is blocked by a piece of food or another object can quickly stop breathing, lose consciousness, and die. You

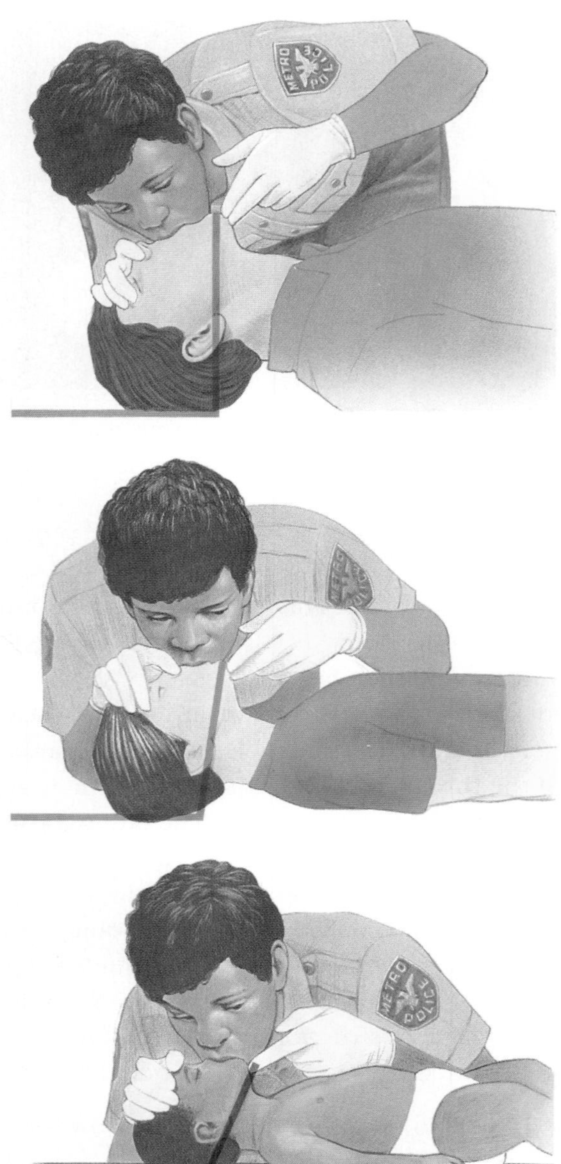

Figure 8-12 There are only minor differences in rescue breathing for adults, children, and infants. Often, the older the victim, the greater the head tilt needed to help open the airway.

must be able to recognize that the airway is obstructed and give care immediately. This is why checking the airway comes first in the ABCs of the initial assessment. If you mistake an obstructed airway for a heart attack or some other serious condition, you might be slow to give the right kind of care or could even give the wrong kind.

A person who is choking may have either a complete or partial airway obstruction. A victim with a **complete airway obstruction** is not able to breathe at all. With a partial airway obstruction, the victim's ability to breathe depends on how much air can get past the obstruction into the lungs.

Partial Airway Obstruction

A person with a **partial airway obstruction** can still move air to and from the lungs. This air allows the person to cough in an attempt to dislodge the object. The person may also be able to move air past the vocal cords to speak. The narrowed airway may cause a wheezing sound as air moves in and out of the lungs. As a natural reaction to choking, the victim may clutch at the throat with one or both hands. This is universally recognized as a distress signal for choking (Fig. 8-13). If the victim is coughing forcefully or speaking, do not interfere with attempts to cough up the object. A person who has enough air to cough forcefully or speak also has enough air entering the lungs to breathe. Stay with the victim and encourage him or her to continue coughing to clear the obstruction. If coughing persists, call for more advanced medical personnel.

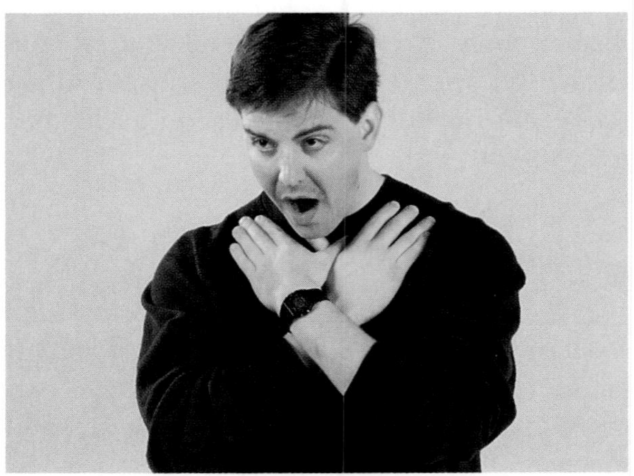

Figure 8-13 Clutching the throat with one or both hands is universally recognized as a distress signal for choking.

Complete Airway Obstruction

A partial airway obstruction can quickly become a complete airway obstruction. A person with a completely blocked airway is unable to speak, cry, breathe, or cough effectively. Sometimes the victim may cough weakly and ineffectively or make high-pitched noises. All of these signs tell you the victim is not getting enough air to the lungs to sustain life. Act immediately. If you have not already done so, have a bystander call for more advanced medical personnel while you begin to give care.

Care for Choking Victims

When someone is choking, you must try to reopen the airway as quickly as possible. Give abdominal thrusts. This technique is also called the **Heimlich maneuver**. **Abdominal thrusts** compress the abdomen, increasing pressure in the lungs and airway. This simulates a cough, forcing trapped air in the lungs to push the object out of the airway like a cork from a bottle of champagne (Fig. 8-14).

Care for a Conscious Choking Adult

To give abdominal thrusts to a conscious choking adult, stand behind the victim and wrap your arms around his or her waist (Fig. 8-15, *A*). The victim may be seated or standing. Make a fist with one hand and place the thumb side against the middle of the victim's abdomen just above the navel and well below the lower tip of the breastbone (Fig. 8-15, *B*). Grab your fist with your other hand and give quick upward

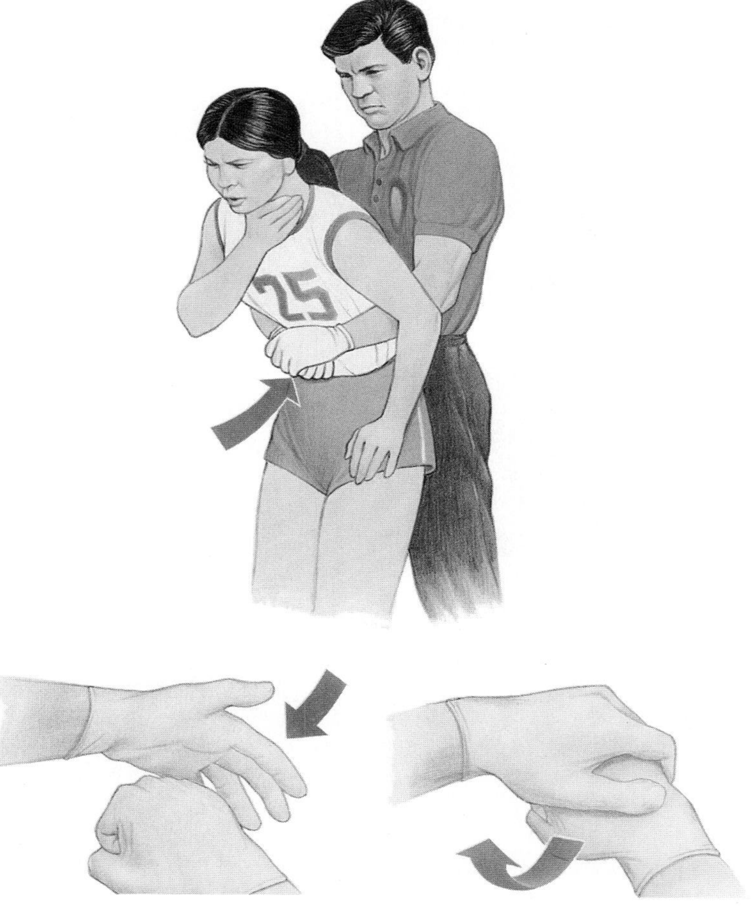

Figure 8-14 Abdominal thrusts simulate a cough, forcing air trapped in the lungs to push the object out of the airway.

A

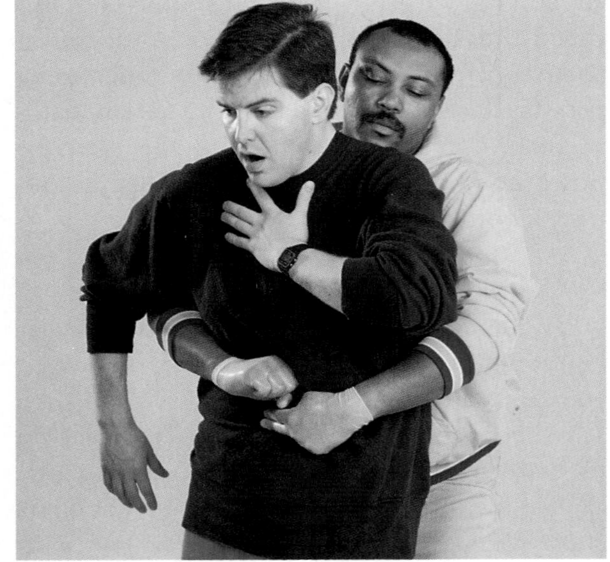

B

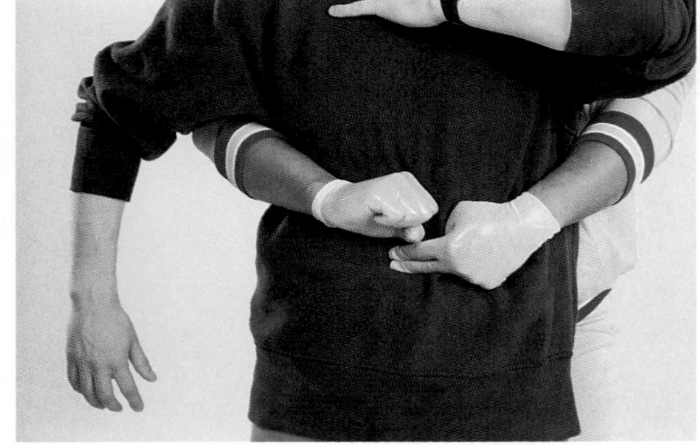

C

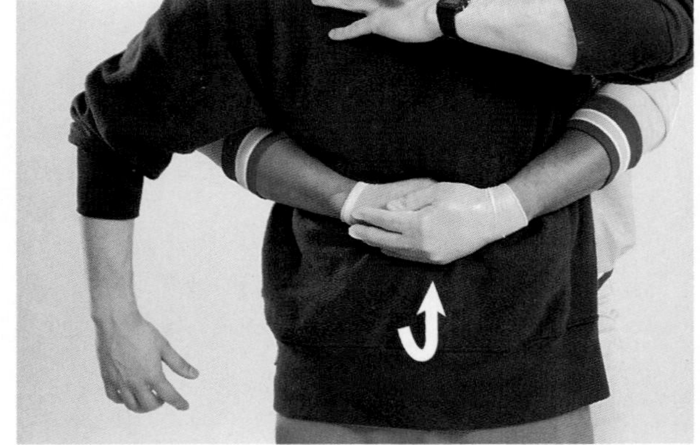

Figure 8-15 **A**, Stand behind the victim and wrap your arms around his waist to give abdominal thrusts. **B**, Place the thumb side of your fist against the middle of the victim's abdomen. **C**, Grasp your fist with your other hand and give quick upward thrusts into the abdomen.

thrusts into the abdomen (Fig. 8-15, *C*). Repeat these thrusts until the object is dislodged or the victim becomes unconscious.

If You Are Alone and Choking

If you are choking and no one is around who can help, you can give yourself abdominal thrusts in two ways: (1) Make a fist with one hand and place the thumb side on the middle of your abdomen slightly above your navel and well below the tip of your breastbone. Grasp your fist with your other hand and give a quick upward thrust. (2) You can also lean forward and press your abdomen over any firm object, such as the back of a chair, a railing, or a sink (Fig. 8-16). Be careful not to lean over anything with a sharp edge or a corner that might injure you.

Care for a Conscious Choking Adult Who Becomes Unconscious

When giving abdominal thrusts to a conscious choking victim, anticipate that the victim will become unconscious if the obstruction is not removed. If he or she becomes unconscious, lower the victim to the floor on his or her back. Take the following steps:

1. Open the airway by grasping the lower jaw and lifting the jaw up.

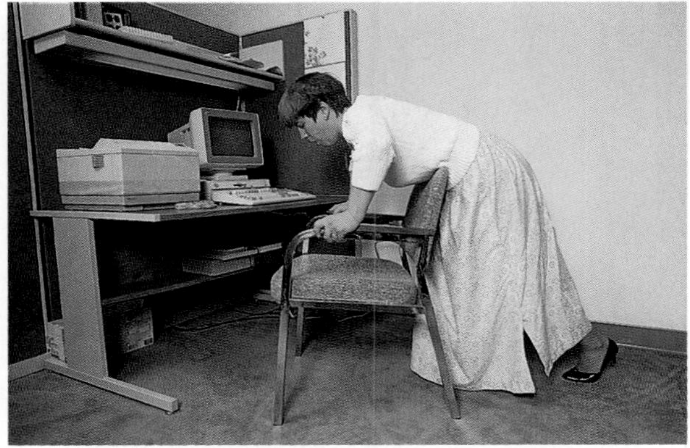

Figure 8-16 To give yourself abdominal thrusts, press your abdomen onto a firm object, such as the back of a chair.

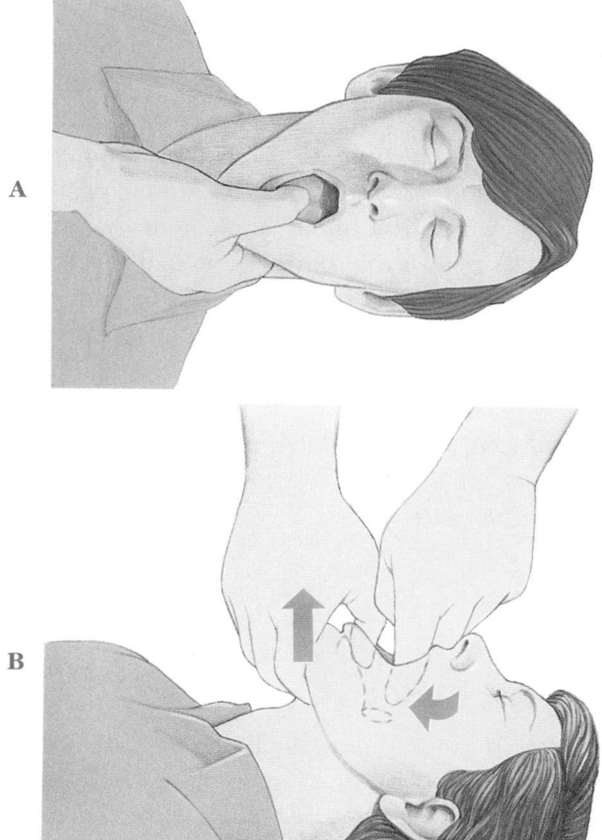

Figure 8-17 A, To do a finger sweep, first lift the lower jaw. B, Use a hooking action to sweep the object out of the airway.

2. Attempt to dislodge and remove the object by sweeping it out with your index finger. This action is called a ***finger sweep*** (Fig. 8-17, *A-B*). When doing a finger sweep, use a hooking action to remove the object. Be careful not to push the object deeper into the victim's throat.
3. Try to open the victim's airway using the head-tilt/chin-lift.
4. Give 2 slow breaths. Often, the throat muscles relax enough after the person becomes unconscious to allow air past the obstruction and into the lungs.

If air does not go in,

5. Reposition (retilt) the head.
6. Give 2 slow breaths.

If air still does not go in, assume the airway is still obstructed.

7. Give up to 5 abdominal thrusts. To give abdominal thrusts to an unconscious victim, straddle one of the victim's thighs. Place the heel of one hand on the victim's abdomen, just above the navel and well below the lower tip of the breastbone. Place the other hand on top of the first. The fingers of both hands should point directly toward the victim's head (Fig. 8-18). Give quick upward thrusts into the abdomen.
8. Do a finger sweep.

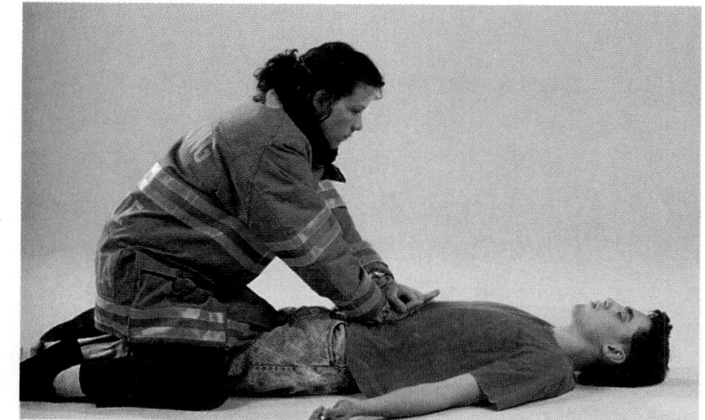

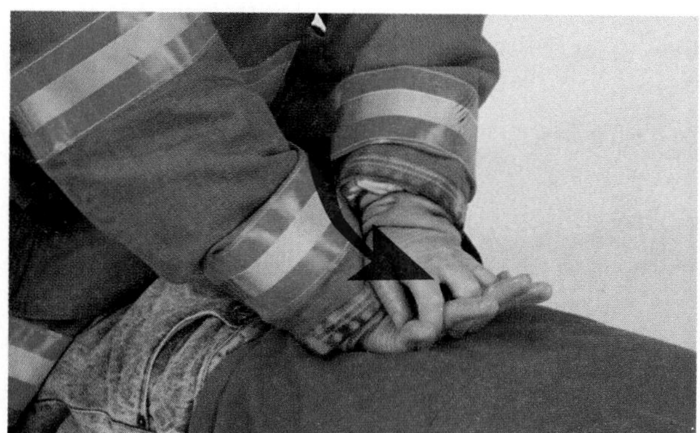

Figure 8-18 **A**, To give abdominal thrusts to an unconscious victim, straddle the victim's thighs. **B**, Position your hands with your fingers pointing toward the victim's head. Give quick upward thrusts.

9. Give 2 slow breaths. If the breaths do not go in, reposition the head and repeat 2 breaths. Repeat this sequence beginning with step 7, until the object is expelled, you can breathe air into the victim, or other trained personnel arrive and take over.

Care for an Unconscious Choking Adult

During the initial assessment, you may discover that an unconscious adult victim is not breathing and that the 2 slow breaths you give will not go in. If this happens, take the following steps:

1. Reposition the head.
2. Give 2 slow breaths again. You may not have tilted the victim's head back far enough the first time. If the breaths will not go in, assume the victim's airway is obstructed.
3. Give up to 5 abdominal thrusts.
4. Do a finger sweep.
5. Open the airway.
6. Give 2 slow breaths.

If breaths do not go in, go back to step 1 and repeat all steps until the object is dislodged, you can breathe air into the victim, or other trained personnel arrive and take over.

If your first attempts to clear the airway are unsuccessful, do not stop. The longer the victim goes without oxygen, the more the muscles will relax, making it more likely that you will be able to clear the airway enough to deliver breaths successfully.

Once you are able to breathe air into the victim's lungs, complete the initial assessment by checking the victim's pulse and checking and caring for any severe bleeding. If there is no pulse, begin CPR (see Chapter 10). If the victim has a pulse but is not breathing on his or her own, continue rescue breathing.

If the victim starts breathing on his or her own, monitor both breathing and pulse until more advanced medical personnel arrive and take over. Maintain an open airway; look, listen, and feel for breathing; and keep checking the pulse.

When to Stop Thrusts

Stop giving thrusts immediately if the object is dislodged or if the person begins to breathe or cough. Watch that the person is breathing freely again. Even after the object is coughed up, the person may still have breathing problems that you do not immediately identify. You should also realize that both abdominal thrusts and chest thrusts (described in the next section) may cause internal injuries. *Therefore, whenever thrusts are used to dislodge an object, the person should be taken to the nearest hospital emergency department for follow-up care, even if he or she seems to be breathing without difficulty.*

Special Considerations for Choking Victims

In some instances, abdominal thrusts are not the best method of care for choking victims. Some choking victims need chest thrusts. For example, if you cannot reach far enough around the victim to give effective abdominal thrusts, you should give chest thrusts. You should also give chest thrusts instead of abdominal thrusts to noticeably pregnant choking victims.

Chest Thrusts for a Conscious Victim

To give **chest thrusts** to a conscious victim, stand behind the victim and place your arms under the victim's armpits and around the chest. As in giving abdominal thrusts, make a fist with one hand, placing the thumb side against the center of the victim's breastbone. Be sure that your thumb is centered on the breastbone, not on the ribs. Also make sure that your fist is not near the lower tip of the breastbone. Grab your fist with your other hand and thrust inward (Fig. 8-19). Repeat these thrusts until the object is dislodged or the victim becomes unconscious.

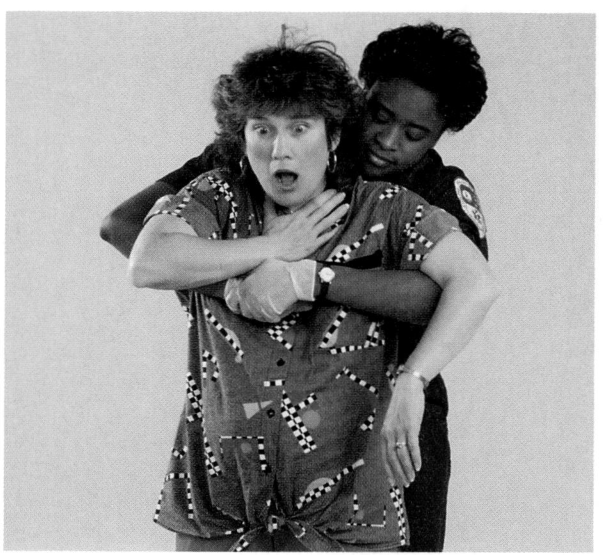

Figure 8-19 Give chest thrusts if you cannot reach around the victim to give abdominal thrusts or if the victim is noticeably pregnant.

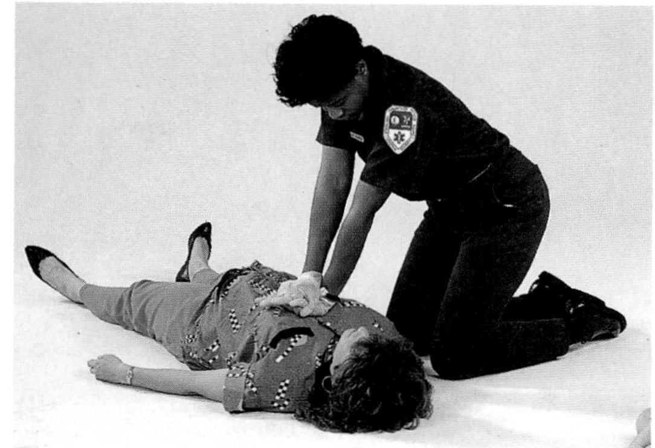

Figure 8-20 Positioning for Chest Thrusts for an Unconscious Victim

Chest Thrusts for an Unconscious Victim

With a noticeably pregnant unconscious victim or any victim to whom you cannot effectively deliver abdominal thrusts, give chest thrusts. Kneel next to the victim. Place the heel of one hand on the center of the victim's breastbone and your other hand on top of it (Fig. 8-20). Give up to 5 quick thrusts. Each thrust should compress the chest 1½ to 2 inches. After giving 5 chest thrusts, continue your steps as you normally would for an unconscious choking victim. Repeat the sequence if the object was not expelled.

Children and Infants

Choking emergencies are common in children and infants and are caused by small objects, such as beads, toys, and uninflated balloons, and by food, such as hot dogs, round candy, nuts, and grapes. Emergency care for a choking child is similar to the care for a choking adult. The only significant difference involves the child's size. Obviously, you cannot use the same force when giving abdominal thrusts to a child to expel the object. Care for choking infants includes a combination of chest thrusts given with two fingers and back blows. Abdominal thrusts are not used for a choking infant because of their potential for causing injury.

Care for a Conscious Choking Child

If you suspect that a child is choking, begin the initial assessment by asking, "Are you choking?" If you have not already done so, call more advanced medical personnel for help. Continue care as you would for an adult.

Give abdominal thrusts. Stand or kneel behind the child. Wrap your arms around the child's waist. Make a fist with one hand. Place the thumb side of your fist against the middle of the child's abdomen just above the navel and well below the lower tip of the breastbone. Grasp your fist with your other hand and give quick upward thrusts into the abdomen (Fig. 8-21, *A-B*). Repeat the thrusts until the obstruction is cleared or the child becomes unconscious.

If the child coughs up the object or starts to breathe or cough, continue to watch the child to ensure that he or she is breathing again. Even though the child may be breathing well, he or she may have other problems that require a doctor's attention. The child should be examined by more advanced medical personnel.

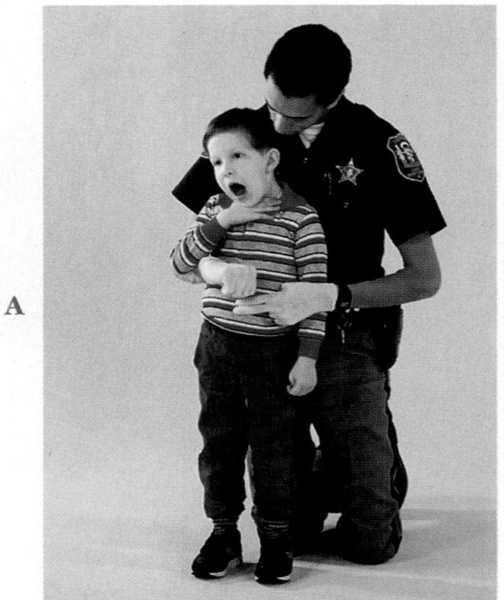

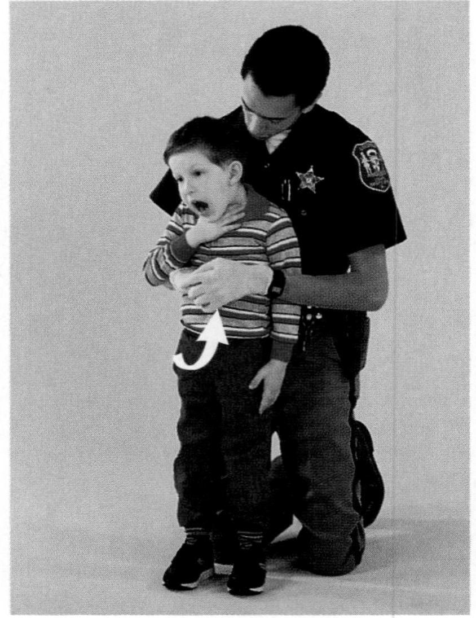

Figure 8-21 To give abdominal thrusts to a child, **A**, stand or kneel behind the child. Wrap your arms around the child's waist. Make a fist with one hand. Place the thumb side of your fist against the middle of the child's abdomen, just above the navel and well below the tip of the breastbone. **B**, Grasp your wrist with your other hand and give quick upward thrusts into the abdomen.

Care for an Unconscious Choking Child

If, during the initial assessment, you determine that an unconscious child has a complete airway obstruction, continue care as follows:

1. Reposition the head.
2. Give 2 slow breaths again. You may not have tilted the child's head back far enough the first time. If the breaths will not go in, assume the child's airway is obstructed.
3. Give up to 5 abdominal thrusts.
4. Do a finger sweep if you see the object.
5. Open the airway.
6. Give 2 slow breaths (Fig. 8-22).

If your breaths still do not go in, go back to step 1 and repeat all the steps until the obstruction is removed, the child starts to breathe or cough, or more advanced medical personnel arrive and take over.

Care for a Conscious Choking Infant

If, during the initial assessment, you determine that a conscious infant cannot breathe, cough, or cry, give care for a complete airway obstruction. Begin by giving 5 back blows followed by 5 chest thrusts.

Start by positioning the infant face-up on your forearm. Place your other arm on top of the infant, using your thumb and fingers to hold the infant's jaw while sandwiching the infant between your forearms (Fig. 8-23, *A*). Turn the infant over so that he or she is facedown on your forearm (Fig. 8-23, *B*). Lower your arm onto your thigh so that the infant's head is lower than his or her chest. Give 5 firm back blows with the heel of your hand between the infant's shoulder blades (Fig. 8-23, *C*). Support the infant's head and neck by firmly holding the jaw between your thumb and forefinger.

To give chest thrusts, you need to turn the infant back over. Start by placing your free hand and forearm along the infant's head and back so that the infant is sandwiched between your hands and forearms. Continue to support the infant's head between your thumb and fingers from the front while you cradle the back of the head with your other hand (Fig. 8-24, *A*).

Turn the infant onto his or her back. Lower your arm that is supporting the infant's back

A

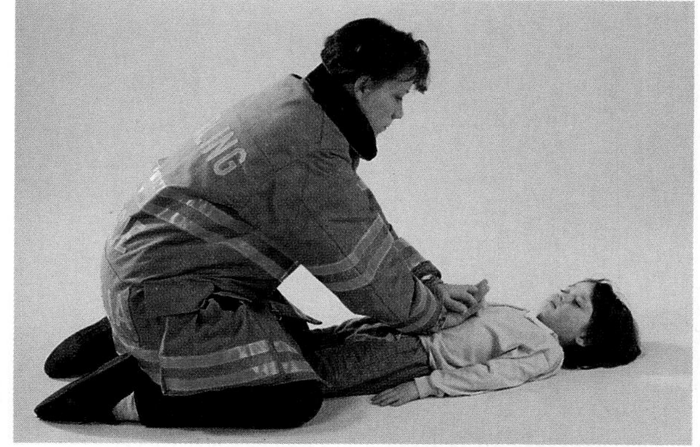

B

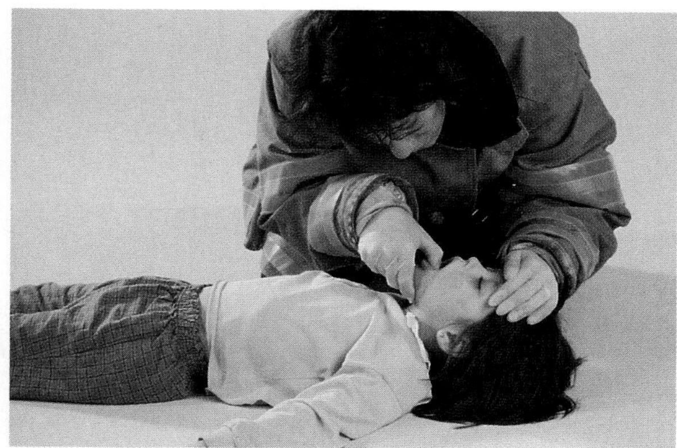

C

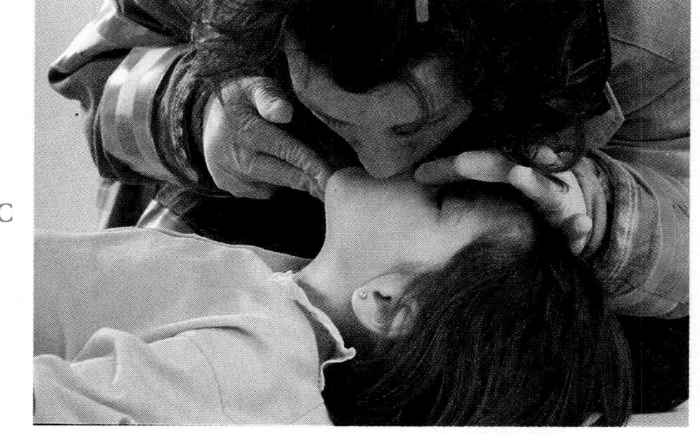

Figure 8-22 To care for an unconscious child with a complete airway obstruction, **A**, give 5 abdominal thrusts. **B**, Do a finger sweep if you see the object. **C**, Open the airway and give 2 slow breaths.

onto your thigh. The infant's head should be lower than his or her chest (Fig. 8-24, *B*). Give 5 chest thrusts (Fig. 8-24, *C*).

To locate the correct place to give chest thrusts, imagine a line running across the infant's chest between the nipples (Fig. 8-25, *A*). Place the pad of your ring finger on the breastbone just under this imaginary line. Then place the pads of the two fingers next to the ring finger just under the nipple line. Raise the ring finger (Fig. 8-25, *B*) off the chest. If you feel the notch at the end of the infant's breastbone, move your fingers up a little bit.

Use the pads of the two fingers to compress the breastbone. Compress the breastbone ½ to 1 inch, then let the breastbone return to its normal position. Keep your fingers in contact with the infant's breastbone. Compress 5 times. You can give back blows and chest thrusts effectively whether you stand up or sit. If the infant is large or your hands are too small to adequately support the infant, you may prefer to sit. Place the infant in your lap to give back blows and chest thrusts. The infant's head should be lower than the chest (Fig. 8-26).

Keep giving back blows and chest thrusts until the object is coughed up or the infant begins to breathe or cough. Summon more advanced medical personnel if you have not already done so. Even if the infant seems to be breathing well, he or she should be examined by more advanced medical personnel.

Care for an Unconscious Choking Infant

If, during the initial assessment, you determine that an unconscious infant is not breathing and that the 2 slow breaths you give will not go in, position your hands and continue care as follows:

1. Reposition the head.
2. Give 2 slow breaths again. If the breaths will not go in, assume the infant's airway is obstructed.
3. Give 5 back blows.
4. Give 5 chest thrusts.
5. Do a foreign body check (see following).
6. Open the airway.
7. Give 2 slow breaths. If the breaths do not go in, go back to step 1 and repeat steps un-

A

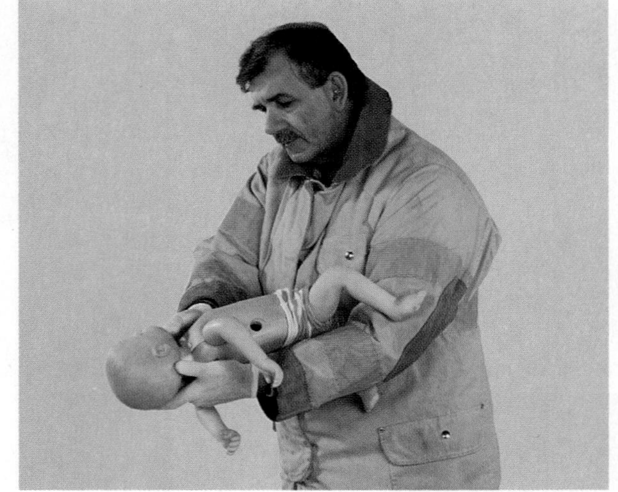

B

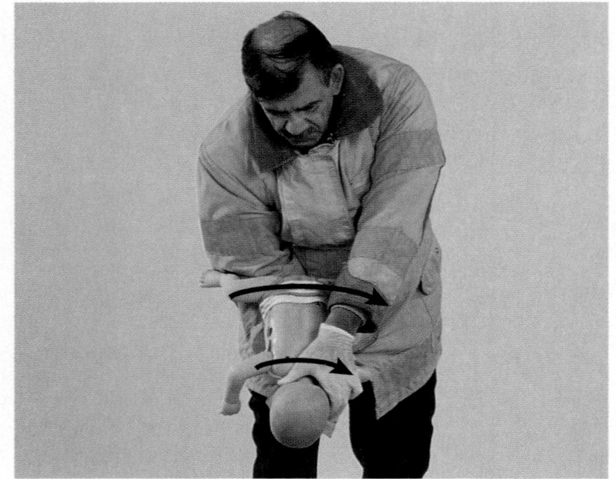

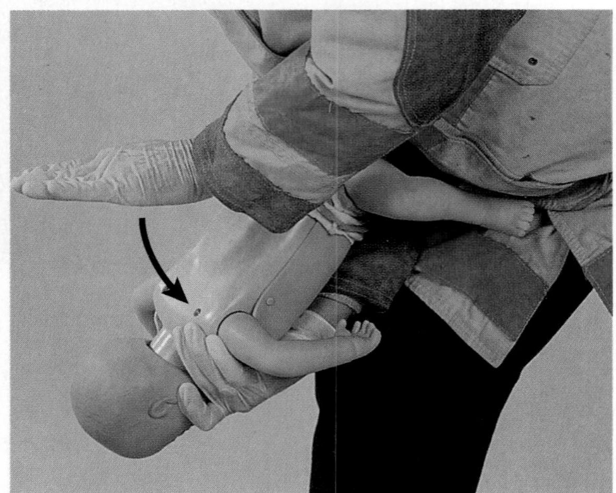

C

Figure 8-23 To give back blows, **A**, sandwich the infant between your forearms. Support the infant's head and neck by holding the jaw between your thumb and forefinger. **B**, Turn the infant over so that he is facedown on your forearm. **C**, Give 5 firm back blows with the heel of your hand while supporting your arm that is holding the infant on your thigh.

til the obstruction is removed, the infant starts to breathe or cough, or more advanced medical personnel arrive and take over.

To do a foreign-body check—

- Stand or kneel beside the infant's head.
- Open the infant's mouth, using your hand that is nearer the infant's feet. Put your thumb into the infant's mouth and hold both the tongue and the lower jaw between the thumb and fingers. Lift the jaw upward (Fig. 8-27, *A*).
- Look for an object. If you can see it, try to remove it by doing a finger sweep with the little finger (Fig. 8-27, B).

If you are able to breathe air into the infant's lungs, finish the initial assessment. Give 2 slow breaths as you did for rescue breathing, and check the infant's brachial pulse. Next, check and care for any severe bleeding. If the infant has no pulse, begin CPR, which you will learn in Chapter 10. If the infant has a pulse and is not breathing on his or her own, continue rescue breathing.

A

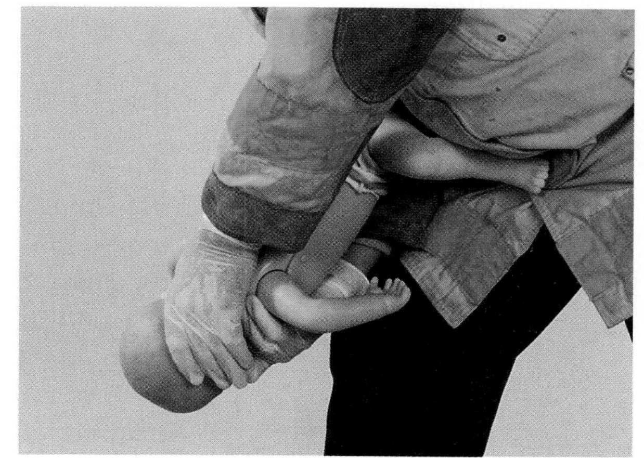

B

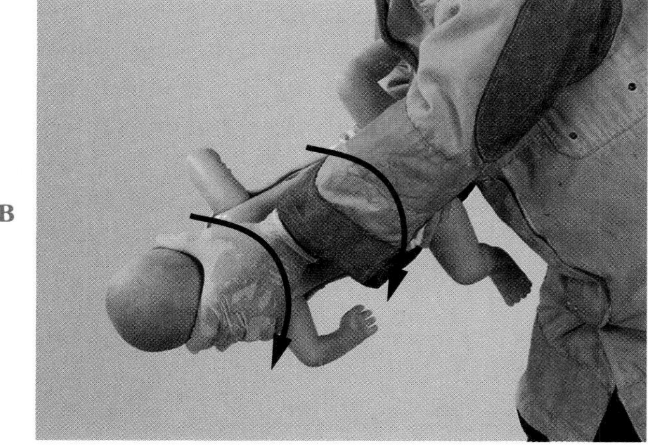

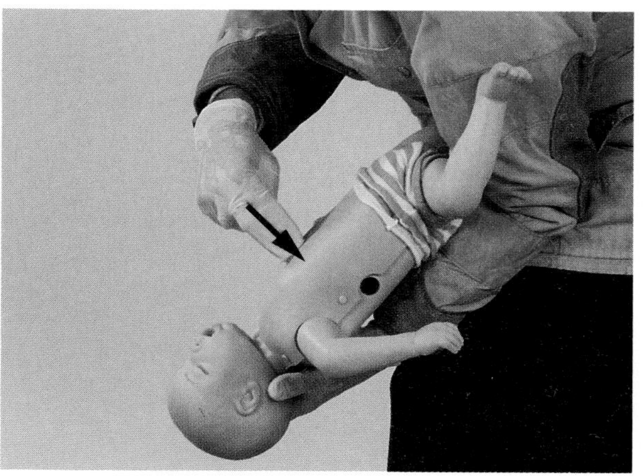

C

Figure 8-24 To give chest thrusts, **A**, sandwich the infant between your forearms. Continue to support the infant's head. **B**, Turn the infant onto his back and support your arm on your thigh. The infant's head should be lower than the chest. **C**, Give 5 chest thrusts.

A

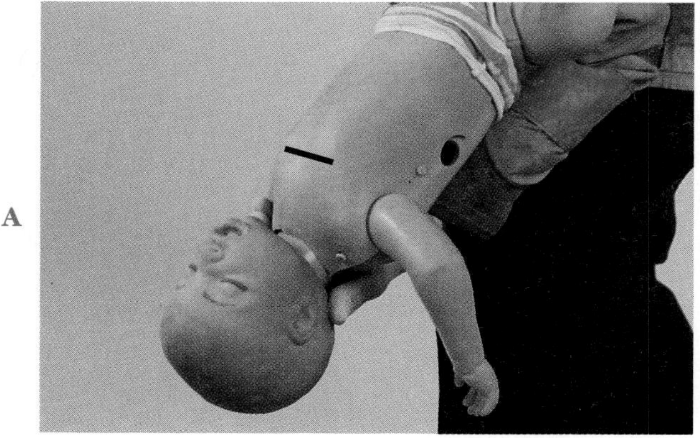

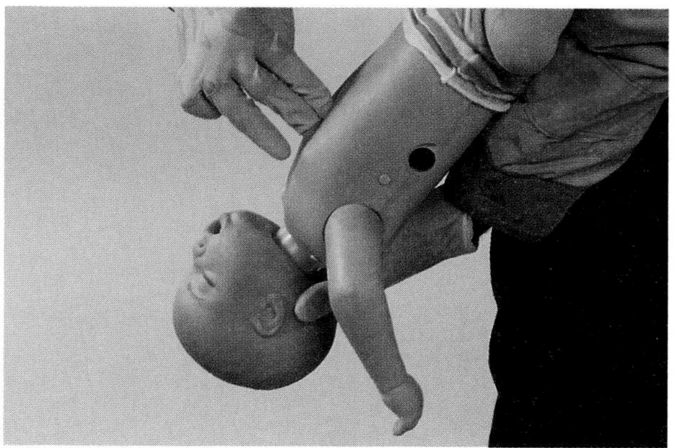

B

Figure 8-25 To locate the correct place to give chest thrusts, **A**, imagine a line running across the infant's chest between the nipples. **B**, Place the pad of your ring finger on the breastbone just under this imaginary line. Place the pads of the two fingers next to the ring finger just under the nipple line. Raise the ring finger.

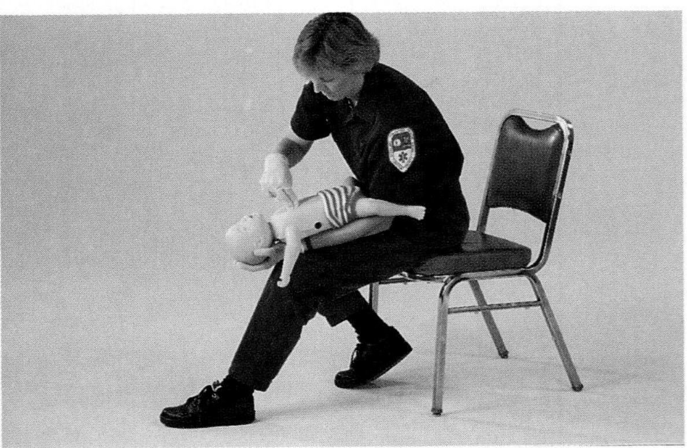

Figure 8-26 If you cannot adequately support the infant, put him on your lap with the head lower than the chest.

If the infant starts to breathe on his or her own, complete a physical examination, continue to maintain an open airway, and monitor breathing and pulse until more advanced personnel arrive and take over.

◆ SUMMARY

In this chapter, you learned how to recognize and provide care for breathing emergencies. You now know to look for a breathing emergency in the initial assessment because such an emergency can be life threatening. You learned the signs and symptoms of respiratory distress and arrest and the appropriate care for each condition. You also learned the basic techniques for rescue breathing and for special situations. Finally, you learned how to care for choking victims, both conscious and unconscious. By knowing how to care for breathing emergencies, you are now better prepared to care for other emergencies. You will learn about cardiac emergencies in Chapter 10.

Use the activities in Unit 8 of the workbook to help you review the material in this chapter.

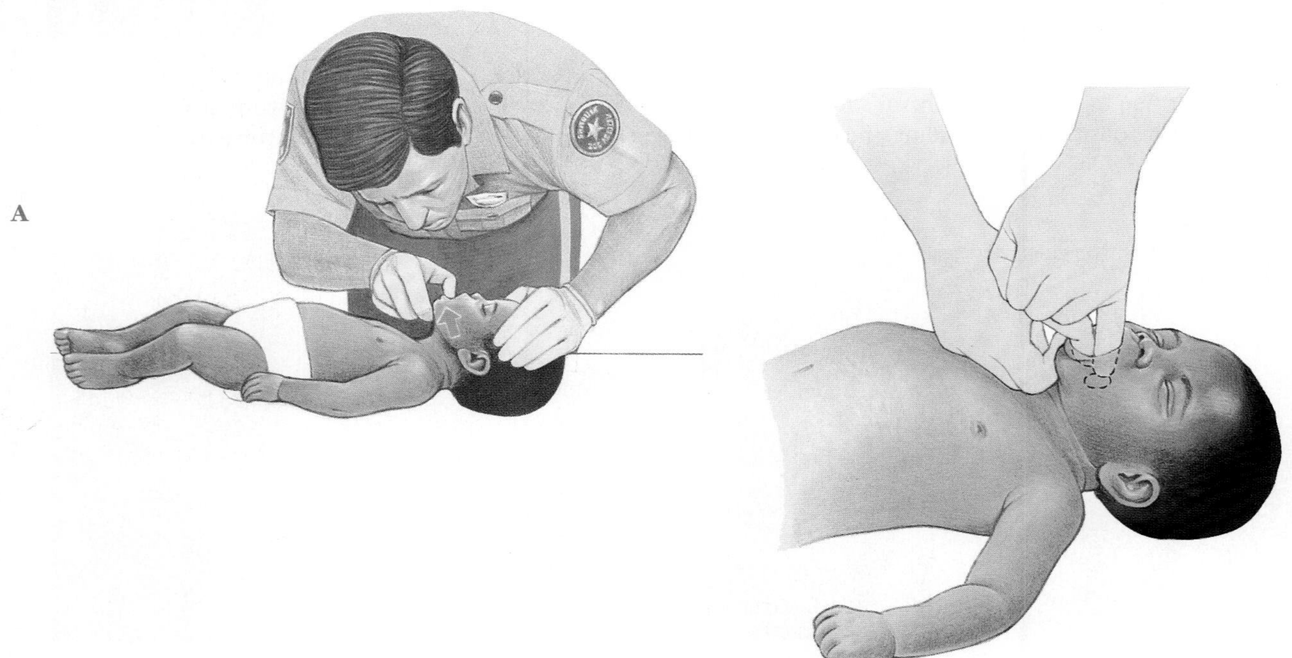

Figure 8-27 To do a finger sweep on an infant, **A**, put your thumb into the infant's mouth and hold the tongue and lower jaw between the thumb and fingers. Lift the jaw upward. **B**, If you see an object, try to remove it by doing a finger sweep using the little finger.

Rescue Breathing for an Adult or Child

Skill Summary

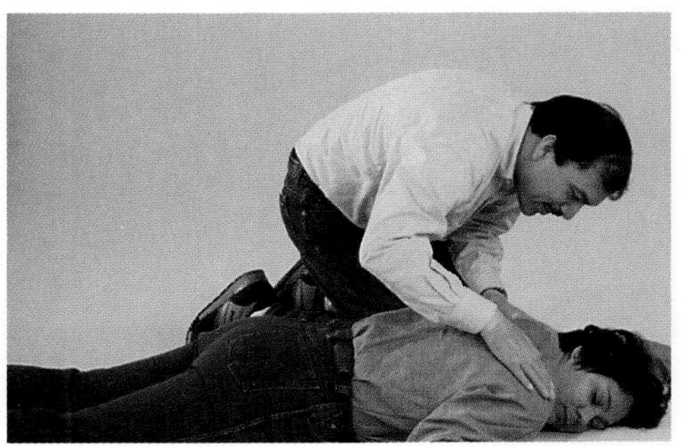

1. Check for consciousness.

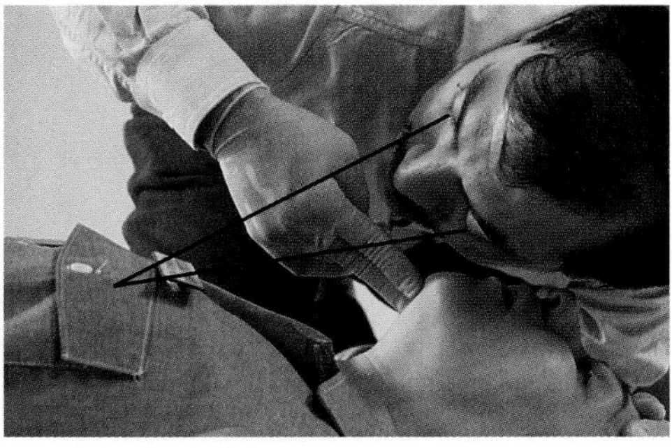

2. Open airway—check for breathing.

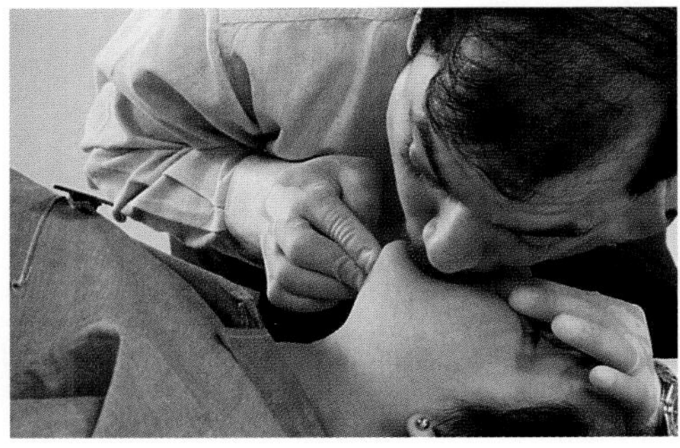

3. No breathing—give 2 slow breaths.

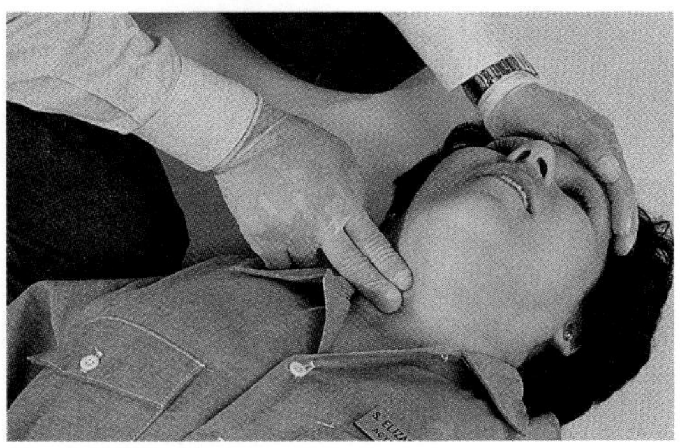

4. Check for pulse (carotid).

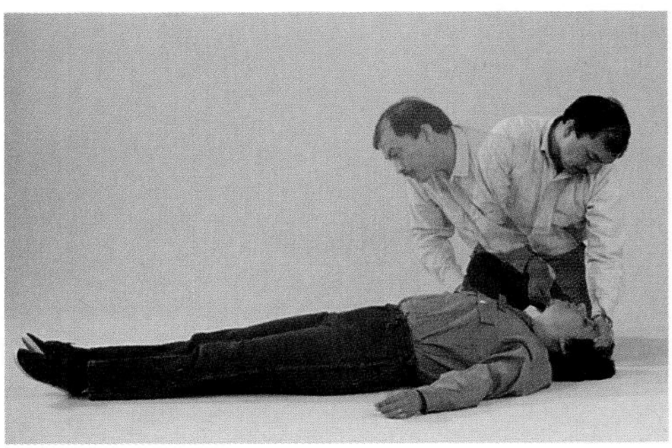

5. Check for severe bleeding.

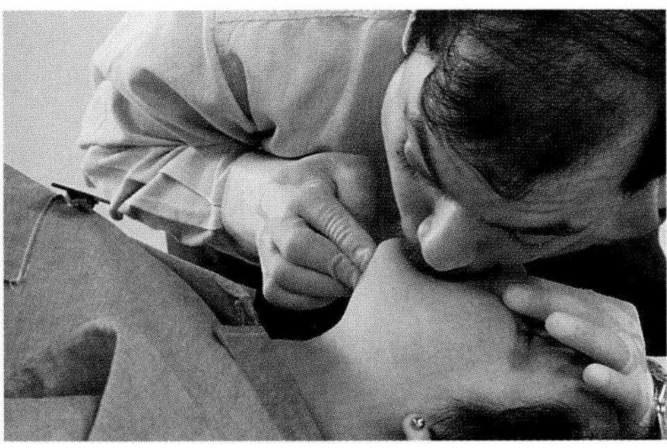

6. Pulse present, no breathing—begin rescue breathing. Give 1 slow breath every 5 seconds for an adult (1 slow breath every 3 seconds for a child).

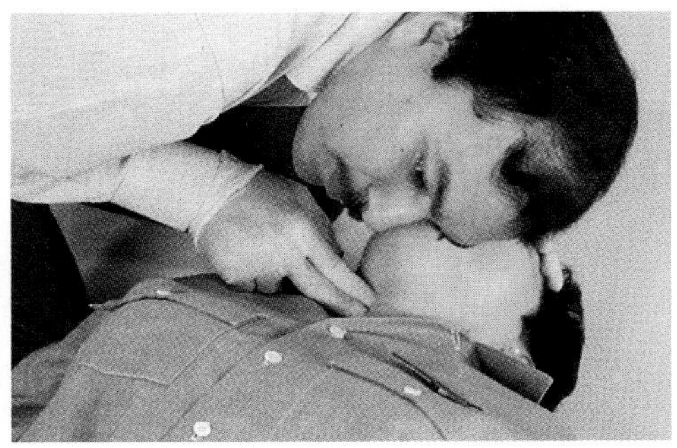

7. Recheck breathing and pulse after each minute.

Rescue Breathing for an Infant

Skill Summary

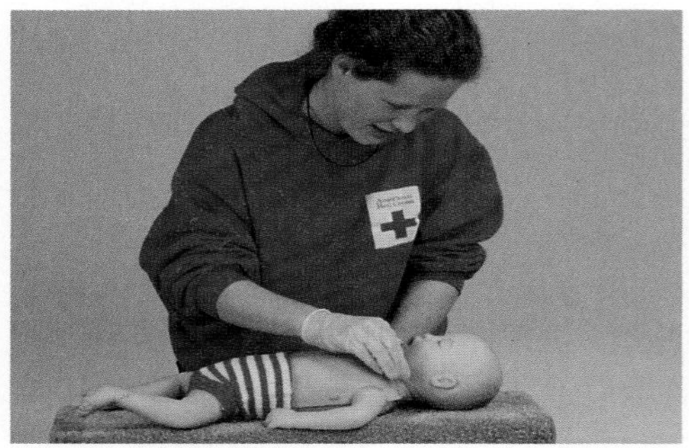

1. Check for consciousness.

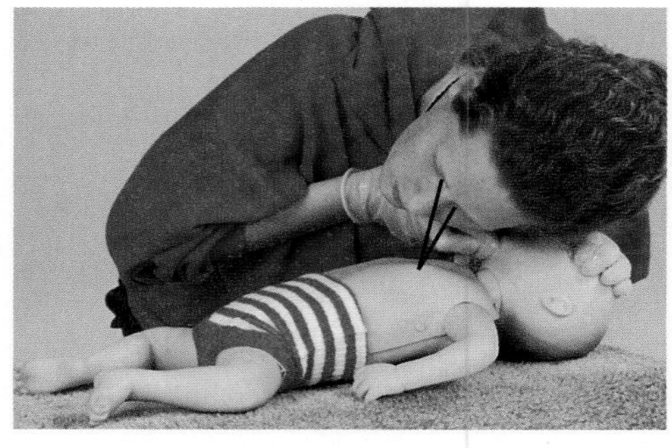

2. Open airway—check for breathing.

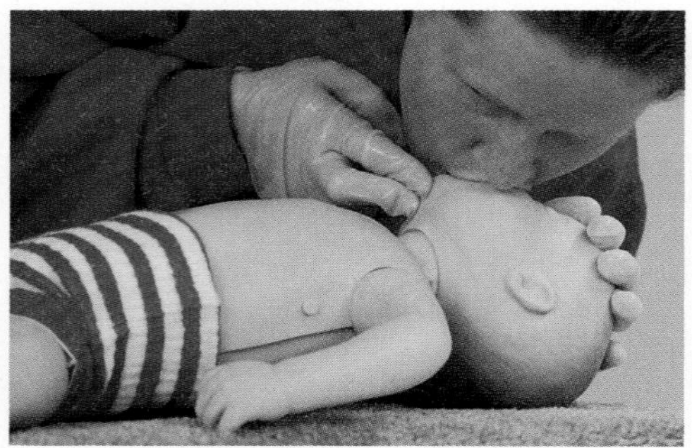

3. No breathing—give 2 slow breaths.

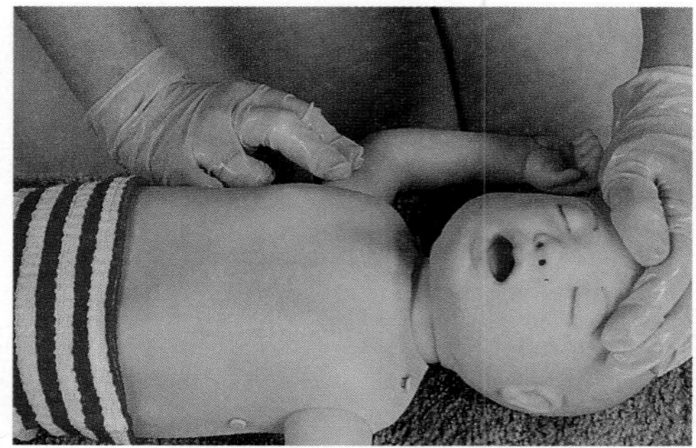

4. Check for pulse (brachial).

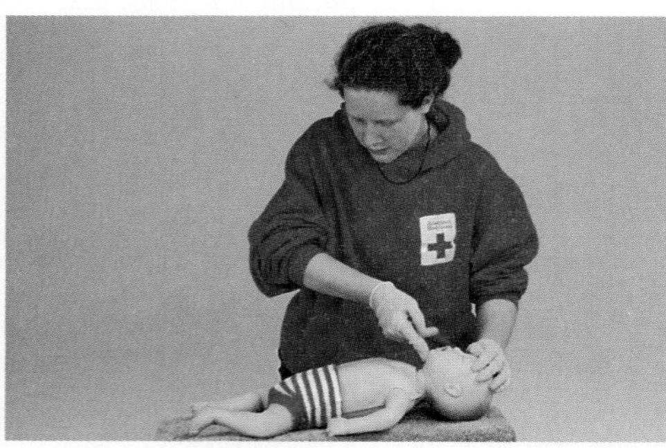

5. Check for severe bleeding.

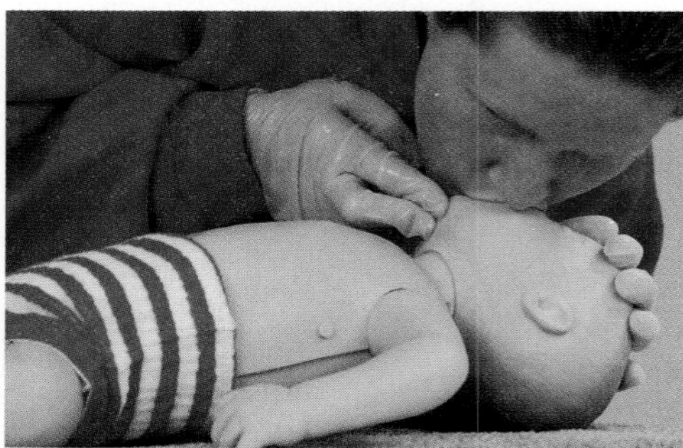

6. Pulse present, no breathing—begin rescue breathing. Give 1 slow breath every 3 seconds.

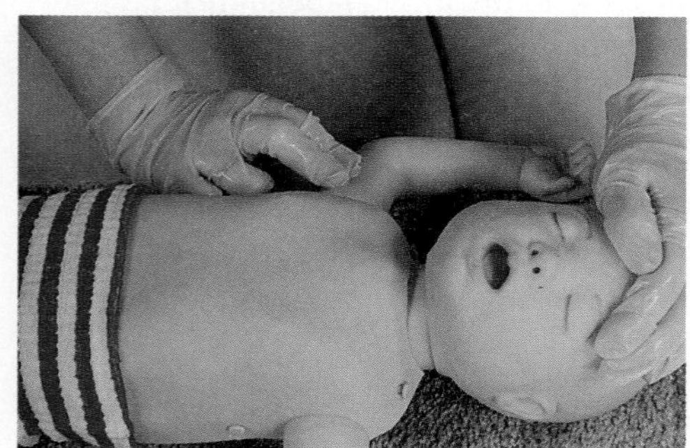

7. Recheck breathing and pulse after each minute.

Unconscious Adult or Child With a Complete Airway Obstruction

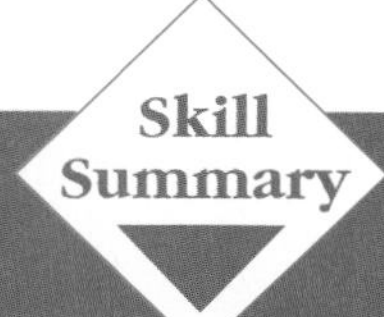

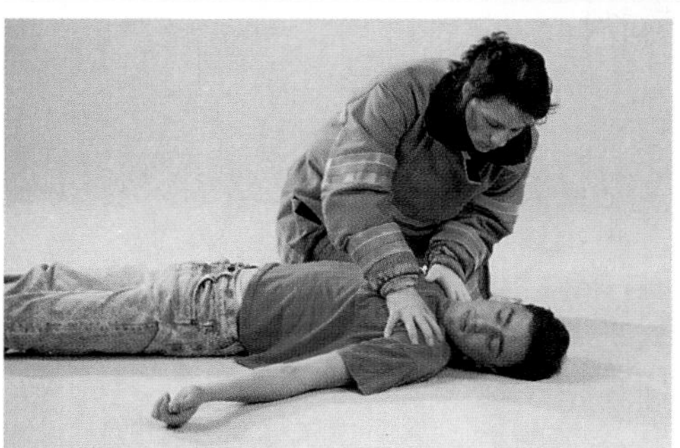

1. Check for consciousness.

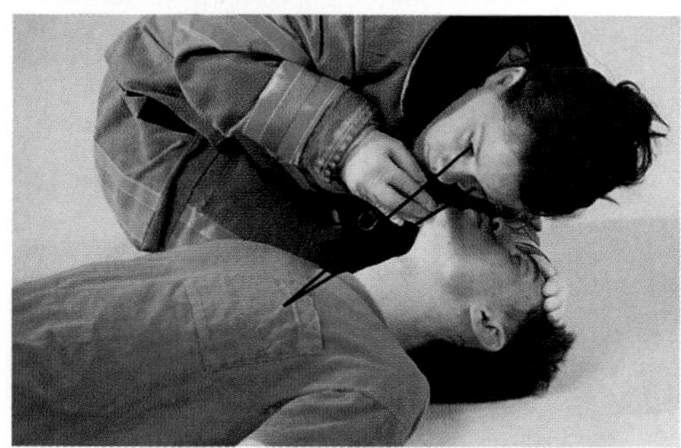

2. Open airway and check for breathing.

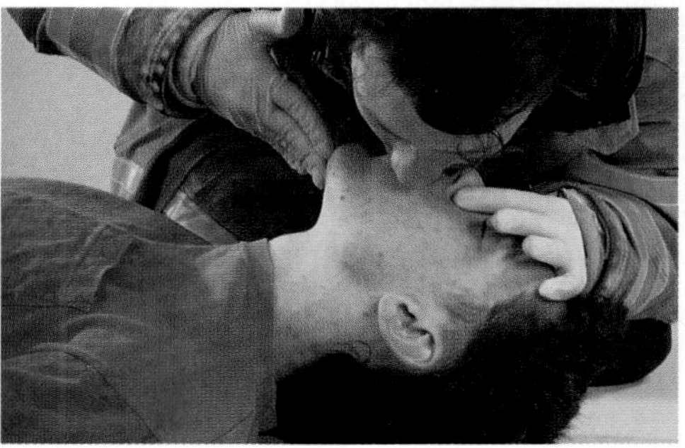

3. Give 2 slow breaths.

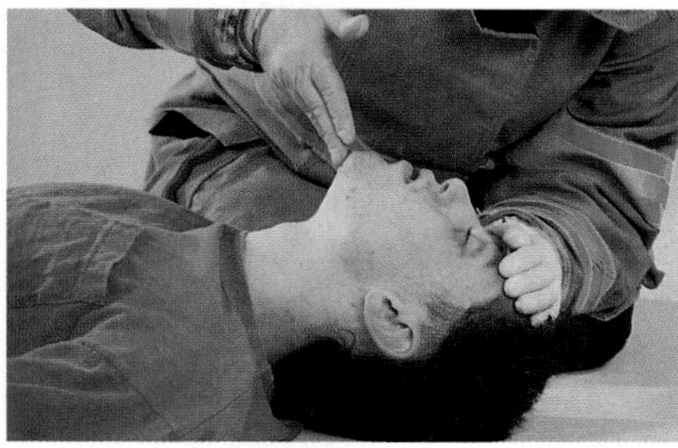

4. *If breaths do not go in,* retilt victim's head and reattempt 2 slow breaths.

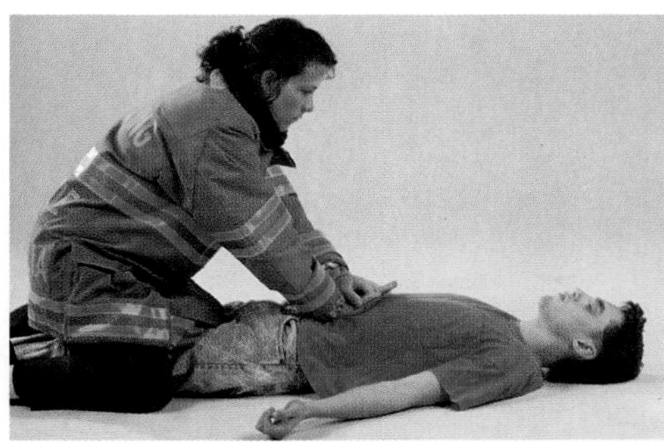

5. Give up to 5 abdominal thrusts.

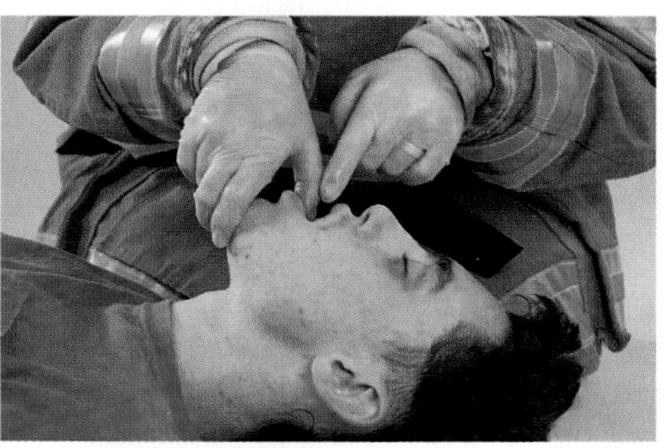

6. Do finger sweep. (For child, sweep only if you see object.)

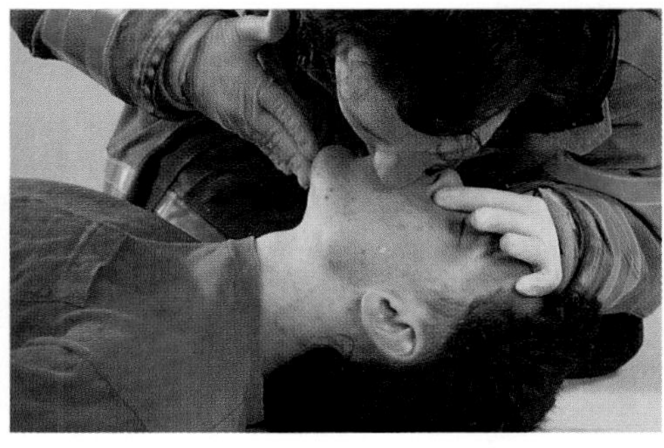

7. Open airway and give 2 slow breaths.

If breaths still do not go in, go back to step 4 and repeat steps until the obstruction is removed, the victim begins to breathe or cough, or more advanced medical personnel arrive and take over.

Conscious Adult or Child With a Complete Airway Obstruction

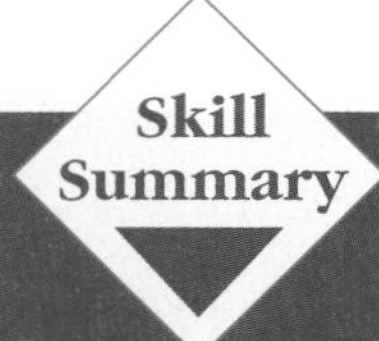

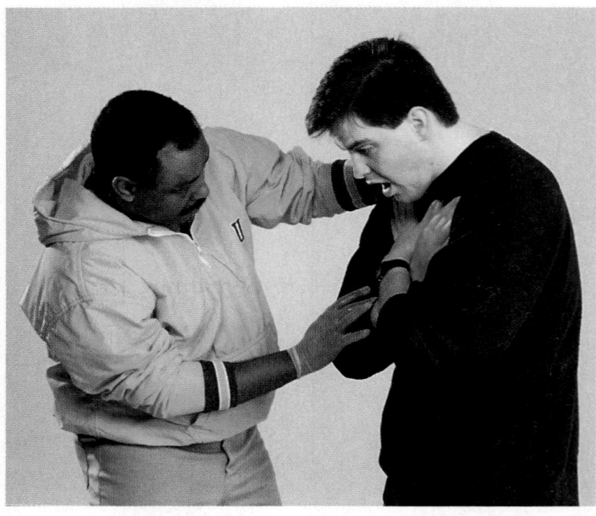

1. Determine if person is choking.

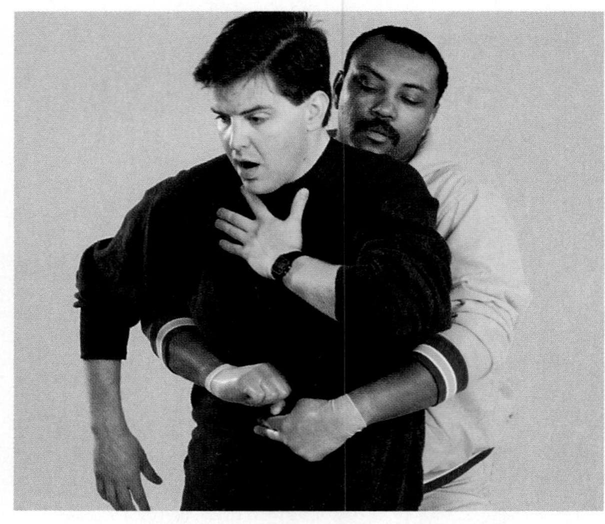

2. Position yourself to give abdominal thrusts.

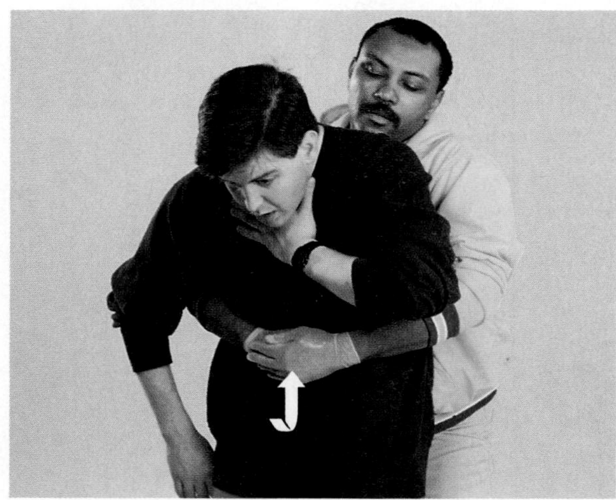

3. Give abdominal thrusts.

Repeat thrusts until object is expelled or victim becomes unconscious.

Unconscious Infant With a Complete Airway Obstruction

Skill Summary

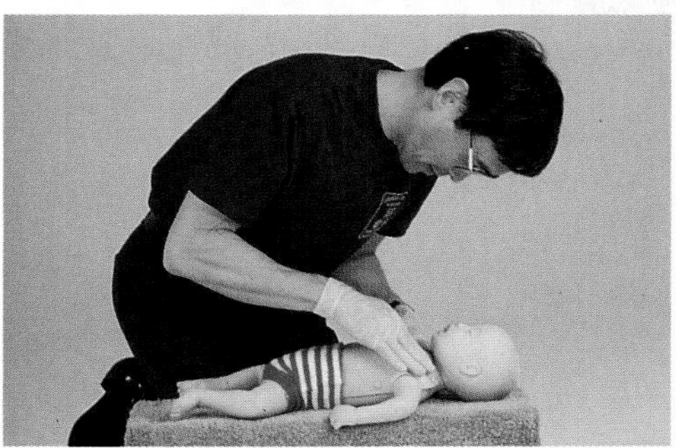

1. Check for consciousness.

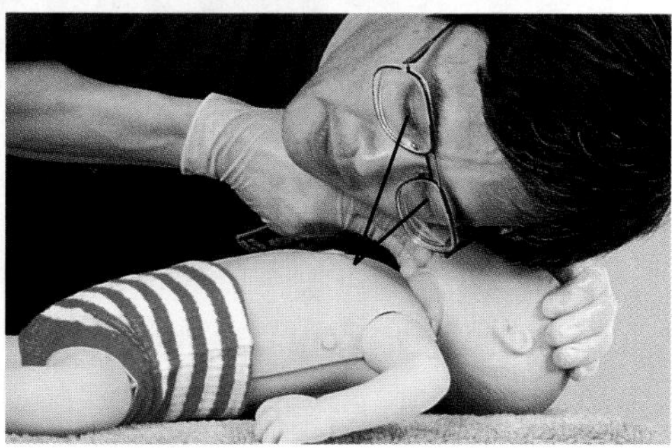

2. Open airway and check for breathing.

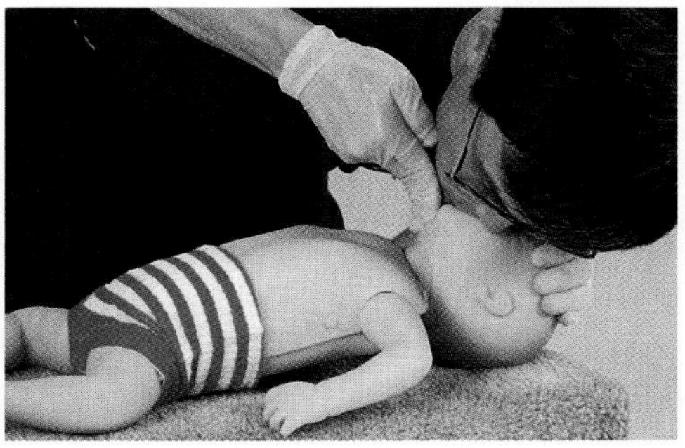

3. Give 2 slow breaths.

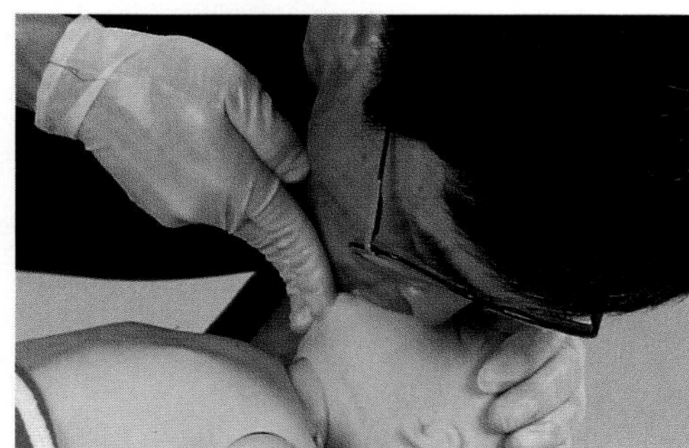

4. *If breaths do not go in,* retilt infant's head and reattempt breaths.

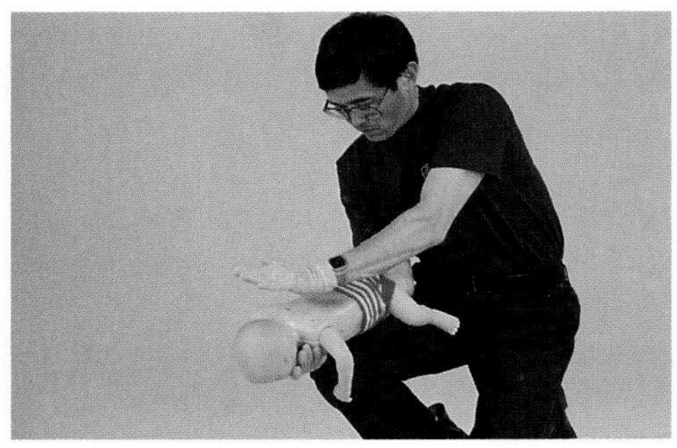

5. Give 5 back blows.

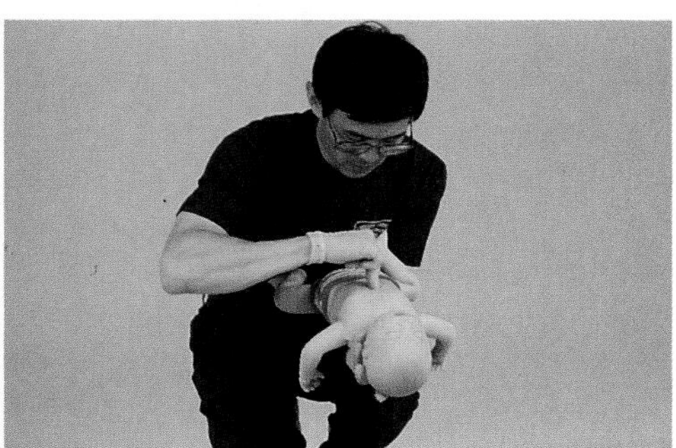

6. Give 5 chest thrusts.

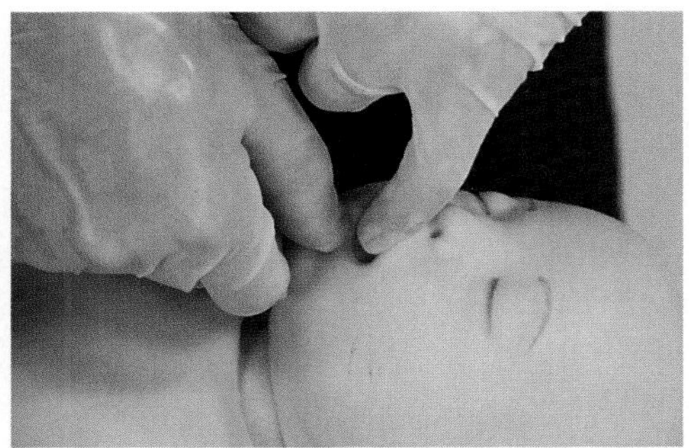

7. Do a foreign body check. Sweep out object if visible.

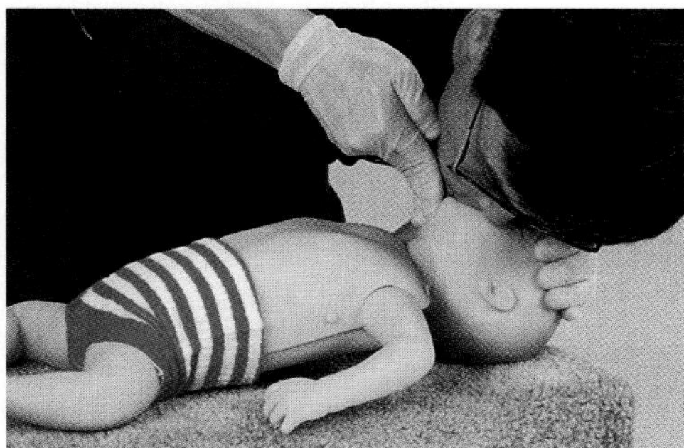

8. Open airway and give 2 slow breaths.

If breaths still do not go in, go back to step 4 and repeat steps until the obstruction is removed, the victim begins to breathe, cough, or cry, or more advanced medical personnel arrive and take over.

Breathing Devices

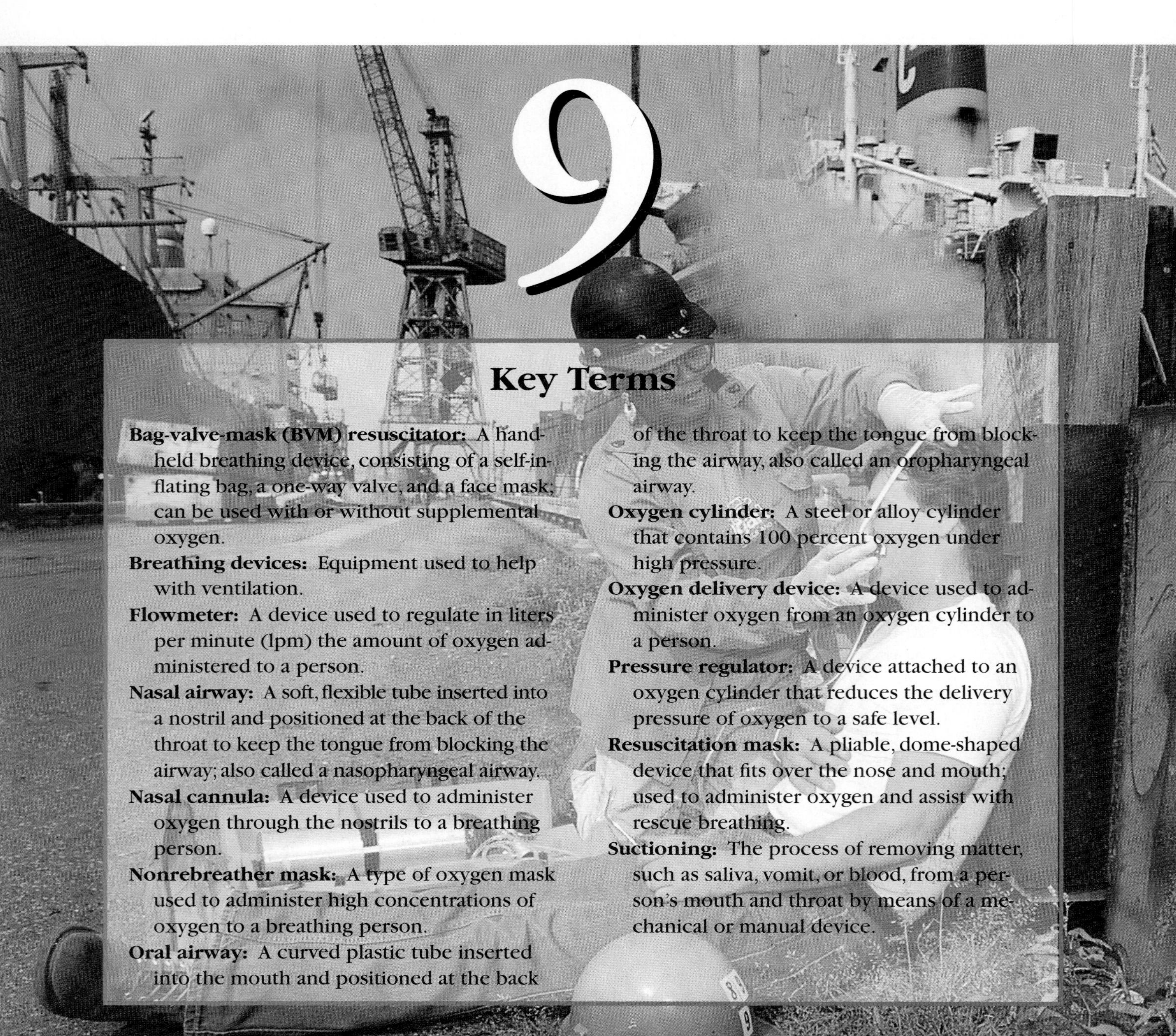

Key Terms

Bag-valve-mask (BVM) resuscitator: A hand-held breathing device, consisting of a self-inflating bag, a one-way valve, and a face mask; can be used with or without supplemental oxygen.

Breathing devices: Equipment used to help with ventilation.

Flowmeter: A device used to regulate in liters per minute (lpm) the amount of oxygen administered to a person.

Nasal airway: A soft, flexible tube inserted into a nostril and positioned at the back of the throat to keep the tongue from blocking the airway; also called a nasopharyngeal airway.

Nasal cannula: A device used to administer oxygen through the nostrils to a breathing person.

Nonrebreather mask: A type of oxygen mask used to administer high concentrations of oxygen to a breathing person.

Oral airway: A curved plastic tube inserted into the mouth and positioned at the back of the throat to keep the tongue from blocking the airway, also called an oropharyngeal airway.

Oxygen cylinder: A steel or alloy cylinder that contains 100 percent oxygen under high pressure.

Oxygen delivery device: A device used to administer oxygen from an oxygen cylinder to a person.

Pressure regulator: A device attached to an oxygen cylinder that reduces the delivery pressure of oxygen to a safe level.

Resuscitation mask: A pliable, dome-shaped device that fits over the nose and mouth; used to administer oxygen and assist with rescue breathing.

Suctioning: The process of removing matter, such as saliva, vomit, or blood, from a person's mouth and throat by means of a mechanical or manual device.

◆ Knowledge Objectives ◆

After reading this chapter and completing the class activities, you should be able to —

- Describe how to measure and insert an oral (oropharyngeal) airway and a nasal (nasopharyngeal) airway.
- State the importance of having a suction unit ready for immediate use when providing emergency medical care.
- Describe the techniques of suctioning.
- Describe how to use a barrier shield device when providing breaths.
- Describe how to ventilate a victim with a resuscitation mask and bag-valve-mask device.
- *Identify when it is appropriate to administer supplemental oxygen.
- *Describe the steps required to administer supplemental oxygen.
- *List precautions to take when using supplemental oxygen.

* signifies an Enrichment section objective.

◆ Skill Objectives ◆

After reading this chapter and completing the class activities, you should be able to —

- Demonstrate how to measure and insert an oral (oropharyngeal) and nasal (nasopharyngeal) airway.
- Demonstrate the techniques of suctioning.
- Demonstrate how to ventilate a victim with a resuscitation mask and a bag-valve-mask.
- *Demonstrate how to prepare the equipment and administer supplemental oxygen to a breathing and nonbreathing victim.
- Make appropriate decisions about care when given an example of an emergency in which a person is having difficulty breathing.

1. A 45-year-old man is experiencing chest pain. He states that it started about 30 minutes ago as a mild, squeezing sensation. Now the pain is severe and he is gasping for breath. You recognize that these signs and symptoms suggest a serious condition. You complete an initial assessment, physical exam, and SAMPLE history. While waiting for an ambulance to arrive, you help him get into the most comfortable position, keep him from getting chilled or overheated, and ask him to remain still. You open a nearby window to circulate fresh air into the stuffy room. Is there anything else that you could do to help?

2. You are called to assist a co-worker with an unknown medical emergency. You find a 60-year-old, unconscious woman who has vomited and is not breathing. You know what must be done, but the sight of vomit causes you to hesitate. You overcome your reluctance, sweep out her mouth, and begin mouth-to-mouth breathing. Is there anything that could have been used to make this incident less difficult?

◆ INTRODUCTION

What do both of these situations have in common? Both are examples of situations in which ***breathing devices,*** used to help with **ventilation,** the process of providing air to a victim's lungs, would have been desirable and could have enhanced the care you were providing. Although most of the care you give will not require the use of breathing devices, in some situations, they can be used effectively as part of your care. Breathing devices include those used to—

- Help clear and maintain an open airway.
- Ventilate a victim.
- Supply supplemental oxygen.

These devices include suction equipment, oral and nasal airways, barrier shields, resuscitation masks, bag-valve-masks, and supplemental oxygen. Such devices can contribute significantly to the survival and recovery of a seriously ill or injured person.

In this chapter, you learn when and how to use various breathing devices to increase the effectiveness of the care you give a person who is injured or has suddenly become ill.

◆ BREATHING DEVICES

Many different breathing devices are commonly used in the out-of-hospital setting. Which breathing aids are available will depend on your local standards and protocols. This chapter focuses on those breathing devices that you are likely to have immediately available or be asked to assist with in providing care. It is important to remember that *you should not delay care because a specific breathing device is not available.* Instead, you should start basic care, adding any breathing devices when they become available. *Whenever you use any breathing device to ventilate a victim, always wear gloves.*

In general, breathing devices provide several advantages. They can help you—

- Clear and maintain an open airway.
- Perform rescue breathing.
- Increase the oxygen concentration in a person's bloodstream.
- Limit the potential for disease transmission.

With all breathing devices, give the same number of breaths as you would for mouth-to-mouth rescue breathing.

Suctioning

Sometimes injury or sudden illness results in foreign matter, such as mucus, water, or blood, collecting in a victim's airway. One method of clearing the airway is to roll the person onto his or her side and sweep the mouth with gloved fingers. A more effective method is to suction the airway clear. ***Suctioning*** is the process of removing foreign matter by means of a mechanical or manual device. A variety of manual and mechanical devices are used to suction the airway.

Manual suction devices are lightweight, compact, and relatively inexpensive (Fig. 9-1, *A*). Mechanical suction devices use either battery-powered pumps or oxygen-powered aspirators and are normally found on ambulances (Fig. 9-1, *B*). Attached to the end of any suction device is a **suction tip**. These come in various sizes and shapes. Some are rigid and others flexible.

Whether you are using a manual or mechanical suction device, perform these six steps:

1. Turn the victim's head to one side. (If you suspect spinal injury, roll the victim's body onto one side, keeping the neck and body from twisting.)
2. Open the victim's mouth.
3. Sweep large debris out of the mouth with your finger before suctioning.
4. Measure the distance of insertion from the victim's earlobe to the corner of the mouth (Fig. 9-2, *A*). You measure to prevent inserting the device past the back of the mouth.

A 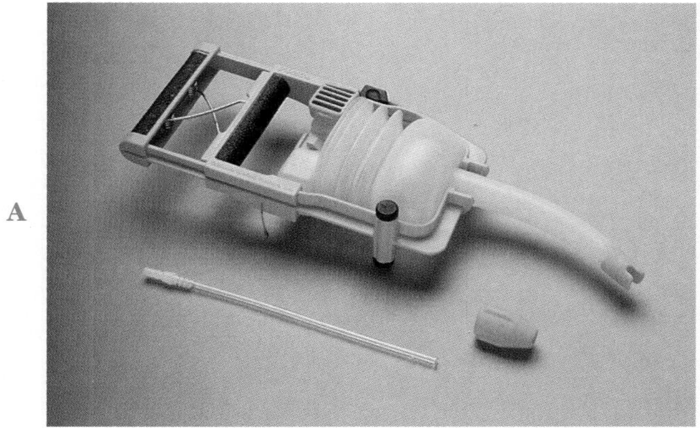 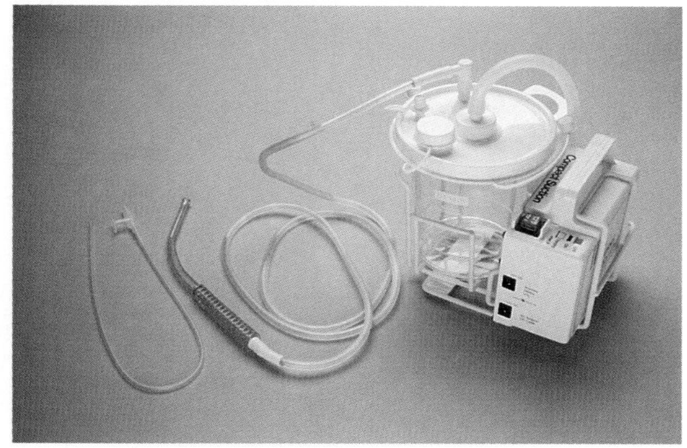 B

Figure 9-1 **A**, Manual suction devices are lightweight and compact. **B**, Mechanical suction devices use either a battery-powered pump or an oxygen-powered aspirator.

5. Insert the suction tip into the back of the mouth (Fig. 9-2, *B*).
6. Suction for no more than 15 seconds at a time as you remove the tip from the victim's mouth.

Airways

As you may remember from Chapter 8, the tongue is the most common cause of airway obstruction in an unconscious person. Keeping the tongue from blocking the air passage is a high priority. Breathing devices known as oral and nasal airways can help you accomplish this task. As their names imply, one type of airway is inserted into the mouth and the other is inserted into the nose.

An ***oral (oropharyngeal) airway*** is inserted into the mouth of an unconscious victim who does not have a gag reflex. A ***nasal (nasopharyngeal) airway*** is inserted into a nostril and may be used on responsive victims who need help to keep the tongue from obstructing the airway. When properly positioned, either of these airways keep the tongue out of the back of the throat, thereby keeping the airway open. An improperly placed airway device can compress the tongue into the back of the throat, further blocking the airway.

Airways come in a variety of sizes (Fig. 9-3, *A-B*). The curved design fits the natural contour of the mouth, nose, and throat. Once you have positioned the device, you can use a resuscitation mask or bag-valve-mask resuscitator, de-

A 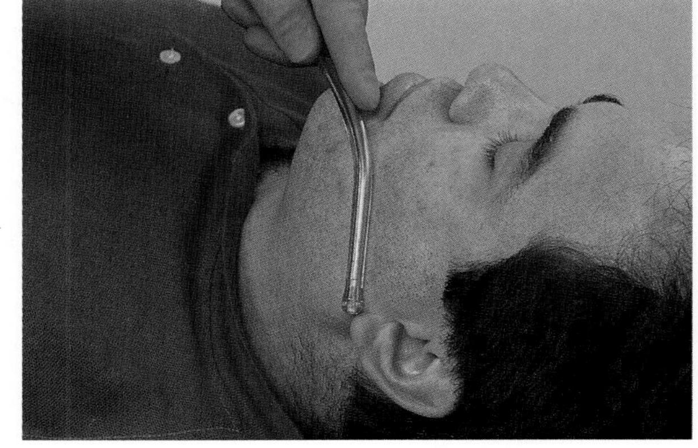 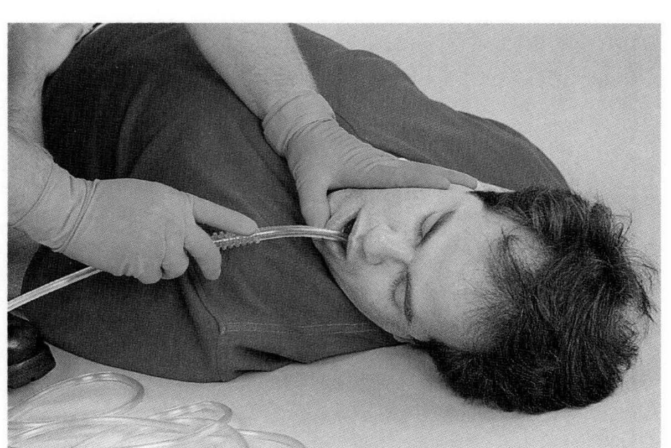 B

Figure 9-2 **A**, Measure the distance of insertion from the victim's earlobe to the corner of the mouth. **B**, Insert the suction tip into the back of the mouth.

A 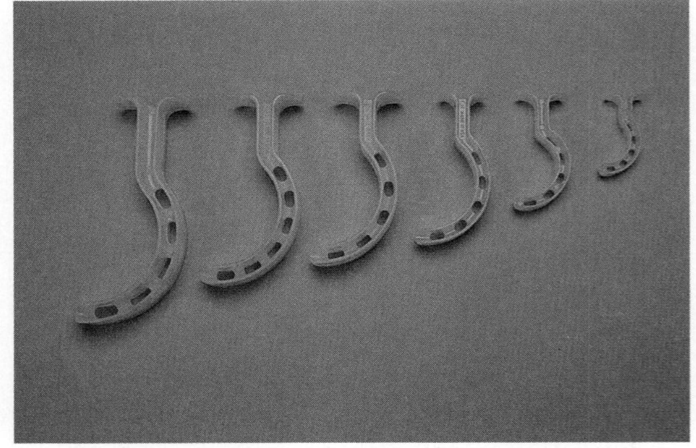 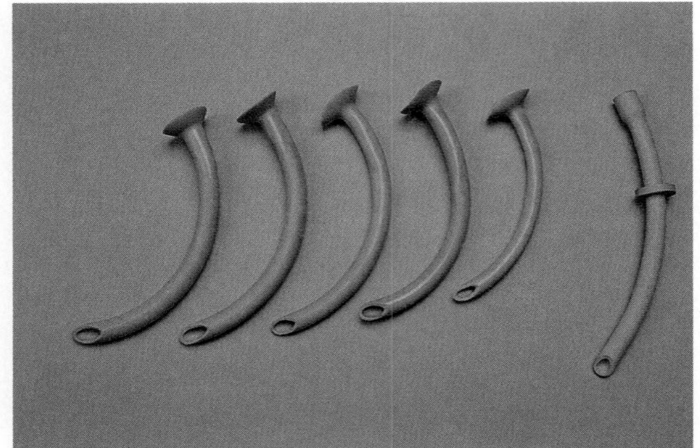 B

Figure 9-3 **A,** Oral airways come in a variety of sizes. **B,** Nasal Airways

scribed later in this chapter, to ventilate a nonbreathing person.

Inserting an Oral Airway

When preparing to insert an oral airway, first be sure the victim is unconscious. Next, select the proper size of airway. Measure the device on the victim to see that it extends from the victim's earlobe to the corner of the mouth (Fig. 9-4). Grasp the victim's lower jaw and tongue and lift upward. With the victim's jaw raised, insert the oral airway with the curved end (tip) along the roof of the mouth (Fig. 9-5, *A*). As the tip of the device approaches the back of the throat, resistance will be felt. Rotate it a half turn to drop it into the back of the victim's throat (Fig. 9-5, *B*). The oral airway should drop into the throat without resistance. The flange end should rest on the victim's lips (Fig. 9-5, *C*). If the victim begins gagging as the device is positioned in the back of the throat, remove the device.

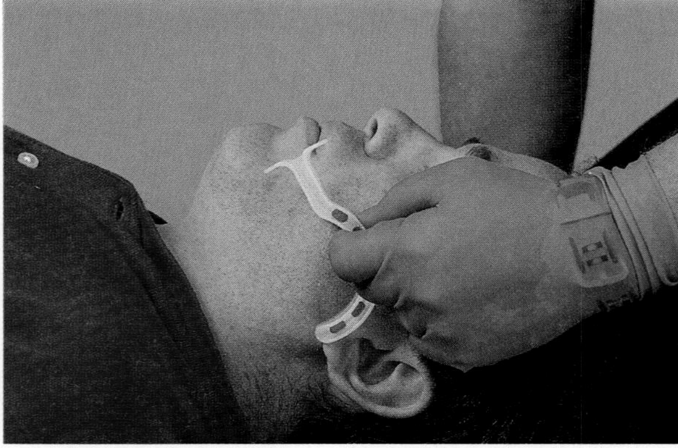

Figure 9-4 Measure the oral airway to see that it extends from the victim's earlobe to the corner of the mouth.

Inserting a Nasal Airway

When using a nasal airway, select an airway of the proper size. Measure the device on the victim to see that it extends from the victim's earlobe to the tip of the nose (Fig. 9-6). Also make sure that the diameter of the nasal airway is not larger than the diameter of the nostril. Lubricate the airway with a water-soluble lubricant. Insert the nasal airway into a nostril, with the bevel toward the **septum** (the wall of tissue that separates the nostrils) (Fig. 9-7, *A*). Advance the airway gently, straight in, not upward, until the flange rests on the nose (Fig. 9-7, *B*). If you feel even minor resistance, do not force the airway. If you cannot get the airway to pass easily, remove it and try the other nostril. Unlike the oral airway, the nasal airway does not cause the victim to gag. Do not use a nasal airway on a victim with a suspected skull fracture.

Barrier Shields

One of the most readily available, breathing devices for first responders is a barrier shield.

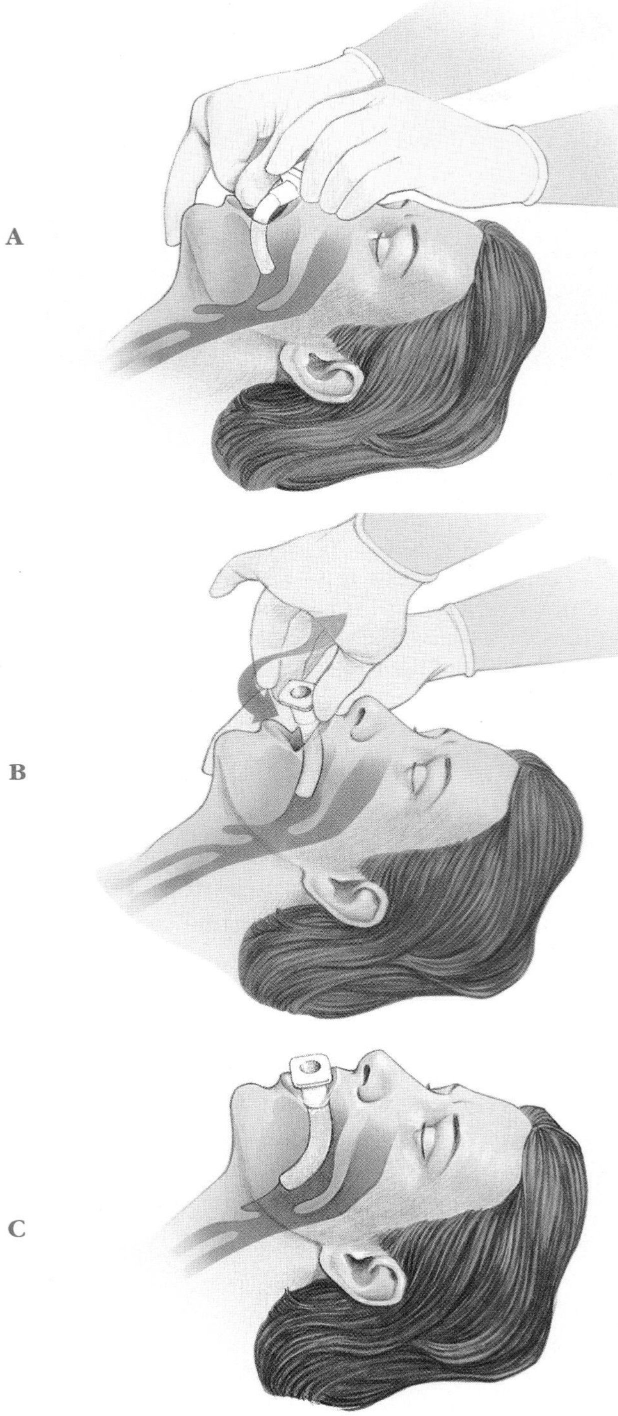

Figure 9-5 **A**, Open the victim's airway using the head-tilt/chin-lift. Insert the oral airway with the curved end along the roof of the mouth. **B**, As the device approaches the back of the throat, rotate it a half turn. **C**, The device should drop into the throat without resistance. The flange end rests on the victim's lower lip.

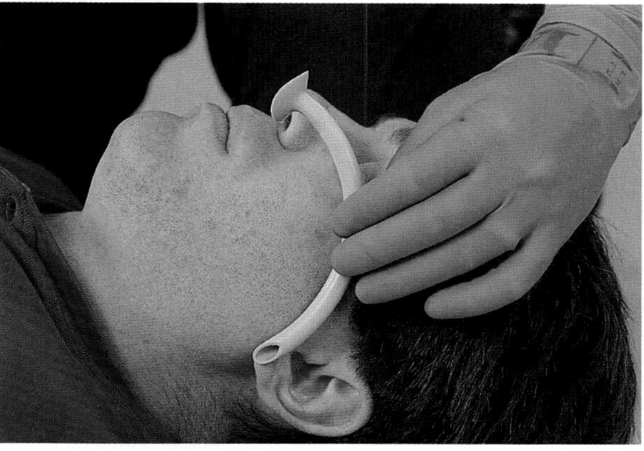

Figure 9-6 Measure the nasal airway on the victim to see that it extends from the victim's earlobe to the tip of the nose.

These lightweight devices have one-way valves that reduce the risk of disease transmission during rescue breathing. Barrier shields have a plastic cover that lies across the victim's face. These devices enable you to ventilate, or give air to, the victim in the same way as in mouth-to-mouth rescue breathing (Fig. 9-8).

Resuscitation Masks

Resuscitation masks are pliable, dome-shaped devices that fit over a person's mouth and nose, aiding **ventilation.** Several types of resuscitation masks are available, varying in size, shape, and features (Fig. 9-9).

Resuscitation masks offer you several advantages. These include —

- Increasing the flow of air to the lungs by allowing air to travel through a person's mouth and nose at the same time.
- Providing an adequate seal for giving breaths, even when a person has facial injuries.
- Providing an effective and easily accessible alternative to other methods of ventilation, such as mouth-to-mouth or mouth-to-nose breathing or bag-valve-mask resuscitation.
- Allowing easy delivery of supplemental oxygen to either a breathing or a nonbreathing person.

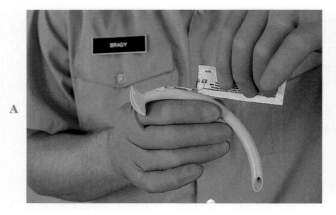

A

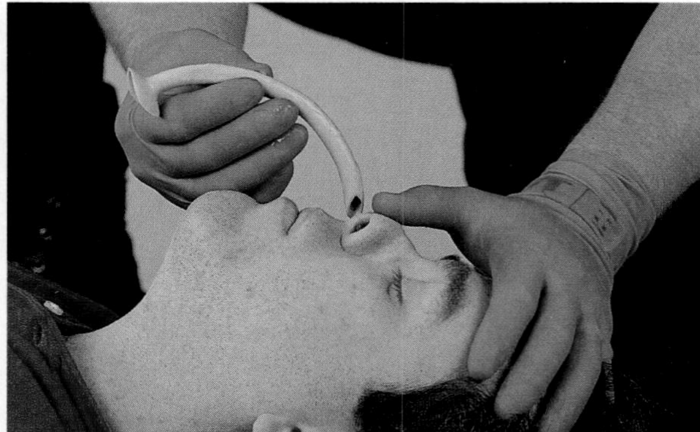

B

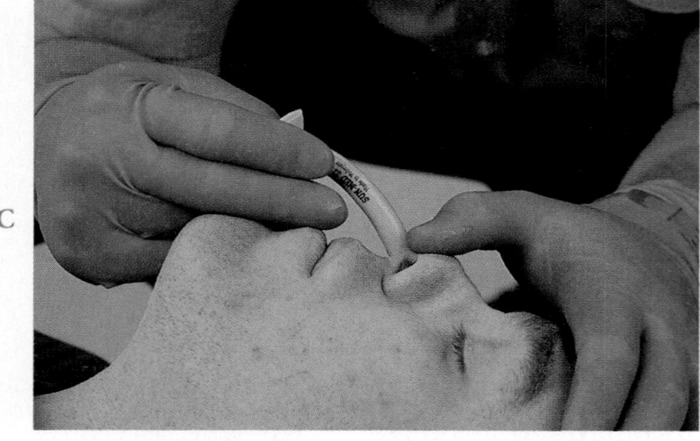

C

Figure 9-7 **A,** Lubricate the nasal airway with a water-soluble lubricant. **B,** Insert the nasal airway into the nostril with the bevel toward the victim's septum. **C,** Advance the airway gently, straight in, not upward, until the flange rests on the nose.

- Reducing the possibility of disease transmission by providing a barrier between the rescuer and the victim.

Selecting a Resuscitation Mask

For a resuscitation mask to be most effective, it should meet the following criteria:

- Be made of a transparent, pliable material that allows you to make a tight seal on the person's face when you perform rescue breathing or supply supplemental oxygen
- Have a one-way valve for preventing the victim's exhaled air from contacting the rescuer
- Have a standard 15-mm or 22-mm coupling assembly (the diameter of the opening that receives the one-way valve)
- Have an inlet for the delivery of supplemental oxygen
- Work well under a variety of environmental conditions, such as extreme heat or cold
- Be easy to assemble, use, and clean if not disposable

Figure 9-10 shows the features of an effective resuscitation mask.

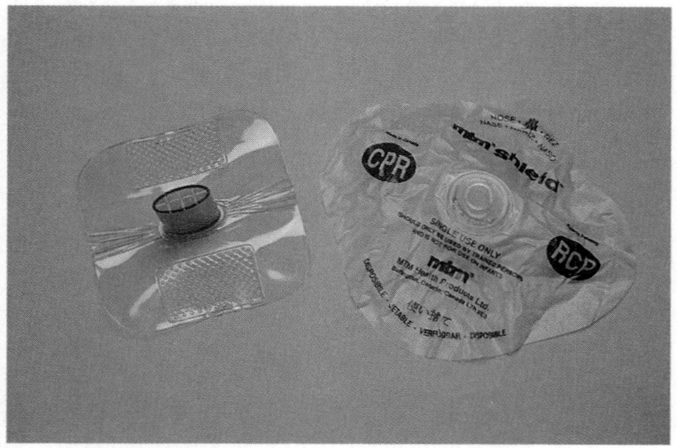

Figure 9-8 Barrier Shields

Using a Resuscitation Mask

When using a resuscitation mask, begin by attaching the one-way valve to the mask. Next, place the mask so that it covers the person's mouth and nose. Position one rim of the mask

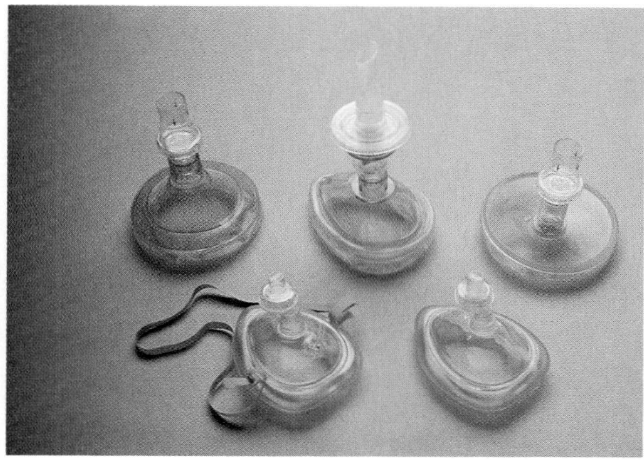

Figure 9-9 Resuscitation masks vary in size, shape, and features.

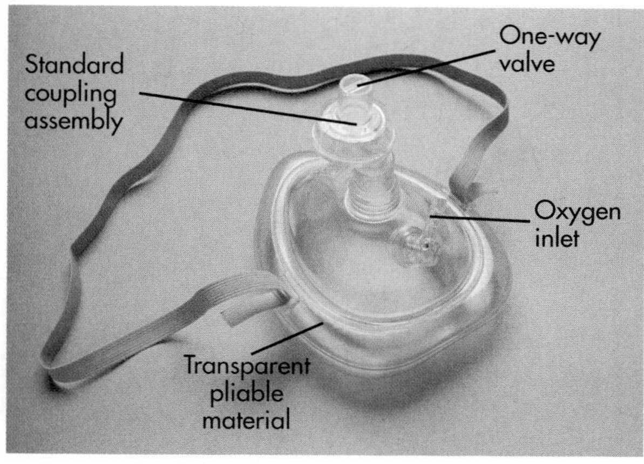

Figure 9-10 A resuscitation mask should meet specific criteria.

between the lower lip and chin. The opposite end of the mask should cover the nose. Figure 9-11, *A-B* shows how to assemble and position the resuscitation mask.

When you use a resuscitation mask to give rescue breathing, you must maintain a good seal to prevent air from leaking at the edges of the mask. Use both hands to hold the mask in place and to maintain an open airway. You do this by following three steps. They involve—

1. Tilting the person's head back.
2. Lifting the jaw upward.
3. Keeping the person's mouth open.

Figure 9-12, *A-B* shows two methods for using a resuscitation mask.

If you suspect the victim has a head, neck, or back injury, use the two-handed jaw-thrust technique without head tilt, described in Chapter 8. This technique can also be used with a resuscitation mask (Fig. 9-13). However, because the success of the two-handed jaw thrust technique depends on one's hand size and strength, some people will find it difficult to perform a two-handed jaw thrust using a resuscitation mask.

Bag-Valve-Mask Resuscitators

There may be times when you will have a bag-valve-mask resuscitator available or be asked to assist with one. A ***bag-valve-mask (BVM) re-***

A

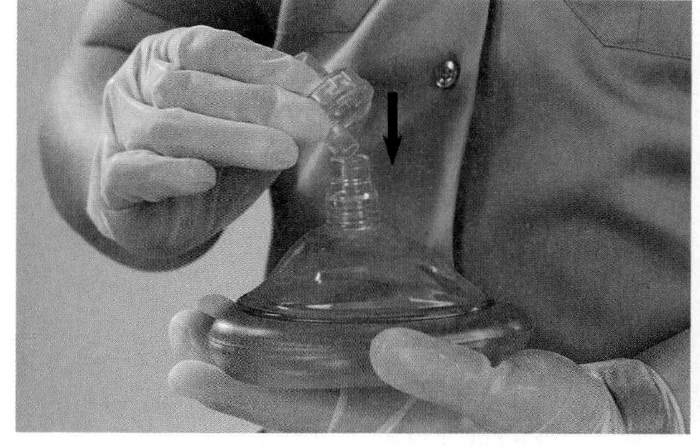

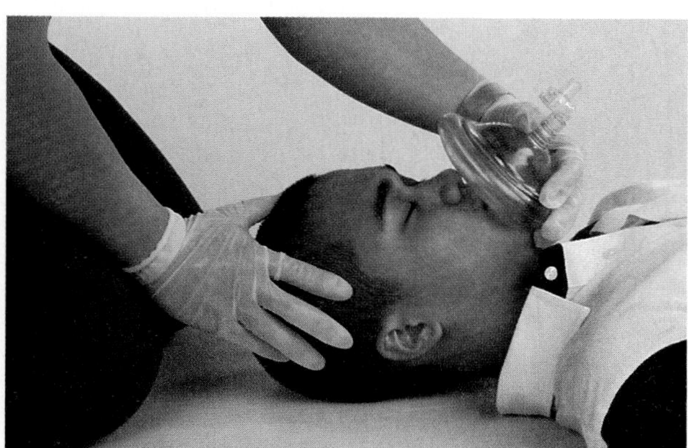

B

Figure 9-11 To use a resuscitation mask, **A,** begin by attaching the one-way valve to the mask. **B,** Position the mask to cover the mouth and nose.

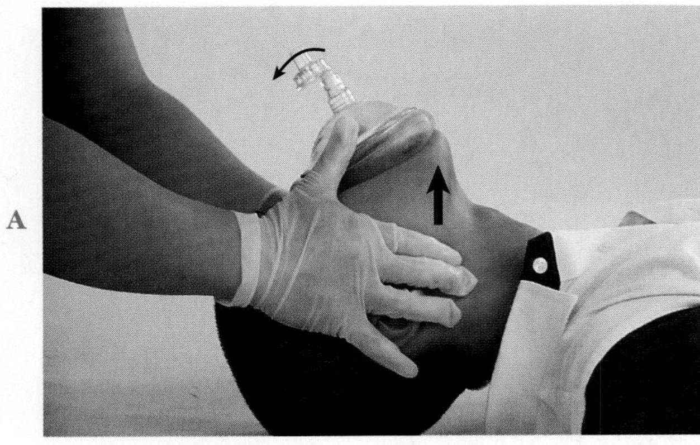

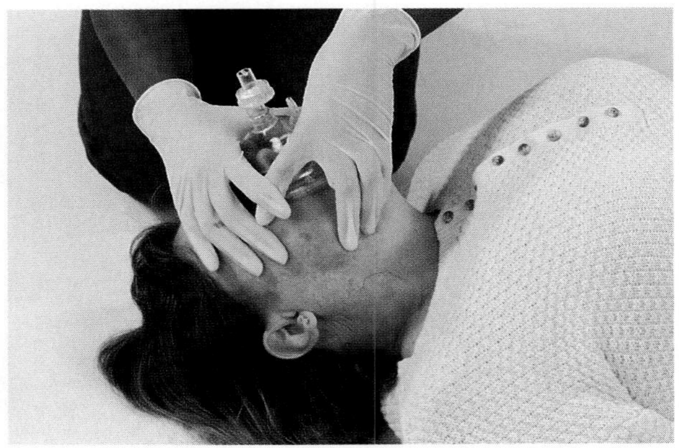

Figure 9-12 **A,** Tilt the head back and lift the jaw to open the airway. **B,** Holding the mask from the side is an alternative method for using a resuscitation mask, for example, during one-rescuer CPR.

suscitator is a hand-held device, like the resuscitation mask, primarily used to give breaths to a nonbreathing person. It is also used to assist breathing of a person who is in respiratory distress.

The device has three main components: a bag, a valve, and a mask. The bag is self-inflating. Once compressed, it reinflates automatically. The one-way valve allows air to move from the bag to the victim but prevents the victim's exhaled air from entering the bag. The mask is similar to the resuscitation mask described earlier in this chapter. An oxygen reservoir bag should be attached to the BVM when supplemental oxygen is administered (Fig. 9-14).

The principle of the BVM is simple. By placing the mask on the victim's face and squeezing the bag, you open the one-way valve, forcing air into the victim's lungs. When you release the bag, the valve closes and air from the atmosphere refills the bag. At approximately the same time, the victim exhales. This exhaled air is diverted into the atmosphere through the closed one-way valve.

Using a Bag-Valve-Mask Resuscitator

In the hands of a well-practiced rescuer, the BVM resuscitator is effective. But studies have shown that without consistent practice, single rescuers have a difficult time maintaining a

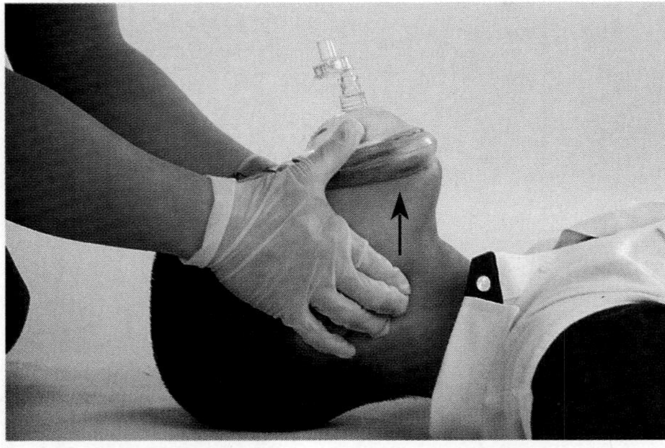

Figure 9-13 If you suspect a head or spine injury, lift the jaw but do not tilt the head back.

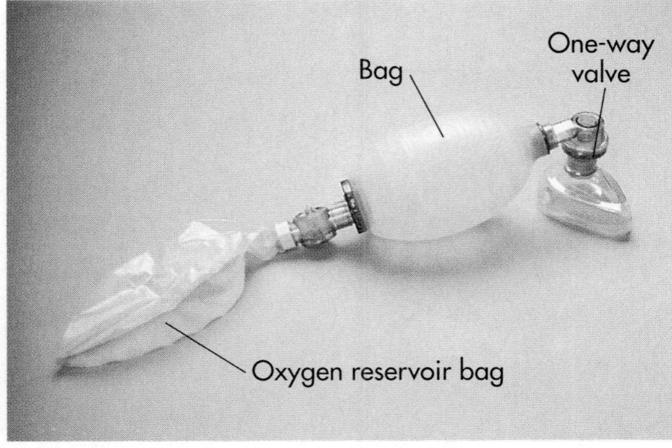

Figure 9-14 A bag-valve-mask (BVM) resuscitator consists of a bag, valve, and mask. An oxygen reservoir bag should be attached at the end of the bag when delivering supplemental oxygen.

Oxygen-Powered Resuscitators

Oxygen-powered resuscitators, commonly called demand valves, have been controversial for several years. The points of controversy are whether these devices are as easy to use and whether they are as safe as other oxygen delivery devices. As the name *demand* valve implies, the victim can get oxygen on demand automatically.

A demand valve works in much the same way as a bag-valve-mask (BVM) resuscitator. However, instead of using a self-inflating bag as the ventilation source, the demand valve uses pressurized oxygen. The demand valve consists of a mask, a one-way valve, and an oxygen source. The mask is basically the same as that of the BVM. The one-way valve is designed to open and allow oxygen to flow to the breathing victim when the victim inhales. The rescuer must depress a button to force oxygen into the lungs of a nonbreathing person. The use of the demand valve to ventilate a nonbreathing person is commonly called *positive pressure resuscitation.*

There are both advantages and disadvantages to using a demand valve. Advantages include delivery of a high concentration of oxygen (approaching 100 percent), ease of use, and protection from disease transmission. Also, like the resuscitation mask and BVM, the demand valve can deliver oxygen to either breathing or nonbreathing victims.

The disadvantages include higher cost compared with other devices, requirement of a constant source of oxygen, and rapid depletion of a cylinder. In addition, because the oxygen is delivered under higher pressure, complications from overventilation have been reported. These reports resulted in manufacturers designing demand valves that restricted oxygen flow and installing relief valves to eliminate overinflation when ventilating nonbreathing victims. However, the new designs created another problem. This new, restricted-flow demand valve did not always meet the needs of a person in severe respiratory distress. In addition, even with these restrictions, the device should not be used to ventilate nonbreathing children or infants because of the possibility that the device will overinflate the victim.

Some EMS systems have stopped using demand valves. Others use the restricted demand valve for nonbreathing victims, the traditional demand valve for breathing victims, and the newest demand valve that can be used for both breathing and nonbreathing victims.

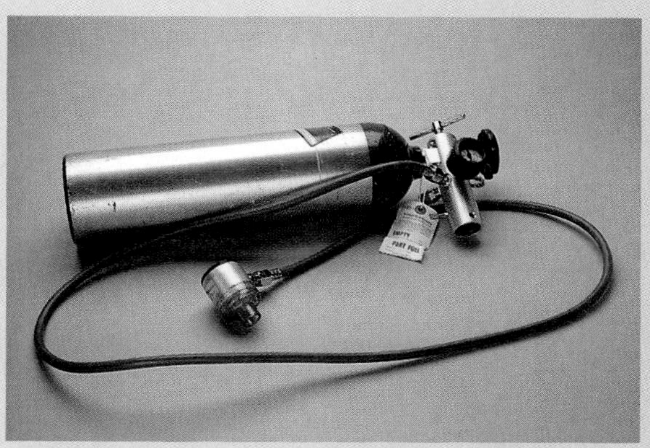

Oxygen-Powered Resuscitator

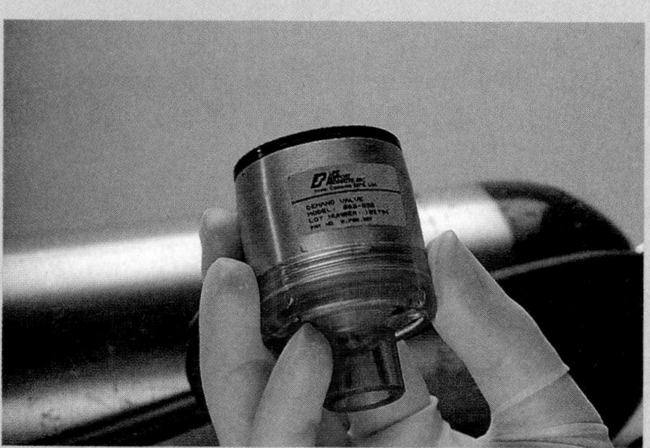

Restricted-Flow Demand Valve

A

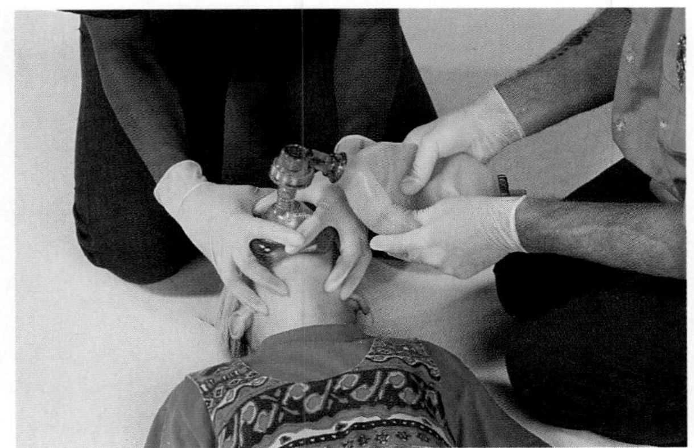

B

Figure 9-15 **A,** Position the mask over the victim's mouth and nose. Hold it in place as you would a resuscitation mask. **B,** Second rescuer squeezes the bag slowly until the chest rises.

tight enough seal and also maintaining an open airway. For this reason, it is best if a BVM is used by two rescuers when possible.

When two rescuers are using a BVM, one rescuer positions the mask and opens the victim's airway. This is done in the same way as previously described for a resuscitation mask. While the first rescuer maintains a tight seal with the mask on the victim's face (Fig. 9-15, *A*), the second rescuer provides ventilation by squeezing the bag until the victim's chest rises (Fig. 9-15, *B*). The bag should always be squeezed smoothly, not forcefully. This two-person technique is preferred because one rescuer can maintain an open airway and a tight mask seal while a second rescuer can provide ventilation.

If you must use a bag-valve-mask resuscitator by yourself, begin by assembling the bag, valve, and mask. Next, position the mask so that it covers the victim's mouth and nose in the same way previously described for a resuscitation mask. Open the airway. With one hand, hold the mask in place by making a C-clamp with your index finger and thumb around the mask. Maintain an open airway, using your other fingers to lift the jaw. You can use your knees to help hold the victim's head in this tilted position.

With one hand, press down on the mask to maintain a tight seal and help open the victim's mouth. With your other hand, squeeze the bag slowly until the victim's chest rises (Fig. 9-16). People with small hands or poor grip strength may find it necessary to compress the bag against their thigh to adequately ventilate the victim.

Advantages and Disadvantages

Using the bag-valve-mask resuscitator has distinct advantages and disadvantages.

Advantages:

- It delivers a higher concentration of oxygen than that delivered during mouth-to-mouth or mouth-to-mask rescue breathing.
- It limits the potential for disease transmission.
- It is very effective when used by two rescuers.

Disadvantages:

- It is a difficult skill for one person to master.

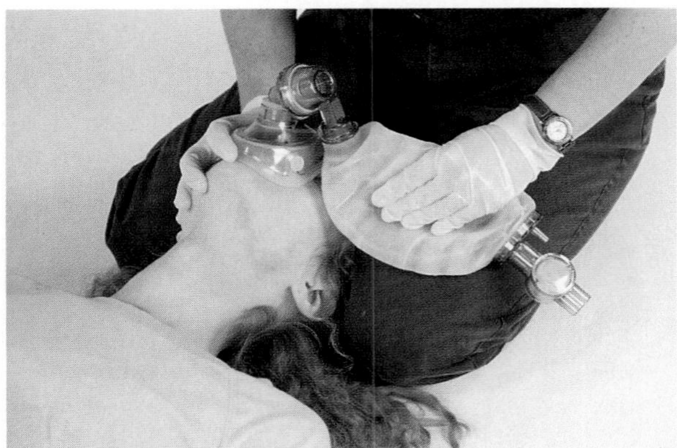

Figure 9-16 If you are alone and need to use a BVM, it may help you to compress the bag against the thigh.

- Without regular practice, you cannot stay proficient.
- It may take longer to assemble than other breathing devices.
- It is not a device readily available to you.

◆ SUMMARY

Breathing devices can make the emergency care you provide safer, easier, and more effective. Suction equipment helps clear the airway of substances, such as water, blood, saliva, or vomit. Always help maintain an open airway by keeping the tongue away from the back of the throat. The use of supplemental oxygen can relieve pain and breathing discomfort. Barrier shields, resuscitation masks, and BVMs are the most appropriate devices for first responders to use when ventilating a victim. They can significantly increase the oxygen concentration that an ill or injured person needs, help ventilate a nonbreathing person, and reduce the likelihood of disease transmission.

Breathing devices, such as the ones discussed in this chapter, are appropriate for almost all types of injury or illness in which breathing may be impaired. Knowing how to use these devices will enable you to provide more effective care until advanced medical personnel arrive.

Use the activities in Unit 9 of the workbook to help you review the material in this chapter.

You Are the Responder

1. A 40-year-old man is experiencing chest pain and difficulty breathing. He is slightly cyanotic (skin has a bluish color), gasping for air, and breathing 26 times per minute. What breathing devices could you use to help this person?
2. The same person collapses, vomits, and stops breathing. How would you change your care for this person?

ENRICHMENT

◆ SUPPLEMENTAL OXYGEN

As you may recall, the normal concentration of oxygen in the air is approximately 21 percent. Under normal conditions, this is more than enough oxygen to sustain life. However, when serious injury or sudden illness occurs, the body does not function properly and can benefit from additional, or supplemental, oxygen. Without adequate oxygen, hypoxia will result. **Hypoxia** is a condition in which insufficient oxygen reaches the cells. When hypoxia occurs, it causes signs and symptoms that include increased breathing and heart rates, cyanosis, changes in consciousness, restlessness, and chest pain.

For example, a person experiencing difficulty breathing and chest pain because of a heart attack or angina can have this pain and breathing discomfort reduced by the delivery of additional oxygen. **Supplemental oxygen** delivered to the victim's lungs can help meet the increased demand for oxygen for all body tissues.

If a heart attack victim suddenly suffers cardiac arrest, then you must use rescue breathing to force air into the victim's lungs. Whether you perform rescue breathing using the mouth-to-mouth or mouth-to-mask method, the oxygen concentration you deliver to the victim is only 16 percent. This is adequate to sustain life in a healthy person. But, since chest compressions only circulate one-third normal blood flow under the best of conditions, body tissues are receiving only the bare minimum of oxygen required for short-term survival.

Using a bag-valve-mask resuscitator alone only improves this situation slightly, since it delivers atmospheric air (21 percent oxygen). A higher oxygen concentration helps to counter the effects of severe illness or injury to the body. Administering supplemental oxygen allows a substantially higher oxygen concentration, in some cases nearly 100 percent, to be delivered to the person (Fig. 9-17).

To deliver supplemental oxygen, you must have—

- An oxygen cylinder.
- A pressure regulator with flowmeter.
- A delivery device.

Figure 9-18 shows an oxygen delivery system.

Oxygen Cylinders

It is easy to recognize an ***oxygen cylinder*** because of its distinctive green color and yellow diamond marking that says *oxidizer.* These cylinders are made of steel or an alloy. Depending on their size, cylinders used in the out-of-hospital setting can hold between 350 and 625 liters of oxygen. These cylinders have internal pressures of approximately 2000 pounds per square inch (psi).

Pressure Regulators

The pressure inside the oxygen cylinder is far too great for a person to simply open the cylinder and administer the oxygen. Instead, a device must be attached to the cylinder to reduce the delivery pressure of the oxygen to a safe level. This regulating device is called a ***pressure regulator***. The pressure regulator reduces the pressure from approximately 2000 psi inside the cylinder to less than 70 psi.

A pressure regulator has a gauge that indicates how much pressure is in the cylinder. By checking the gauge, you can determine if a cylinder is full (2000 psi), nearly empty (200 psi), or somewhere in between.

A pressure regulator has three metal prongs that fit into the valve at the top of the oxygen

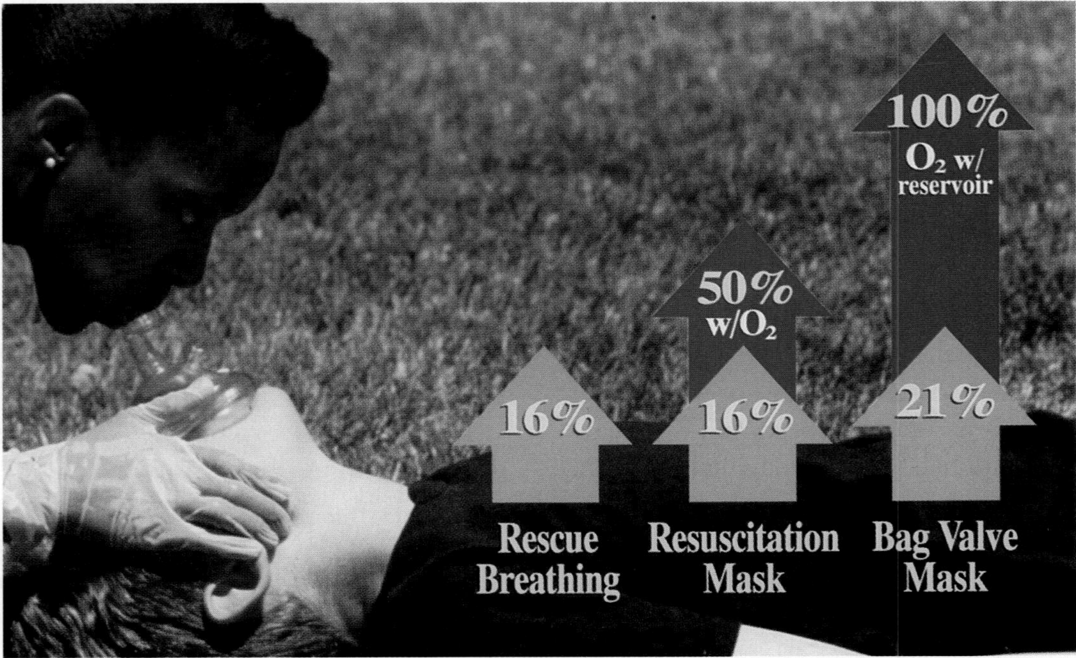

Figure 9-17 Breathing devices and supplemental oxygen can greatly increase the concentration of oxygen that a victim receives.

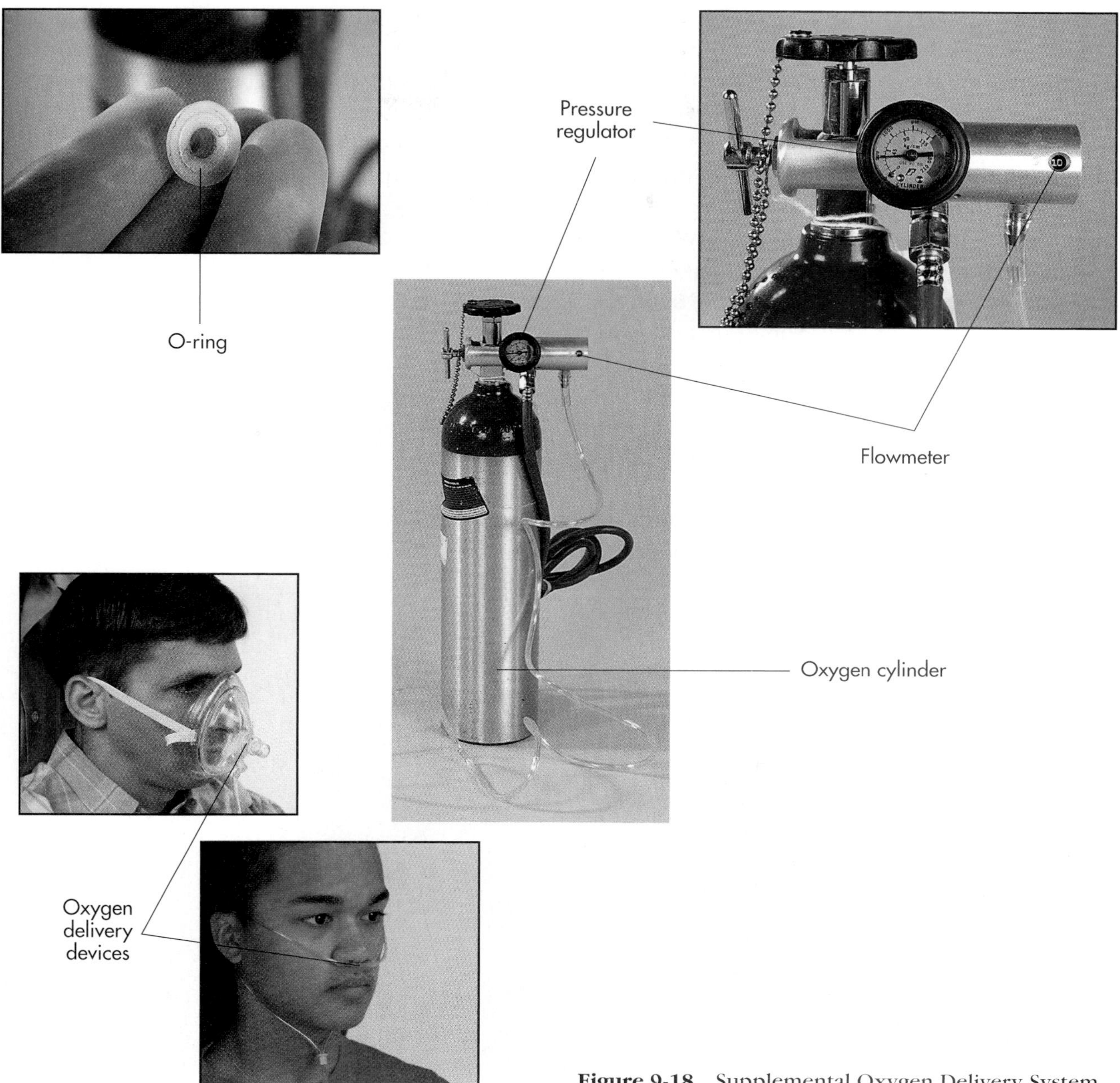

Figure 9-18 Supplemental Oxygen Delivery System

cylinder. The largest of these prongs must have a doughnut-shaped gasket, commonly called an O-ring, attached. This gasket provides a tight seal between the oxygen cylinder and the pressure regulator.

Flowmeter

A ***flowmeter*** controls the amount of oxygen administered in liters per minute (lpm). Flowmeters normally deliver from 1 to 15 lpm, but some of the newer flowmeters can deliver as much as 25 lpm.

Oxygen Delivery Devices

Some ***oxygen delivery devices*** can deliver oxygen to breathing victims only or nonbreathing victims only. Two devices, the resuscitation mask and the BVM, can deliver oxygen to both. For this reason, these devices are the most appropriate for you to use. Regardless of the device being used, a section of tubing is attached to the device at one end and to the flowmeter at the other end to create an oxygen-enriched environment for the victim.

A resuscitation mask is capable of delivering approximately 50 percent oxygen to a breathing person when the oxygen is delivered at 6 or more lpm. This is substantially higher than the normal 21 percent that the victim is getting from the atmosphere. Some resuscitation masks have elastic straps attached to the mask. The elastic strap can be placed over the victim's head and tightened to help keep the mask securely in place (Fig. 9-19, *A*). If the mask does not have a strap, either you or the victim can hold it in place. When a resuscitation mask is used on a nonbreathing victim, it will deliver an oxygen concentration of approximately 35 percent. The oxygen concentration is reduced because oxygen mixes with your exhaled air as you perform mouth-to-mask rescue breathing.

The bag-valve-mask resuscitator with an oxygen reservoir is capable of supplying a minimum oxygen concentration of 90 percent when used at 15 or more lpm. The BVM can be held against the victim's face, allowing a breathing victim to inhale the supplemental oxygen (Fig. 9-19, *B*). A victim breathing at a rate of less than 10 breaths per minute or more than 30 per minute should have his or her breathing assisted. You assist breathing by squeezing the bag as the victim breathes.

Some devices, such as the nasal cannula, can be used to administer oxygen only to breathing victims. A ***nasal cannula*** is a device that delivers oxygen through the victim's nostrils (Fig. 9-19, *C*). It is a plastic tube with two small prongs that are inserted into the nose. The use of a nasal cannula is limited, since it is normally

A

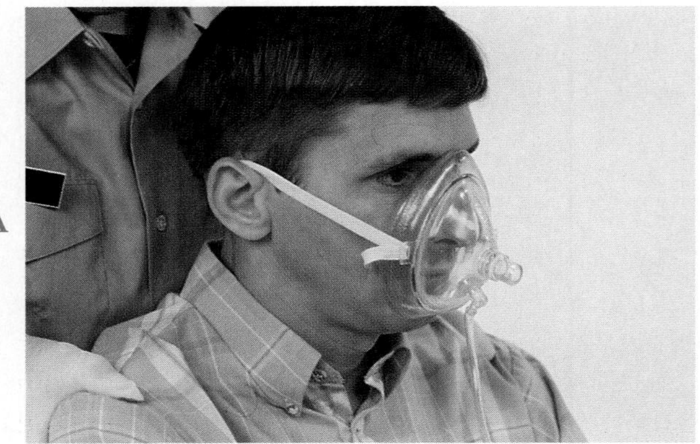

B

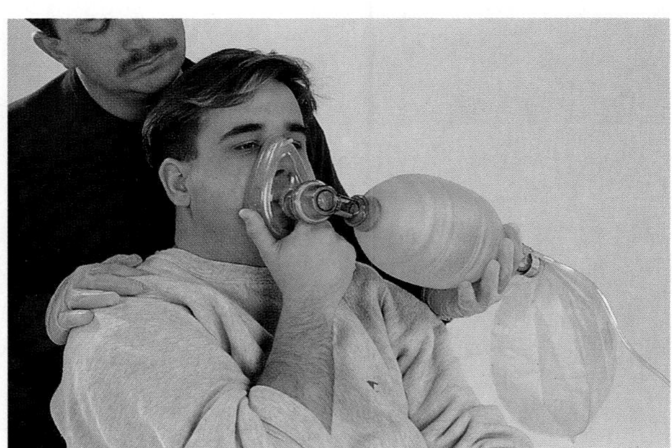

C

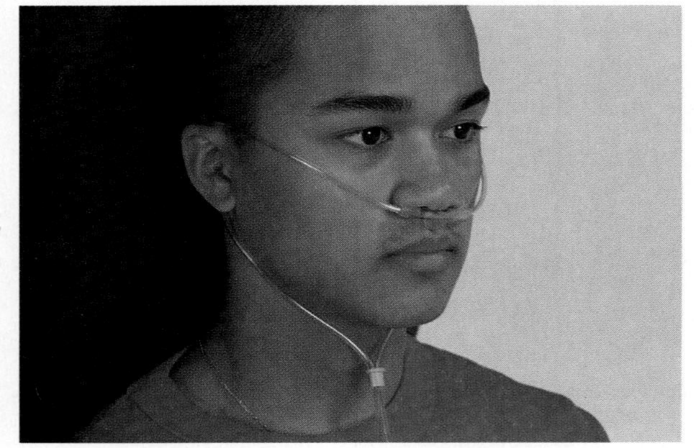

Figure 9-19 Common oxygen delivery devices include, **A,** a resuscitation mask, **B,** a BVM, and **C,** a nasal cannula.

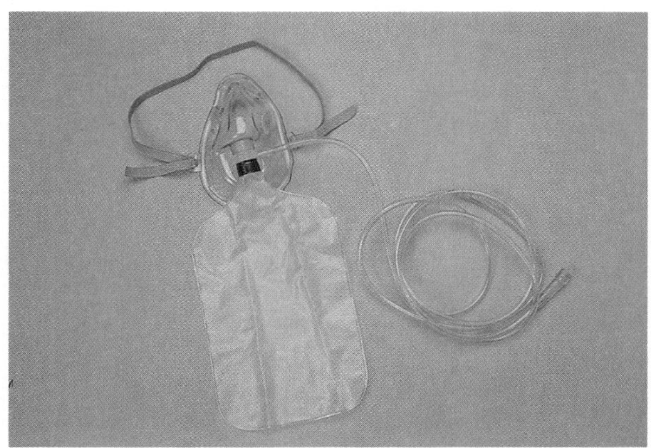

Figure 9-20 Nonrebreather Mask

used at a flow rate of 1 to 4 lpm. Under these conditions, it only delivers a peak oxygen concentration of approximately 36 percent. Flow rates above 4 lpm are not commonly used because they tend to quickly dry out mucous membranes, which can cause nosebleeds and headaches.

Because of its limitations, the nasal cannula is commonly used for people who cannot tolerate a mask or are using oxygen on a long-term basis and are not experiencing difficulty breathing. This device is not appropriate for victims experiencing serious respiratory distress, since they are generally breathing through the mouth and need a device that can supply a greater concentration of oxygen. In addition, the nasal cannula can be ineffective if the victim has a nasal airway obstruction, a nasal injury, or a bad cold causing blocked sinus passages. It should be used if the victim cannot tolerate a mask over his or her face.

A ***nonrebreather mask*** (Fig. 9-20) is the most effective method for delivering high concentrations of oxygen to conscious breathing victims in the out-of-hospital setting. The nonrebreather mask consists of a face mask with an attached oxygen reservoir bag and a one-way valve between the mask and bag to prevent the victim's exhaled air from mixing with the oxygen in the reservoir bag. As the victim breathes, he or she inhales oxygen from the bag. Flutter valves on the side of the mask allow exhaled air to escape freely. When using the nonrebreather mask with a high **flow rate** of oxygen, up to 90 percent oxygen can be delivered to the victim. The mask should not be used with flow rates lower than 10 lpm.

Before placing the nonrebreather mask on the victim, be sure that the oxygen regulator is securely attached to the regulator. Attach the oxygen tubing of the nonrebreather mask to the oxygen cylinder. Next, inflate the attached reservoir bag by placing your finger over the one-way valve in the mask. Apply the mask to the victim. The nonrebreather mask can feel restrictive to some victims, so be sure the victim can breathe comfortably with the mask on. As the victim begins to breathe, you will need to readjust the flow rate so that the reservoir bag does not completely collapse when the victim breathes in. The flow rate should be between 10 and 15 lpm. Nonrebreather masks come in different sizes for adults, children, and infants, so be sure you have selected the proper size for the victim you are caring for. A properly sized mask should fit snugly around the nose to ensure maximum

Table 9-1 Oxygen Delivery Devices

Device	Common flow rate	Oxygen concentration	Function
Nasal cannula	1-4 lpm	24-36 percent	Breathing victims only
Resuscitation mask	6 lpm	35-55 percent	Breathing and nonbreathing
Nonrebreather mask	10 lpm	90+ percent	Breathing victims only
Bag-valve-mask resuscitator	15 lpm	90 percent	Breathing and nonbreathing

A

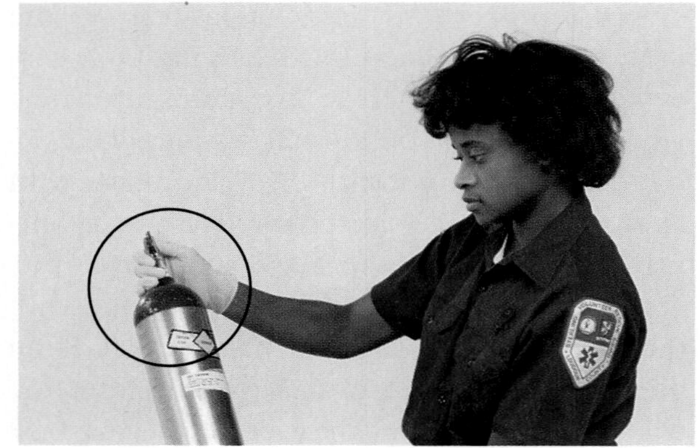

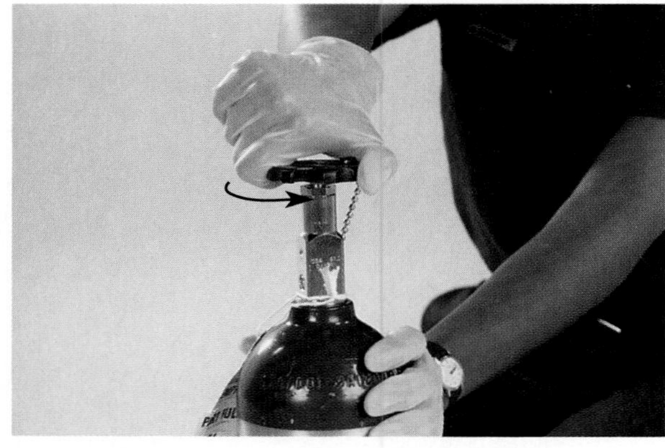

B

Figure 9-21 **A,** An oxygen cylinder is usually green, with a yellow diamond indicating oxygen. **B,** When preparing oxygen equipment, clear the cylinder valve by turning it counterclockwise.

A

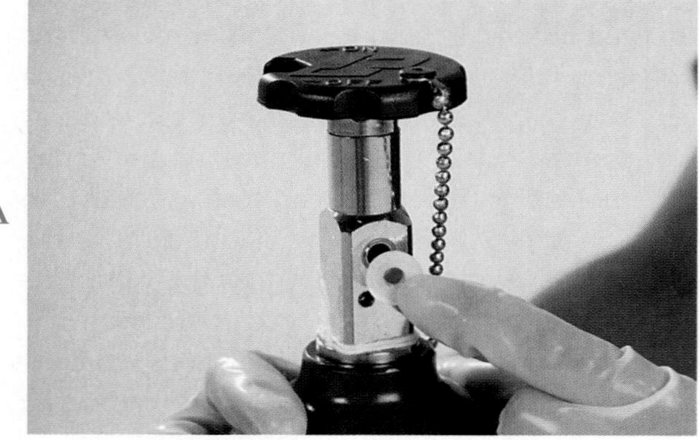

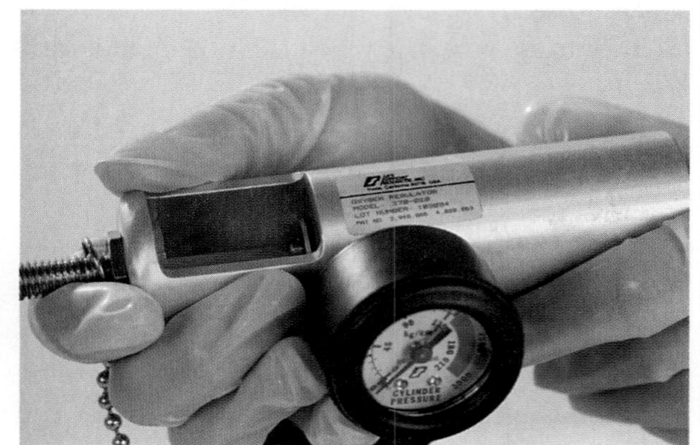

B

C

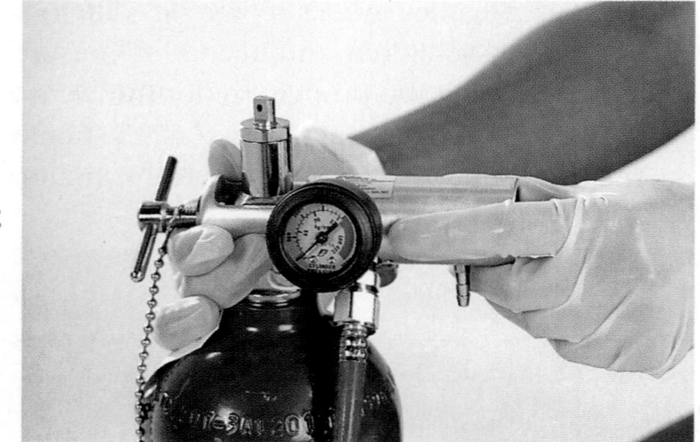

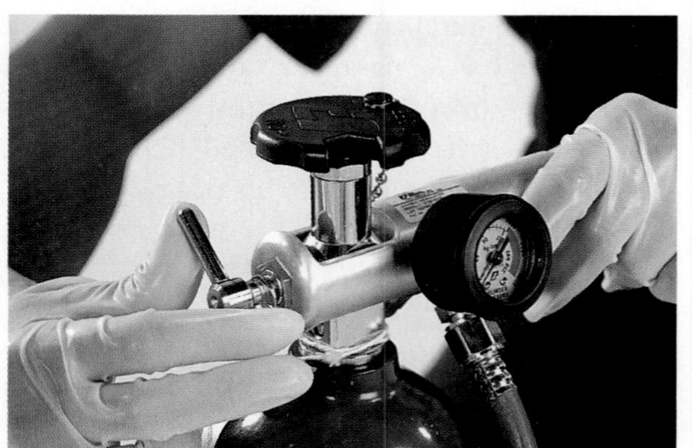

D

Figure 9-22 To attach the pressure regulator to the oxygen cylinder, **A,** insert the gasket into the opening of the cylinder. **B,** Check to see that the pressure regulator is for use with oxygen. **C,** Seat the three prongs of the regulator inside the cylinder. **D,** Hand tighten the screw until the regulator is snug.

oxygen delivery. Always monitor the victim's respirations and other vital signs while you are using a nonrebreather mask.

It is sometimes difficult to remember how many liters of oxygen to deliver. To eliminate confusion over how many liters of oxygen to deliver per minute, remember this general rule: *one to four and ten or more.* For a nasal cannula, administering 1 to 4 lpm is appropriate. When using a mask that covers the victim's face, you can safely administer 10 or more lpm. Table 9-1 provides an overview of each of the delivery devices presented.

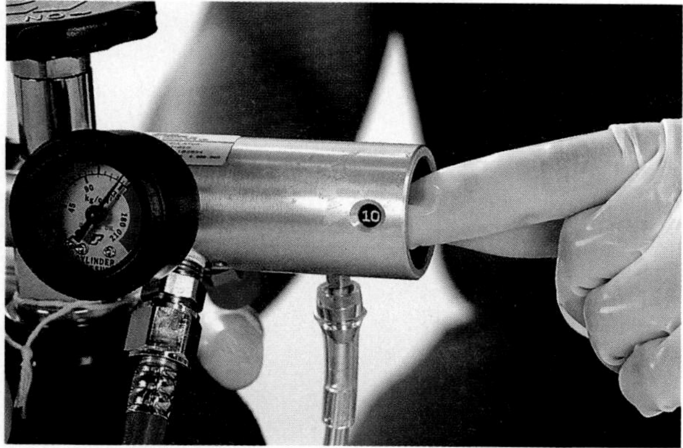

Figure 9-23 Turn the flowmeter clockwise to the desired flow rate.

Administering Oxygen

Whether you are administering oxygen to a breathing or a nonbreathing person, the steps for preparing the equipment remain the same. Begin by examining the cylinder to be certain that it is labeled *oxygen* (Fig. 9-21, *A*). Next, check to see that the cylinder is full. Full cylinders come with a protective covering holding the plastic gasket (O-ring) in place. Remove this covering and save the gasket. Slightly open the cylinder valve for 1 second (Fig. 9-21, *B*). Doing so will remove any dirt or debris from the cylinder valve. Insert the gasket into the large opening of the cylinder (Fig. 9-22, *A*).

Next, examine the pressure regulator. Check to see that it is labeled *oxygen* pressure regulator (Fig. 9-22, *B*). Attach the pressure regulator to the cylinder, seating the three prongs inside the cylinder (Fig. 9-22, *C*). Hand tighten the screw until the regulator is snug (Fig. 9-22, *D*). Open the cylinder valve one full turn.

Check the pressure gauge to determine how much pressure is in the cylinder. A full cylinder should have approximately 2000 psi. Attach the chosen delivery device to the oxygen port near the flowmeter. Some devices, such as the resuscitation mask and the BVM, require that you attach a section of the tubing between the flowmeter and the device. Other devices, such as the nasal cannula, have this section of tubing already attached.

Turn on the flowmeter to the desired flow rate (Fig. 9-23). Listen and feel to make sure that oxygen is flowing into your delivery device. Then, place the delivery device on the victim.

Precautions

When administering oxygen, safety is a primary concern. Remember the following precautions:

- *Do not* operate oxygen equipment around an open flame or sparks. Oxygen causes fire to burn more rapidly.
- *Do not* stand oxygen cylinders upright unless they can be well secured. If the cylinder falls, it could damage the regulator or possibly loosen the cylinder valve.
- *Do not* use grease, oil, or petroleum products to lubricate any pressure regulator parts. Oxygen does not mix with these products, and a severe chemical reaction could cause an explosion.
- Always check to see that oxygen is properly flowing from the delivery device before placing the device over the person's face.

Airway Management

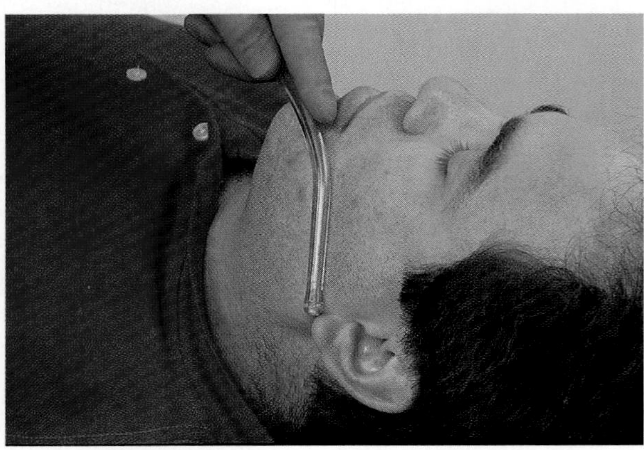

1a Measure distance of insertion from victim's ear-lobe to corner of mouth.

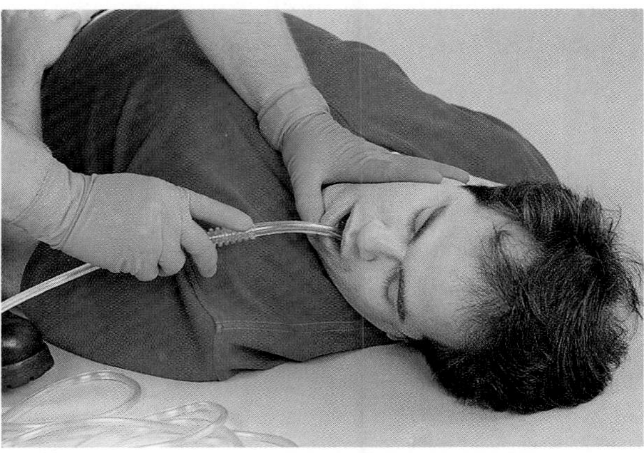

1b Insert suction tip into back of mouth.

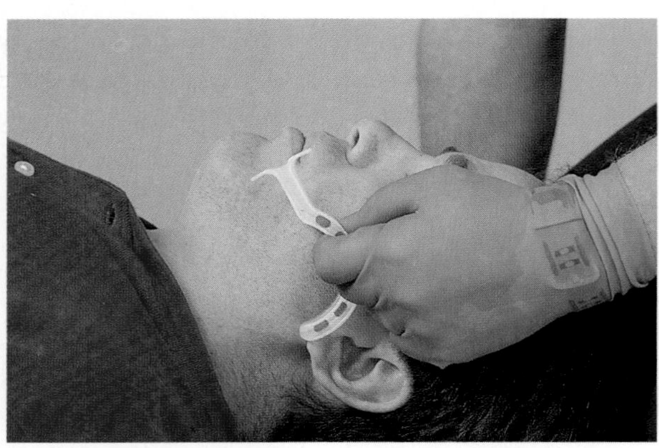

2a Measure oral airway from corner of victim's mouth to earlobe.

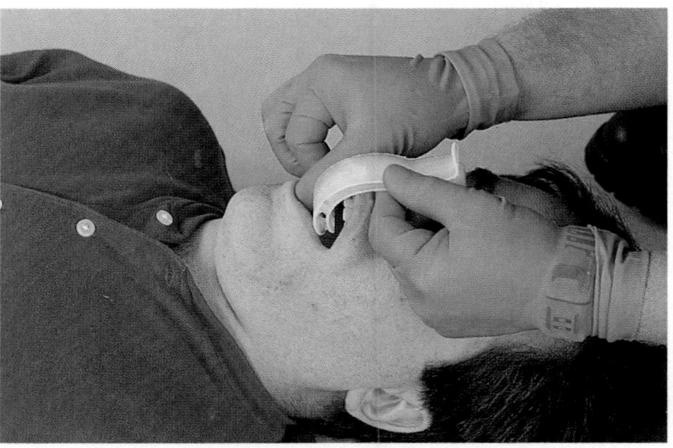

2b Open victim's mouth using cross-fingered technique, and insert oral airway.

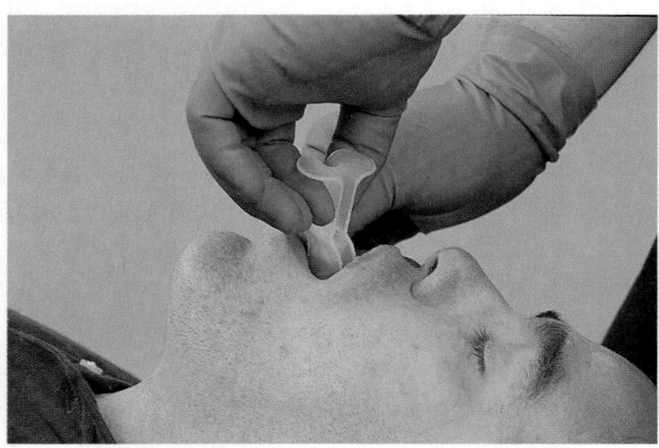

3. When resistance is felt, rotate oral airway so that curved tip drops in place.

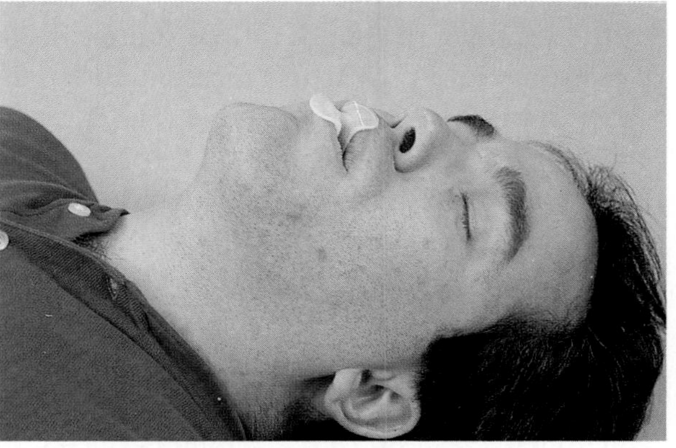

4. Properly inserted airway will have flange resting on victim's lips.

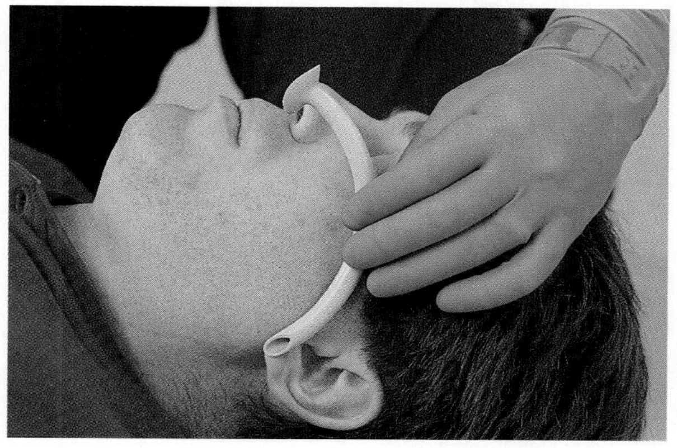

5a Measure nasal airway on victim to see that it extends from earlobe to tip of nose.

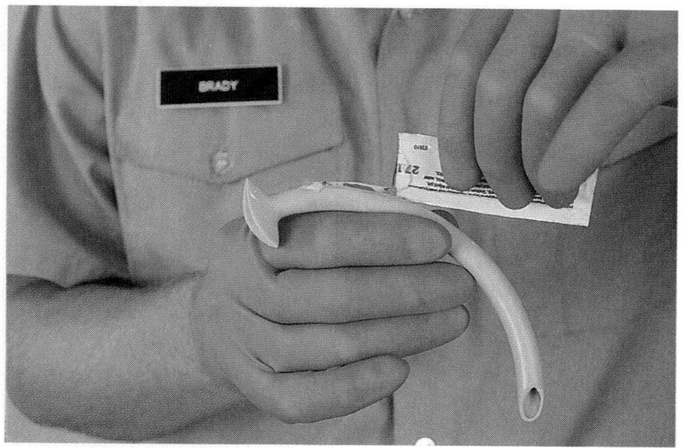

5b Lubricate airway with water-soluble lubricant.

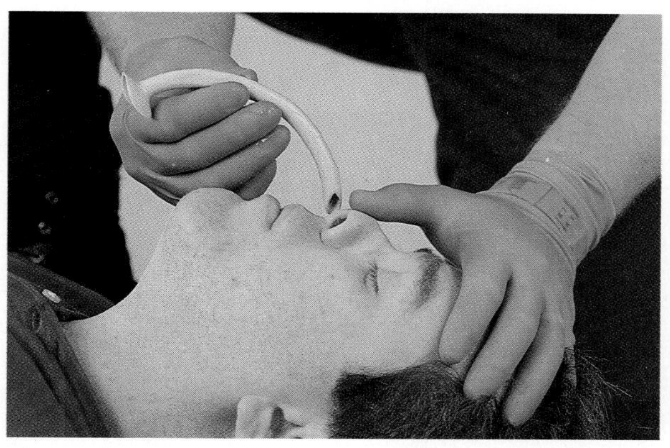

6a Insert airway gently into nostril with bevel toward victim's septum.

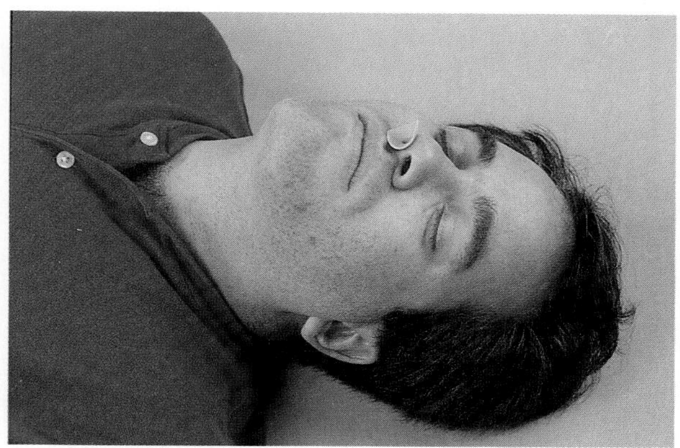

6b Advance airway gently, straight in, not upward, until flange rests on nose.

Using a Resuscitation Mask for Rescue Breathing (one rescuer)

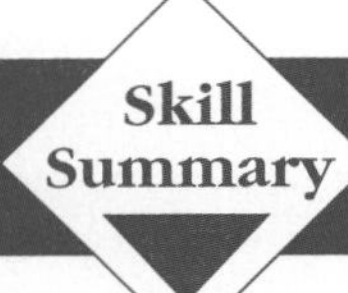

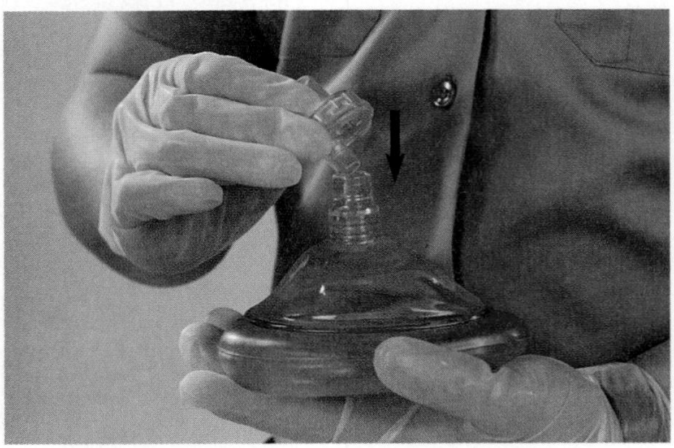

1. Assemble the mask.

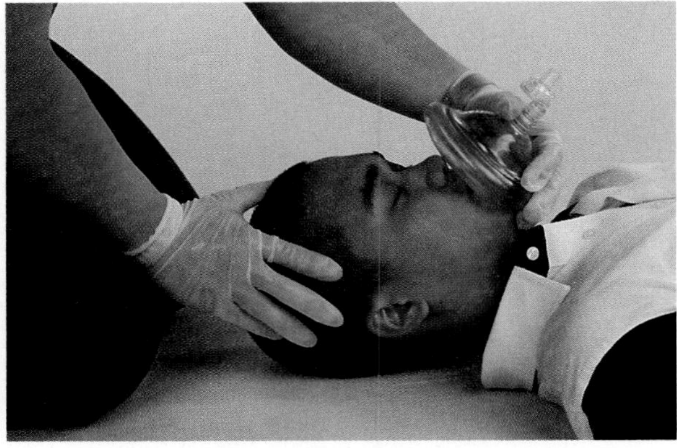

2. Kneel behind victim's head. Position the mask.

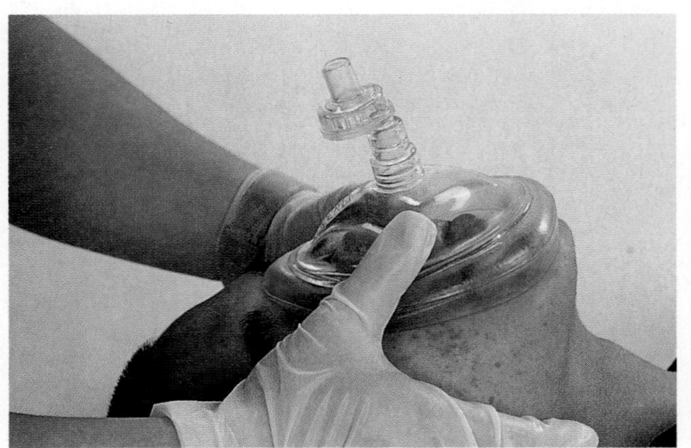

3. Seal the mask. Tilt the head back and lift the jaw to open the airway.

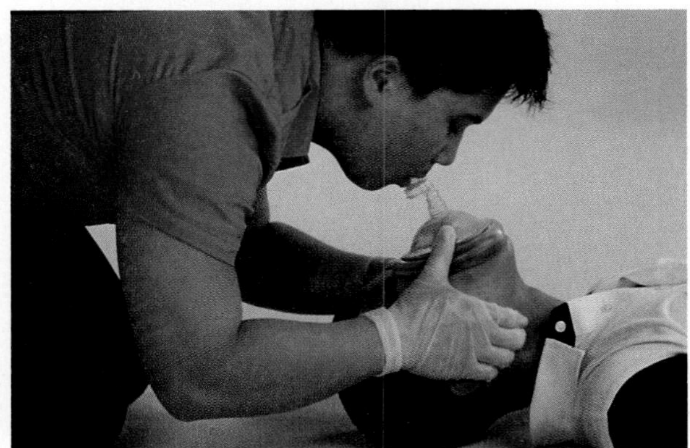

4. Begin rescue breathing.

Using a Bag-Valve-Mask Resuscitator for Rescue Breathing (two rescuers)

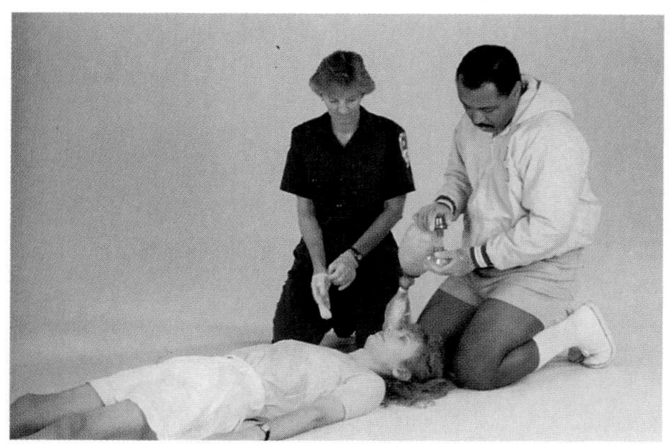

1. First rescuer assembles BVM.

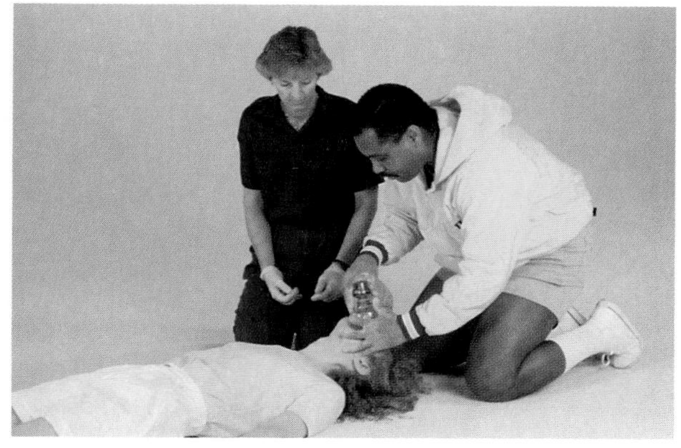

2. First rescuer positions mask.

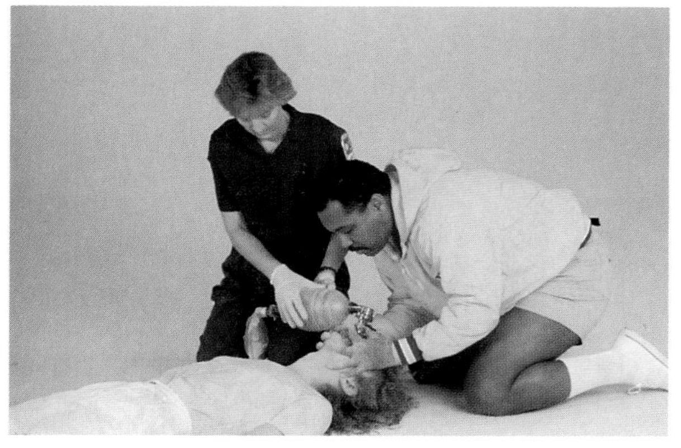

3. First rescuer tilts head, lifts jaw, and applies pressure to mask.

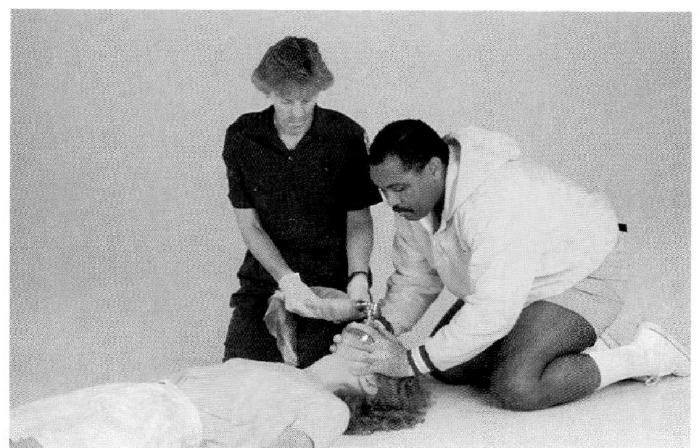

4. Second rescuer begins ventilation.

Give the same number of ventilations as you would for mouth-to-mouth rescue breathing.

Oxygen Delivery

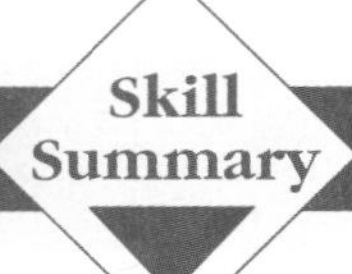

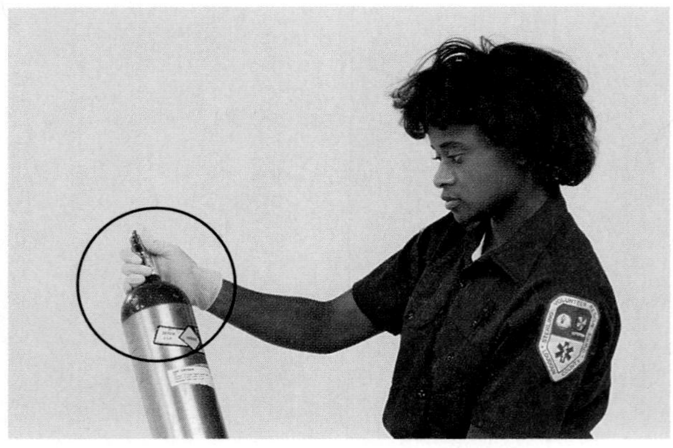

1. Check cylinder.

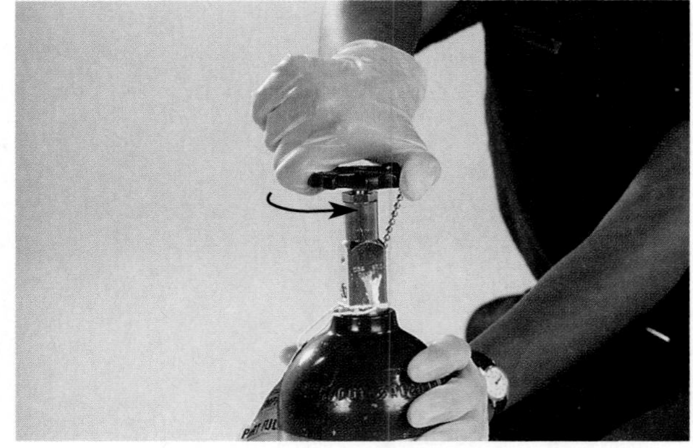

2. Clear valve.

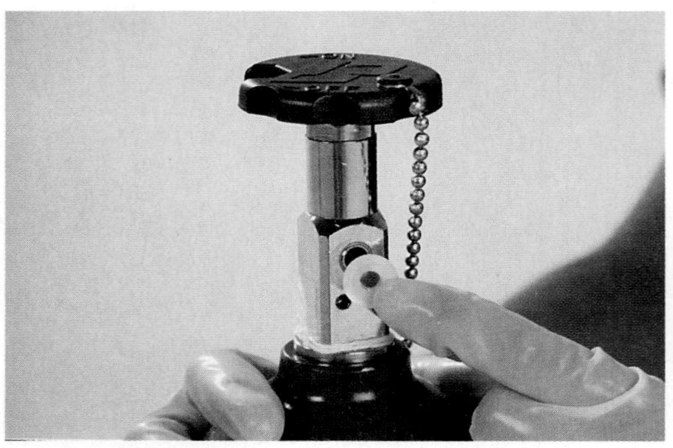

3. Insert gasket into cylinder.

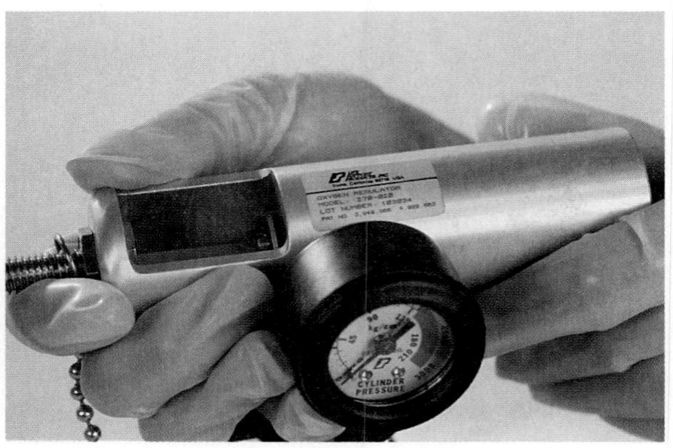

4. Check pressure regulator.

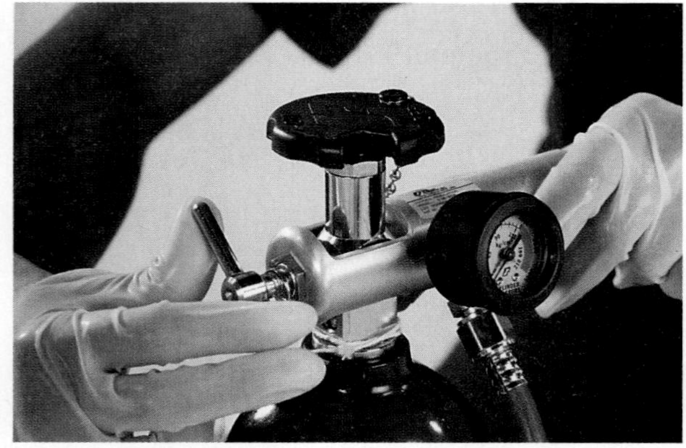

5. Attach pressure regulator.

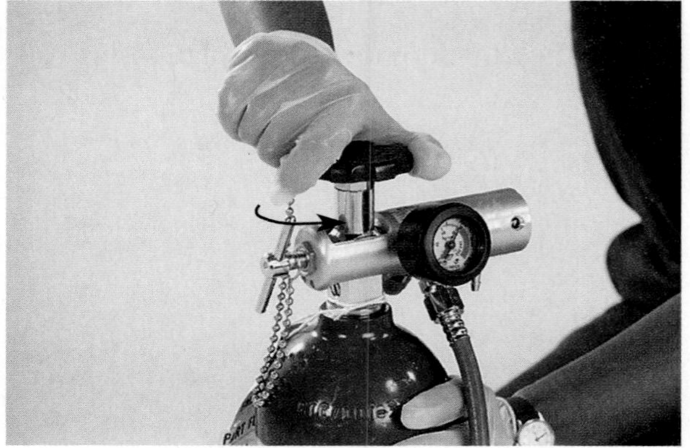

6. Open cylinder one full turn.

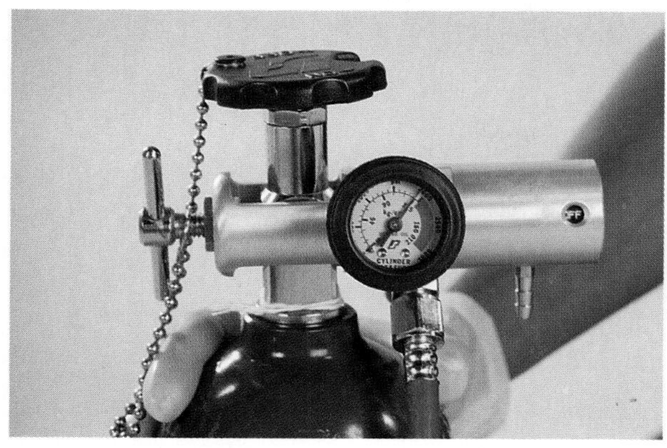

7. Check pressure gauge.

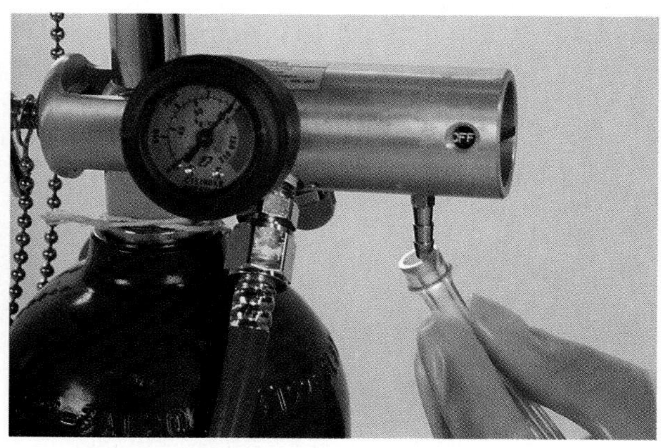

8. Attach delivery device to flowmeter.

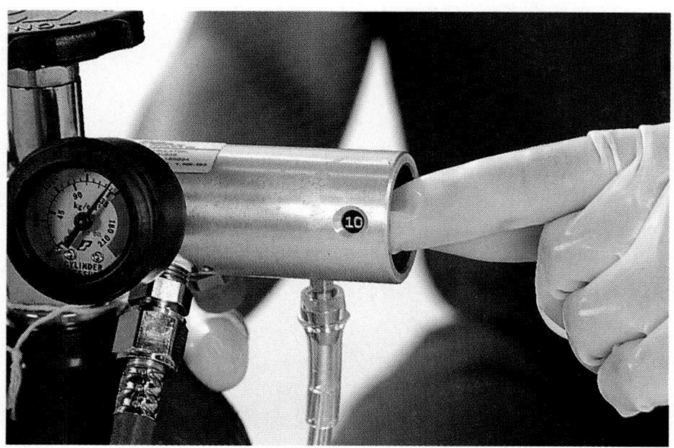

9. Adjust flowmeter.

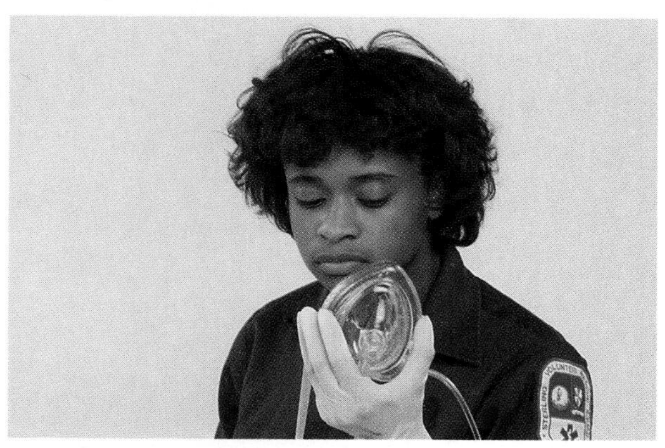

10. Verify oxygen flow.

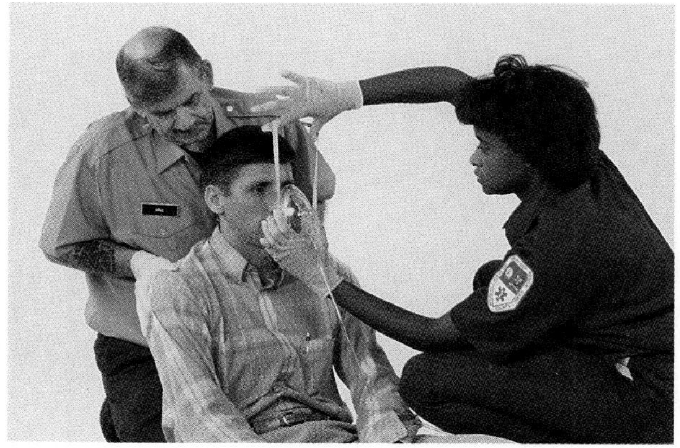

11. Place delivery device on victim.

CAUTION: When breaking down the equipment, remove the delivery device from the victim's face, turn off the flowmeter, close the cylinder, and then turn on the flowmeter to bleed the line. Finally, remove the regulator from the cylinder so that other participants may practice the complete skill.

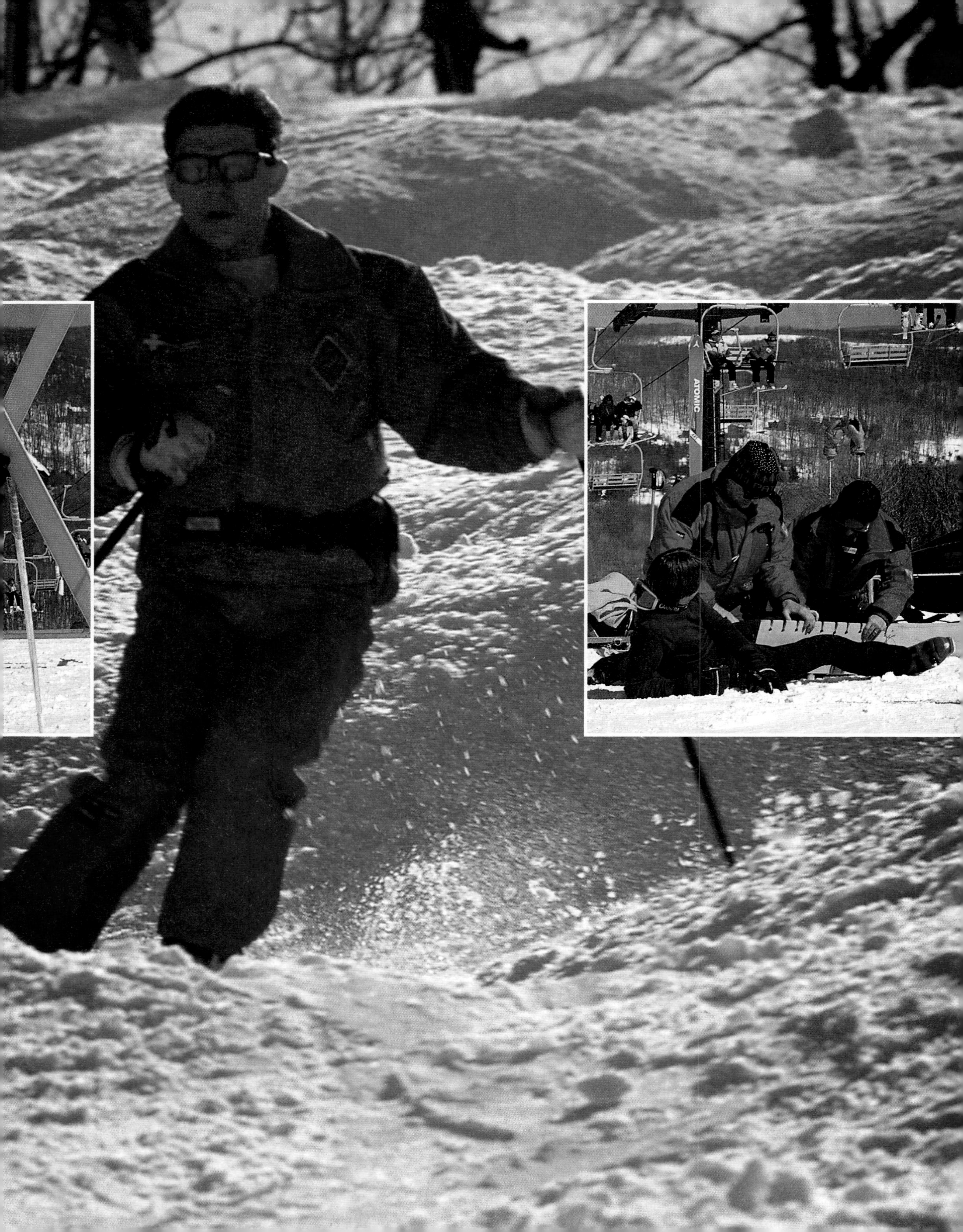
ATOMIC

Module Four

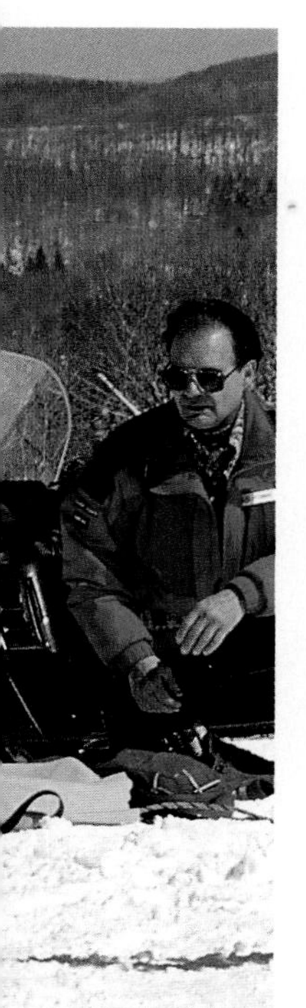

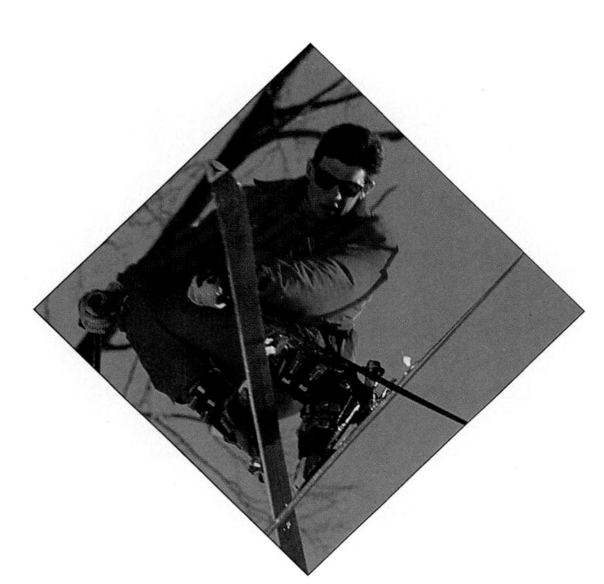

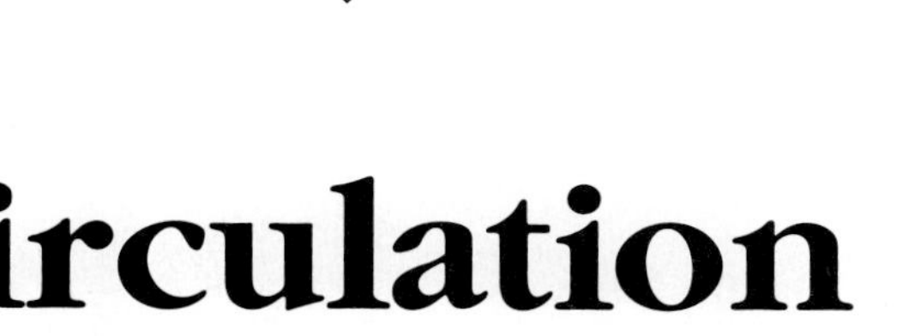

Circulation

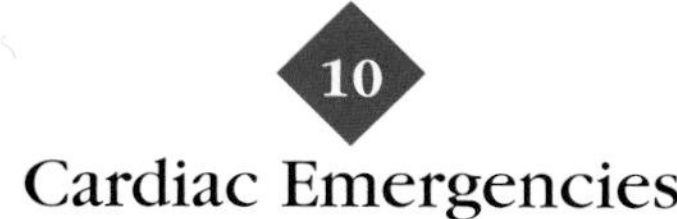

10

Cardiac Emergencies

Cardiac Emergencies

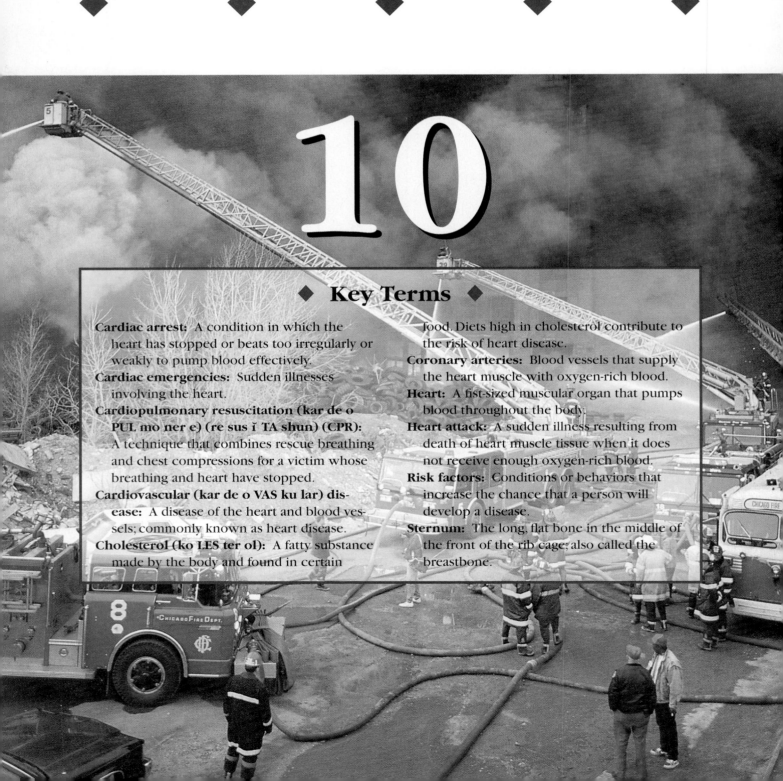

Key Terms

Cardiac arrest: A condition in which the heart has stopped or beats too irregularly or weakly to pump blood effectively.

Cardiac emergencies: Sudden illnesses involving the heart.

Cardiopulmonary resuscitation (kar de o PUL mo ner e) (re sus ĭ TA shun) (CPR): A technique that combines rescue breathing and chest compressions for a victim whose breathing and heart have stopped.

Cardiovascular (kar de o VAS ku lar) disease: A disease of the heart and blood vessels; commonly known as heart disease.

Cholesterol (ko LES ter ol): A fatty substance made by the body and found in certain food. Diets high in cholesterol contribute to the risk of heart disease.

Coronary arteries: Blood vessels that supply the heart muscle with oxygen-rich blood.

Heart: A fist-sized muscular organ that pumps blood throughout the body.

Heart attack: A sudden illness resulting from death of heart muscle tissue when it does not receive enough oxygen-rich blood.

Risk factors: Conditions or behaviors that increase the chance that a person will develop a disease.

Sternum: The long, flat bone in the middle of the front of the rib cage; also called the breastbone.

◆ Knowledge Objectives ◆

After reading this chapter and completing the class activities, you should be able to—

- List the signs and symptoms of a heart attack.
- Describe how to care for a victim who may be experiencing a heart attack.
- Identify risk factors for cardiovascular disease that can be controlled.
- List the reasons for the heart to stop beating.
- Describe the components of cardiopulmonary resuscitation.
- List the steps of one-rescuer CPR for an adult, child, and infant.
- Describe how to perform chest compressions on an adult, child, and infant.
- Explain when it is appropriate to stop CPR.
- Describe how to perform two-rescuer CPR.

◆ Attitude Objectives ◆

After reading this chapter and completing the class activities, you should be able to—

- Value the importance of leading a healthy lifestyle to reduce the risks of cardiovascular disease.
- Accept that despite the best efforts of everyone involved, victims of cardiac arrest do not often survive.

◆ Skill Objectives ◆

After reading this chapter and completing the class activities, you should be able to—

- Demonstrate the proper technique for chest compressions on an adult, child, and infant.
- Demonstrate how to perform one-rescuer CPR for an adult, child, and infant.
- Demonstrate how to perform two-rescuer CPR.

◆ INTRODUCTION

In the initial assessment, you identify and care for immediate threats to a victim's life. Your priorities are to care for the victim's airway, breathing, and circulation (the ABCs). In Chapter 7, you learned how to open a victim's airway and assess breathing. In Chapter 8, you learned how to provide rescue breathing for a victim who has a pulse but is not breathing.

In this chapter, you will learn how to recognize and provide care for ***cardiac emergencies***, sudden illnesses involving the heart. You will learn the care for a victim with persistent chest pain and for a victim whose heart stops

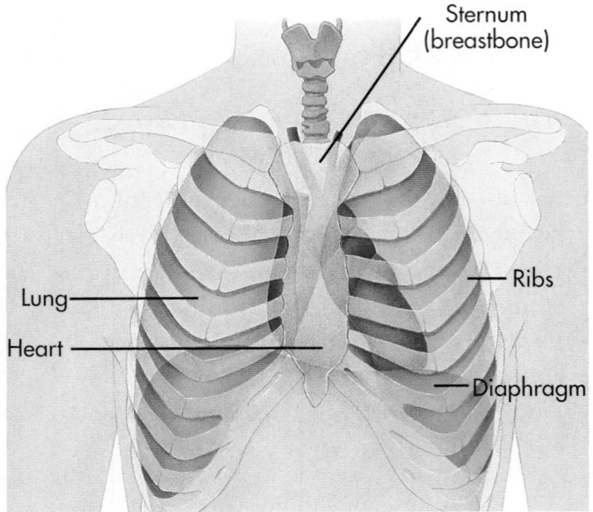

Figure 10-1 The heart is located in the middle of the chest, behind the lower half of the sternum.

beating. The condition in which the heart stops, known as ***cardiac arrest***, sometimes results from a heart attack. To provide care for a cardiac arrest victim, you need to learn how to perform cardiopulmonary resuscitation (CPR). Properly performed, CPR can keep a victim's vital organs supplied with oxygen-rich blood until more highly trained personnel arrive to provide advanced care.

This chapter also identifies the important risk factors for cardiovascular disease. It is as important to prevent heart attack and cardiac arrest as it is to learn how to recognize them when they occur and provide appropriate care. Learn to modify your behavior to prevent cardiovascular disease.

◆ HEART ATTACK

The ***heart*** is a muscular organ, about the size of an adult fist, that functions like a pump. It lies between the lungs, in the middle of the chest, behind the lower half of the ***sternum*** (breastbone). The heart is protected by the ribs and sternum in front and by the spine in back (Fig. 10-1). It has four chambers and is separated into right and left halves. The right side of the heart has the chambers known as the **right atrium,** which receives oxygen-poor blood from the veins of the body, and **right ventricle,** which pumps this oxygen-poor blood to the lungs where waste products are removed and oxygen absorbed. The now oxygen-rich blood returns to the left side of the heart, where it enters the **left atrium** and goes on to the **left ventricle,** where it is pumped to all parts of the body. One-way valves direct the flow of blood as it moves through each of the heart's four chambers (Fig. 10-2). For the circulatory system to be effective, the respiratory system must also be working so that the blood can pick up oxygen in the lungs.

Like all living tissue, the cells of the heart need a continuous supply of oxygen. The ***coronary arteries*** supply the heart muscle with oxygen-rich blood (Fig. 10-3, *A*). If heart muscle tissue is deprived of this blood, it dies, and the victim often develops specific signs and symptoms. If too much tissue dies, the heart is not able to pump effectively. When heart tissue dies, the resulting sudden illness is called a ***heart attack***.

A heart attack interrupts the heart's electrical system. This interruption may result in an irregular heartbeat, which prevents blood from circulating effectively.

Common Causes of Heart Attack

Heart attack is usually the result of cardiovascular disease. ***Cardiovascular disease***—disease of the heart and blood vessels—is the leading cause of death for adults in the United States. It is estimated that approximately 70 million Americans suffer some form of cardiovascular disease. Nearly one million deaths each year are attributed to cardiovascular disease. Of these, approximately 500,000 result from heart attack, and most of them are sudden deaths.

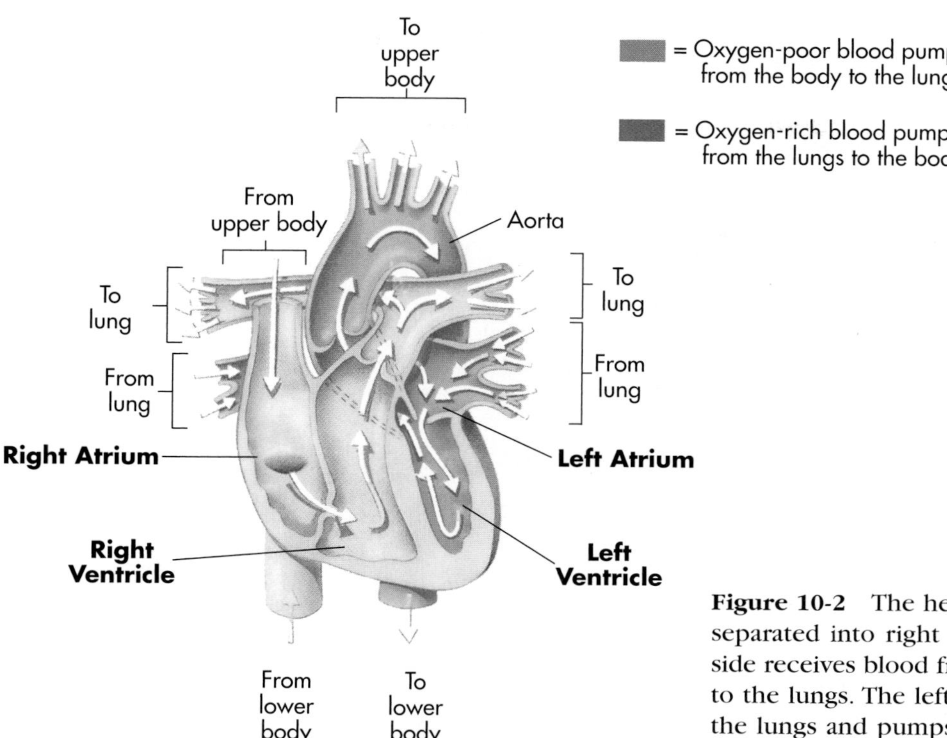

Figure 10-2 The heart has 4 chambers and is separated into right and left halves. The right side receives blood from the body and sends it to the lungs. The left side receives blood from the lungs and pumps it out through the body. One-way valves direct the flow of blood through the heart.

Cardiovascular disease develops slowly. Deposits of ***cholesterol,*** a fatty substance made by the body, and other material may gradually build up on the inner walls of the arteries. This condition, called **atherosclerosis,** causes these vessels to progressively narrow. When coronary arteries narrow, a heart attack may occur (Fig. 10-3, *B*). Atherosclerosis can also involve arteries in other parts of the body, such as the brain. Diseased arteries in the brain can lead to **stroke**, a disruption of blood flow to a part of the brain.

Because atherosclerosis develops gradually, it can go undetected for many years. Even with significantly reduced blood flow to the heart muscle, there may be no signs and symptoms of heart trouble. Most people with atherosclerosis are unaware of it. As the narrowing progresses, some people experience symptoms such as chest pain, an early warning sign that the heart is not receiving enough oxygen-rich blood. Others may suffer a heart attack or even cardiac arrest without any previous warning. Fortunately, this process can be slowed or stopped by lifestyle changes, such as forming healthy eating habits. Later in this chapter, you will learn ways to promote a lifestyle that is healthy for your heart.

Signs and Symptoms of Heart Attack

The most prominent symptom of a heart attack is persistent chest pain or discomfort (Table 10-1). However, it may not always be easy for you to distinguish between the pain of a heart attack and chest pain caused by indigestion, muscle spasms, or other conditions. Brief, stabbing chest pain or pain that feels more intense when the victim bends or breathes deeply is usually not caused by a heart attack.

The pain of heart attack can range from mild discomfort to an unbearable crushing sensation in the chest. The victim may describe it as

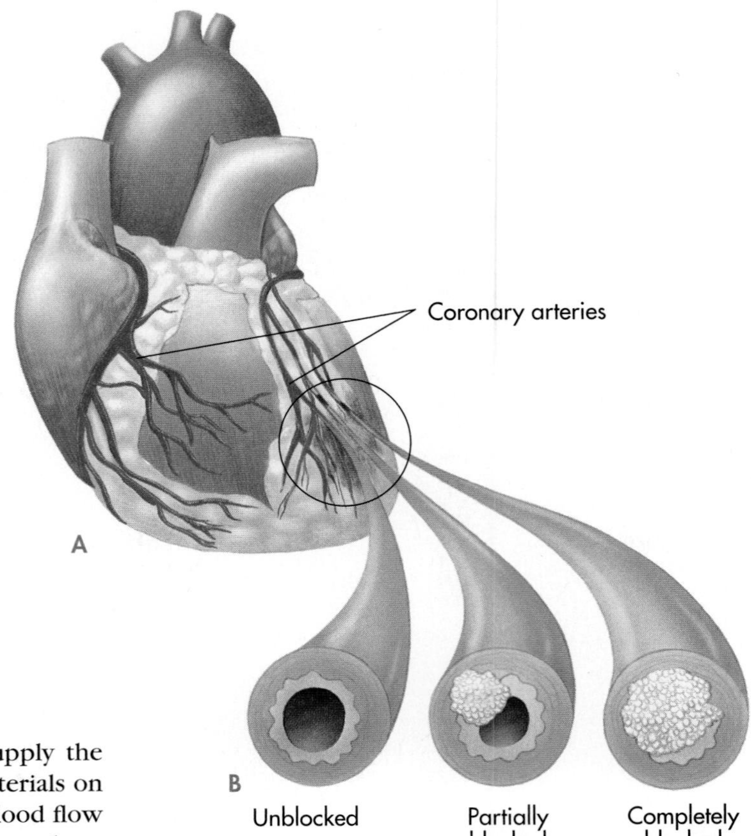

Figure 10-3 **A**, The coronary arteries supply the heart muscle with blood. **B**, Buildup of materials on the inner walls of these arteries reduces blood flow to the heart muscle and may cause a heart attack.

Table 10-1 Signs and Symptoms of a Heart Attack

Signs and symptoms	Characteristics
Persistent chest pain or discomfort	Persistent pain or pressure in the chest that is not relieved by resting, changing position, or oral medication Pain may range from discomfort to an unbearable crushing sensation Pain may radiate to the shoulders, arms, neck, or back
Difficulty breathing	Victim's breathing is noisy Victim feels short of breath Victim breathes faster than normal
Changes in pulse rate	Pulse may be faster or slower than normal or may be irregular
Skin appearance	Victim's skin may be pale, ashen, or bluish in color Victim's face may be moist, or victim may sweat profusely

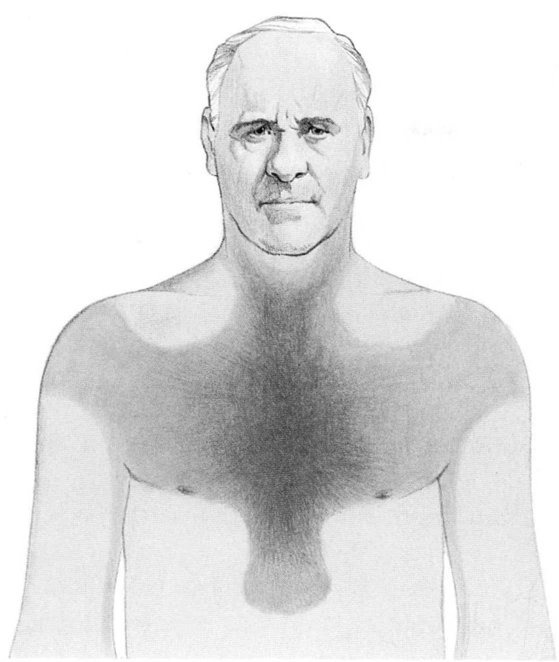

Figure 10-4 Heart attack pain is most often felt in the center of the chest, behind the sternum. It may spread to the shoulder, arm, neck, or jaw.

an uncomfortable pressure, squeezing, tightness, aching, constricting, or a heavy sensation in the chest. Often, the victim feels pain in the center of the chest behind the sternum. It may spread to the shoulder, arm, neck, or jaw (Fig. 10-4). The pain is constant and usually not relieved by resting, changing position, or taking oral medication. Any severe chest pain, chest pain that lasts longer than 10 minutes, or chest pain that is accompanied by other heart attack signs and symptoms should receive emergency medical care immediately.

Although a heart attack is often dramatic, heart attack victims can have relatively mild symptoms. The victim often mistakes the symptoms for indigestion. Some heart attack victims feel little or no chest pain or discomfort.

Some people with cardiovascular disease may experience chest pain or pressure that comes and goes and is not generally caused by a heart attack. This type of pain is called **angina pectoris**. Angina pectoris develops when the heart needs more oxygen-rich blood than it gets, such as during physical activity or emotional stress. This lack of oxygen can cause a constricting chest pain that may spread to the neck, jaw, and arms.

Pain associated with angina usually lasts less than 10 minutes. A victim who knows he or she has angina will often have a prescribed medication to help relieve the pain. Reducing the heart's demand for oxygen, such as by stopping physical activity and by taking prescribed medication, often relieves angina. Administering oxygen to victims experiencing angina helps relieve chest pain. Angina can progress to a heart attack if the pain is not relieved.

Another sign of a heart attack is difficulty breathing. The victim may be breathing faster than normal because the body tries to get much-needed oxygen to the heart. Depending on the victim's general condition, the victim's pulse may be faster or slower than normal or irregular. The victim's skin may be pale, ashen, or bluish, particularly around the face. The face may also be moist from perspiration. Some heart attack victims sweat profusely. These signs result from the stress the body experiences when the heart does not work effectively.

Since any heart attack may lead to cardiac arrest, it is important to recognize the signs and symptoms of heart attack and act immediately. Prompt action may prevent cardiac arrest. A heart attack victim whose heart is still beating has a far better chance of living than a victim whose heart has stopped. Most people who die from a heart attack die within 1 to 2 hours after the first signs and symptoms appear. Many could have been saved if bystanders or the victim had been aware of the signs and symptoms of a heart attack and acted promptly. Since most heart attacks result from blood clotting within arteries, early treatment of an attack with medication that dissolves clots has been helpful in minimizing damage to the heart.

Many heart attack victims delay seeking care. Nearly half of them wait 2 or more hours before going to the hospital. Victims often do

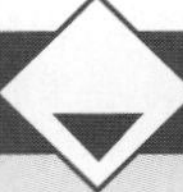

How the Heart Functions

Too often we take our hearts for granted. The heart is extremely reliable. The heart beats about 70 times each minute, or more than 100,000 times a day. During the average lifetime, the heart will beat nearly 3 billion times. The heart moves about a gallon of blood per minute through the body. This is about 40 million gallons in an average lifetime. The heart moves blood through about 60,000 miles of blood vessels.

not realize they are having a heart attack. They may dismiss the symptoms as indigestion or muscle soreness.

Remember, the key symptom of a heart attack is persistent chest pain. If the victim states that chest pain is severe or chest discomfort has been present for more than 10 minutes, summon more advanced medical personnel immediately and begin to care for the victim.

Care for Heart Attack

The most important step in providing care is to recognize that any of the signs and symptoms listed below may be those of a heart attack. You must take immediate action if any of these appear. A heart attack victim may deny the seriousness of the symptoms he or she is experiencing. Do not let this influence you. If you think there is a possibility that a person is having a heart attack, you must act. First, have the victim stop what he or she is doing and rest comfortably. Many heart attack victims find it easier to breathe while sitting (Fig. 10-5). Then, summon more advanced medical personnel.

Continue with your history. Talk to bystanders and the victim, if possible, to get more information. If the victim is experiencing persistent chest pain, ask him or her the following:

- When did the pain start?
- What brought it on?
- Does anything lessen it?
- What does it feel like?
- Where does it hurt?

Care for a Heart Attack

Recognize the signals of a heart attack.

Convince the victim to stop activity and rest.

Help the victim to rest comfortably.

Try to obtain information about the victim's condition.

Comfort the victim.

Administer oxygen if available and you are trained to do so.

Call for advanced medical personnel.

Assist with medication, if prescribed.

Monitor vital signs.

Be prepared to give CPR if the victim's heart stops beating.

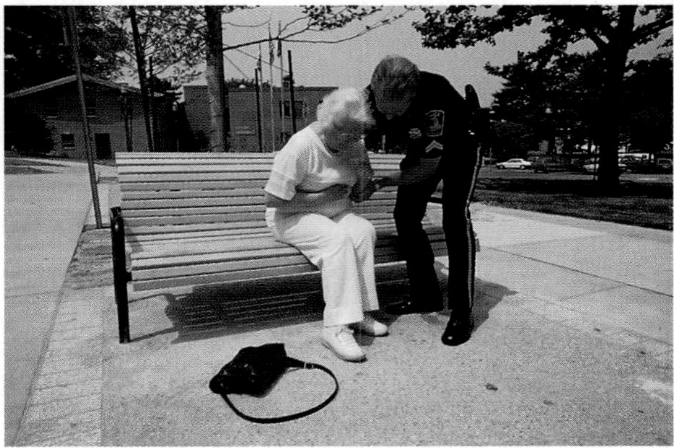

Figure 10-5 The heart attack victim should rest in a position that helps breathing.

Ask the victim if he or she has a history of heart disease. Some victims who have heart disease have prescribed medications for chest pain. Although you should not administer the medication, you can help by getting any medication for the victim. A medication often prescribed for angina is nitroglycerin, a small tablet that is dissolved under the tongue. Sometimes nitroglycerin patches are placed on the chest or the person uses a nitroglycerin spray by mouth. Once absorbed into the body, nitroglycerin enlarges the blood vessels to make it easier for blood to reach heart muscle tissue. The pain is relieved because the heart does not have to work so hard and oxygen delivery to the heart is increased.

Administer oxygen if it is available and you are trained to administer it. Ensure that advanced medical personnel have been summoned. Surviving a heart attack often depends on how soon the victim receives **advanced cardiac life support (ACLS),** the use of special equipment and medications to maintain breathing and circulation for the victim of a cardiac emergency.

Be calm and reassuring when caring for a heart attack victim. Comforting the victim helps reduce anxiety and eases some of the discomfort. Continue to monitor the vital signs until advanced medical personnel arrive. Watch for any changes in appearance or behavior. Since the heart attack may cause cardiac arrest, be prepared to give CPR.

◆ CARDIAC ARREST

When a person suffers a cardiac arrest, time is a critical factor. The longer the time until CPR is started, the less the chance that the victim will survive.

What Is Cardiac Arrest?

Cardiac arrest is the condition that occurs when the heart stops beating or beats too irregularly or weakly to circulate blood effectively. Without a heartbeat, breathing soon ceases. The condition when the heart stops beating and breathing stops is referred to as **clinical death**. Cardiac arrest is a life-threatening emergency because the vital organs of the body are no longer receiving oxygen-rich blood. Approximately 300,000 people die annually from cardiac arrest before reaching a hospital.

Common Causes of Cardiac Arrest

Cardiovascular disease is the most common cause of cardiac arrest. Other causes include drowning, suffocation, certain drugs, severe injuries to the chest, severe loss of blood, and electrocution. Stroke and other types of brain damage can also stop the heart.

Signs of Cardiac Arrest

A victim in cardiac arrest is not breathing and does not have a pulse. The victim's heart has either stopped beating or is beating so weakly or irregularly that it cannot produce a pulse. The absence of a pulse is the primary sign of cardiac arrest. No matter how hard you try, you will not be able to feel a pulse. If you cannot feel a carotid pulse, no blood is reaching the brain. The victim will be unconscious and breathing will stop.

Although cardiac arrest can result from a heart attack, cardiac arrest can also occur suddenly, independent of a heart attack. Therefore the victim may not have shown the signs and symptoms of a heart attack before the cardiac arrest. Death resulting from sudden cardiac arrest is called **sudden death**.

Care for Cardiac Arrest

A victim who is not breathing and has no pulse is clinically dead. However, the cells of the brain and other vital organs will continue to live for a few minutes until the oxygen in the bloodstream is depleted. This victim needs

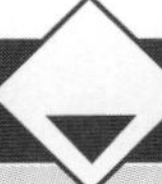

The Shock of Your Life

Each year, more than 300,000 Americans collapse in cardiac arrest in their homes and on the streets. Ninety-five percent will not survive, but the development of a simple, computerized electric-shocking device offers an opportunity to increase survival.

In two thirds of all cardiac arrests, the heartbeat flutters chaotically before it stops, a condition called ventricular fibrillation. The electrical impulses that cause the heart muscle to pump are no longer synchronized and fail to create the strong pumping action needed to circulate the blood.

Electric-shocking devices, or defibrillators, were introduced onto mobile coronary units in 1966.[1] The machines allowed emergency personnel to monitor the heart's electrical rhythm. A doctor attached electrodes to the victim and reviewed the heart's rhythm. If necessary, an electric shock was delivered to the heart to try to restore its proper rhythm. Outside the hospital, paramedics eventually took the place of doctors in evaluating rhythms and administering shocks. Because there were too few trained personnel across the United States, cardiac arrest victims were not always able to get the lifesaving help they needed.

Fortunately, a new, easy-to-use type of Automatic External Defibrillator (AED) allows emergency medical technicians, first responders, and

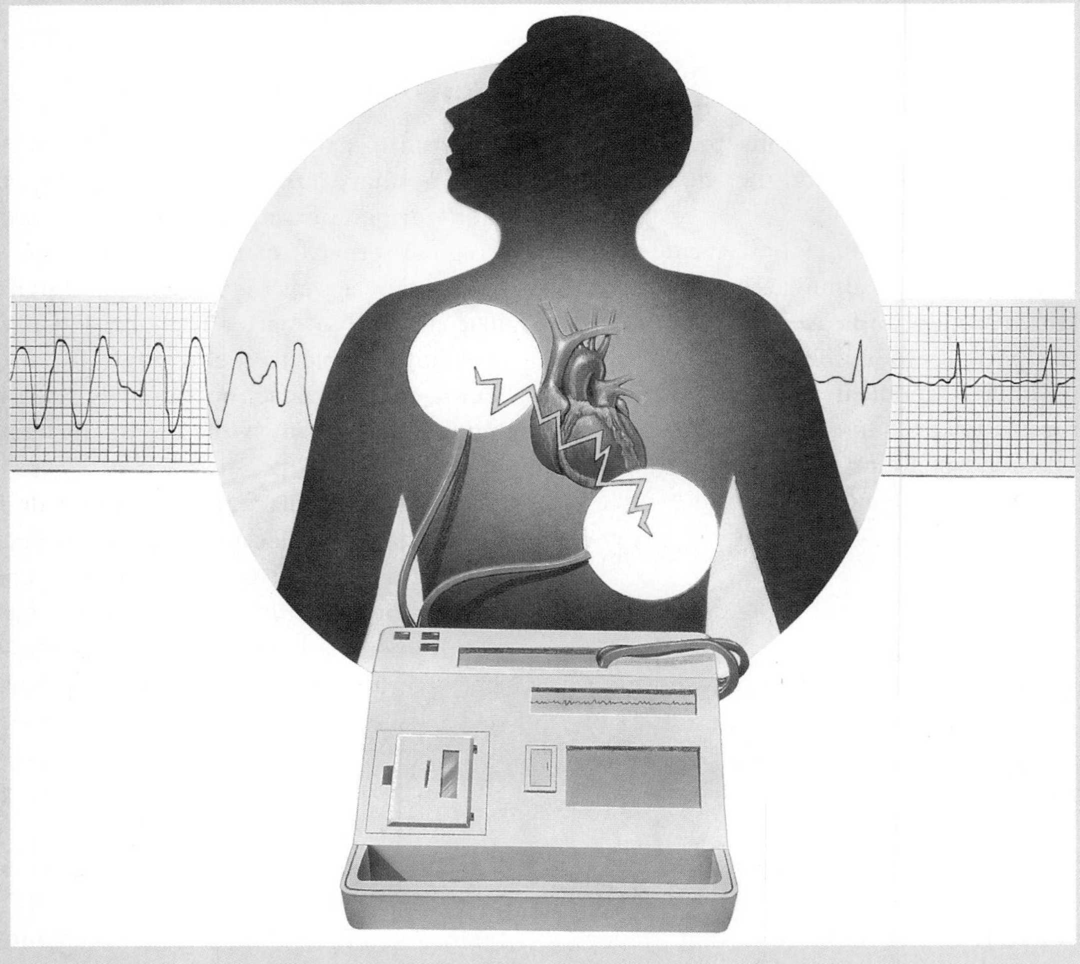

even citizen responders to provide the lifesaving shocks. With the new defibrillators, a computer chip, rather than an advanced medical professional, analyzes the heart's rhythm. Typically, the first responder places the two electrodes on the victim's chest and then presses two buttons—first "ANALYZE," then, when indicated, "SHOCK." The machine does the rest.

AEDs monitor the heart's electrical activity through two electrodes placed on the chest. On a heart monitor, ventricular fibrillation looks like a chaotic, wavy line, whereas a normal heartbeat shows a pattern of evenly spaced, well-defined spiked points. The computer chip determines the need for a shock by looking at the pattern, size, and frequency of the electrocardiogram waves.

If the rhythm resembles ventricular fibrillation, the machine readies an electrical charge. When the electrical charge disrupts the irregular heartbeat, it is called defibrillation. This allows the heart's natural electrical system to begin to fire off electrical impulses correctly so that the heart can beat normally.

When first responders are trained to use AEDs, they can drastically reduce the amount of time it takes to administer a shock in a cardiac emergency, researchers say. By extending training to first responders, communities increase the numbers of emergency personnel trained to use AEDs. In Eugene and Springfield, Oregon, AEDs were placed on every fire truck, and all fire fighters were trained to use them. Researchers saw these communities' survival rates for cardiac arrest increase by 18 percent in the first year.[2]

Most states recognize defibrillator training for EMTs. AEDs also are being introduced in areas that hold large groups of people, such as convention centers, stadiums, large businesses, and industrial complexes. Some health experts hope that someday AEDs will be as commonplace as fire alarms.

REFERENCES

1. Pantridge JF, Geddes JS: A mobile intensive care unit in the treatment of myocardial infarction, *Lancet* 2:271, 1967.
2. Graves JR, Austin D Jr, Cummins RO: *Rapid zap: automated defibrillation,* Englewood Cliffs, NJ, 1989, Prentice-Hall.

cardiopulmonary resuscitation (CPR). The term *cardia* refers to the heart, and *pulmonary* refers to the lungs. CPR is a combination of rescue breathing and chest compressions. Chest compressions are a method of making the blood circulate when the heart is not beating. Given together, rescue breathing and chest compressions artificially take over the functions of the lungs and heart.

CPR increases a cardiac arrest victim's chances of survival by keeping the brain supplied with oxygen until the victim receives advanced medical care. Without CPR, the brain will begin to die within 4 to 6 minutes. The irreversible damage caused by brain cell death is known as **biological death** (Fig. 10-6). Be aware that at best, CPR only generates about one third of the normal blood flow to the brain.

CPR alone is not enough to help someone survive cardiac arrest. Call for advanced medical personnel immediately when a victim suffers cardiac arrest. Trained emergency personnel can provide advanced cardiac life support (ACLS). Acting as an extension of a hospital emergency department, EMTs and paramedics can administer medications or use a defibrillator as part of their emergency care (Fig. 10-7).

A **defibrillator** is a device that sends an electric shock through the chest to the heart to start the heart beating effectively again. Defibrillation given as soon as possible is the key to helping some victims survive cardiac arrest. Immediate CPR must be combined with early defibrillation and other forms of ACLS to give the victim of cardiac arrest the best chance for survival.

First responders in some communities are trained to use new defibrillators called **automated external defibrillators (AEDs)**. To-

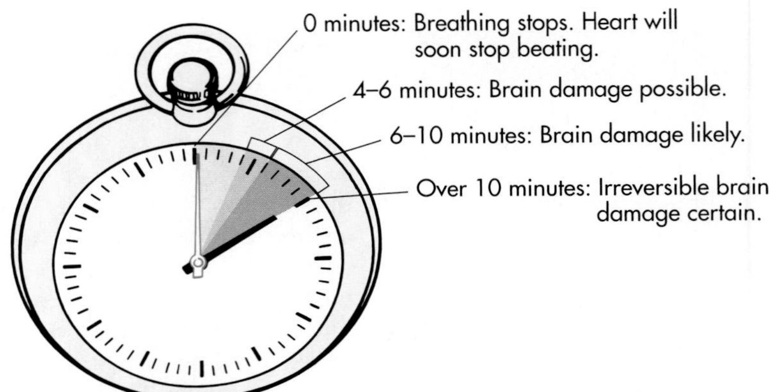
0 minutes: Breathing stops. Heart will soon stop beating.
4–6 minutes: Brain damage possible.
6–10 minutes: Brain damage likely.
Over 10 minutes: Irreversible brain damage certain.

Figure 10-6 Clinical death is a condition in which the heart and breathing stop. Without resuscitation, clinical death will result in biological death. Biological death is the irreversible death of brain cells.

day, AEDs are available for use by trained individuals in places such as factories, stadiums, and other places where large numbers of people gather. Soon, automated external defibrillators may be used even more commonly. Appendix A is an instructional unit on AEDs.

In all cases of cardiac arrest, it is very important to start CPR promptly and continue it until a defibrillator is available. Prompt, effective CPR can help extend the time in which defibrillation can be successful. When a defibrillator is not available, CPR should be continued. Effective rescue breathing and chest compressions can help keep the brain, heart, and other vital organs supplied with oxygen-rich blood. Any delay in starting CPR, or unnecessary delays in continuing it, reduces the victim's chance for survival.

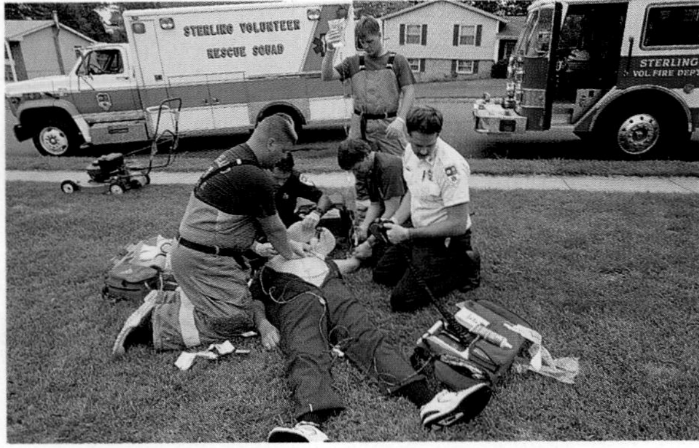
STERLING VOLUNTEER RESCUE SQUAD
STERLING VOL. FIRE DEPT

Figure 10-7 Use of a defibrillator and other advanced measures may restore a heartbeat in a victim of cardiac arrest.

Unfortunately, CPR and defibrillation do not always work. Even in the best of situations, in which CPR is started promptly and advanced medical personnel arrive quickly, victims of cardiac arrest do not often survive. In some situations, victims will survive the initial event and be admitted to the hospital, only to succumb to cardiac arrest within hours or days. Controlling your emotions and accepting death are not easy. Remember that any attempt to resuscitate is worthwhile. Since performing CPR and summoning more advanced medical personnel are not the only factors that determine whether a cardiac arrest victim survives, you should feel assured that you did everything you could to help.

◆ CPR FOR ADULTS

CPR is a combination of chest compressions and ventilations. Ventilations place oxygen into the victim's lungs, and chest compressions help to move the oxygen throughout the body.

Chest Compressions

It is not entirely understood why giving CPR circulates blood. The theory is most widely held today is that chest compressions create pressure within the chest cavity that moves blood through the circulatory system. For chest compressions to be most effective, the victim should be flat on his or her back on a firm surface. The victim's head should be on the same level as the heart or lower. CPR is much less effective if the victim is on a soft surface, such as a sofa or mattress, or is sitting up in a chair.

Finding the Correct Hand Position

Using the correct hand position allows you to give the most effective compressions without causing injury. The correct position for your hands is over the lower half of the sternum (breastbone). At the lowest point of the sternum is an arrow-shaped piece of hard tissue called the **xiphoid**. You should avoid pressing directly on the xiphoid, which can break and injure underlying tissues.

To locate the correct hand position for chest compressions—

- Find the lower edge of the victim's rib cage with your hand that is closer to the victim's feet. Slide your middle and index fingers up the edge of the rib cage to the notch where the ribs meet the sternum (Fig. 10-8, *A*). Place your middle finger on this notch. Place your index finger next to your middle finger.
- Place the heel of your other hand on the sternum next to your index finger (Fig. 10-8, *B*). The heel of your hand should rest along the length of the sternum.
- Once the heel of your hand is in position on the sternum, place your other hand directly on top of it (Fig. 10-8, *C*).

Use the heel of your hand to apply pressure on the sternum. Try to keep your fingers off the chest by interlacing them or holding them upward. Applying pressure with your fingers can cause inefficient chest compressions or unnecessary damage to the chest.

Positioning the hands correctly provides the most effective compressions. Correct hand position also decreases the chance of pushing the xiphoid into the delicate organs beneath it, although this rarely occurs.

If you have arthritis or a similar condition in your hands or wrists, you may use an alternative hand position. Find the correct hand position, as above, then grasp the wrist of the hand on the chest with the other hand (Fig. 10-9).

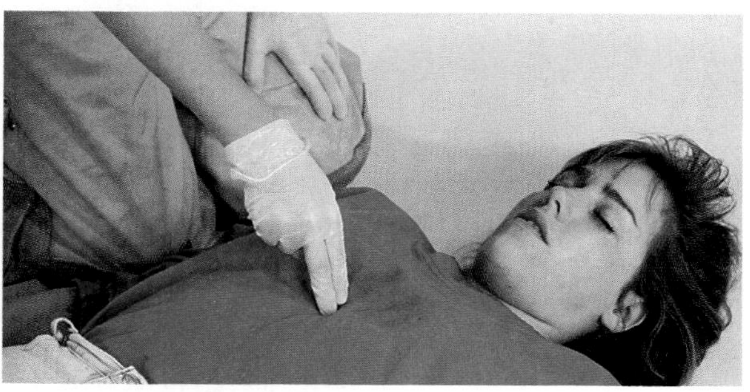
A

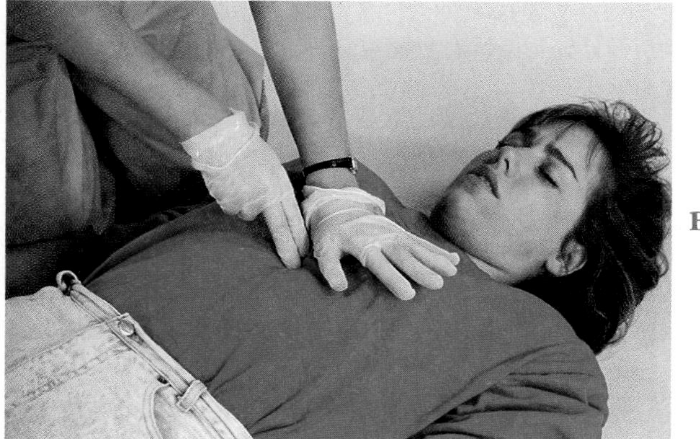
B

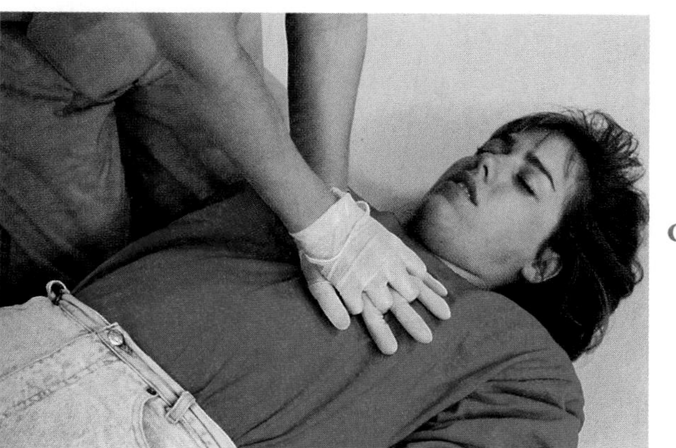
C

Figure 10-8 To locate compression position, **A**, find the notch where the lower ribs meet the sternum. **B**, Place the heel of your hand on the sternum, next to your index finger. **C**, Place your other hand over the heel of the first hand. Use the heel of your bottom hand to apply pressure on the sternum.

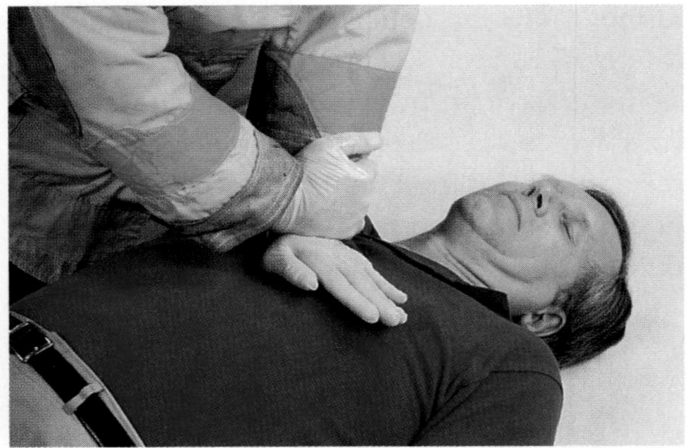

Figure 10-9 Grasping the wrist of the hand positioned on the chest is an alternate hand position for giving chest compressions.

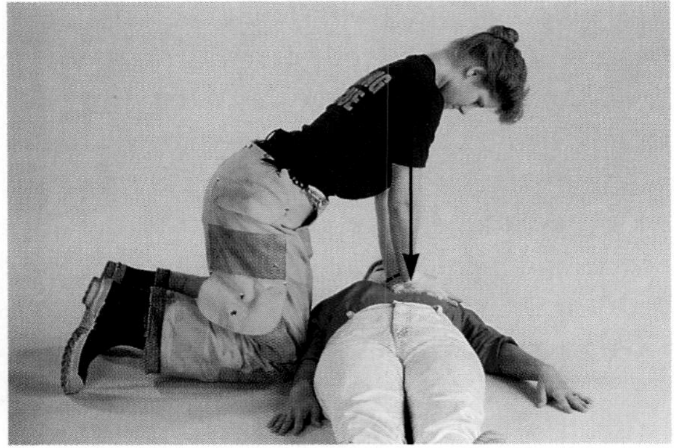

Figure 10-10 With your hands in place, position yourself so that your shoulders are directly over your hands, arms straight and elbows locked.

The victim's clothing will not necessarily interfere with your ability to position your hands correctly. If you can find the correct position without removing thin clothing, such as a T-shirt, do so. Sometimes a layer of thin clothing will help keep your hands from slipping, since the victim's chest may be moist with sweat. However, if you are not sure that you can find the correct hand position, bare the victim's chest. You should not be overly concerned about being able to find the correct position if the victim is obese, since fat does not accumulate over the sternum.

Position of the Rescuer

Your body position is important when giving chest compressions. Compressing the chest straight down provides the best blood flow. The correct body position is also less tiring for you.

Kneel at the victim's chest with your hands in the correct position. Straighten your arms and lock your elbows so that your shoulders are directly over your hands (Fig. 10-10). When you press down in this position, you are pushing straight down onto the victim's sternum. Locking your elbows keeps your arms straight and prevents you from tiring quickly.

Compressing the chest requires little effort in this position. When you press down, the weight of your upper body creates the force needed to compress the chest. Push with the weight of your upper body, not with the muscles of your arms. Push straight down. Do not rock back and forth. Rocking results in less effective compressions and uses unnecessary energy. If your arms and shoulders tire quickly, you are not using the correct body position. After each compression, release the pressure on the chest without losing contact with it and allow the chest to return to its normal position before you start the next compression (Fig. 10-11).

Compression Technique

Each compression should push the sternum down from 1½ to 2 inches. The downward and upward movement should be smooth, not jerky. Maintain a steady down-and-up rhythm, and do not pause between compressions. When you press down, the chambers of the heart empty. When you come up, release all pressure on the chest, which lets the chambers of the heart fill with blood between compressions.

Keep your hands in their correct position on the sternum. If your hands slip, find the notch as you did before and reposition your hands.

Give compressions at the rate of 80 to 100 per minute. As you do compressions, count aloud, "One and two and three and four and five and six and . . ." up to 15. Counting aloud will help you pace yourself. Push down as you

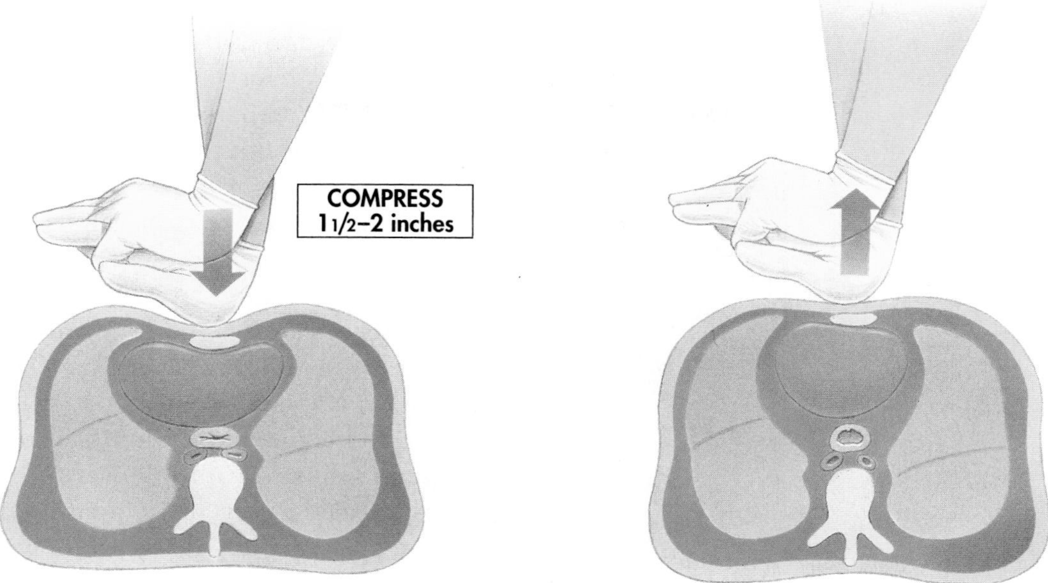

Figure 10-11 Push straight down with the weight of your body, then release, allowing the chest to return to the normal position.

say the number and come up as you say "and." You should be able to do the 15 compressions in about 10 seconds. Even though you are compressing the chest at a rate of 80 to 100 times per minute, you will actually perform only 60 compressions in a minute. You only perform 60 because you must take the time to do rescue breathing, giving 2 slow breaths between each group of 15 compressions.

Compression/Breathing Cycles

When you give CPR, do cycles of 15 compressions and 2 breaths. You should be positioned midway between the chest and the head to move easily between compressions and breaths (Fig. 10-12). For each cycle, give 15 chest compressions, then open the airway with a head-tilt/chin-lift and give 2 slow breaths. This cycle should take about 15 seconds. When you are alone and using a resuscitation mask, the cycle may take a little longer. For each new cycle of compressions and breaths, use the correct hand position by first finding the notch at the lower end of the sternum.

After doing 4 cycles of continuous CPR, check to see if the victim has a pulse. These 4 cycles should take about 1 minute. Check the pulse at the end of the fourth cycle of 15 compressions and 2 breaths (Fig. 10-13). Tilt the victim's head to open the airway, and take time to check the carotid pulse. If there is no pulse, continue CPR, beginning with compressions. Check the pulse again every few minutes. If you find a pulse, check for breathing. Give rescue breathing if necessary. If the victim is breathing, keep his or her airway open and continue to monitor breathing and pulse closely. The Skill Summaries at the end of this chapter provide a guide for step-by-step practice of CPR.

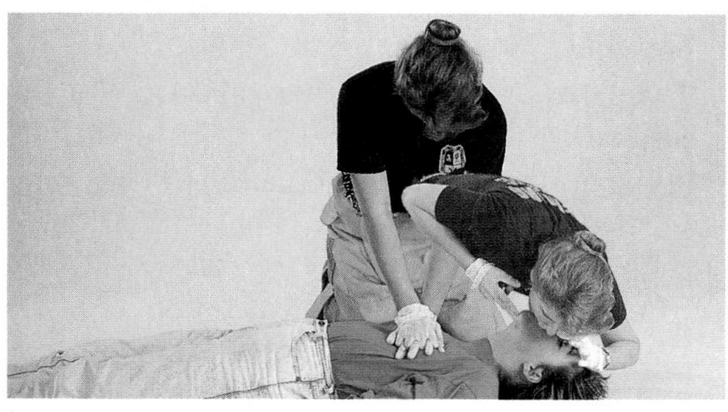

Figure 10-12 Give 15 compressions, then give 2 breaths.

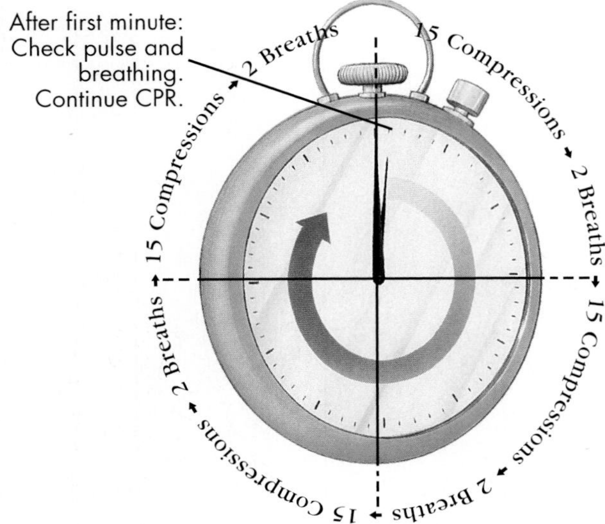

Figure 10-13 Check the pulse at the end of the fourth cycle of 15 compressions and 2 breaths and again every few minutes.

When to Stop CPR

Once you begin CPR, try not to interrupt the blood flow you are creating artificially. However, you can stop CPR —

- If another trained person takes over CPR for you. (Continue to assist by calling advanced medical personnel for help if this has not already been done.)
- If advanced medical personnel arrive and take over care of the victim.
- If the person's heart starts beating.
- If the scene suddenly becomes unsafe.
- If a defibrillator is available and someone trained in its use and authorized to use it is present.
- If you are presented with a valid Do Not Resuscitate (DNR) order.
- If you are exhausted and unable to continue.

◆ CARDIAC EMERGENCIES IN INFANTS AND CHILDREN

A child's heart is usually healthy. Unlike adults, children do not often initially suffer a cardiac emergency. Instead, the child suffers a respiratory emergency. Then a cardiac emergency develops.

The most common cause of cardiac emergencies in children is respiratory problems. Other causes for both infants and children include injuries (from motor vehicle crashes, near-drowning, smoke inhalation, electrocution, burns, poisoning, airway obstruction, firearms, and falls) and heart defects existing at birth. Rarely, a cardiac emergency results from a medical condition or illness such as severe **croup** (a respiratory infection that occurs mainly in children and infants), severe asthma, or certain respiratory infections.

Most cardiac emergencies in infants and children are preventable. One way to prevent them in this age group is to prevent injuries. Another is to make sure that infants and children receive proper medical care. A third is to recognize the early signs of a respiratory emergency. These signs include —

- Agitation.
- Drowsiness.
- Change in skin color (to pale, blue, or ashen).
- Increased difficulty breathing.
- Increased heart and breathing rates.

If you recognize that an infant or child is in respiratory distress or respiratory arrest, provide the care you learned in Chapter 8 for those emergencies. If the infant or child is in cardiac arrest, start CPR immediately. In either event, summon more advanced medical personnel.

◆ CPR IN INFANTS AND CHILDREN

The CPR technique for infants and children is similar to the CPR technique for adults. As in rescue breathing, you need to modify the techniques to accommodate the smaller body size and faster breathing and heart rates. Figure 10-14 compares the adult, child, and infant CPR techniques.

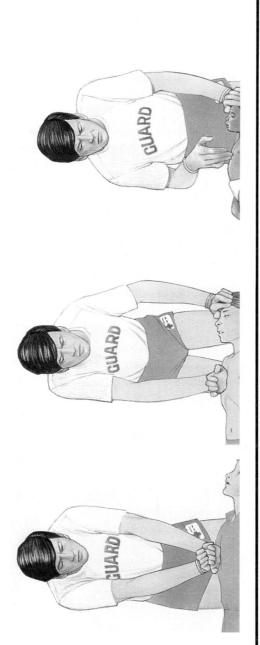

HAND POSITION:	Two hands on lower ½ of sternum	One hand on lower ½ of sternum	Two fingers on lower ½ of sternum (one finger-width below nipple line)
COMPRESS:	1½-2 inches	1-1½ inches	½-1 inch
BREATHE:	Slowly until chest gently rises (about 1.5 seconds per breath)	Slowly until chest gently rises (about 1.5 seconds per breath)	Slowly until chest gently rises (about 1.5 seconds per breath)
CYCLE:	15 compressions 2 breaths	5 compressions 1 breath	5 compressions 1 breath
RATE:	15 compressions in about 10 seconds	5 compressions in about 3 seconds	5 compressions in about 3 seconds

Figure 10-14 The technique for chest compressions differs for adults, children, and infants.

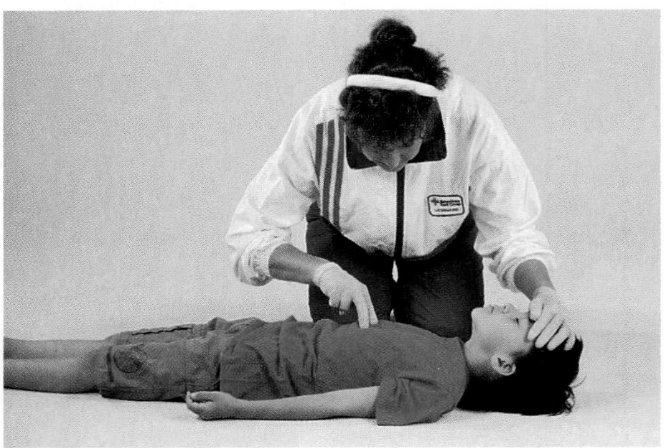

Figure 10-15 While kneeling beside the child, maintain an open airway with one hand and find the correct hand position with the other.

CPR for Children

To find out if a child needs CPR, begin with the initial assessment. If you determine that there is no pulse, begin CPR.

To give compressions, kneel beside the child's chest with your knees against the child's side. Maintain an open airway with one hand and find the correct hand position with the other (Fig. 10-15). To locate hand position on a child, slide your middle finger up the lower edge of the ribs until you locate the notch where the ribs meet the sternum (breastbone). Place the index finger next to it. The two fingers should be resting on the lower end of the sternum (Fig. 10-16, *A*).

Visually mark the place where you put your index finger. Lift your fingers off the sternum and put the heel of the same hand on the sternum immediately above where you had your index finger (Fig. 10-16, *B*). Keep your fingers off the child's chest. Only the heel of your hand should rest on the sternum.

When you compress the chest, use only the hand that is on the child's sternum. *You do not use both hands to give chest compressions to a child*. Push straight down, making sure your shoulder is directly over your hand (Fig. 10-17). Each compression should push the sternum down from 1 to 1½ inches. The down-and-up movement should be smooth, not jerky. Release the pressure on the chest completely, but do not lift your hand off the child's chest (Fig. 10-18).

When you give CPR to a child, do cycles of 5 compressions and 1 breath at a rate of about 100 compressions per minute. While giving compressions with one hand, keep your other hand on the child's forehead to help maintain an open airway. After giving 5 compressions, remove your compression hand from the chest, lift the chin, and give 1 slow breath. The breath should last about 1½ seconds. Always use a chin-lift with a head-tilt to ensure that the

A

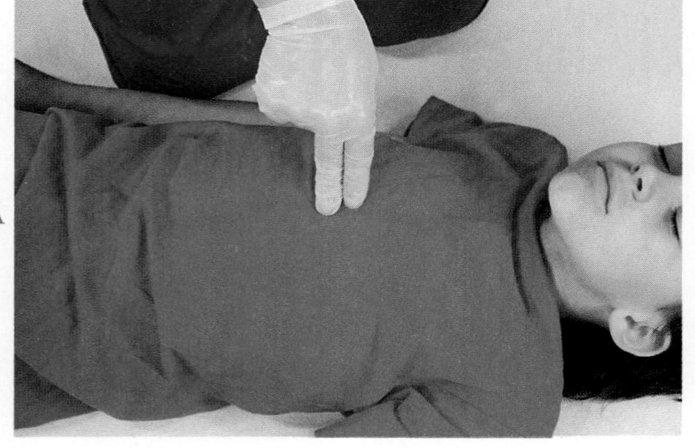

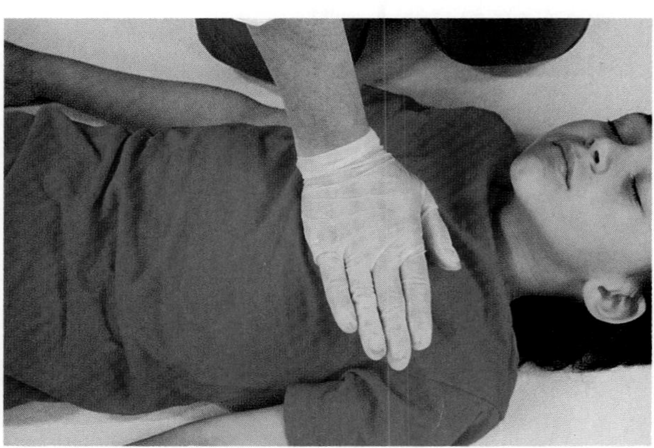

B

Figure 10-16 To locate compression position, **A**, find the notch where the lower rib meets the sternum with your middle finger. Place the index finger next to it so that both fingers rest on the lower end of the breastbone. **B**, Place the heel of the same hand on the breastbone immediately above where you had your index finger.

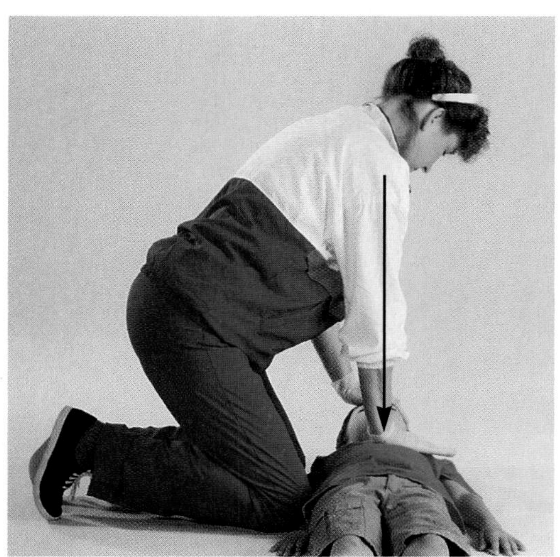

Figure 10-17 When you compress the chest, use the heel of your hand. Push straight down, making sure your shoulder is directly over your hand.

child's airway is open unless you suspect a head, neck, or back injury. After giving the breath, place your hand in the same position as before and continue compressions. You do not have to measure your hand position each time by sliding your fingers up the rib cage unless you lose your place.

Keep repeating the cycle of 5 compressions and 1 breath (Fig. 10-19). Each cycle of 5 compressions and 1 breath should take about 5 seconds. After you do about 1 minute of continuous CPR (about 12 cycles), recheck the child's pulse for about 5 seconds. If there is no pulse, continue CPR, beginning with compressions. Repeat the pulse check every few minutes.

If you do find a pulse, then check for breathing for about 5 seconds. If the child is breathing, keep the airway open and monitor breathing and pulse closely. Check the pulse once every minute. Cover the child, and keep the child warm and as quiet as possible. If the child is not breathing, give rescue breathing and keep checking the pulse. Do not keep your fingers on the carotid artery between pulse checks.

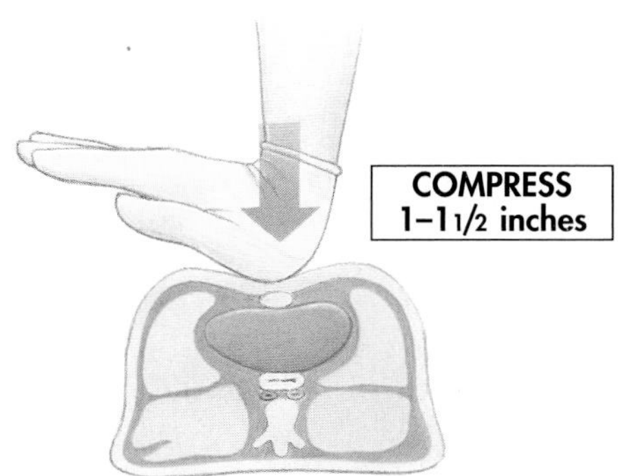

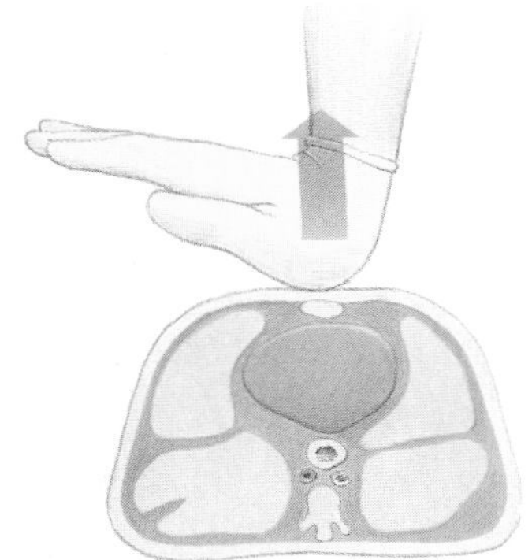

Figure 10-18 Push straight down with the weight of your body and then release, allowing the chest to return to its normal position.

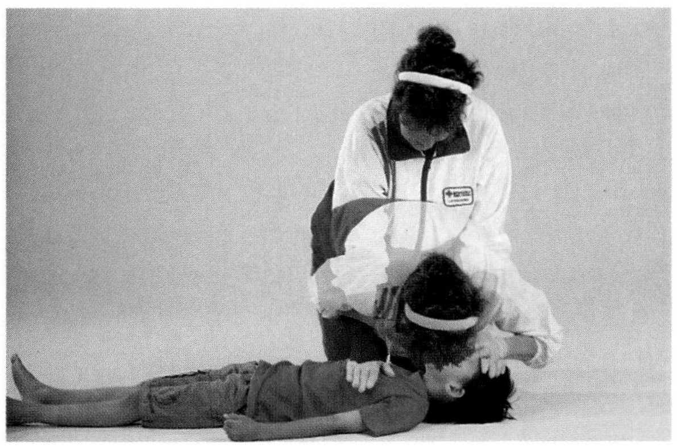

Figure 10-19 Give 5 compressions and then 1 breath.

CPR for Infants

To find out if an infant needs CPR, begin with an initial assessment to check the ABCs. To check the pulse in an infant, locate the brachial

A

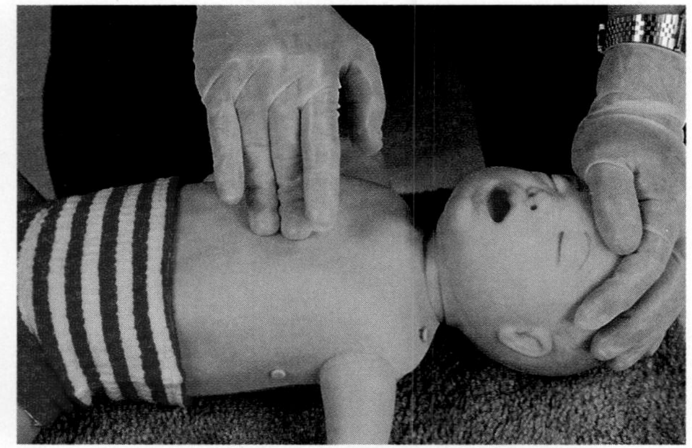

B

C

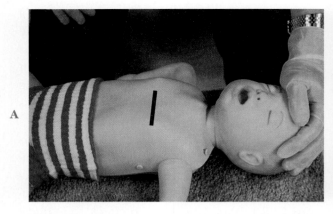

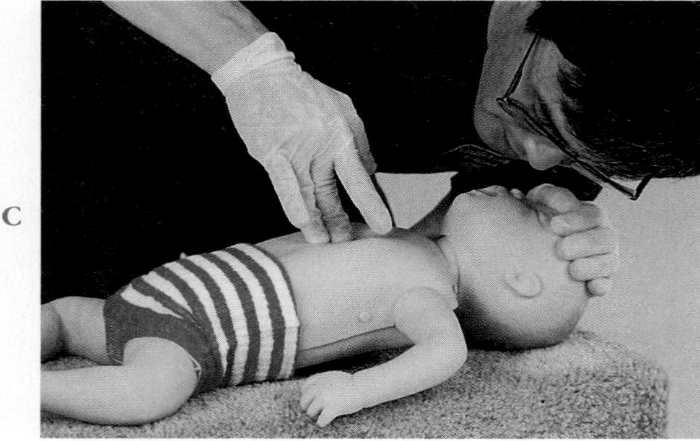

Figure 10-20 To locate compression position, **A**, imagine a line running across the chest between the infant's nipples. **B**, Place the pads of the middle and ring fingers next to your index finger on the breastbone. Raise the index finger. **C**, Use the pads of the remaining two fingers to compress the chest.

pulse in the arm. If the infant has no pulse, begin CPR.

Position the infant faceup on a firm, flat surface. The infant's head must be on the same level as the heart or lower. Stand or kneel, facing the infant from the side. Keep one hand on the infant's head to maintain an open airway. Use your other hand to give compressions.

To find the correct place to give compressions, imagine a line running across the chest between the infant's nipples (Fig. 10-20, *A*). Place your index finger on the sternum (breastbone) just below this imaginary line. Then place the pads of the two fingers next to your index finger on the sternum. Raise the index finger (Fig. 10-20, *B*). If you feel the notch at the end of the infant's sternum, move your fingers up a little bit.

Use the pads of two fingers to compress the chest (Fig. 10-20, *C*). Compress the chest ½ to 1 inch, then let the sternum return to its normal position. When you compress, push straight down. The down-and-up movement of your compressions should be smooth, not jerky. Keep a steady rhythm. Do not pause between compressions. When you are coming up, release pressure on the infant's chest completely, but do not let your fingers lose contact with the chest (Fig. 10-21). Keep your fingers in the compression position. Use your other hand to keep the airway open using a head-tilt.

When you give CPR, do cycles of 5 compressions and 1 breath (Fig. 10-22). Compress at a rate of at least 100 compressions per minute. The rate is slightly faster than the rate of compressions for an adult or a child. When you complete 5 compressions, give 1 slow breath, covering the infant's nose and mouth with your mouth. The breath should take about 1½ seconds. Keep repeating cycles of 5 compressions and 1 breath. A complete cycle of 5

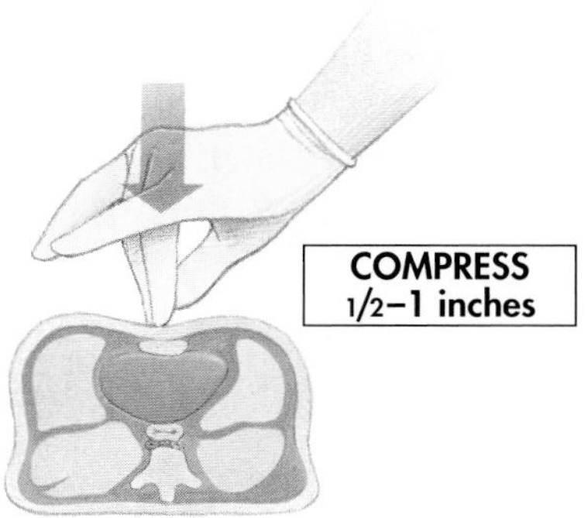

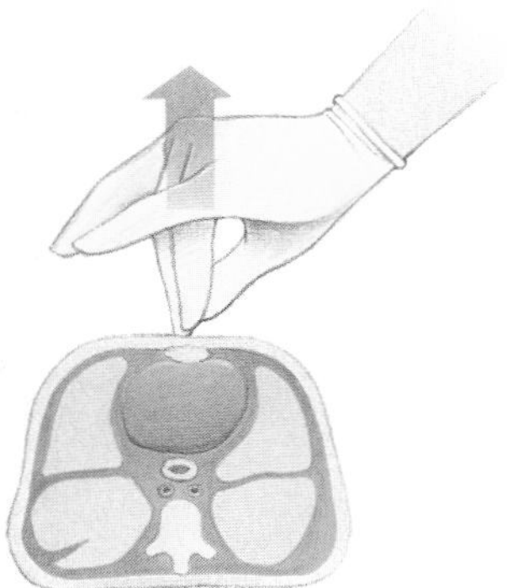

Figure 10-21 Push straight down with your fingers and then release the pressure on the chest completely.

compressions and 1 breath should take about 5 seconds.

Recheck the pulse after about 1 minute of continuous CPR (about 12 cycles). Check the brachial pulse for about 5 seconds with the hand that was giving compressions. If there is no pulse, continue CPR, starting with compressions. Repeat the pulse check every few minutes.

If you do find a pulse, then check breathing for about 5 seconds. If the infant is breathing, keep the airway open and monitor breathing and pulse closely. Check the pulse once every minute. Maintain normal body temperature. If the infant is not breathing, give rescue breathing.

◆ TWO-RESCUER CPR

When two professional rescuers are available, they often give two-rescuer CPR. They share the responsibility for performing rescue breathing and chest compressions (Fig. 10-23). You should be able to perform two-rescuer CPR in each of the following situations:

1. CPR is *not* being given and two or more rescuers arrive on the scene at the same time and begin CPR together.
2. One rescuer is giving CPR and a second rescuer is available to begin two-rescuer CPR.

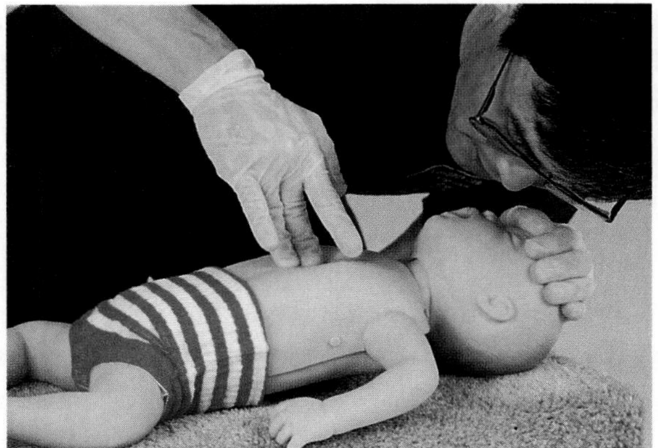

Figure 10-22 Give 5 compressions and then 1 breath.

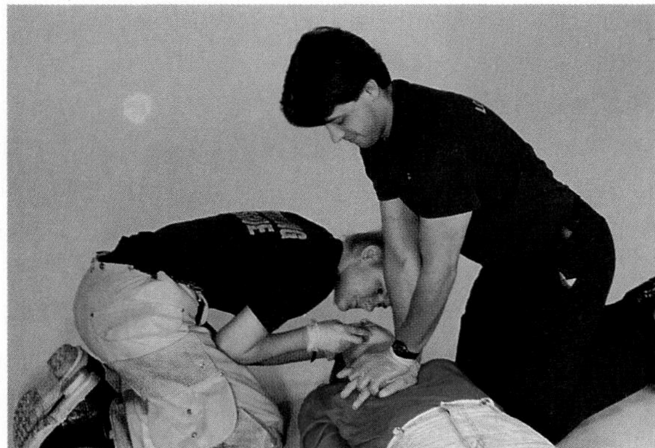

Figure 10-23 During two-rescuer CPR, the rescuers share the responsibility for performing rescue breathing and chest compressions.

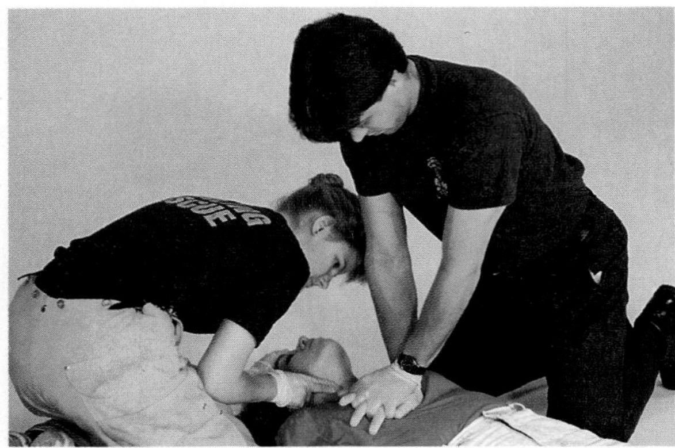

Figure 10-24 The ventilator periodically checks the effectiveness of compressions by feeling for the carotid pulse while the compressor gives chest compressions.

3. Either rescuer tires and the rescuers change position.

Two-Rescuer Techniques

In two-rescuer CPR for an adult, the victim is given breaths more often than in one-rescuer CPR. Instead of the single-rescuer cycle of 15 compressions and 2 breaths, a two-rescuer CPR cycle involves 5 compressions and 1 breath (a ratio of 5 to 1). Compressions are stopped at the upstroke of the fifth compression, and the rescuer giving breaths immediately gives 1 slow breath. The other rescuer then continues giving compressions.

Chest compressions are given at a rate of 80 to 100 per minute and at a depth of 1½ to 2 inches, the same as in one-rescuer CPR. The rescuer performing compressions uses the same counting rhythm as for one-rescuer CPR: "One and, two and, three and, four and, five" —(breath)—"One and, two and, three and, four and, five."

During two-rescuer CPR, the person giving breaths frequently checks the effectiveness of the compressions by feeling for the carotid pulse while chest compressions are being performed (Fig. 10-24). He or she advises whether the compressions are effective. If the victim has lost a significant amount of blood, a carotid pulse may not be felt, even though compressions are effective.

The rescuer performing rescue breathing also does a pulse check after the first minute of compressions and repeats the check every few minutes after that to determine if circulation has returned. He or she says, "Pulse check," and the rescuer performing compressions stops after the fifth compression. The same rescuer checks the pulse for about 5 seconds. If there is no pulse, they continue CPR, starting with compressions.

When Two Rescuers Arrive on the Scene at the Same Time

If CPR is not being performed when you arrive, one rescuer should do a initial assessment and, if appropriate, begin CPR. The other rescuer should manage other responsibilities at the scene, such as scene safety, communications, and setting up equipment and supplies. Then the second rescuer can assist with CPR.

Two Rescuers Beginning CPR Together

When both rescuers are available to begin CPR at the same time, the first rescuer does an initial assessment. While the first rescuer is doing the initial assessment, the second rescuer gets into position to give chest compressions and locates the correct hand position. He or she should begin chest compressions when the first rescuer says, "No pulse, begin CPR." Both rescuers continue CPR together.

When CPR Is in Progress by One Rescuer

When a person is giving CPR and a second rescuer arrives, that rescuer should ask whether advanced medical personnel have been summoned. If not, he or she should summon them or send someone else to call. Then the second rescuer should either replace the first rescuer or assist him or her in giving two-rescuer CPR.

If the second rescuer is going to assist with two-rescuer CPR, he or she enters immediately after the first rescuer has completed a cycle of 15 compressions and 2 breaths.

The second rescuer gets into position at the victim's chest and finds the correct hand position. The first rescuer remains at the victim's head and checks the pulse. If there is still no pulse, the first rescuer signals to begin CPR. The second rescuer, at the chest, begins chest compressions. Both rescuers continue giving two-rescuer CPR.

Changing Positions

If a rescuer becomes tired, he or she can change position with the other rescuer. When the rescuers change, the rescuer at the victim's head completes 1 breath and then moves immediately to the chest. The rescuer at the chest moves immediately to the head. Both rescuers move quickly into position without changing sides. The sequence for changing positions is the following:

1. The rescuer performing compressions says to change positions. He or she begins the cycle of compressions by saying,"Change and, two and, three and, four and, five."
2. Change positions. The rescuer at the head gives the ventilation at the end of the "change" cycle and moves to the chest. He or she locates the correct hand position and waits for the other rescuer to signal before beginning compressions. The rescuer now at the victim's head checks for a pulse for 5 seconds. If there is no pulse, he or she says, "No pulse, continue CPR."
3. They continue two-rescuer CPR, giving 5 compressions and 1 breath. The rescuer at the head periodically assesses the effectiveness of the compressions by checking for a pulse during compressions.

Skill Summaries for all two-rescuer skills are at the end of this chapter.

◆ PREVENTING CARDIOVASCULAR DISEASE

Although a heart attack seems to strike suddenly, the conditions that lead to it may develop over years. Many Americans' lifestyles may gradually be endangering their hearts, which can eventually result in cardiovascular disease. Potentially harmful behaviors frequently begin early in life. For example, many children develop tastes for "junk" foods that are high in cholesterol and have little or no nutritional value. Sometimes children are not encouraged to exercise.

Several studies have shown that coronary artery disease actually begins in the teenage years, when most smoking begins. Teenagers are more likely to begin smoking if their parents smoke. Smoking contributes to cardiovascular disease, as well as to other diseases.

Risk Factors of Heart Disease

Scientists have identified many factors that increase a person's chances of developing heart disease. These are known as ***risk factors***. Some risk factors for heart disease cannot be changed. For instance, men have a somewhat higher risk for heart disease than do women. Having a history of heart disease in your family also increases your risk.

But people can control many risk factors for heart disease. Smoking, diets high in fats, high blood pressure, obesity, and lack of routine exercise are all linked to increased risk of heart disease. When one risk factor, such as high blood pressure, is combined with other risk factors, such as obesity or cigarette smoking, the risk of heart attack or stroke is greatly increased.

Controlling Risk Factors

Controlling your risk factors involves adjusting your lifestyle to minimize the chance of future cardiovascular disease. The three major risk factors you can control are cigarette smoking, high blood pressure, and high blood cholesterol levels.

Cigarette smokers are more than twice as likely to have a heart attack as nonsmokers and 2 to 4 times as likely to have cardiac arrest. The earlier a person starts using tobacco, the greater the risk to his or her future health. Giving up smoking will rapidly reduce the risk of heart disease. After a number of years, the risk becomes almost the same as if the person had never smoked. If you do not smoke, do not start. If you do smoke, quit.

Uncontrolled high blood pressure can damage blood vessels in the heart, kidneys, and other organs. You can often control high blood pressure by losing excess weight and by changing your diet. When these measures are not enough, medications can be prescribed. It is important to have regular checkups to guard against high blood pressure and its harmful effects.

Diets high in saturated fats and cholesterol increase the risk of heart disease. These diets raise the level of cholesterol in the blood and increase the chance that cholesterol and other fatty materials will be deposited on blood vessel walls and cause atherosclerosis.

Some cholesterol is essential for the body. The amount of cholesterol in the blood is determined by how much your body produces and by the food you eat. Foods high in cholesterol include egg yolks and organ meats, such as liver.

More important to an unhealthy blood cholesterol level is saturated fat. **Saturated fats** raise blood cholesterol level by interfering with the body's ability to remove cholesterol from the blood. Saturated fats are found in beef, lamb, veal, pork, ham, coconut oil, palm oil, whole milk, and whole milk products.

Rather than eliminating saturated fats and cholesterol from your diet, limit your intake. This is easier than you think. Moderation is the key. Make changes whenever you can by substituting low-fat milk or skim milk for whole milk, margarine for butter, trimming visible fat from meat, and broiling or baking rather than frying. Read labels carefully. A "cholesterol-free" product may be high in saturated fat.

Two additional ways to help prevent heart disease are to control your weight and exercise regularly. You store excess calories in your diet as fat. In general, overweight people have a shorter life expectancy. Obese middle-aged men have nearly 3 times the risk of a fatal heart attack as do normal-weight middle-aged men.

Routine exercise has many benefits, including increased muscle tone and weight control. Exercise can also help you survive a heart attack because the increased circulation of blood through the heart develops additional channels for blood flow. If the primary channels that supply the heart are blocked in a heart attack, these additional channels can supply the heart tissue with oxygen-rich blood.

Results of Managing Risk Factors

Managing your risk factors for cardiovascular disease really works. During the past 20 years, deaths from cardiovascular disease have decreased more than 30 percent in the United States. As a result, as many as 250,000 lives may have been saved each year. Also, deaths from stroke have declined 50 percent.

Why did deaths from these causes decline? Probably they declined as a result of improved detection and treatment, as well as lifestyle changes. People are becoming more aware of their risk factors for heart disease and are taking action to control them. If you take action, you can improve your chances of living a long and healthy life. If you suffer a cardiac arrest, your chances of survival are poor. Begin today to reduce your risk of cardiovascular disease. Completing the Healthy Lifestyles Awareness Inventory, Appendix B in this textbook, will help you evaluate your risk for cardiovascular disease and other conditions that may cause sudden illness.

◆ SUMMARY

It is important to recognize signs and symptoms that may indicate a heart attack. If you think someone is suffering from a heart attack or if you are unsure, summon more advanced medical personnel without delay. Provide care by helping the victim rest in the most comfortable position until help arrives.

When heartbeat and breathing stop, it is called cardiac arrest. A person who suffers a cardiac arrest is clinically dead, since no oxygen is reaching the cells of vital organs. Irreversible brain damage will occur from lack of oxygen. By starting CPR immediately, you can help keep the brain supplied with oxygen. By summoning more advanced medical personnel, you can increase the cardiac arrest victim's chances for survival.

If the victim does not have a pulse, start CPR. Always remember these simple guidelines for CPR:

- Use the correct hand position.
- Compress down and up smoothly.
- Give 15 compressions in approximately 10 seconds.
- Give 2 slow breaths.
- Repeat this cycle of compressions and breaths 3 more times (4 times in all).
- Check for the return of a pulse.
- If there is no pulse, continue CPR, beginning with compressions.
- Check for the return of a pulse every few minutes.
- If the victim's pulse returns, stop CPR and check to see if the person has started to breathe.
- If the victim is still not breathing, begin rescue breathing.

If two rescuers are available, begin two-rescuer CPR as soon as possible. If either rescuer tires, quickly change positions and continue. Once you start CPR, do not stop unnecessarily.

Use the activities in Unit 10 of the workbook to help you review the material in this chapter.

You Are the Responder

You arrive on the scene of an emergency to find a bystander giving CPR. You confirm that 9-1-1 has been called and the victim is in cardiac arrest. You take over CPR. Advanced medical personnel have not yet arrived. You are tiring and do not think you can continue. What do you do?

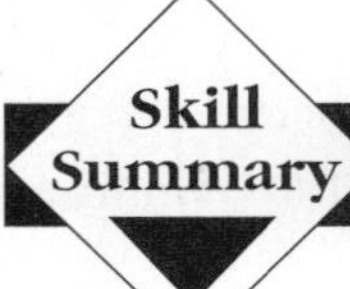

CPR for an Adult

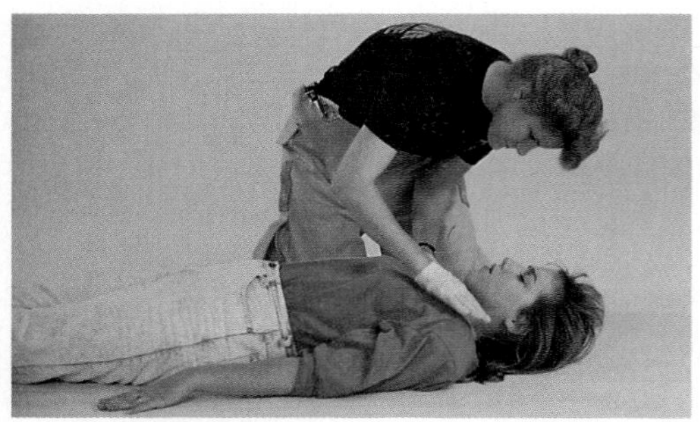

1. Check for consciousness.

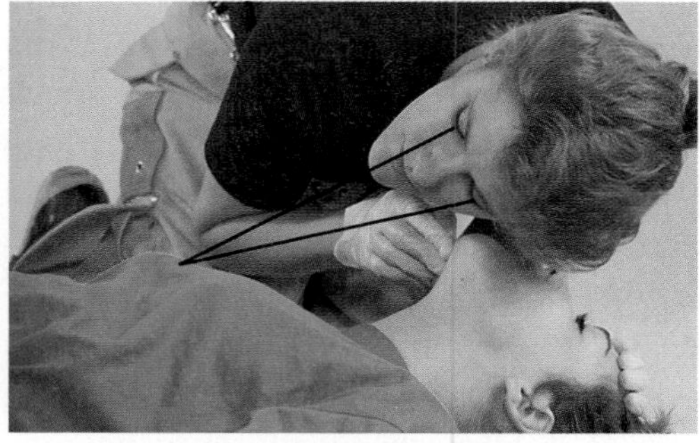

2. Open airway and check for breathing.

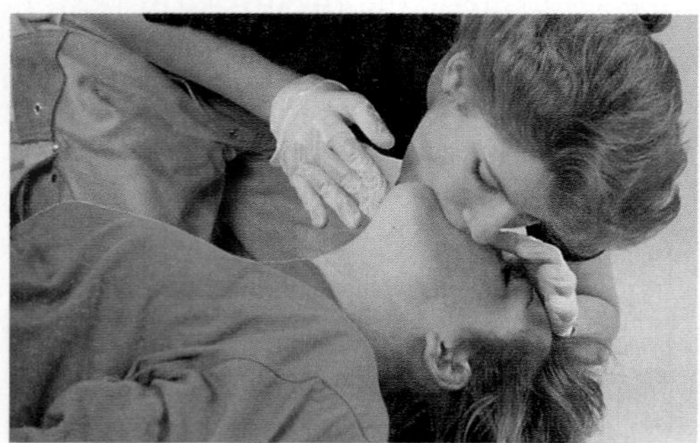

3. Give 2 slow breaths.

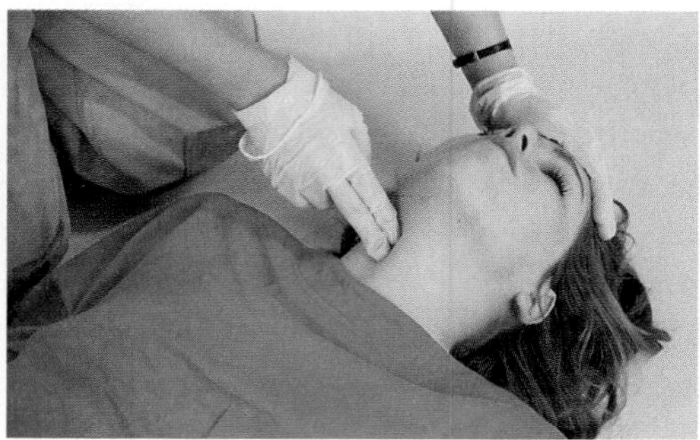

4. Check for pulse and severe bleeding.

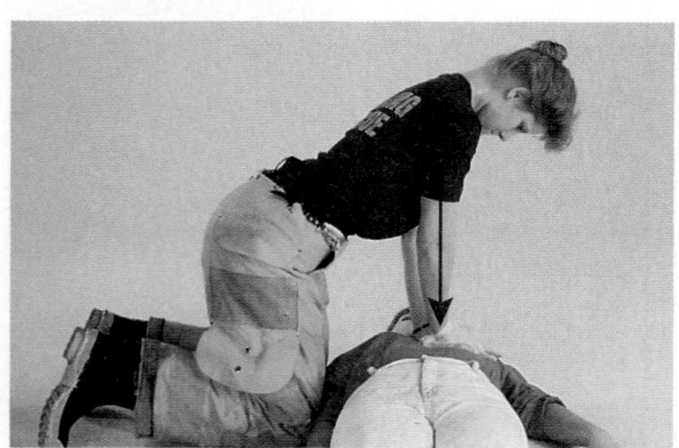

5. Begin CPR by giving 15 compressions.

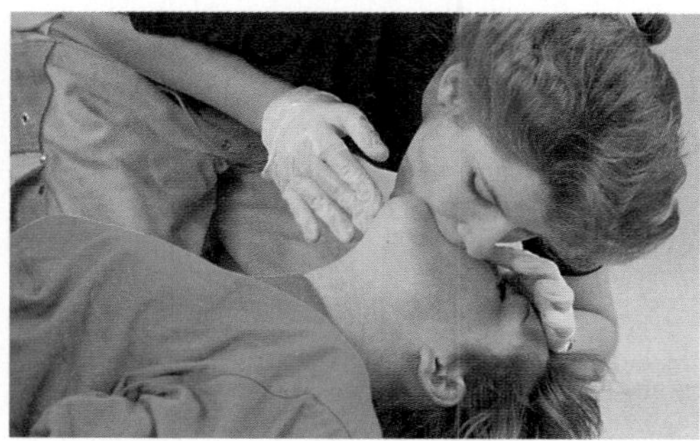

6. Then give 2 slow breaths.

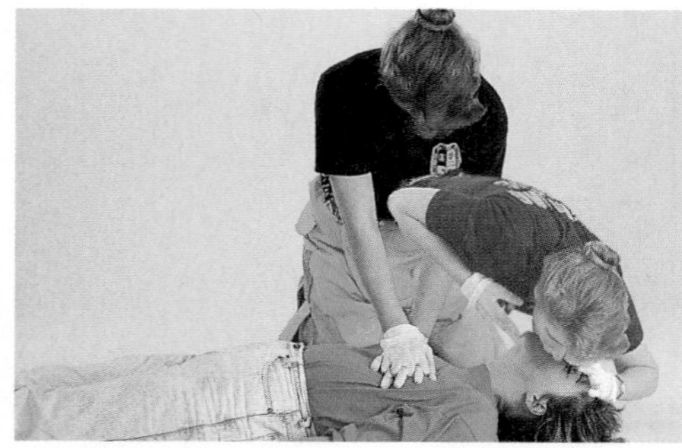

7. Repeat cycles of 15 compressions and 2 breaths.

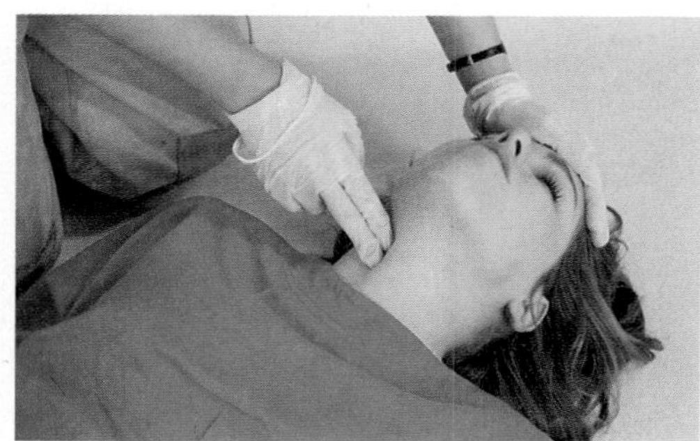

8. After about 1 minute, recheck pulse for about 5 seconds.

If there is still no pulse, continue CPR, beginning with compressions.

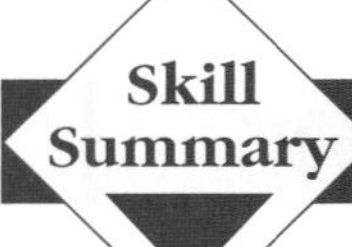

CPR for a Child

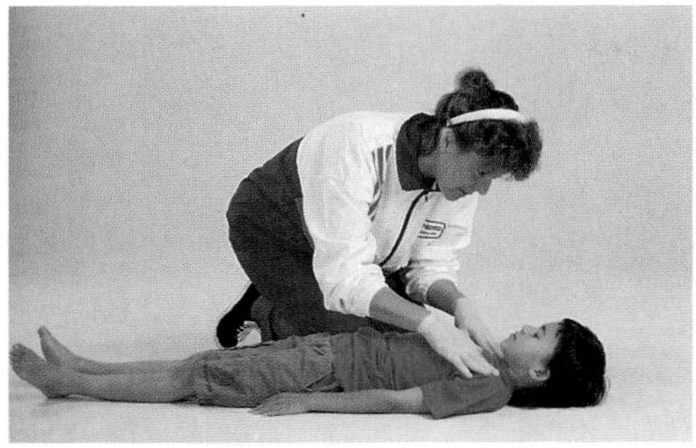

1. Check for consciousness.

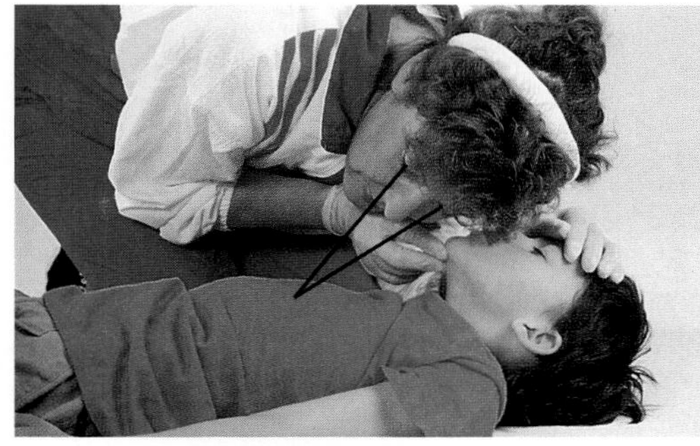

2. Open airway and check for breathing.

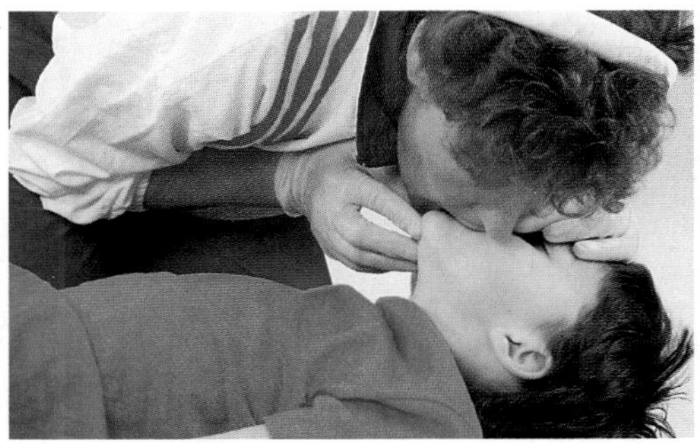

3. Give 2 slow breaths.

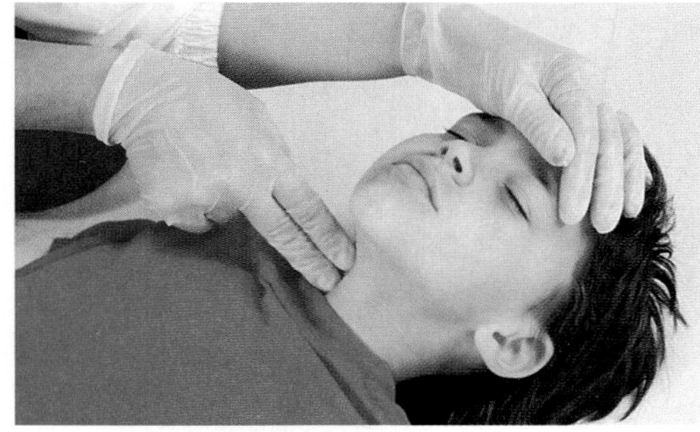

4. Check for pulse and severe bleeding.

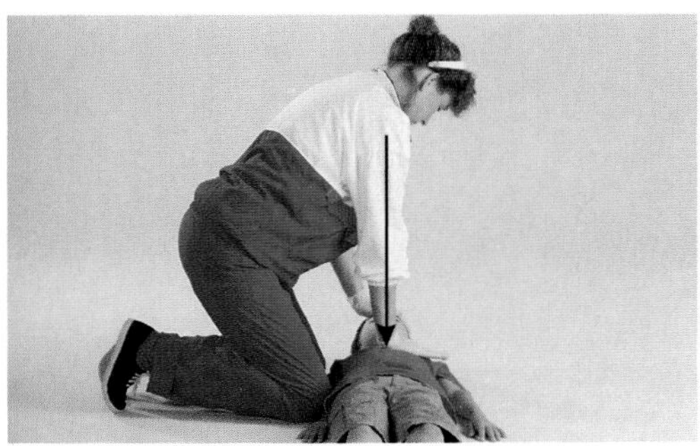

5. Begin CPR by giving 5 compressions.

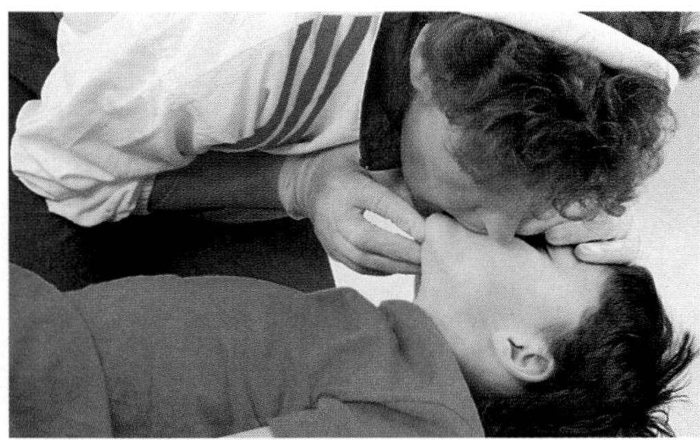

6. Then give 1 slow breath.

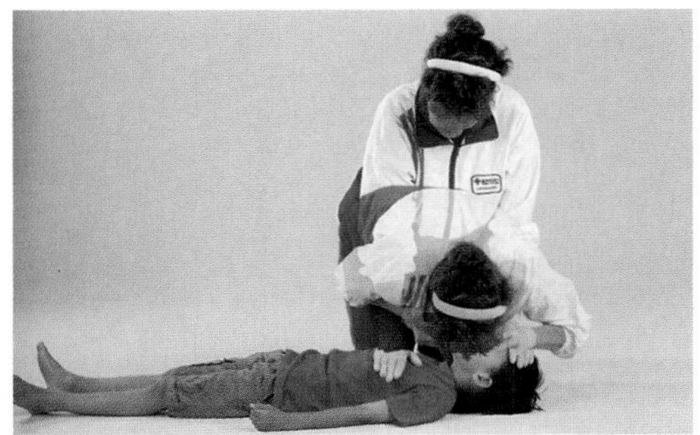

7. Repeat cycles of 5 compressions and 1 breath.

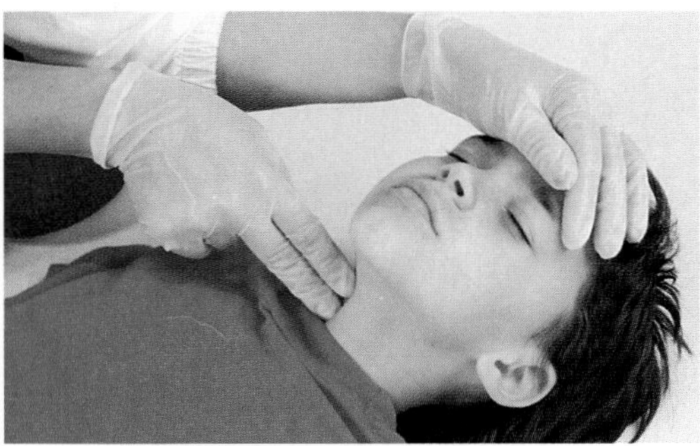

8. After about 1 minute, recheck pulse for about 5 seconds.

If there is still no pulse, continue CPR, beginning with compressions.

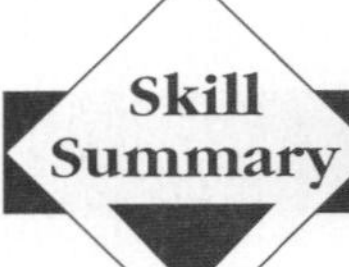

CPR for an Infant

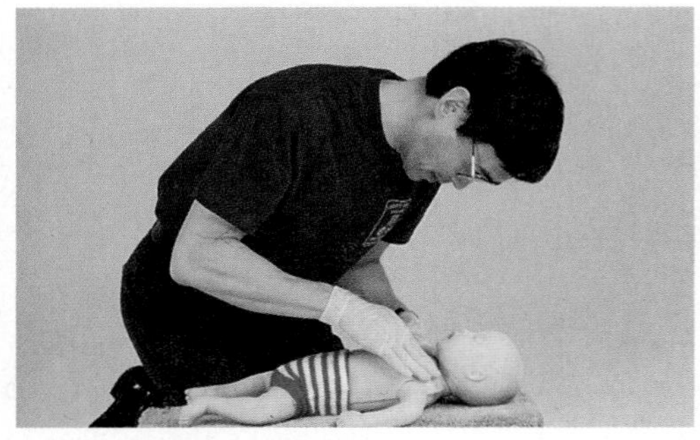

1. Check for consciousness.

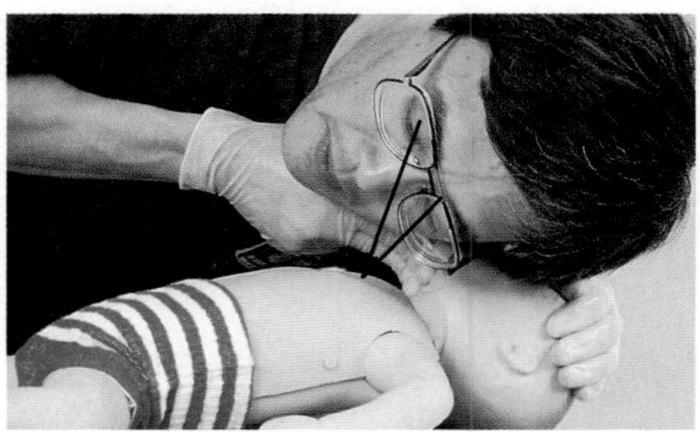

2. Open airway and check for breathing.

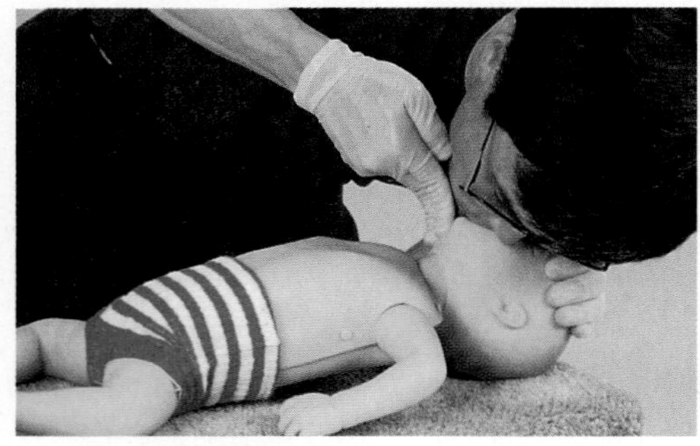

3. Give 2 slow breaths.

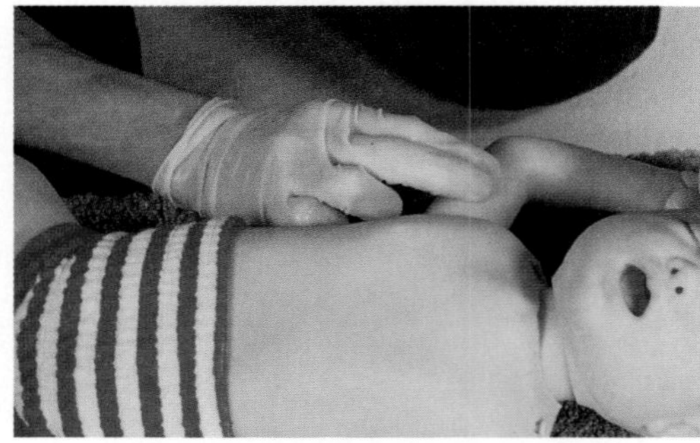

4. Check for pulse and severe bleeding.

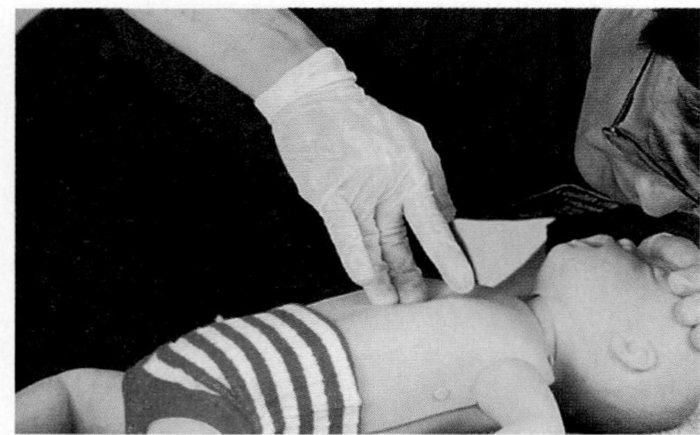

5. Begin CPR by giving 5 compressions.

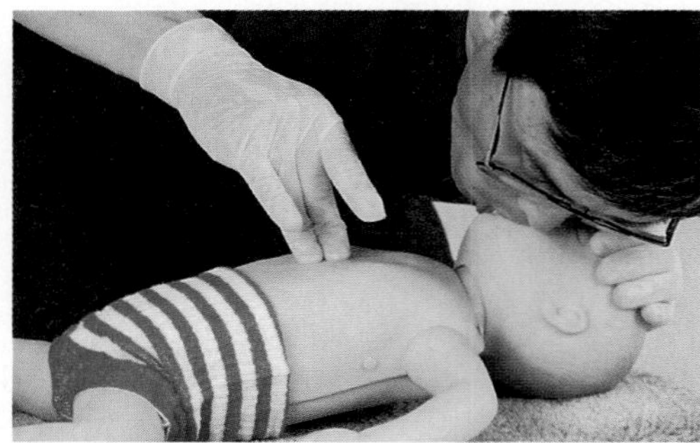

6. Then give 1 slow breath.

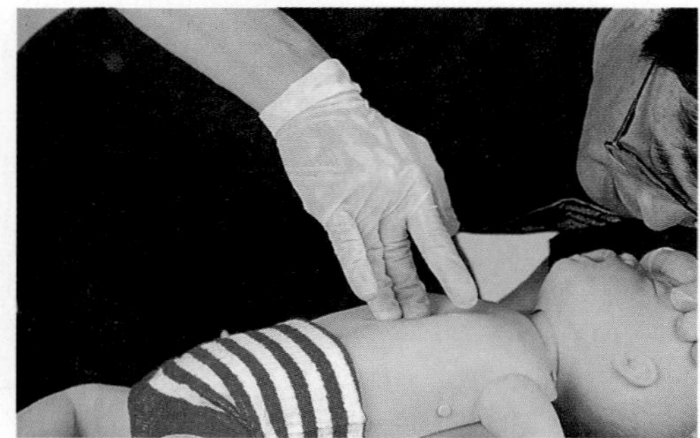

7. Repeat cycles of 5 compressions and 1 breath.

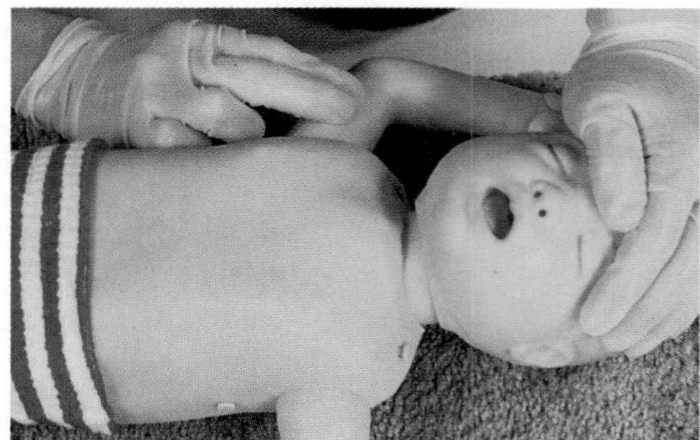

8. After about 1 minute, recheck pulse for about 5 seconds.

If there is still no pulse, continue CPR, beginning with compressions.

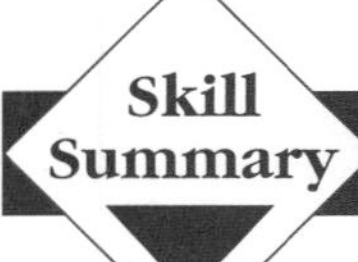

Two-Rescuer CPR—Beginning Together

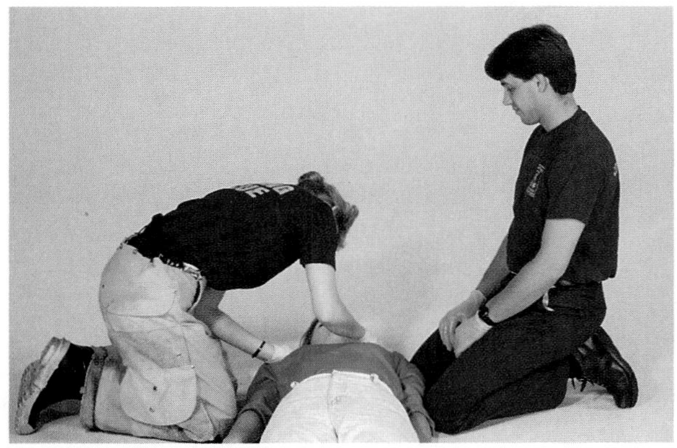

1. First rescuer checks consciousness.

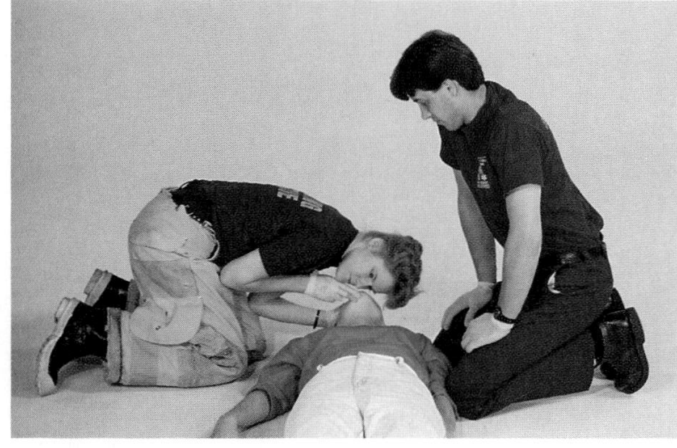

2. First rescuer opens airway and checks breathing.

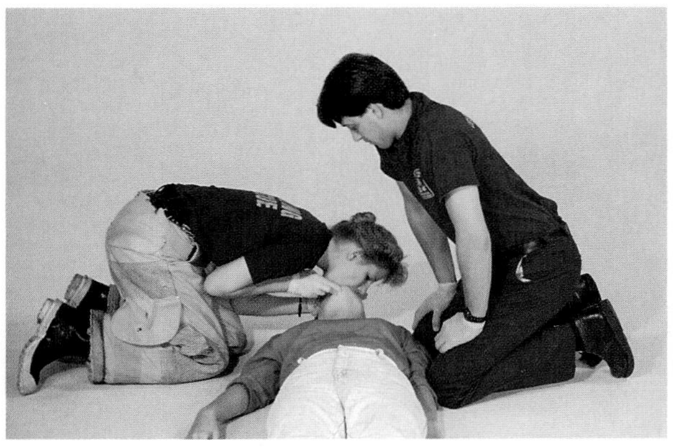

3. First rescuer gives 2 slow breaths.

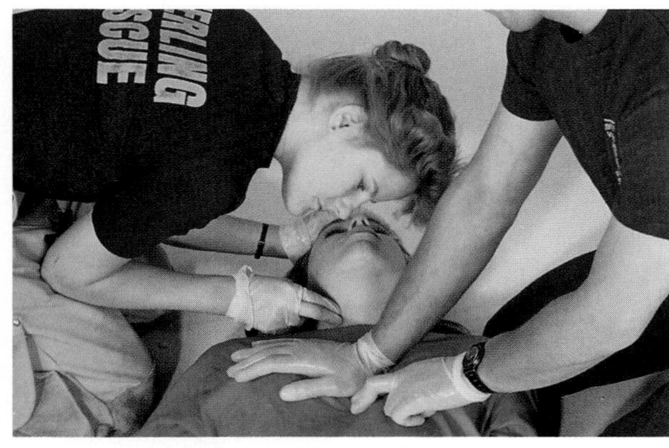

4. First rescuer checks pulse. Second rescuer locates proper hand placement.

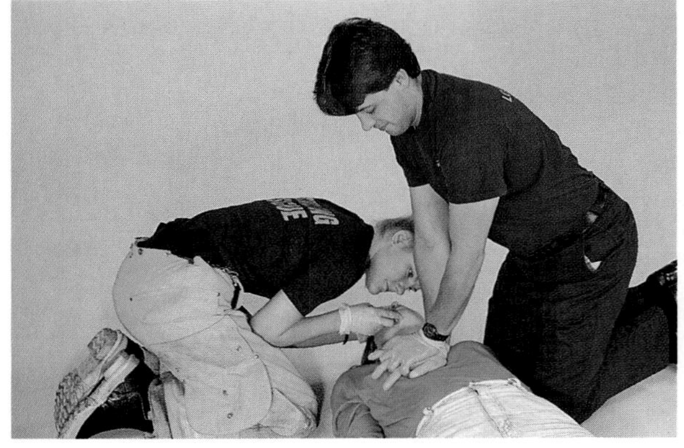

5. Second rescuer does 5 chest compressions.

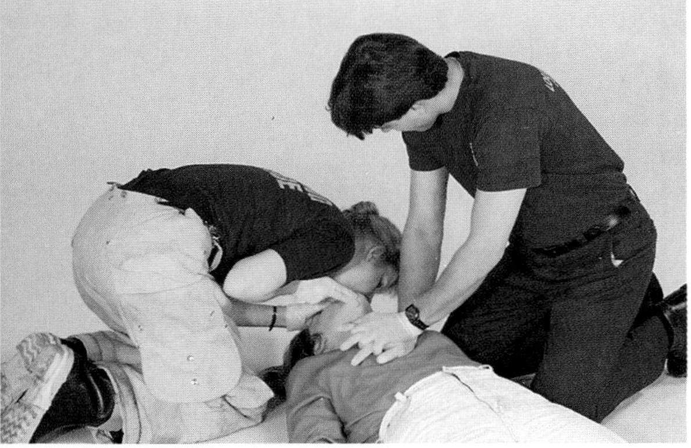

6. First rescuer gives 1 slow breath. Two rescuers repeat cycles of CPR.

After about 1 minute of CPR, the first rescuer checks pulse. If there is still no pulse, both rescuers continue CPR, beginning with compressions.

Two Rescuers—Changing Positions

Skill Summary

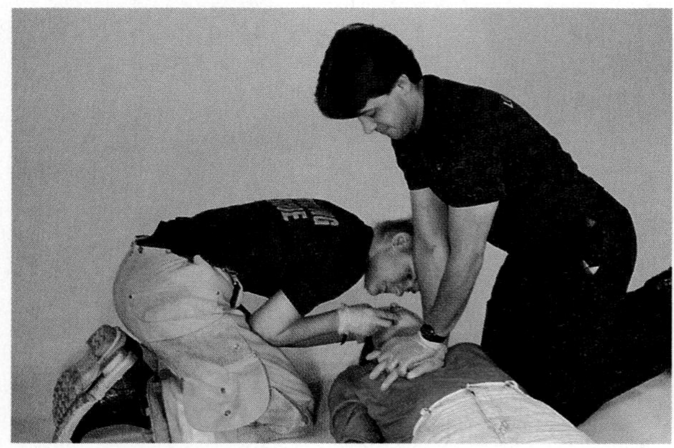

1. Rescuer at chest calls, "Change" and finishes compressions.

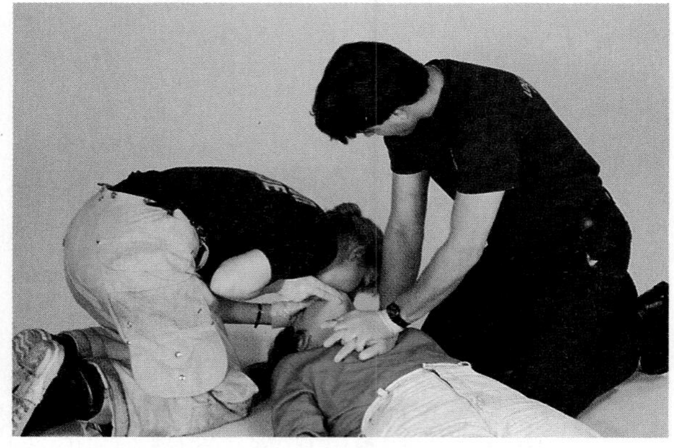

2. Rescuer at head gives breath.

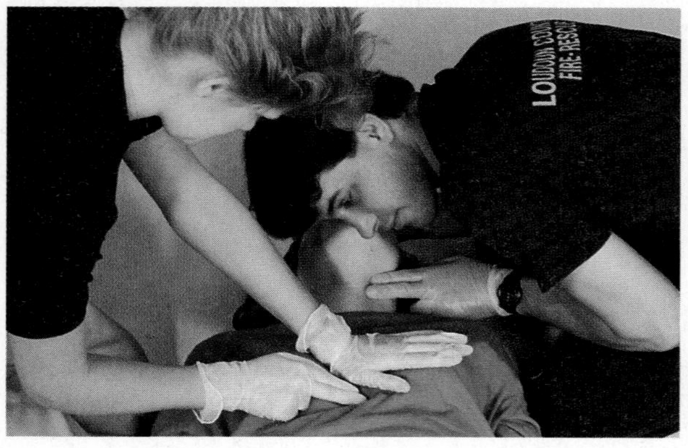

3. Rescuers change positions. The new ventilator rechecks pulse.

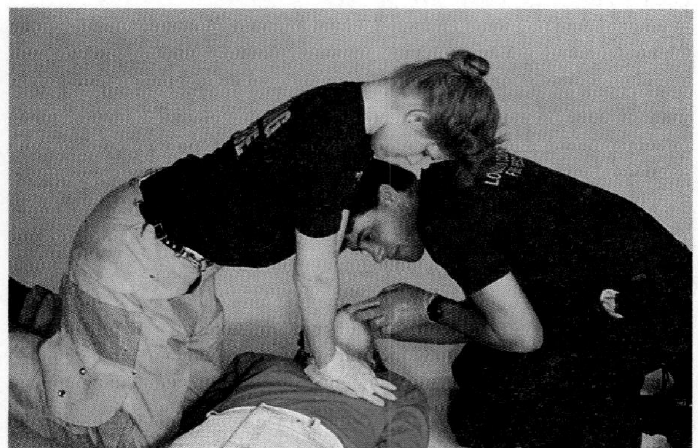

4. Compressor continues with chest compressions.

Repeat cycles of CPR. After about 1 minute of CPR, the first rescuer rechecks pulse. If there is still no pulse, both rescuers continue CPR, beginning with compressions.

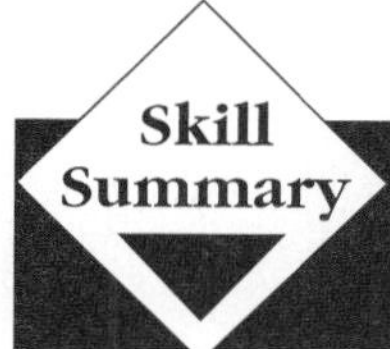

Entry of a Second Rescuer When One-Person CPR Is in Progress

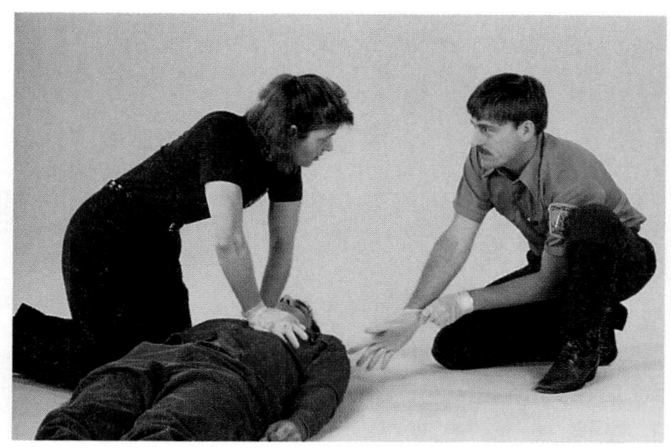

1. Second rescuer identifies himself or herself.

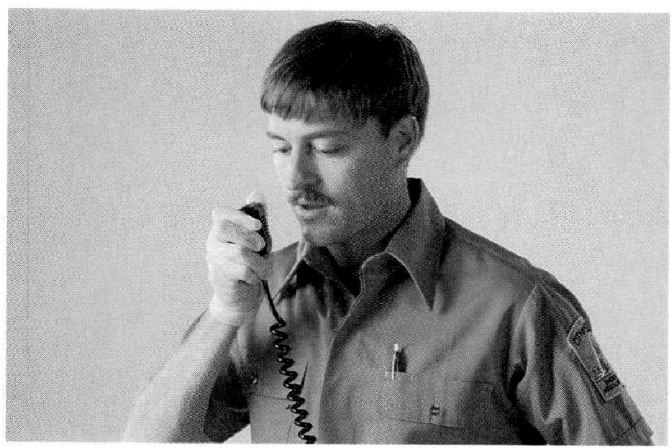

2. Second rescuer summons advanced medical personnel (if necessary).

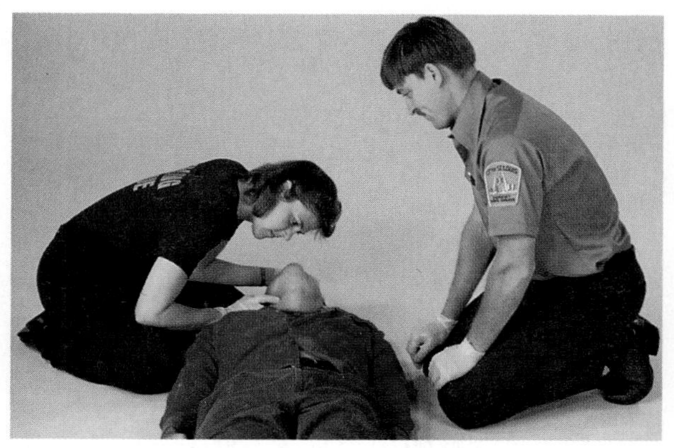

3. First rescuer completes CPR cycle and checks pulse. Second rescuer gets into position.

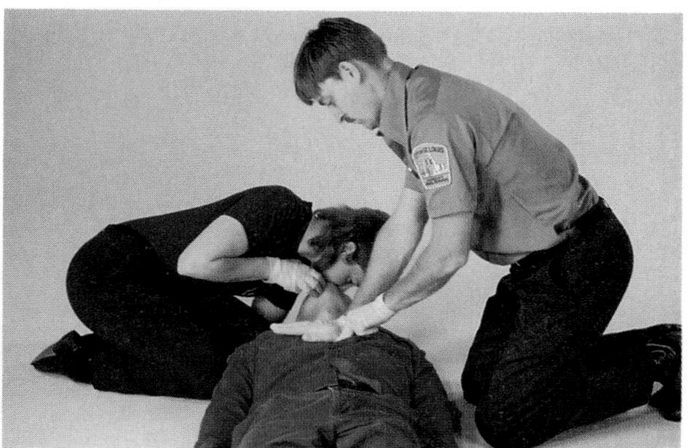

4. Second rescuer locates proper hand placement and does 5 chest compressions.

Repeat cycles of CPR. After about 1 minute of CPR, the first rescuer rechecks pulse. If there is still no pulse, both rescuers continue CPR, beginning with compressions.

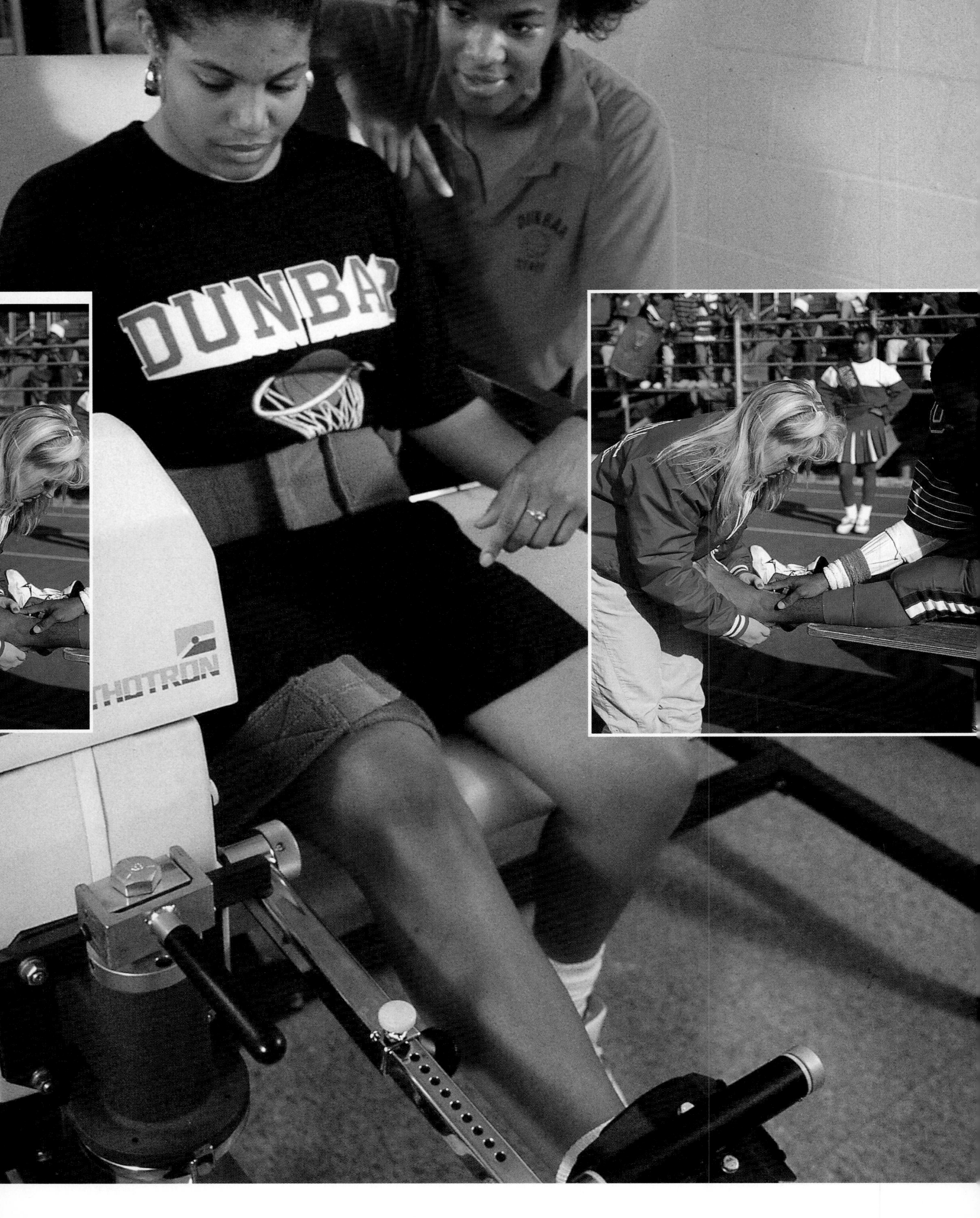
DUNBAR

Module Five

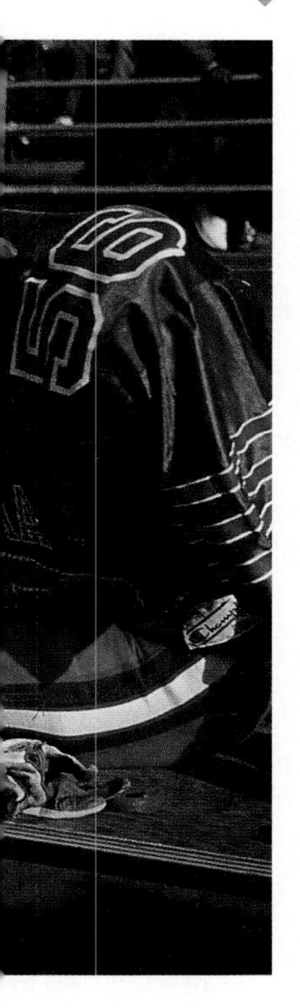

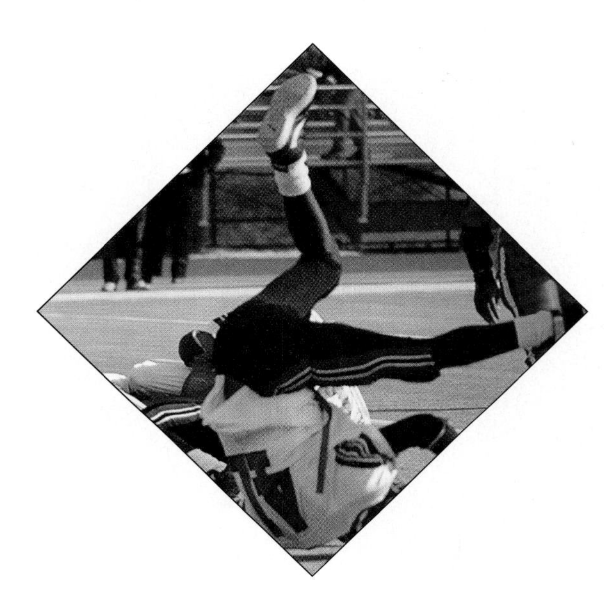

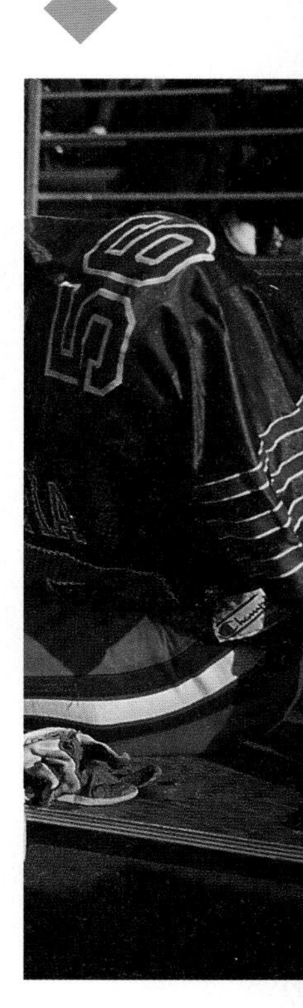

Illness and Injury

Bleeding and Shock

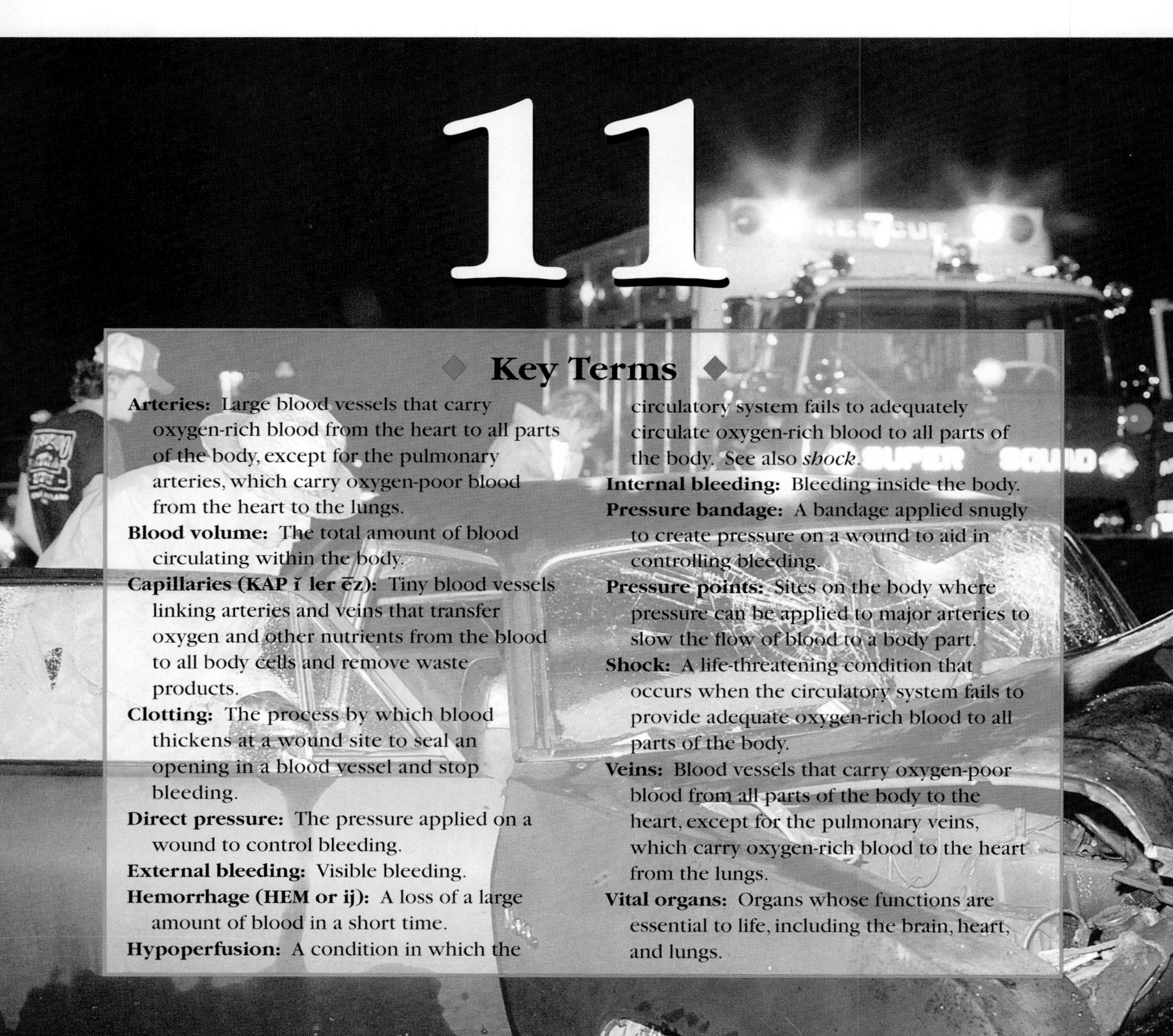

Key Terms

Arteries: Large blood vessels that carry oxygen-rich blood from the heart to all parts of the body, except for the pulmonary arteries, which carry oxygen-poor blood from the heart to the lungs.

Blood volume: The total amount of blood circulating within the body.

Capillaries (KAP ĭ ler ēz): Tiny blood vessels linking arteries and veins that transfer oxygen and other nutrients from the blood to all body cells and remove waste products.

Clotting: The process by which blood thickens at a wound site to seal an opening in a blood vessel and stop bleeding.

Direct pressure: The pressure applied on a wound to control bleeding.

External bleeding: Visible bleeding.

Hemorrhage (HEM or ij): A loss of a large amount of blood in a short time.

Hypoperfusion: A condition in which the circulatory system fails to adequately circulate oxygen-rich blood to all parts of the body. See also *shock*.

Internal bleeding: Bleeding inside the body.

Pressure bandage: A bandage applied snugly to create pressure on a wound to aid in controlling bleeding.

Pressure points: Sites on the body where pressure can be applied to major arteries to slow the flow of blood to a body part.

Shock: A life-threatening condition that occurs when the circulatory system fails to provide adequate oxygen-rich blood to all parts of the body.

Veins: Blood vessels that carry oxygen-poor blood from all parts of the body to the heart, except for the pulmonary veins, which carry oxygen-rich blood to the heart from the lungs.

Vital organs: Organs whose functions are essential to life, including the brain, heart, and lungs.

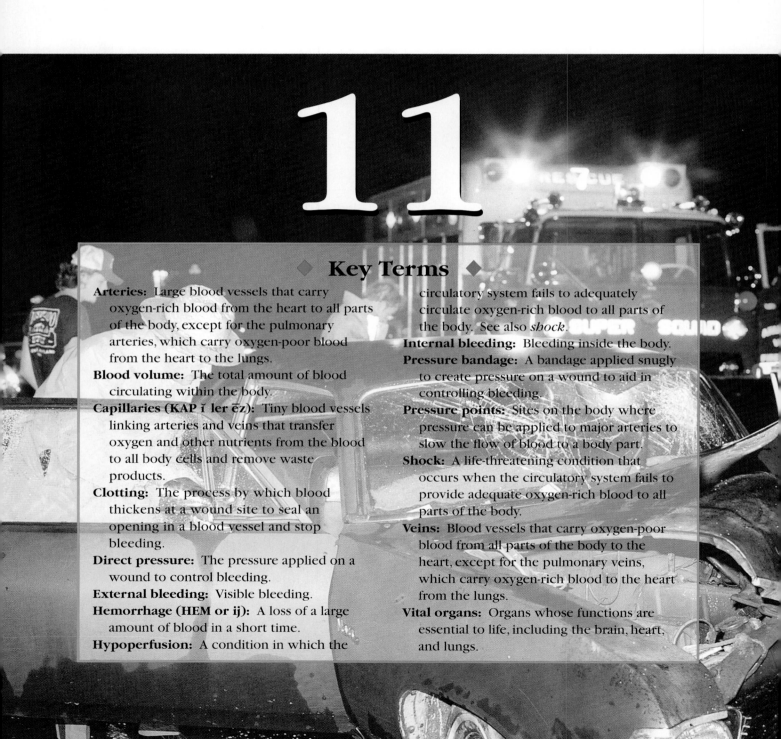

◆ Knowledge Objectives ◆

After reading this chapter and completing the class activities, you should be able to—

- Describe the components of blood.
- Explain the functions of blood and blood vessels.
- Differentiate among arterial, venous, and capillary bleeding.
- Describe how to care for external bleeding.
- Explain the use of body substance isolation (BSI) with bleeding.
- List the signs of internal bleeding.
- Describe how to care for a victim who exhibits the signs and symptoms of internal bleeding.
- List conditions that can result in shock.
- List signs and symptoms of shock.
- Describe how to provide care to minimize shock.

◆ Skill Objectives ◆

After reading this chapter and completing the class activities, you should be able to—

- Make appropriate decisions about care when given an example of an emergency in which a person is bleeding.
- Make appropriate decisions about care when given an example of an emergency in which shock is likely to occur.

You are summoned to assist a worker who has been injured in a machinery incident. She is bleeding severely from a large wound in her thigh. What care would you provide first? If the wound continues to bleed even after you have applied a pressure bandage and additional dressings, what further care would you provide?

◆ INTRODUCTION

Bleeding is the loss of blood from arteries, veins, or capillaries. A large amount of bleeding occurring in a short time is called a ***hemorrhage***. Bleeding is either internal or external. Internal bleeding is often difficult to recognize. External bleeding is usually obvious because it is typically visible. Uncontrolled bleeding, whether internal or external, is a life-threatening emergency.

As you learned in previous chapters, severe bleeding can result in death. Check for and control severe bleeding during the initial assessment once you have checked for a pulse. You may not identify internal bleeding until you perform a more detailed check during the physical exam and history.

You also learned that both medical emergencies and injuries can cause life-threatening conditions, such as cardiac and respiratory arrest and severe bleeding. Medical emergencies and injuries also can become life threatening in another way—as a result of shock. When the body experiences injury or sudden illness, it responds in a number of ways. Survival depends on the body's ability to adapt to the physical stresses of illness or injury. When the body's measures to adapt fail, the victim can progress into a life-threatening condition called shock, which complicates the effects of injury or sudden illness.

In this chapter, you will learn how to recognize and care for both internal and external bleeding. You will also learn to recognize the signs and symptoms of shock and to provide care to minimize it.

◆ BLOOD AND BLOOD VESSELS

The circulatory system consists of the heart, blood, and blood vessels. The blood vessels create a closed system, in which blood is pumped from the heart and circulated to the cells and back to the lungs and heart. When bleeding occurs, the system is disrupted.

Blood Components

Blood consists of liquid and solid components and comprises approximately 8 percent of the body's total weight. The liquid part of the blood is called **plasma**. The solid components are the red and white blood cells and cell fragments called **platelets.**

Plasma makes up about half of the ***blood volume,*** the total amount of blood circulating within the body. Composed mostly of water, plasma maintains the blood volume that the circulatory system needs to function normally. Plasma also contains nutrients essential for energy production, growth, and cell maintenance and carries waste products for elimination.

White blood cells are a key disease-fighting component of the immune system. They defend the body against invading microorganisms. They also aid in producing antibodies that help the body resist infection.

Red blood cells account for most of blood's solid components. They are produced in the marrow in the hollow center of large bones, such as the large bone of the arm (humerus) and of the thigh (femur). Red blood cells number nearly 260 million in each drop of blood. The red blood cells transport oxygen from the lungs to the body cells and carbon dioxide from the cells to the lungs. Red blood cells outnumber white blood cells approximately 1000 to 1.

Platelets are disk-shaped cell fragments in the blood. Platelets are an essential part of the blood's clotting mechanism because they tend to bind together. ***Clotting*** is the process by which whole blood thickens at a wound site. Platelets help stop bleeding by forming blood clots at wound sites. Blood clots form the framework for healing. Until blood clots form, bleeding must be controlled artificially.

Blood Functions

The blood has three major functions:

- Transporting oxygen, nutrients, and wastes
- Protecting against disease by producing antibodies and defending against infections
- Helping to maintain constant body temperature by circulating throughout the body

Blood Vessels

Blood is channeled through blood vessels. There are three major types of blood vessels: arteries, capillaries, and veins (Fig. 11-1). Most ***arteries*** carry oxygen-rich blood away from the heart. The pulmonary arteries carry oxygen-poor blood from the heart to the lungs. Arteries become narrower the farther they extend from the heart until they connect to the capillaries. ***Capillaries*** are microscopic blood vessels linking arteries and veins that transfer oxygen and other nutrients from the blood to the cells. Capillaries pick up waste products, such as carbon dioxide, from the cells and transfer them to the veins. The ***veins*** carry waste products from the cells back to the heart where

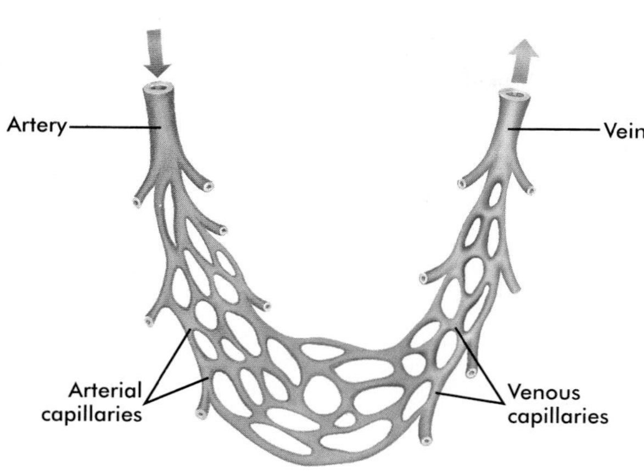

Figure 11-1 Blood flows through the three major types of blood vessels: arteries, veins, and capillaries.

waste products are pumped through the arteries to the kidneys and lungs and eliminated from the body.

Because the blood in the arteries is closer to the pumping action of the heart, blood in the arteries travels faster and under greater pressure than blood in the capillaries or veins. Blood flow in the arteries pulses with the heartbeat; blood in the veins flows more slowly and evenly.

◆ WHEN BLEEDING OCCURS

When bleeding occurs, the body begins a complex chain of events. The brain, heart, and lungs immediately attempt to compensate for blood loss to maintain the flow of oxygen-rich blood to the body, particularly to the vital organs.

Other important reactions also occur. Platelets collect at the wound site in an effort to stop blood loss through clotting. White blood cells try to prevent infection by attacking microorganisms that commonly enter through breaks in the skin. The body manufactures extra red blood cells to help transport more oxygen to the cells.

Blood volume is also affected by bleeding. Normally, excess fluid is absorbed from the bloodstream by the kidneys, lungs, intestines, and skin. However, when bleeding occurs, this excess fluid is reabsorbed into the bloodstream as plasma. This reabsorption helps maintain the critical balance of fluids needed by the body to keep blood volume constant. Bleeding severe enough to critically reduce the blood volume is life threatening. Severe bleeding can be either external or internal (Fig. 11-2).

External Bleeding

External bleeding occurs when a blood vessel is opened externally, such as through a tear in the skin. You can usually see this type of bleeding. Most external bleeding you will encounter will be minor. Minor bleeding, such as occurs with most small cuts, usually stops by itself within 10 minutes when the blood clots. Sometimes, however, the damaged blood vessel is too large or the blood is under too much pressure for effective clotting to occur. In these cases, you will need to recognize and control bleeding promptly. Look for severe bleeding during the check for circulation that is part of the initial assessment.

Recognizing External Bleeding

The signs of severe external bleeding include—

- Blood spurting from a wound.
- Blood that fails to clot after you have taken all measures to control bleeding.

Each type of blood vessel bleeds differently. Bleeding from arteries is often rapid and profuse. It is life threatening. Because arterial blood is under direct pressure from the heart, it usually spurts from the wound, making it difficult for clots to form. Because clots do not form rapidly, arterial bleeding is harder to control than bleeding from veins and capillaries. Its high concentration of oxygen gives arterial blood a bright red color.

Blood: The Beat Goes On

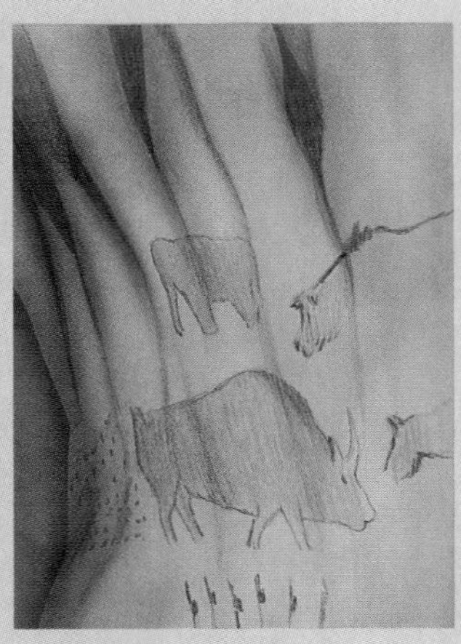

The Ice Age—Prehistoric Man
Primitive man draws a giant mammoth on a cave, with a red ochre marking resembling a heart in its chest.

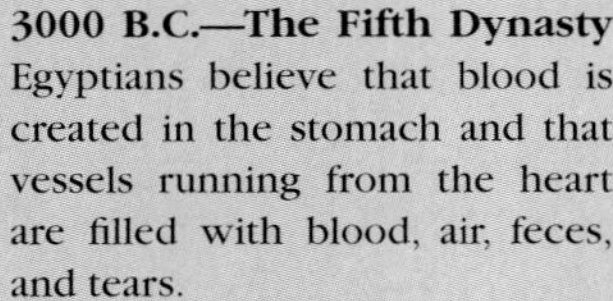

3000 B.C.—The Fifth Dynasty
Egyptians believe that blood is created in the stomach and that vessels running from the heart are filled with blood, air, feces, and tears.

500 B.C.—Greek Civilization
Ancient Greek physicians propound the theory of the humours, associating man's personality and health with four substances in the body—blood, black bile, yellow bile, and phlegm. An imbalance can cause diseases or emotional problems. A practice called bloodletting develops in which physicians open a patient's vein and let him or her bleed to fix an imbalance in the humours.

Circa 200 A.D.—Late Roman Civilization
Galen, doctor of Roman Emperor Marcus Aurelius, theorizes that blood is continuously formed in the liver and then moves in two systems—one that combines with the air and a second that forms from food to nourish the body.

900 to 1400—The Middle Ages
Bloodletting flourishes during the Middle Ages. Astrology's influence grows, leading doctors to use astrological charts to determine when and where to open a vein. Medical schools sprout up in England, France, Belgium, and Italy.

1628—The Renaissance Period
Dr. William Harvey cuts into live frogs and snakes to observe the heart. Through his studies, Harvey determines that blood circulates through the heart, the lungs and rest of the body.

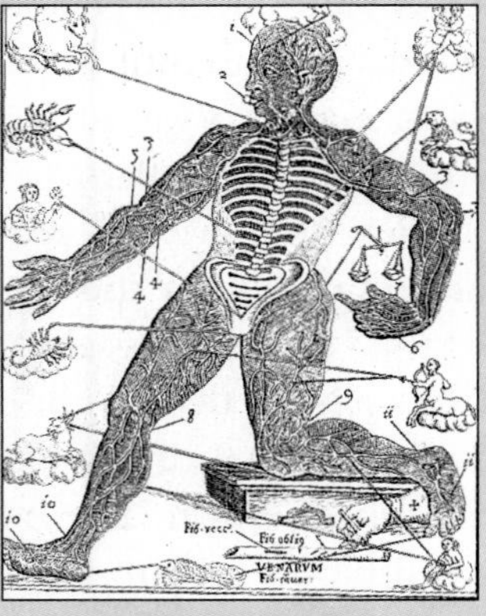

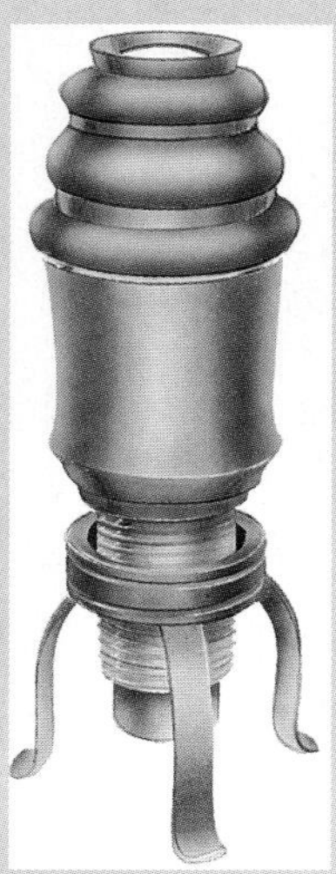

1661
The invention of the microscope allows Italian-born physician Malpighi to see the tiny capillaries that link veins and arteries.

1665
The first blood transfusion mixes the blood of one dog with another. Transfusions range from successful to disastrous. One scientist proposes a transfusion between unhappily married people to try to reconcile the couple. After a man who receives sheep's blood dies, transfusion is outlawed in France.

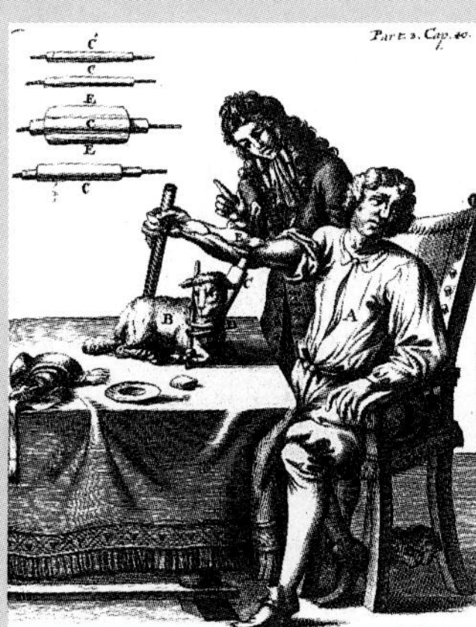

Early 1900s—The Twentieth Century
Dr. Karl Landsteiner discovers that all human blood is not compatible and names the blood types. His work helps make blood transfusions commonplace.

1944
When kidneys fail, poisons are released into the bloodstream that can cause vomiting, coma, and eventually death. Dr. Willem Kolff, a Dutch physician, develops one of the first artificial kidneys by sending the blood through a cellophane tubing that filters out the poisons.

1953
Dr. John H. Gibbon invents a heart-lung machine to recirculate blood and provide oxygen during open-heart surgery, enabling more complex surgical techniques to develop.

1967
The first heart transplant is attempted by Dr. Christiaan Barnard in Cape Town, South Africa. Louis Washansky, a 54-year-old grocer receives the heart of a woman hit by a speeding car. Washansky survives 18 days.

1982
Dr. William DeVries implants the first artificial heart in Barney Clark. The Seattle dentist survives 112 days, and the Jarvik-7 beats 12,912,499 times before Clark dies. In the 1980s, five artificial hearts are implanted. The longest survival period lasts 620 days. The body continues to treat the artificial heart as a "foreign body" and rejects it.

The Future
Through the ages, medical science has made extensive progress in saving lives. Two to three million Americans receive blood transfusions each year. More than 5,000 Americans are living with another person's heart inside their chest. About 160,000 Americans are kept alive with an artificial kidney or a kidney transplant. The early medical experiments of yesterday have become commonplace lifesaving procedures today.

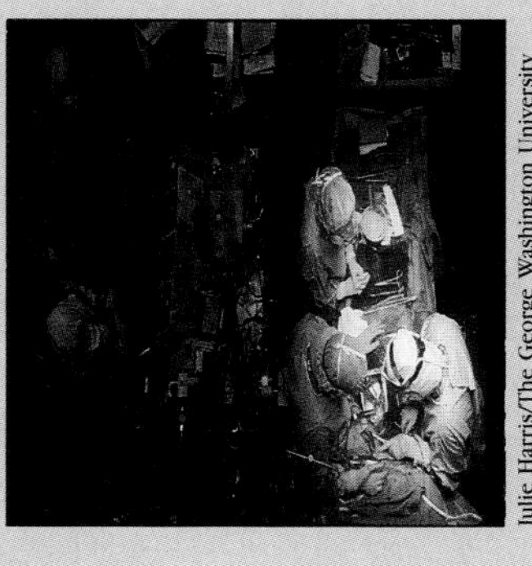

Julie Harris/The George Washington University

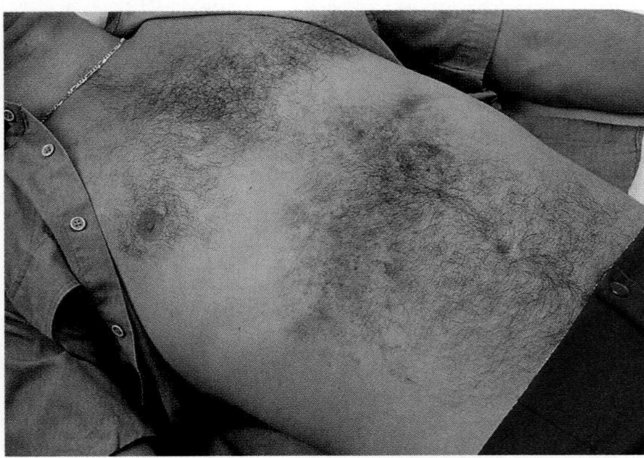

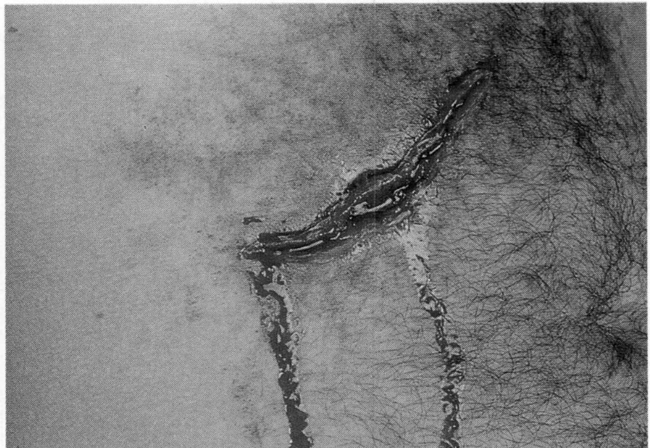

Figure 11-2 Severe bleeding can be internal or external.

Veins are damaged more often than arteries because they are closer to the skin's surface. Venous bleeding (bleeding from the veins) is easier to control than arterial bleeding. Venous blood is under less pressure than arterial blood and flows from the wound at a steady rate without spurting. Only damage to veins deep in the body, such as those in the trunk or thigh, produces profuse bleeding that is hard to control. Because it is oxygen-poor, venous blood is dark red or maroon.

Capillary bleeding is usually slow because the vessels are small and the blood is under low pressure. It is often described as "oozing" from the wound. Clotting occurs easily with capillary bleeding. The blood is dark red in color.

Controlling External Bleeding

External bleeding is usually easy to control. Generally, you can control it by applying pressure with your gloved hand on the wound. Doing so is called applying ***direct pressure***. Pressure on the wound restricts the blood flow through the wound and allows normal clotting to occur. Elevating the injured area also slows the flow of blood and encourages clotting. You can maintain pressure on a wound by snugly applying a bandage to the injured area. A bandage applied to control bleeding is called a ***pressure bandage.*** The combination of pressure and elevation will control most bleeding.

In a few cases, direct pressure and elevation may not control severe bleeding. In these cases, you will have to take other measures. In an effort to further slow bleeding, you can compress the artery supplying the area against an underlying bone at specific sites on the body. These sites are called ***pressure points*** (Fig. 11-3, *A*).

The main pressure points used to control bleeding in the arms and legs are over the brachial and femoral arteries (Fig. 11-3, *B*). A **tourniquet,** a tight band placed around an arm or leg to constrict blood vessels to stop blood flow to a wound, is rarely used as part of emergency care because it too often does more harm than good. It is only used as a last resort to save a life and may result in the loss of the limb below the injury.

To control external bleeding, follow these general steps:

1. Follow BSI precautions. Wear gloves and other equipment if there is a large quantity of blood or a chance for blood to splatter.
2. Place pressure directly on the wound with a sterile gauze pad or any clean cloth, such as a washcloth, towel, or handkerchief. Using gauze or a clean cloth keeps the wound free of germs. Place your fingers or hand over the gauze pad and apply firm pressure (Fig. 11-4, *A*). If you do not have gauze or cloth available, apply pressure with your own gloved hand or have the injured person apply pressure with his or her hand.

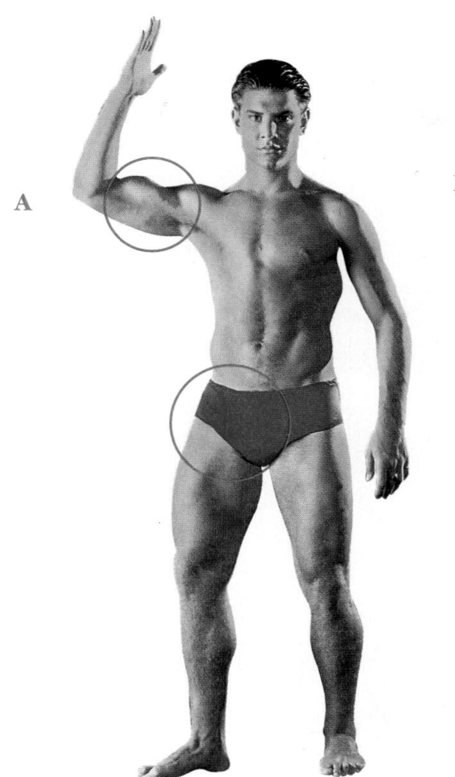

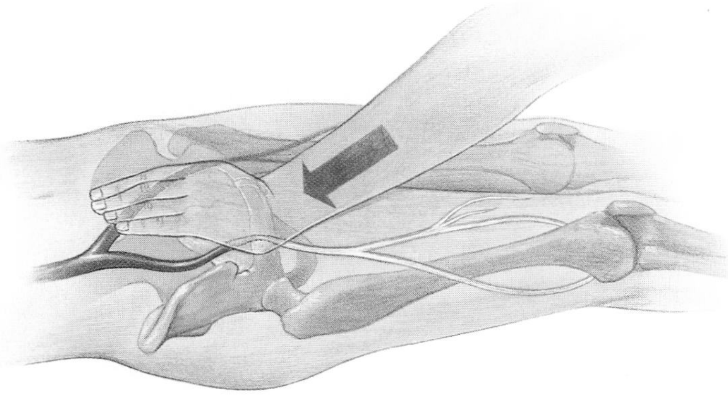

Figure 11-3 **A,** Pressure points are specific sites on the body where arteries lie close to the bone and the body's surface. **B,** Blood flow to an area can be controlled by applying pressure at one of these sites, compressing the artery against the bone.

3. Elevate the injured area above the level of the heart if the victim does not have a painful, swollen deformity (Fig. 11-4, *B*).
4. Apply a pressure bandage. This bandage will hold the gauze pads or cloth in place while maintaining direct pressure (Fig. 11-4, *C*). If blood soaks through, add dressings and bandages. Do not remove any blood-soaked dressings or bandages. The use of pressure bandages is discussed in detail in Chapter 12.
5. If bleeding continues, apply pressure at a pressure point to slow the flow of blood (Fig. 11-4, *D*).

Continue to monitor the victim's airway and breathing. Observe the victim closely for signs that indicate a worsening condition. If bleeding is severe, administer supplemental oxygen to the victim if it is available and you are trained to use it. Summon more advanced medical personnel if this has not already been done. If bleeding is not severe, provide care as needed.

Preventing Disease Transmission

To reduce the risk of disease transmission when controlling bleeding, you should always follow the BSI precautions you learned in Chapter 3. These include—

- Avoiding contacting the victim's blood, directly or indirectly, by using barriers, such as gloves and protective eyewear.
- Avoiding eating and drinking and touching your mouth, nose, or eyes while providing care or before washing your hands.
- Always washing your hands thoroughly after providing care, even if you wore gloves or used other barriers.

Refer to Chapter 3 for a more detailed discussion of preventing disease transmission.

Internal Bleeding

Internal bleeding is the escape of blood from arteries, veins, or capillaries into spaces in

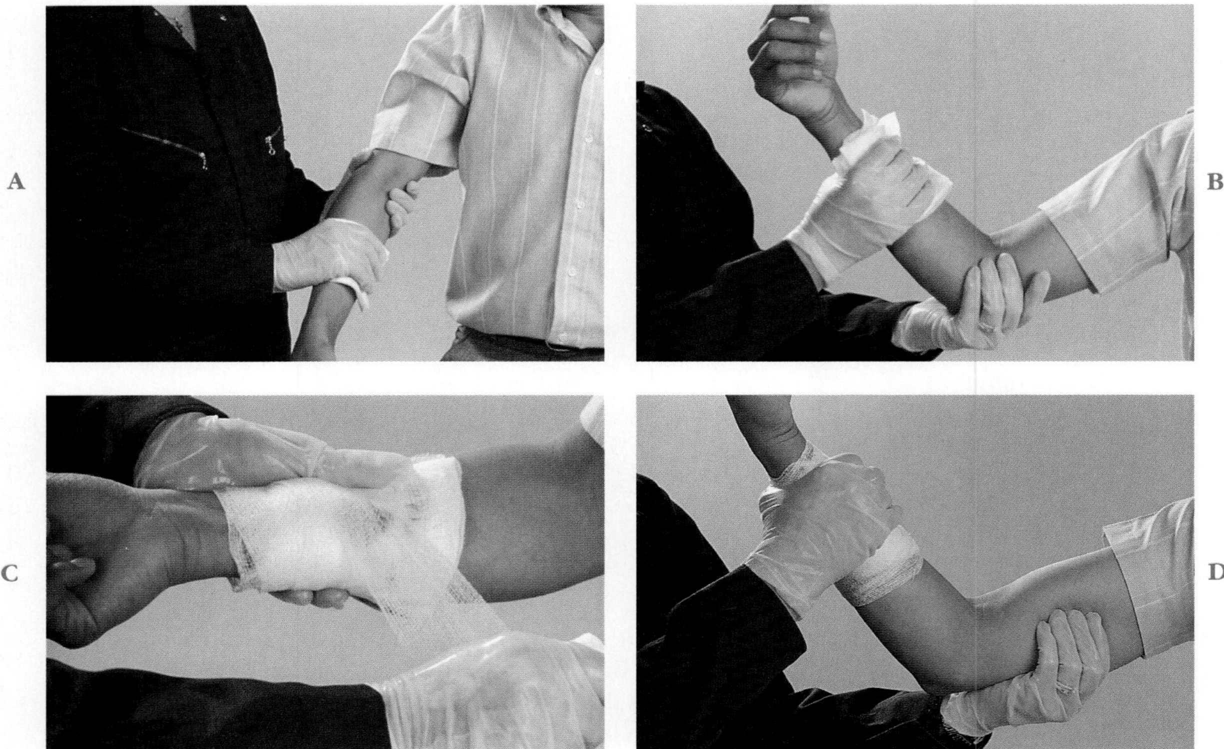

Figure 11-4 **A,** Apply direct pressure to the wound using a sterile gauze pad or clean cloth. **B,** Elevate the injured area above the level of the heart if you do not suspect a fracture. **C,** Apply a pressure bandage. **D,** If necessary, slow the flow of blood by applying pressure to the artery with your hand at the appropriate pressure point.

the body. Internal capillary bleeding, indicated by mild bruising, is just beneath the skin and is not serious. Deeper bleeding involves arteries and veins and may result in severe blood loss.

Severe internal bleeding usually occurs in injuries caused by a violent blunt force, such as when the driver is thrown against the steering wheel in a car crash or someone falls from a height. Internal bleeding may also occur when a sharp object, such as a knife, penetrates the skin and damages internal structures.

Recognizing Internal Bleeding

Because internal bleeding is more difficult to recognize than external bleeding, you should always suspect internal bleeding in any serious injury. For example, if you find a motorcycle rider thrown from a bike, you may not see any serious external bleeding, but you should consider that the violent forces involved indicate the likelihood of internal injuries. Internal bleeding also can occur from a fractured bone that ruptures an organ or lacerates a blood vessel.

The body's inability to adjust to severe internal bleeding will eventually produce signs and symptoms that indicate shock. These signs and symptoms are not always obvious and may take time to appear. These signs and symptoms include—

- Discoloration of the skin (bruising) in the injured area.
- Soft tissues, such as those in the abdomen, that are tender, swollen, or firm.
- Anxiety or restlessness.
- Rapid, weak pulse.
- Rapid breathing.
- Skin that feels cool or moist or looks pale, ashen, or bluish.
- Nausea and vomiting.
- Excessive thirst.

- Declining level of consciousness (LOC).
- Drop in blood pressure.

Controlling Internal Bleeding

How you control internal bleeding depends on the severity and the site of the bleeding. For minor internal bleeding, such as a bruise on an arm, apply ice or a chemical cold pack to the injured area to help reduce pain and swelling. When applying ice, always remember to place something, such as a gauze pad or a towel, between the source of cold and the skin to prevent skin damage.

If you suspect internal bleeding caused by serious injury, summon more advanced medical personnel immediately. There is little you can do to control this bleeding effectively. The victim must be transported rapidly to the hospital. The victim will often need immediate surgery to correct the problem. While waiting for more advanced medical personnel to arrive, follow the general guidelines for caring for any emergency. These are —

- Do no further harm.
- Monitor the ABCs and vital signs.
- Help the victim rest in the most comfortable position.
- Keep the victim from getting chilled or overheated.
- Reassure the victim.
- Provide care for other conditions.
- Administer oxygen if it is available and you are trained to do so.

◆ SHOCK (HYPOPERFUSION)

11:00 PM. *On an isolated road, an 18-year-old male driver loses control of a motor vehicle and collides with a tree. In the crash, the driver's legs are broken and pinned in the wreckage.*

11:15 PM. *Another car finally approaches. The driver stops and comes forward to help. She finds the occupant conscious, restless, and in obvious pain. She says she will go to call an ambulance at the nearest house about a mile down the road.*

11:25 PM. *When the driver returns, she sees that the victim's condition has changed. He looks ill.*

11:35 PM. *Having been dispatched, you arrive at the scene minutes before the ambulance and engine company. You assess the victim and notice he only responds to loud verbal stimuli, is breathing fast, and looks pale. His skin is cold and moist. His pulse is fast and weak.*

12:00 PM. *Finally, you and the other rescuers free the driver's legs and remove him from the car. You notice that he looks worse. He only responds to painful physical stimuli. His breathing has become very irregular. You know the hospital is still 20 minutes away.*

12:45 AM. *Despite the best efforts of everyone involved, you hear the man was pronounced dead. He was a victim of a progressively deteriorating condition called shock.*

Shock, also known as ***hypoperfusion,*** is a condition in which the circulatory system fails to adequately circulate oxygen-rich blood to all parts of the body. Shock is the inevitable result of any serious injury or illness. When vital organs, such as the heart, lungs, brain, and kidneys, do not receive oxygen-rich blood, they fail to function properly. Improper function triggers a series of responses that produces specific signs and symptoms known as shock. These responses are the body's attempt to maintain adequate blood flow to the vital organs, preventing their failure.

When the body is healthy, three conditions are necessary to maintain adequate blood flow:

- The heart must be working well.
- An adequate amount of blood must be circulating in the body.
- The blood vessels must be intact and able to adjust blood flow.

Injury or sudden illness can interrupt normal body functions. In cases of minor injury or illness, this interruption is brief because the body is able to compensate quickly. With more severe injuries or illnesses, however, the body is unable to adjust. When the body is unable to meet its demands for oxygen because the blood fails to circulate adequately, shock occurs.

Why Shock Occurs

There are different types of shock, as shown in Table 11-1. Although the first responder does not have to be able to identify these different types of shock, it may be helpful to know that there are different ways in which people can develop shock. Each type of shock causes a decrease in the amount of blood that effectively circulates in the body. For instance, shock may be caused by severe bleeding, the heart failing to pump blood properly, severe vomiting, diarrhea, or dehydration, or by the body's inability to control the diameter of blood vessels. Regardless of the cause, when the body cells receive inadequate oxygen, it triggers shock.

How does shock develop? You learned in Chapters 5 and 10 that the heart pumps blood by contracting and relaxing in a consistent, rhythmic pattern. The heart adjusts its speed and the force of its contractions to meet the body's changing demands for oxygen. For instance, when a person exercises, the heart beats faster and more forcefully because the working muscles demand more oxygen (Fig. 11-5).

Similarly, when someone suffers a severe injury or sudden illness that affects the flow of blood, the heart beats faster and stronger at first to adjust to the increased demand for more oxygen (Fig. 11-6). Because the heart is beating faster, breathing must also speed up to meet the body's increased demands for oxygen. You can detect these changes by feeling the pulse and listening to breathing when you check vital signs during the physical exam.

For the heart to do its job properly, an adequate amount of blood must circulate within the body. As you learned earlier in this chapter, this amount is referred to as blood volume. The body can compensate for some decrease in blood volume. Consider what happens when

Table 11-1 Types of Shock

Type	Cause
Anaphylactic	Life-threatening allergic reaction to a substance; can occur from insect stings or from foods and drugs
Cardiogenic	Failure of the heart to effectively pump blood to all parts of the body; occurs with heart attack or cardiac arrest
Hemorrhagic	Severe bleeding or loss of blood plasma; occurs with internal or external wounds or burns
Metabolic	Loss of body fluid; occurs after severe diarrhea or vomiting or a heat illness
Neurogenic	Failure of nervous system to control size of blood vessels, causing them to dilate; occurs with brain or nerve injuries
Psychogenic	Factor, such as emotional stress, causes blood to pool in the body in areas away from the brain, resulting in fainting
Respiratory	Failure of the lungs to transfer sufficient oxygen into the bloodstream; occurs with respiratory distress or arrest
Septic	Poisons caused by severe infections that cause blood vessels to dilate

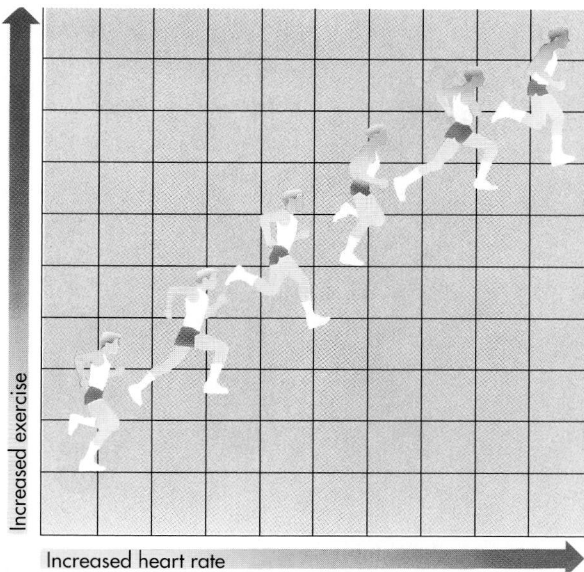

Figure 11-5 The heartbeat changes to meet the body's demands for oxygen.

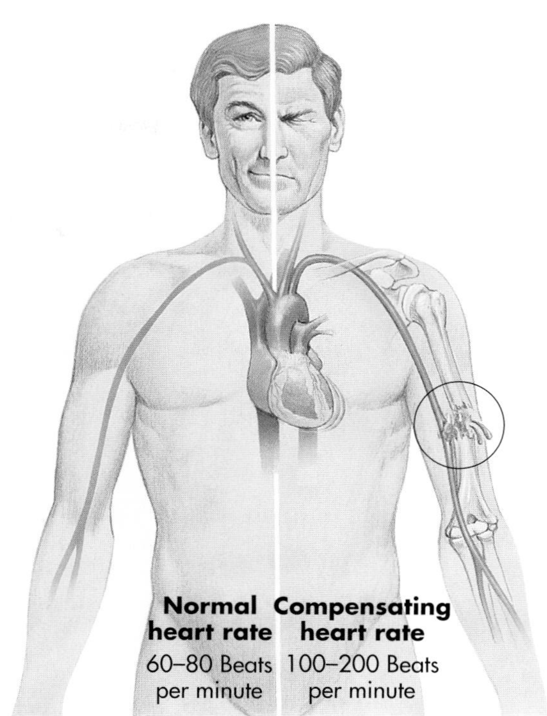

Figure 11-6 The heart beats faster to compensate for significant blood loss.

you donate blood. You can lose one pint of blood over a 10- to 15-minute period without any real stress to the body. Fluid is reabsorbed from the kidneys, lungs, and intestines to replace lost fluid. The body immediately begins to manufacture the blood's solid components. With severe injuries involving greater or more rapid blood loss, however, the body may not be able to adjust adequately. Body cells do not receive enough oxygen, and shock occurs. Any significant fluid loss from the body, such as with prolonged diarrhea or vomiting, can also precipitate shock.

The blood vessels act as pipelines, transporting oxygen and nutrients to all parts of the body and removing wastes. For the circulatory system to function properly, blood vessels must remain intact to maintain blood volume. Normally, blood vessels decrease or increase the flow of blood to different areas of the body by constricting (decreasing their diameter) or dilating (increasing their diameter). This ability ensures that blood reaches the areas of the body that need it most, such as the vital organs. Injuries or illnesses, especially those that affect the brain and spinal cord, can cause blood vessels to lose this ability to change size, causing a drop in blood volume (Fig. 11-7). Blood vessels can also be affected if the nervous system is damaged by infections, drugs, or poisons.

Regardless of the cause, a significant decrease in blood volume affects the function of the heart. The heart will eventually fail to beat rhythmically. The pulse will become irregular or be absent altogether. With some irregular heart rhythms, blood does not circulate at all.

When shock occurs, the body attempts to prioritize its needs for blood by ensuring adequate flow to the vital organs. The body does this by reducing the amount of blood circulating to the less important tissues of the arms, legs, and skin. This is why the skin of a person in shock appears pale or ashen and feels cool. When checking capillary refill, as with infants and children, you may find it to be slow. In later stages of shock, the skin, especially on the lips and around the eyes, may appear blue from a prolonged lack of oxygen. Increased sweating is

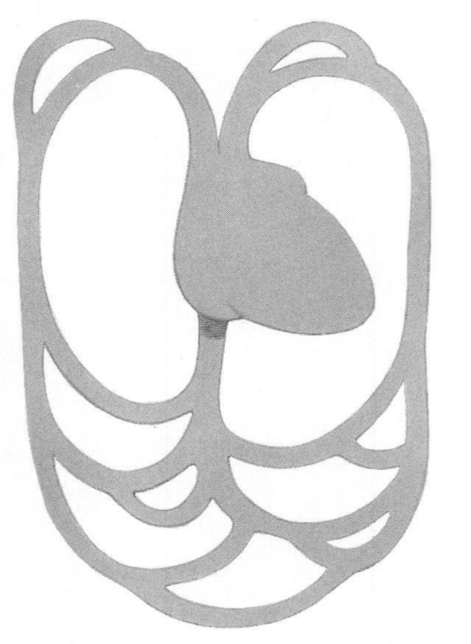

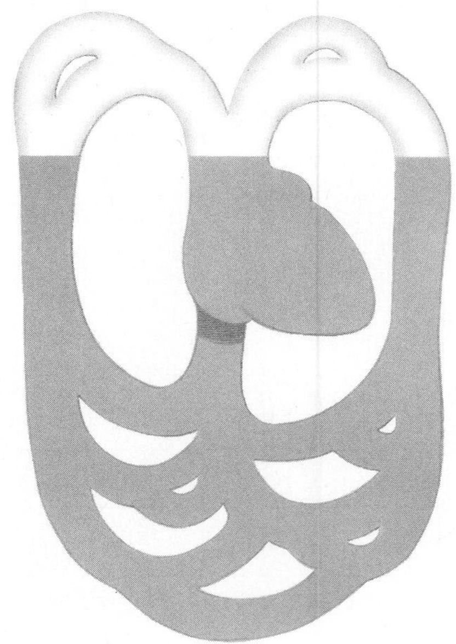

Figure 11-7 Injuries or medical emergencies that cause blood vessels to dilate cause a serious drop in blood volume.

also a natural reaction to stress caused by injury or illness, making the skin feel moist.

Signs and Symptoms of Shock

Although you may not always be able to determine the cause, remember that shock is a life-threatening condition. You should learn to recognize its signs and symptoms (Fig. 11-8).

Shock victims usually show many of the same signs and symptoms. A common one is restlessness or irritability, which is often the first indicator that the body is experiencing a significant problem resulting from inadequate oxygen reaching the brain. More clearly recognizable signs are pale or ashen, cool, moist skin; rapid breathing; a rapid and weak pulse; and changes in the level of consciousness. Often, a recognizable symptom is nausea. Conditions that affect blood volume or cause the blood vessels to work improperly can also cause significant changes in blood pressure.

If the victim does not show the obvious signs and symptoms of specific injury or illness, such as the persistent chest pain of heart attack or obvious external bleeding, it can be difficult to know what is wrong. Remember, you do not have to identify the specific nature of illness or injury to provide care that may help save the victim's life. If the signs and symptoms of shock are present, assume there is a potentially life-threatening injury or illness.

Care for Shock

To care for shock, first, do an initial assessment. The care, such as controlling severe bleeding, that you provide for life-threatening conditions will minimize the effects of shock. If you do not find any life-threatening conditions, perform a physical exam and obtain a SAMPLE history. Always follow the general care steps you learned in Chapter 7 for any emergency:

- Do no harm.
- Monitor the ABCs and provide care for any airway, breathing, or circulation problem you find (Fig. 11-9, *A*).
- Help the victim rest comfortably. Helping the victim rest comfortably is important because

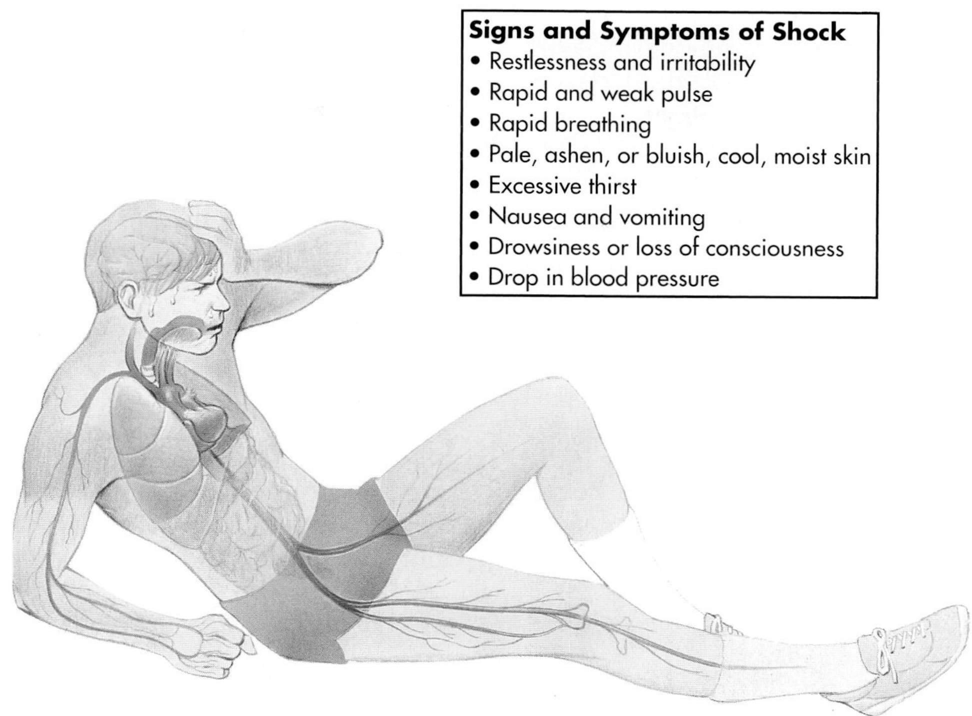

Signs and Symptoms of Shock
• Restlessness and irritability
• Rapid and weak pulse
• Rapid breathing
• Pale, ashen, or bluish, cool, moist skin
• Excessive thirst
• Nausea and vomiting
• Drowsiness or loss of consciousness
• Drop in blood pressure

Figure 11-8 The signs and symptoms of shock may not be obvious immediately. Be alert for these signs and symptoms in cases of injury or sudden illness.

pain can intensify the body's stress and accelerate the progression of shock. Helping the victim rest in a more comfortable position may minimize the pain.

- Keep the victim from getting chilled or overheated (Fig. 11-9, *B*).
- Reassure the victim.
- Provide care for specific conditions.

The general care you provide in any emergency will always help the victim's body adjust to the stresses imposed by any injury or illness, thus reducing the effects of shock.

You can further help the victim manage the effects of shock if you—

- Control any external bleeding as soon as possible to minimize blood loss.
- Elevate the legs about 12 inches to keep blood circulating to vital organs, unless you suspect head, neck, or back injuries or painful, swollen deformities involving the hips or legs (Fig. 11-9, *C*). If you are unsure of the victim's condition, leave him or her lying flat.
- Administer oxygen if it is available and you are trained to do so.
- Do not give the victim anything to eat or drink, even though he or she is likely to be thirsty. The victim's condition may be severe enough to require surgery, in which case, it is better that the stomach is empty.
- Call more advanced medical personnel immediately. Shock cannot be managed effectively by first aid alone. A victim of shock requires advanced life support as soon as possible.

◆ SUMMARY

One of the most important things you can do in any emergency is to recognize and control severe bleeding. External bleeding is easily recognized and should be cared for immediately.

Shock: The Domino Effect

- An injury causes severe bleeding.
- The heart attempts to compensate for the disruption of blood flow by beating faster. The victim first has a rapid pulse. More blood is lost. As blood volume drops, the pulse becomes weak or hard to find.
- The increased work load on the heart results in an increased oxygen demand. Therefore breathing becomes faster.
- To maintain circulation of blood to the vital organs, blood vessels in the arms and legs and in the skin constrict. Therefore the skin appears pale and feels cool. In response to the stress, the body perspires heavily and the skin feels moist.
- Since tissues of the arms and legs are now without oxygen, cells start to die. The brain now sends a signal to return blood to the arms and legs in an attempt to balance blood flow between these body parts and the vital organs.
- Vital organs are now without adequate oxygen. The heart tries to compensate by beating even faster. More blood is lost and the victim's condition worsens.
- Without oxygen, the vital organs fail to function properly. As the brain is affected, the person becomes restless, drowsy, and eventually loses consciousness. As the heart is affected, it beats irregularly, resulting in an irregular pulse. The rhythm then becomes chaotic and the heart fails to pump blood. There is no longer a pulse. When the heart stops, breathing stops.
- The body's continuous attempt to compensate for severe blood loss eventually results in death.

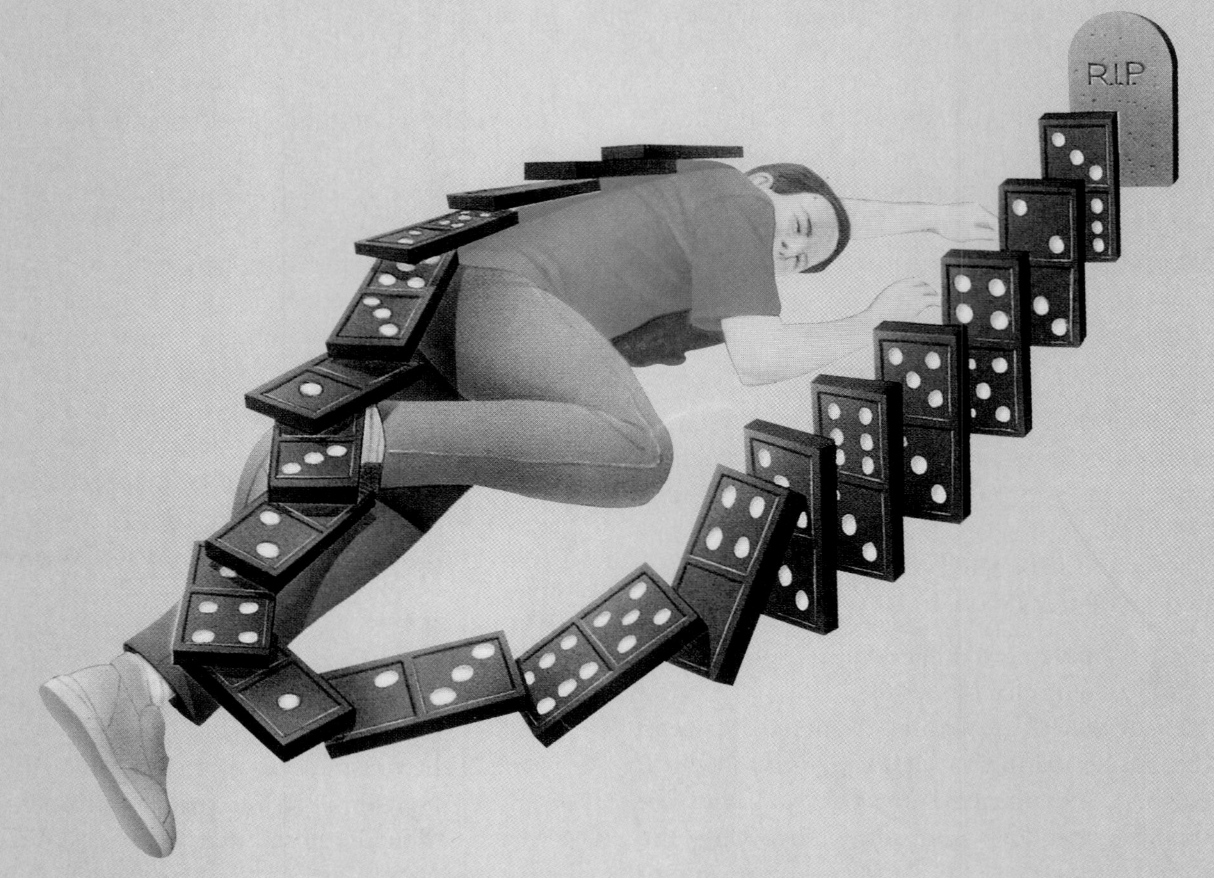

A

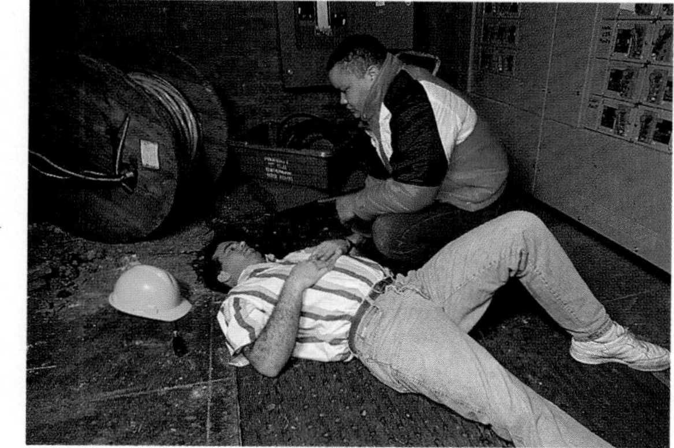

B

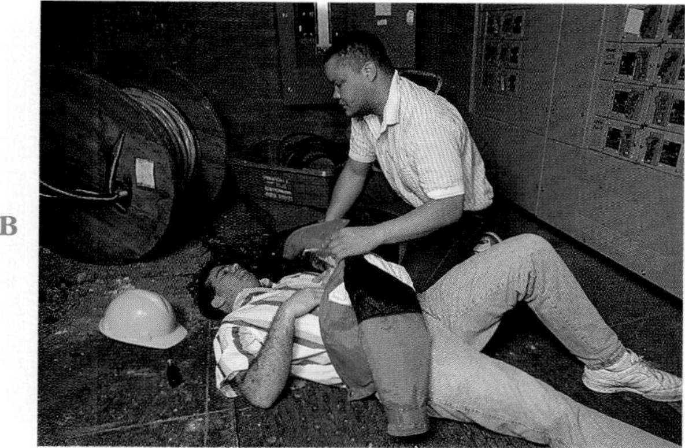

C

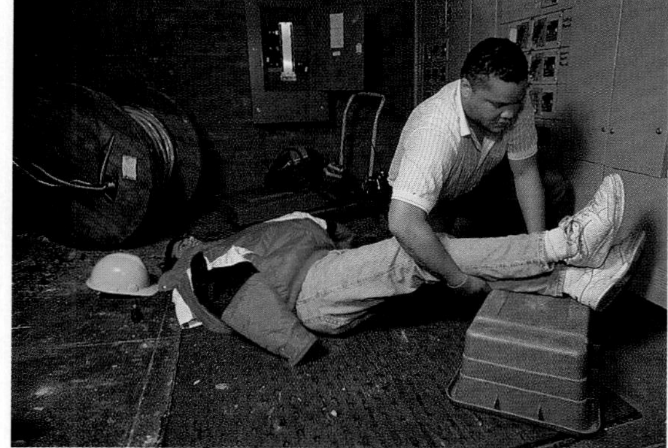

Figure 11-9 **A,** Monitor the victim's ABCs if he or she is in shock. **B,** Keep the victim from getting chilled or overheated. **C,** Elevate the victim's legs to keep blood circulating to the vital organs.

Check and care for severe bleeding during the initial assessment. Severe external bleeding is life threatening. Although internal bleeding is less obvious, it also can be life threatening. Recognize when a serious injury has occurred and suspect internal bleeding. You may not identify internal bleeding until you perform the physical exam and history. When you identify or suspect severe bleeding, request an ambulance so that the victim can be transported quickly to a hospital. Continue to provide care until more advanced medical personnel arrive and take over.

Do not wait for shock to develop before providing care to a victim of injury or sudden illness. Care for life-threatening conditions, such as breathing problems or severe external bleeding, before caring for lesser injuries. Remember that managing shock effectively begins with recognizing a situation in which shock may develop and giving appropriate care. Shock is a factor in serious injuries and illnesses, particularly if there is blood loss or if the normal function of the heart is interrupted. With serious injuries or illnesses, shock is often the final stage before death. You cannot always prevent shock by giving emergency care, but you can usually slow its progress. Summon more advanced medical personnel immediately if you notice signs and symptoms of shock. Shock can often be reversed by advanced medical care, but only if the victim is reached in time.

Use the activities in Unit 11 of the workbook to help you review the material in this chapter.

You Are the Responder

You respond to an industrial incident and find a victim seated on the ground, leaning against a wall. You notice a large amount of blood around the victim. One of the victim's wrists has been cut, and blood continues to flow from the wound. What signs and symptoms would you look for to indicate shock? How would you provide care for this person to minimize shock?

Specific Injuries

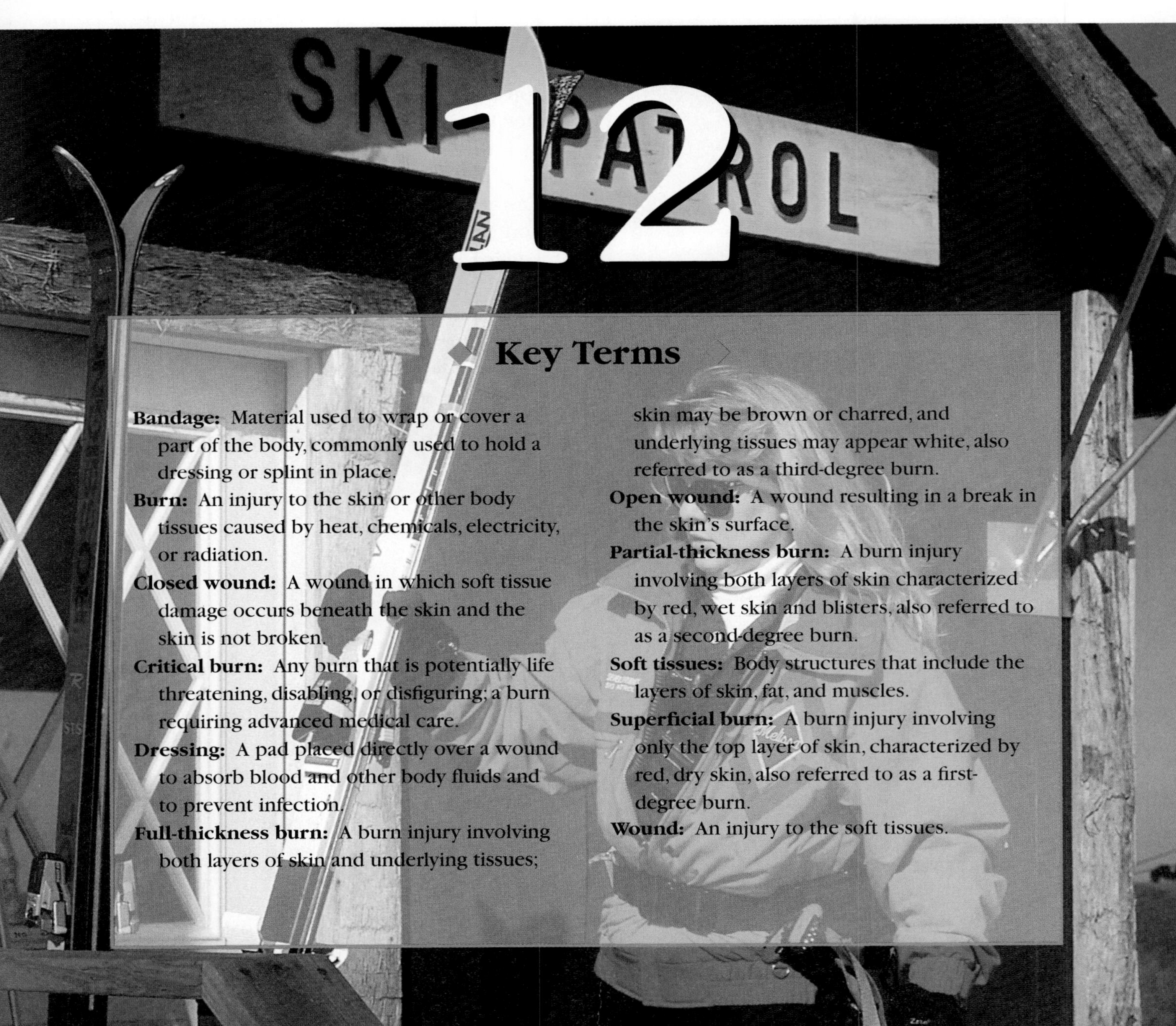

Key Terms

Bandage: Material used to wrap or cover a part of the body, commonly used to hold a dressing or splint in place.

Burn: An injury to the skin or other body tissues caused by heat, chemicals, electricity, or radiation.

Closed wound: A wound in which soft tissue damage occurs beneath the skin and the skin is not broken.

Critical burn: Any burn that is potentially life threatening, disabling, or disfiguring; a burn requiring advanced medical care.

Dressing: A pad placed directly over a wound to absorb blood and other body fluids and to prevent infection.

Full-thickness burn: A burn injury involving both layers of skin and underlying tissues; skin may be brown or charred, and underlying tissues may appear white, also referred to as a third-degree burn.

Open wound: A wound resulting in a break in the skin's surface.

Partial-thickness burn: A burn injury involving both layers of skin characterized by red, wet skin and blisters, also referred to as a second-degree burn.

Soft tissues: Body structures that include the layers of skin, fat, and muscles.

Superficial burn: A burn injury involving only the top layer of skin, characterized by red, dry skin, also referred to as a first-degree burn.

Wound: An injury to the soft tissues.

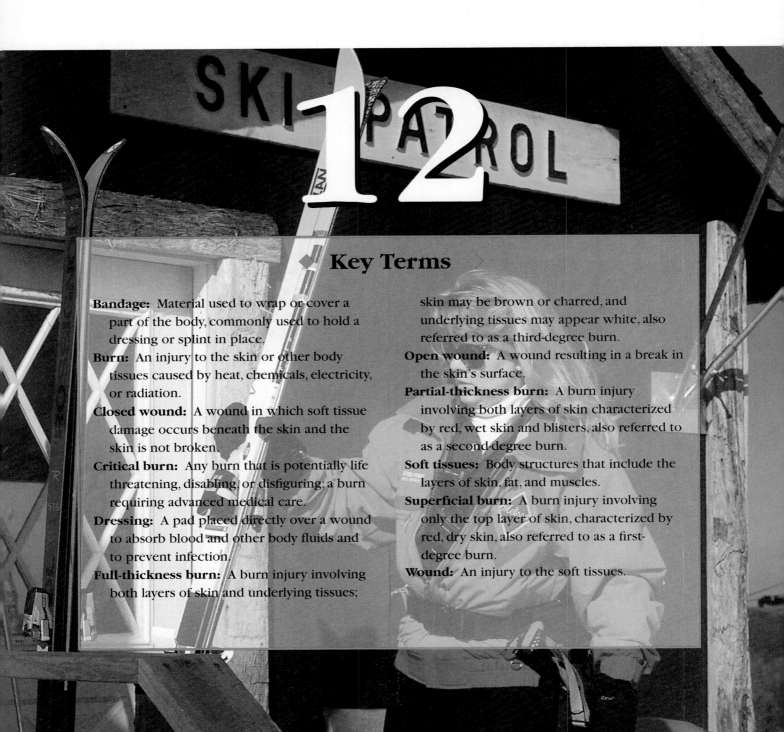

◆ Knowledge Objectives ◆

After reading this chapter and completing the class activities, you should be able to—

- List the types of open soft tissue injuries.
- Describe the emergency medical care for the victim who has the following: a soft tissue injury, a penetrating chest injury, an embedded object, an open wound to the abdomen, an amputation.
- Describe the emergency medical care for burns.
- Explain the functions of dressing and bandaging.
- *Describe the kinds of injuries that might occur as a result of excess mechanical energy, heat, electricity, chemicals, and radiation.
- *Discuss various factors affecting injury statistics.
- *Describe the role a first responder can play in injury prevention.
- List signs of closed wounds.
- Describe the best initial defense against infection of an open wound.
- List the causes of burn injury
- List conditions under which you would summon more advanced medical help for a burn injury.
- Describe how to care for thermal, chemical, electrical, and radiation burns.
- Describe how to care for rib fractures and sucking chest wounds.

*Signifies an Enrichment section objective.

◆ Attitude Objectives ◆

After reading this chapter and completing the class activities, you should be able to—

- Recognize the feelings of a victim with a soft tissue injury or bleeding.
- Acknowledge the need for having a caring attitude toward victims with a soft tissue injury or bleeding.
- *Appreciate the relationship between risky behaviors and the chance of injury.
- *Acknowledge the importance of the first responder's role in injury prevention.

*Signifies an Enrichment section objective.

◆ Skill Objectives ◆

After reading this chapter and completing the class activities, you should be able to—

- Demonstrate the steps in the emergency medical care for open soft tissue injuries, open chest wounds, abdominal wounds, embedded objects, and amputations.
- Demonstrate techniques for controlling severe bleeding.
- Make appropriate decisions about care when given an example of an emergency involving soft tissue injuries.

It is nearly the end of a seemingly endless third shift. For some crew members, it has been a double shift. The work has been exhausting as they struggle against the clock to get a new boiler installed before the deadline. The foreman reminds everyone that there is a bonus if they can complete the task on time.

The most difficult part, the installation, is complete. Now, a final test is needed to see that everything is working. Paul, one of the crew, notices a leaking pipe and climbs up to tighten a connection. He slips and falls, breaking a pipe. Steam and scalding water spew everywhere, burning his chest and arms.

The foreman immediately activates the plant's emergency plan. You, the first responder, arrive quickly and assess the situation. After ensuring the scene is safe for you to approach the victim, you take steps to cool the crew member's burned skin and administer oxygen. Recognizing that more advanced medical care is needed, you send a co-worker to call the emergency number to request an ambulance.

As Paul passes through the hospital's emergency department, he becomes part of the statistics that reflect for one of our nation's most significant health problems — injuries.

◆ INTRODUCTION

An infant falls and bruises his arm while learning to walk; a toddler scrapes his knee while learning to run; a child needs stitches in her chin after she tumbles from the "monkey bars" on the playground; an adolescent gets a black eye in a fist fight; a teenager suffers a sunburn as a result of a weekend at the beach; and an adult cuts her hand while working in a woodshop. What do these injuries have in common? They are all soft tissue injuries.

In the course of growing up and in our daily lives, soft tissue injuries occur often and in many different ways. Fortunately, most soft tissue injuries are minor, requiring little attention. Often, only an adhesive bandage or ice and rest are needed. Some injuries, however, are more severe and require immediate medical attention. In this chapter, you will learn how to recognize and care for soft tissue injuries.

◆ SOFT TISSUE INJURIES

The ***soft tissues*** include the layers of skin, fat, and muscles that protect the underlying body structures (Fig. 12-1). In Chapter 5, you learned that the skin is the largest single organ in the body and that without it the human body could not function. It provides a protective barrier for the body, it helps regulate the body's temperature, and it receives information about the environment through the nerves in the skin.

The skin has two layers. The outer layer of skin, the **epidermis**, provides a barrier to bacteria and other organisms that can cause infection. The deeper layer, the **dermis**, contains the important structures of the nerves, the

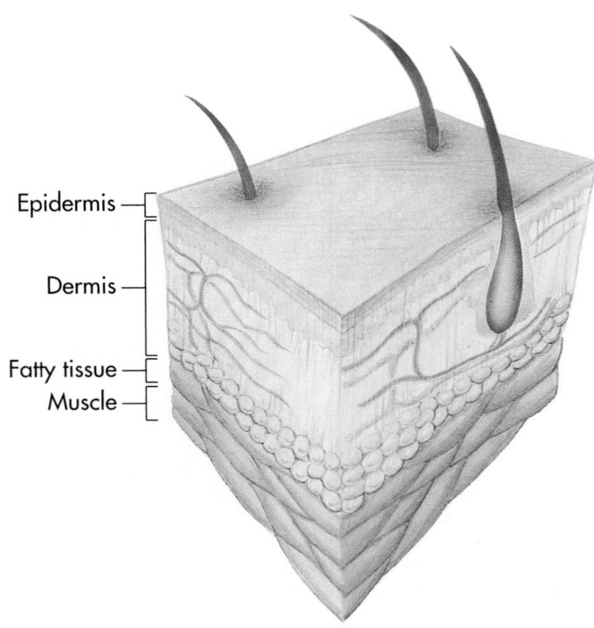

Figure 12-1 The soft tissues include the layers of skin, fat, and muscle.

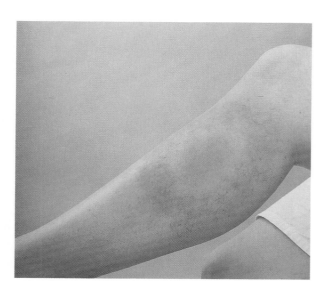

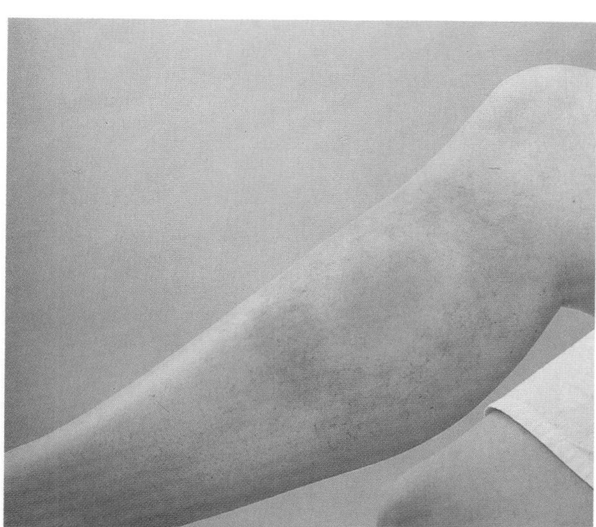
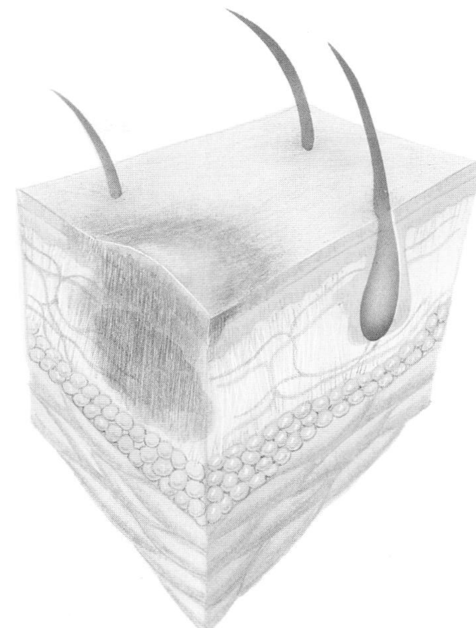

Figure 12-2 The simplest closed wound is a bruise.

sweat and oil glands, and the blood vessels. Because the skin is well supplied with blood vessels and nerves, most soft tissue injuries are likely to bleed and be painful.

Beneath the skin layers lies a layer of fat. This layer helps insulate the body to help maintain body temperature. The fat layer also stores energy. The amount of fat varies in different parts of the body and in each person.

The muscles lie beneath the fat layer and comprise the largest segment of the body's soft tissues. Most soft tissue injuries involve the outer layers of tissue. However, violent forces, such as those that cause deep burns or cause objects to penetrate the skin, can injure all the soft tissue layers. Although the muscles are considered soft tissues, muscle injuries are discussed more thoroughly in Chapter 13 along with other musculoskeletal injuries.

Types of Soft Tissue Injuries

An injury to the soft tissues is called a ***wound***. Soft tissue injuries are typically classified as either closed wounds or open wounds. A wound is closed when the soft tissue damage occurs beneath the surface of the skin, leaving the outer layer intact. A wound is open if there is a break in the skin's outer layer. Open wounds usually result in external bleeding.

Burns are a special kind of soft tissue injury. A burn injury occurs when intense heat, certain chemicals, electricity, or radiation contacts the skin or other body tissues. Burns are classified as either superficial, partial-thickness, or full-thickness. Superficial burns affect only the outer layer of skin. Partial-thickness burns damage both skin layers. Full-thickness burns penetrate the layers of skin and can affect other soft tissues and even bone. Burns are discussed in more detail later in this chapter.

Closed Wounds

Closed wounds occur beneath the surface of the skin. The simplest ***closed wound*** is a bruise, also called a contusion (Fig. 12-2). Bruises result when the body is subjected to a blunt force, such as when you bump your leg on a table or chair. Such a blow usually results in damage to soft tissue layers and blood vessels beneath the skin, causing internal bleeding. When blood and other fluids seep into the

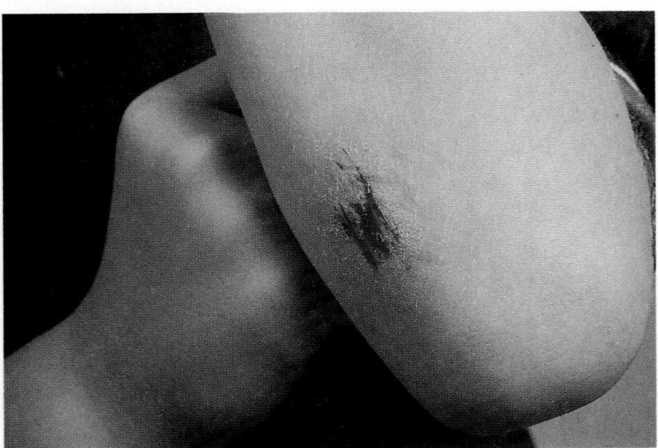

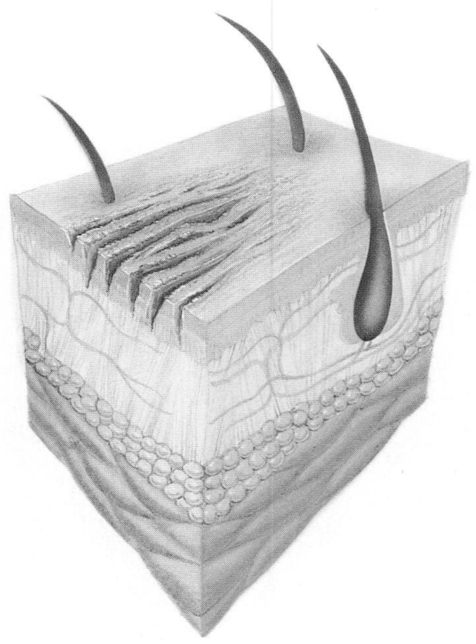

Figure 12-3 Abrasions can be painful, but bleeding is easily controlled.

surrounding tissues, the area discolors (turns black and blue) and swells. The amount of discoloration and swelling varies depending on the severity of the injury. At first, the area may only appear red. Over time, more blood may leak into the area, making the area appear dark red or purple. Violent forces can cause more severe soft tissue injuries involving larger blood vessels, the deeper layers of muscle tissue, and even organs deep within the body. These injuries can result in profuse internal bleeding. With deeper injuries, a first responder may or may not see bruising immediately.

Open Wounds

Open wounds are injuries that break the skin. These breaks can be as minor as a scrape of the surface layers or as severe as a deep penetration. The amount of bleeding depends on the severity of the injury. Any break in the skin provides an entry point for disease-producing microorganisms, or pathogens. There are four main types of open wounds:

- Abrasions
- Lacerations
- Avulsions
- Punctures

An **abrasion** is the most common type of open wound. It is characterized by skin that has been rubbed or scraped away (Fig. 12-3). Rubbed away or scraped skin occurs when a child falls and scrapes his or her hands or knees. An abrasion is sometimes called a rug burn, road rash, or strawberry. Because the scraping of the outer skin layers exposes sensitive nerve endings, an abrasion is usually painful. Bleeding is easily controlled and not severe, since only the capillaries are affected. Because of the way the injury occurs, dirt and other matter can easily become embedded in the skin, making it especially important to clean the wound.

A **laceration** is a cut, usually from a sharp object. The cut may have either jagged or smooth edges (Fig. 12-4). Lacerations are commonly caused by sharp-edged objects, such as knives, scissors, or broken glass. A laceration can also result when a blunt force splits the skin. Such splits occur in areas where bone lies directly under the skin's surface, such as the

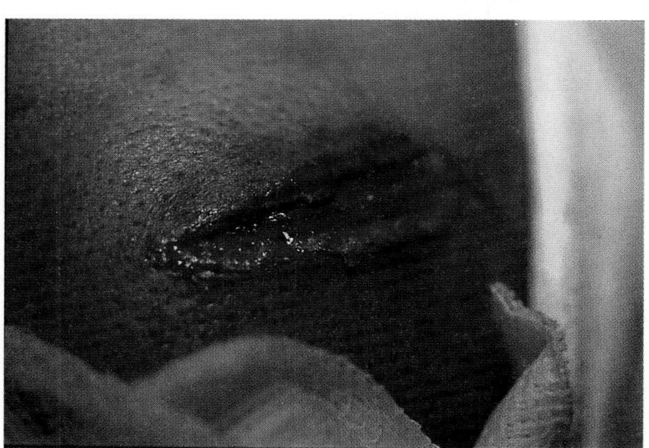

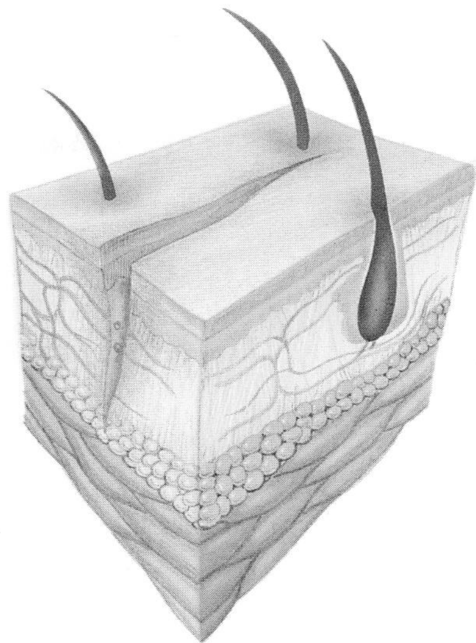

Figure 12-4 A laceration may have jagged or smooth edges.

jaw. Deep lacerations can also affect the layers of fat and muscle, damaging both nerves and blood vessels. Lacerations usually bleed freely and, depending on the structures involved, can bleed profusely. Because the nerves may also be injured, lacerations are not always immediately painful.

An **avulsion** is an injury in which a portion of the skin and sometimes other soft tissue is partially or completely torn away (Fig. 12-5). A partially avulsed piece of skin may remain attached but hangs like a flap. Bleeding is usually heavy because avulsions often involve deeper soft tissue layers. Sometimes a force is

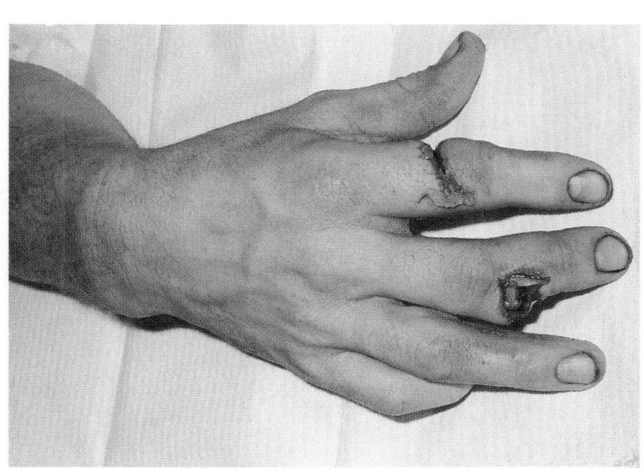

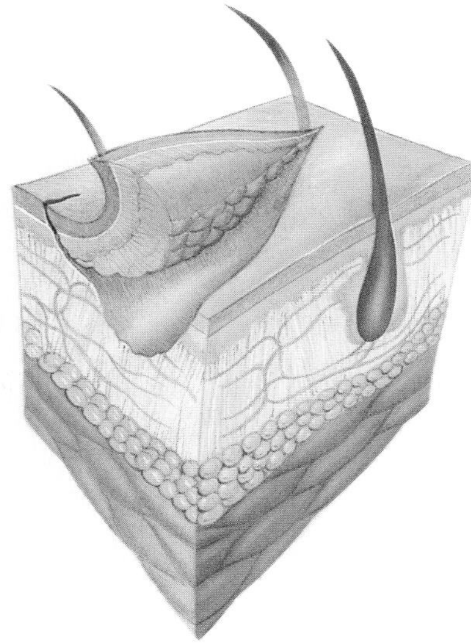

Figure 12-5 In an avulsion, part of the skin and other soft tissue is torn away.

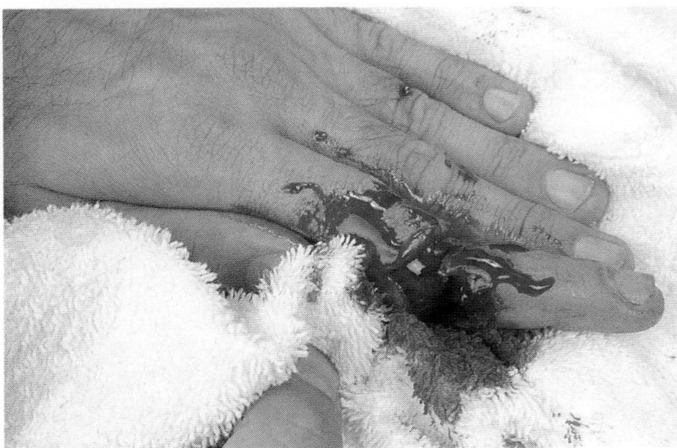

Figure 12-6 In an avulsion, a body part may also be completely severed.

so violent that a body part, such as a finger, may be severed. A complete severing of a part is sometimes called an **amputation** (Fig. 12-6). Although damage to the tissue is severe, bleeding is usually not as bad as you might expect. The blood vessels usually constrict and retract (pull in) at the point of injury, slowing bleeding and making it relatively easy to control with direct pressure. In the past, a completely severed body part could not be successfully reattached. With today's technology, reattachment is often successful, making it important to send the severed part to the hospital with the victim.

A **puncture** wound results when the skin is pierced with a pointed object, such as a nail, a piece of glass, a splinter, or a knife (Fig. 12-7). A bullet wound is also a puncture wound. Because the skin usually closes around the penetrating object, external bleeding is generally not severe. However, internal bleeding can be severe if the penetrating object damages major blood vessels or internal organs. An object that remains in the open wound is called an **embedded object** (Fig. 12-8). An object also may pass completely through a body part, making two open wounds — one at the entry point and one at the exit point.

Although puncture wounds generally do not bleed profusely, they are potentially more dangerous than wounds that do because they are more likely to become infected. Objects penetrating the soft tissues carry microorganisms that cause infections. Of particular danger is the microorganism that causes tetanus, a severe infection.

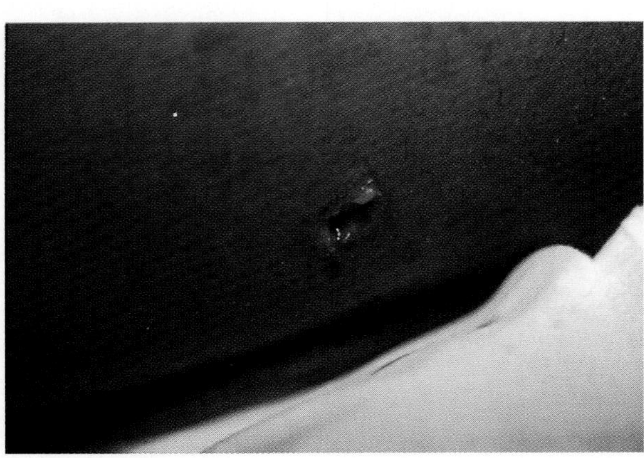

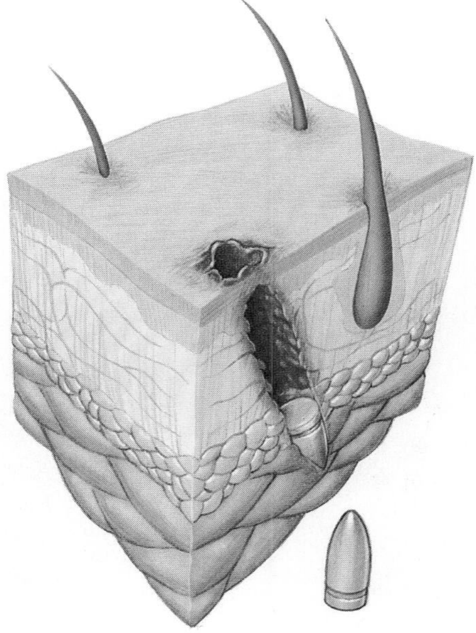

Figure 12-7 A puncture wound results when skin is pierced by a pointed object.

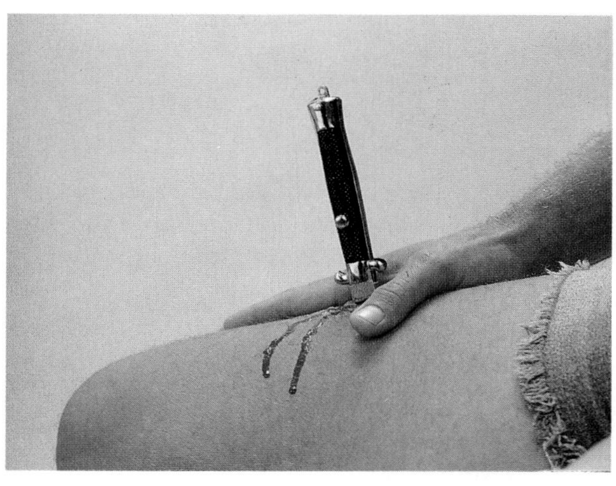

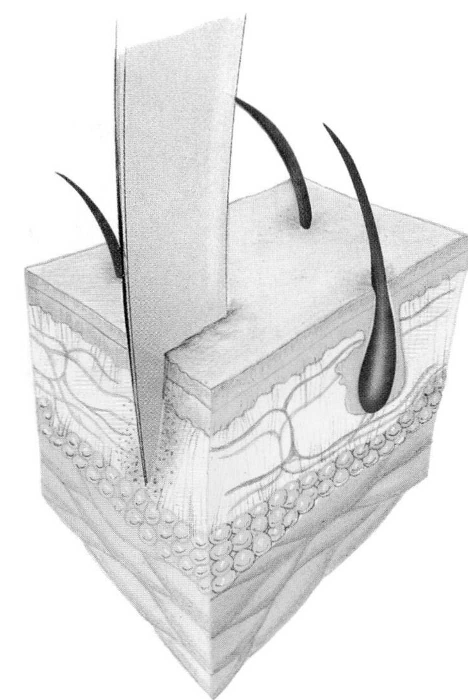

Figure 12-8 An embedded object is an object that remains in a wound.

Dressings and Bandages

All open wounds need some type of covering to help control bleeding and prevent infection. These coverings are commonly referred to as dressings and bandages. There are many different types of both.

Dressings

Dressings are pads placed directly on the wound to absorb blood and other fluids and to prevent infection. To minimize the chance of infection, dressings should be sterile. Most dressings are porous, allowing air to circulate to the wound to promote healing. Standard dressings include varying sizes of cotton gauze, commonly ranging from 2 to 4 inches square. Much larger dressings called **universal dressings** or trauma dressings are used to cover very large wounds and multiple wounds in one body area (Fig. 12-9). Some dressings have non-stick surfaces to prevent the dressing from sticking to the wound.

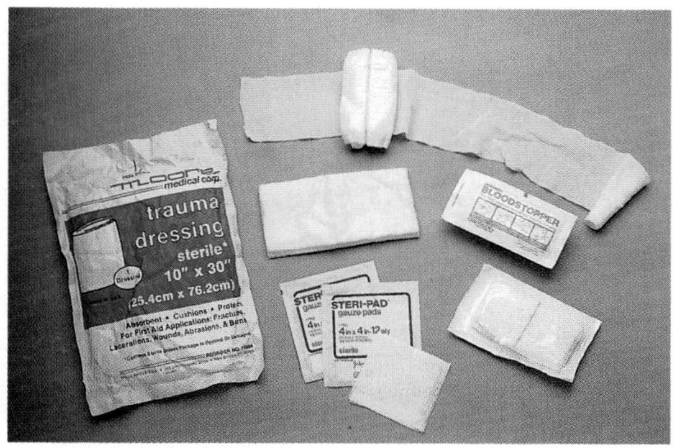

Figure 12-9 Dressings come in various sizes.

A special type of dressing, called an **occlusive dressing**, does not allow air to pass through. Aluminum foil, plastic wrap, and petroleum jelly-soaked gauze are examples of this type of dressing (Fig. 12-10).

Bandages

A ***bandage*** is any material used to wrap or cover any part of the body. Bandages are used

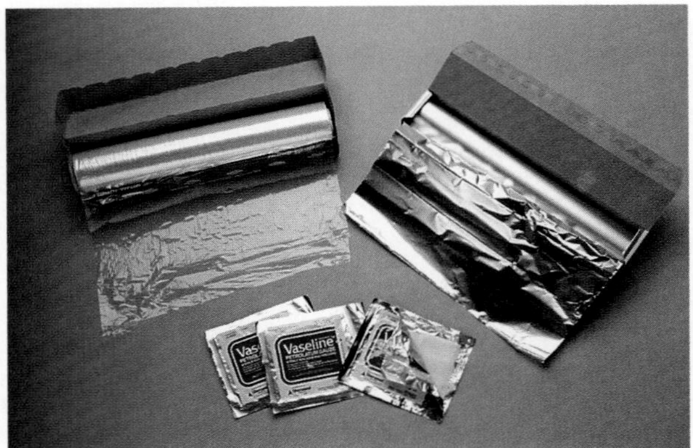

Figure 12-10 Special dressings are designed to prevent air from passing through.

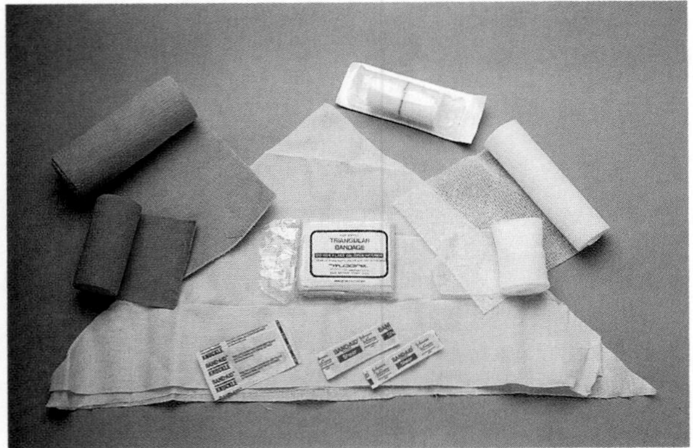

Figure 12-11 Different types of bandages are used to hold dressings in place, apply pressure to a wound, protect the wound from infecting, and provide support to an injured area.

to hold dressings in place, to apply pressure to control bleeding, to help protect a wound from dirt and infection, and to provide support to an injured limb or body part. Many different types of bandages are available commercially (Fig. 12-11). A bandage applied snugly to create pressure on a wound or injury is called a pressure bandage.

A common type of bandage is a commercially made adhesive compress, such as a Band-Aid®. Available in assorted sizes, an adhesive compress consists of a small pad of nonstick gauze (the dressing) on a strip of adhesive tape (the bandage) applied directly to small injuries. Also available is the **bandage compress**, a thick gauze dressing attached to a gauze bandage. This bandage can be tied in place. Because it is specially designed to help control severe bleeding, the bandage compress usually comes in a sterile package.

A **roller bandage** is usually made of gauze or gauze-like material (Fig. 12-12). Some gauze bandages are made of a self-adhering material that easily conforms to different body parts. Kling® roller gauze is one example. Roller bandages are available in assorted widths from ½ to 12 inches and lengths from 5 to 10 yards. A roller bandage is generally wrapped around the body part, over a dressing, using overlapping turns until the dressing is completely covered.

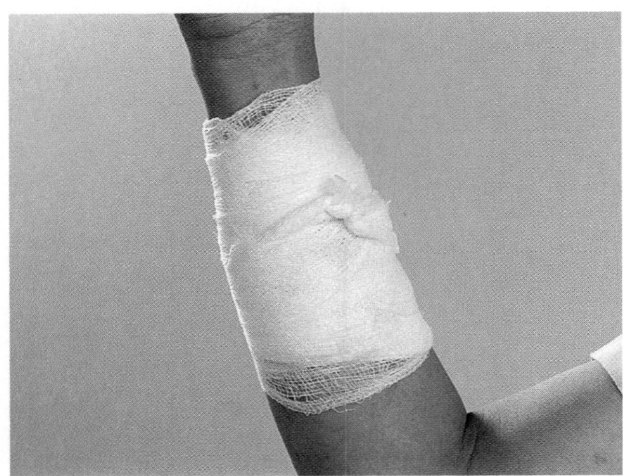

Figure 12-12 Roller bandages are usually made of gauze and are easy to apply.

It can be tied or taped in place. A folded strip of roller bandage may also be used as a dressing or compress. In Chapter 13, you will learn to use roller bandages to hold splints in place.

A special type of roller bandage is an **elastic bandage**, sometimes called an elastic wrap. Elastic bandages are designed to keep continuous pressure on a body part (Fig. 12-13). When properly applied, they can effectively control swelling or support an injured limb. Elastic bandages are available in assorted widths from 2 to 6 inches. They are very effective in managing injuries to muscles, bones, and joints. Elastic

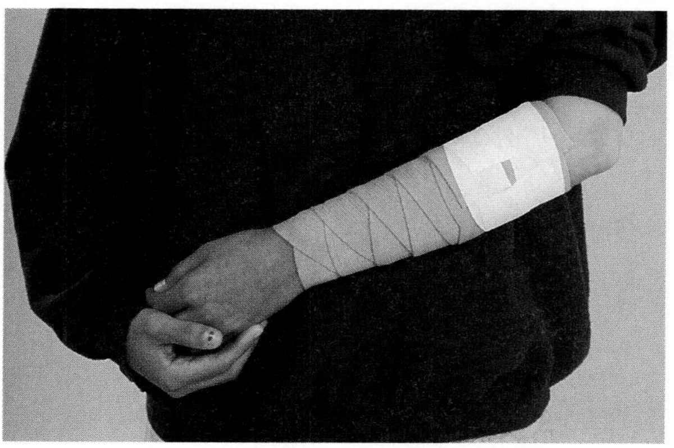

Figure 12-13 Elastic bandages can be applied to control swelling or support an injured extremity.

bandages are frequently used in athletic environments and should be applied only by people who are trained and proficient in their use.

Another commonly used bandage is the **triangular bandage**. Folded, it can hold a dressing or splint in place on most parts of the body (Fig. 12-14). Used as a sling, the triangular bandage can support an injured shoulder, arm, or hand (Fig. 12-15).

To apply a roller bandage, follow these general guidelines:

- If possible, elevate the injured body part above the level of the heart.
- Secure the end of the bandage in place. Wrap the bandage around the body part until the dressing is completely covered and the bandage extends several inches beyond the dressing. Tie or tape the bandage in place (Fig. 12-16, *A-C*).
- Do not cover fingers or toes, if possible. By keeping these parts uncovered, you will be able to tell if the bandage is too tight (Fig. 12-16, *D*). If fingers or toes become cold, numb, or begin to turn pale, ashen, or blue, the bandage is too tight and should be loosened slightly.
- If blood soaks through the bandage, apply additional dressings and another bandage. *Do not remove the blood-soaked ones.*

Elastic bandages can easily restrict blood flow if not applied properly. Restricted blood flow is not only painful but also can cause tissue damage if not corrected. Figure 12-17, *A-D* shows the proper way to apply an elastic bandage.

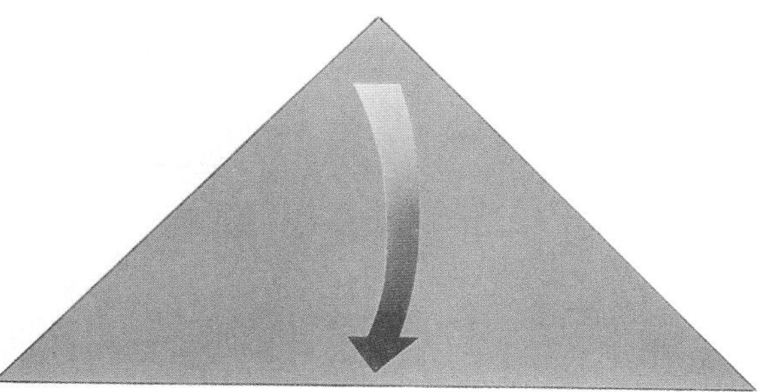

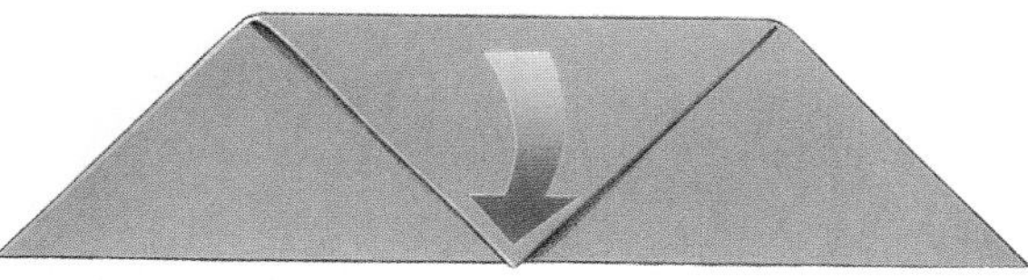

Figure 12-14 A cravat is made by folding a triangular bandage.

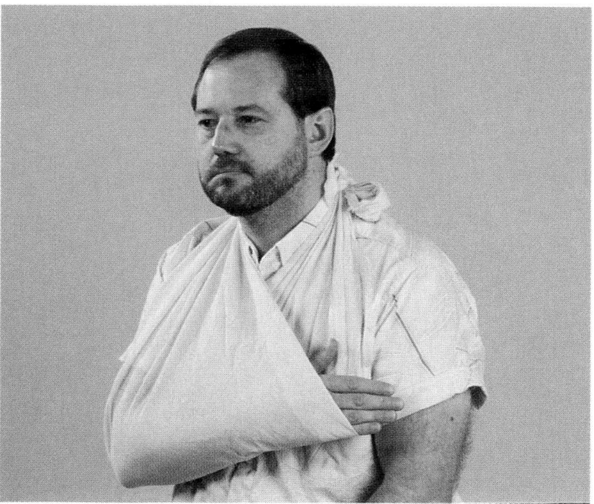

Figure 12-15 A triangular bandage is commonly used as a sling.

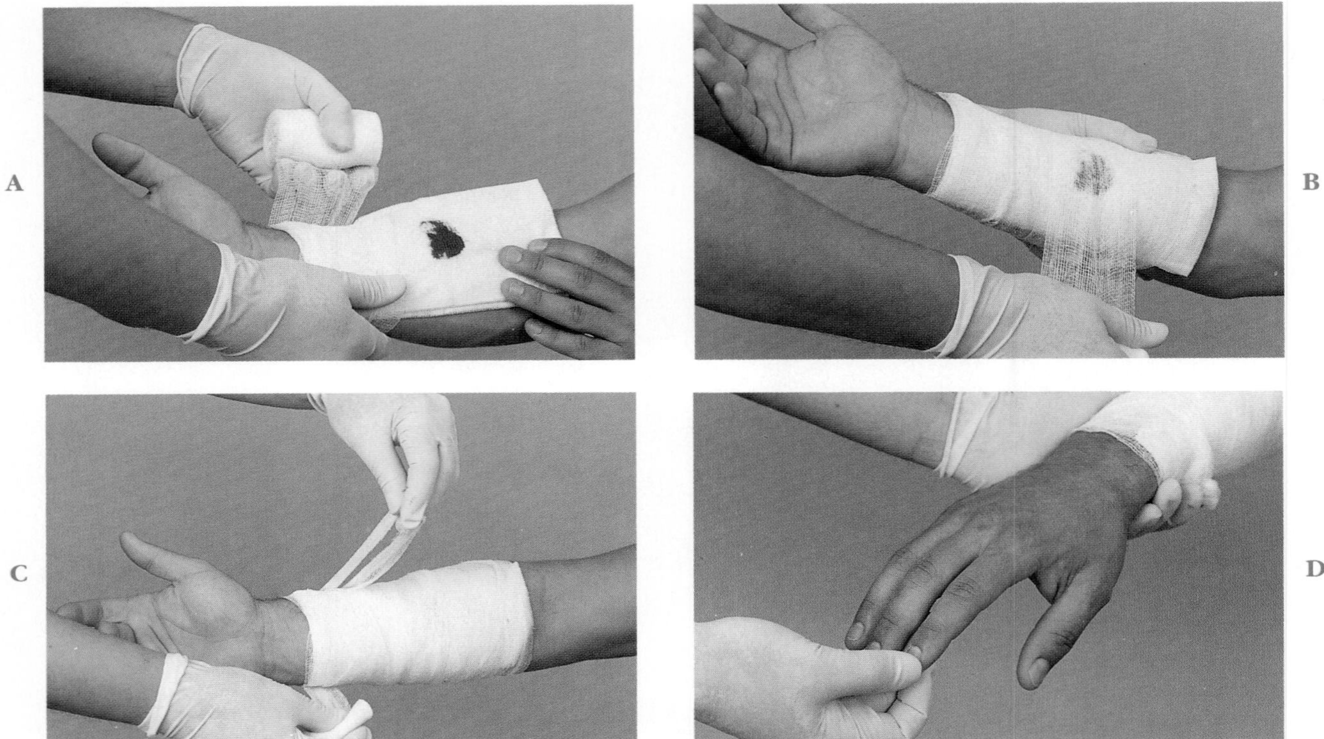

Figure 12-16 **A**, Start by securing the end of the roller bandage in place. **B**, Use overlapping turns to cover the dressing completely. **C**, Tie or tape the bandage in place. **D**, Check the fingers to ensure the bandage is not too tight.

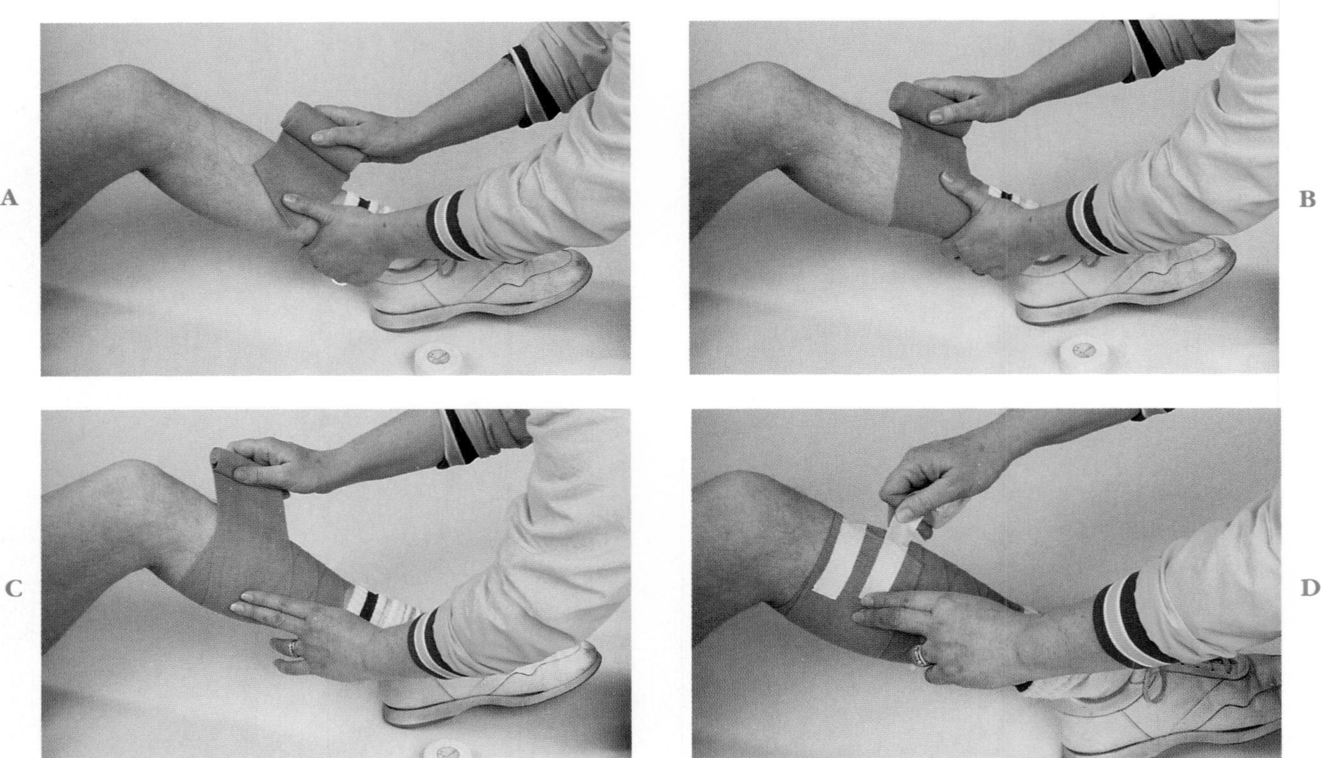

Figure 12-17 **A**, Start the elastic bandage at the point furthest from the heart. **B**, Secure the end of the bandage in place. **C**, Wrap the bandage using overlapping turns. **D**, Tape the end of the bandage in place.

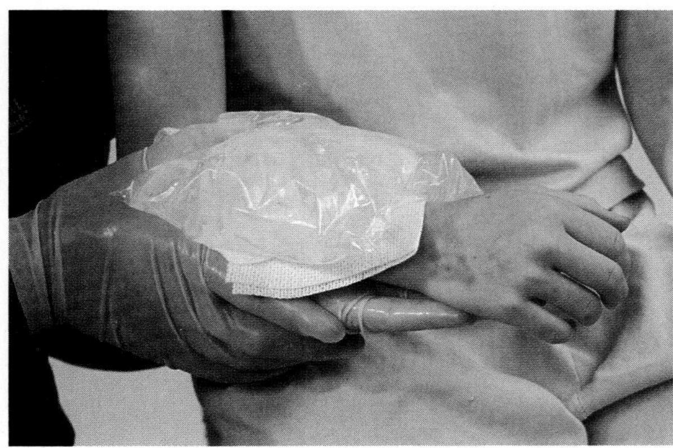

Figure 12-18 For a closed wound, apply ice to help control pain and swelling.

Role of the First Responder

Caring for wounds is not difficult. *Be sure to follow the basic guidelines for bleeding control and BSI.*

Care for Closed Wounds

Most closed wounds do not require special medical care. Direct pressure on the area decreases bleeding. Elevating the injured part helps to control bleeding and reduce swelling. Cold can be effective in helping control both pain and swelling. When applying ice or a chemical cold pack, place a gauze pad, towel, or other cloth between the ice and the skin to protect the skin (Fig. 12-18).

Do not dismiss a closed wound as "just a bruise." Be aware of possible serious injuries to internal organs or other underlying structures, such as the muscles or bones. Take the time to evaluate how the injury happened and whether more serious injuries could be present. If a person complains of severe pain or cannot move a body part without pain or if you think the force that caused the injury was great enough to cause serious damage, call for more advanced medical help immediately. Care for these injuries is described later in this chapter and in Chapter 13.

Care for Major Open Wounds

A major open wound is one with severe bleeding, deep destruction of tissue, or a deeply embedded object. To care for a major open wound, follow these general guidelines:

- *Do not* waste time trying to wash the wound.
- Quickly control bleeding, using direct pressure and elevation. Apply direct pressure by placing a sterile dressing over the wound with your gloved hand. If nothing sterile is

A Stitch in Time . . .

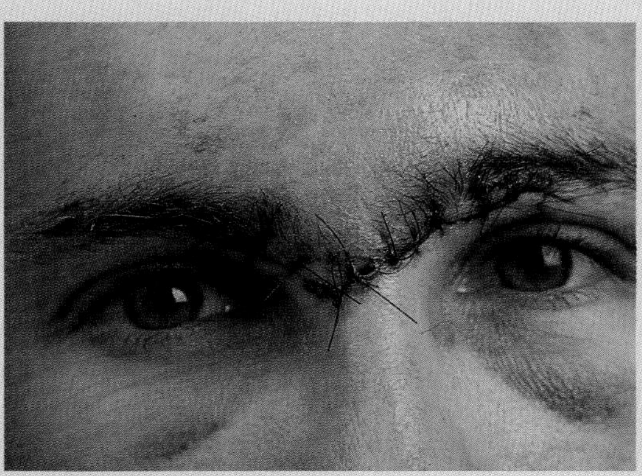

It can be difficult to judge when a wound should be seen by a doctor for stitches. A quick rule of thumb is that stitches are needed when the edges of skin do not fall together or when the wound is more than an inch long. Stitches speed the healing process, lessen the chances of infection, and improve the look of scars. The wound should be stitched within the first few hours following the injury. The following major injuries may require stitches:

- Bleeding from an artery or uncontrollable bleeding
- Deep cuts or avulsions that show the muscle or bone, involve joints near the hands or feet, gape widely, or involve the thumb or the palm of the hand
- Large or deep punctures
- Large or deeply embedded objects
- Human and animal bites
- Wounds that, if left unattended, could leave a conspicuous scar, such as those that involve the lip or eyebrow

If you are caring for a wound and think it may need stitches, it probably does.

available, use any clean covering, such as a towel or a handkerchief. If you do not have a glove and a cloth is not available, have the injured person use his or her hand.

- Continue direct pressure by applying a pressure bandage.
- Summon more advanced medical care.
- Use a pressure point to control bleeding if necessary.
- Wash your hands immediately after completing care.

Care for Minor Wounds

A minor wound is one, such as an abrasion, in which damage is only superficial and bleeding is minimal. To care for a minor wound, follow these general guidelines:

- Cleanse the wound with soap and water.
- Place a sterile or clean dressing over the wound.
- Apply direct pressure for a few minutes to control any bleeding.
- Remove dressing and apply an antibiotic

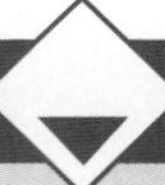

An Ounce of Prevention . . .

A serious infection can cause severe medical problems. One such infection is tetanus, caused by the organism *Clostridium tetani*. This organism, commonly found in soil and feces of cows and horses, can infect many kinds of wounds. This probably explains why the cavalry in the American Civil War had higher rates of tetanus than the infantry. Worldwide, tetanus kills about 50,000 people annually. In the United States in 1994, 51 cases of tetanus were reported.

Tetanus is introduced into the body through a puncture wound, abrasion, laceration, or burn. Because the organism multiplies in an environment that is low in oxygen, puncture wounds and other deep wounds are at particular risk for tetanus infection. It produces a powerful toxin, one of the most lethal poisons known, that affects the central nervous system and specific muscles. People at risk for tetanus include drug addicts, burn victims, and people recovering from surgery. Newborn babies can be infected through the stump of the umbilical cord.

Signs and symptoms of tetanus include difficulty swallowing, irritability, headache, fever, and muscle spasms near the infected area. Later, as the infection progresses, it can affect other muscles, such as those in the jaw, causing the condition called "lockjaw." Once tetanus gets into the nervous system, its effects are irreversible.

The first line of defense against tetanus is to thoroughly clean an open wound. Major wounds should be cleaned and treated at a medical facility. Clean a minor wound with soap and water, and apply an antibiotic ointment and a clean or sterile dressing. If signs of wound infection develop, seek medical attention immediately. Infected wounds of the face, neck, and head should receive *immediate* medical care, since the tetanus toxin can travel rapidly to the brain. A physician will determine whether a tetanus shot or a booster shot is needed, depending on the victim's immunization status. Always contact your personal physician if you are unsure how long it has been since you received a tetanus immunization or booster.

The best way to prevent tetanus is to be immunized against it and then receive periodic booster shots. Immunizations assist the natural function of the immune system by building up antibodies, disease-fighting proteins that help protect the body against specific bacteria. Because the effects of immunization do not last a lifetime, booster shots help maintain the antibodies that protect against tetanus. Booster shots are recommended every 5 to 10 years or whenever a wound has been contaminated by dirt or an object, such as a rusty nail, causes a puncture wound. Most children in this country receive as infants an immunization known as *DPT*, which includes the tetanus toxoid.

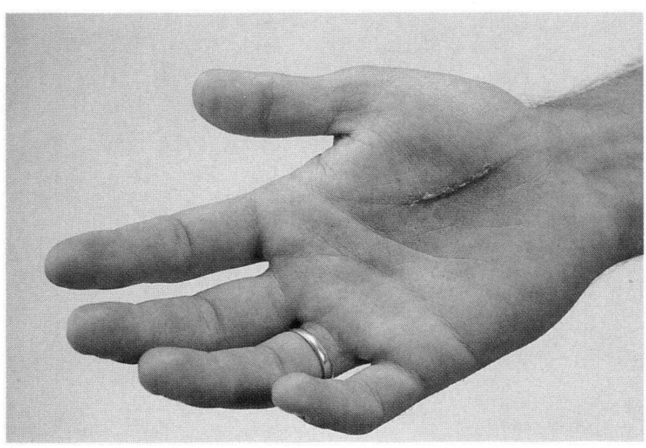

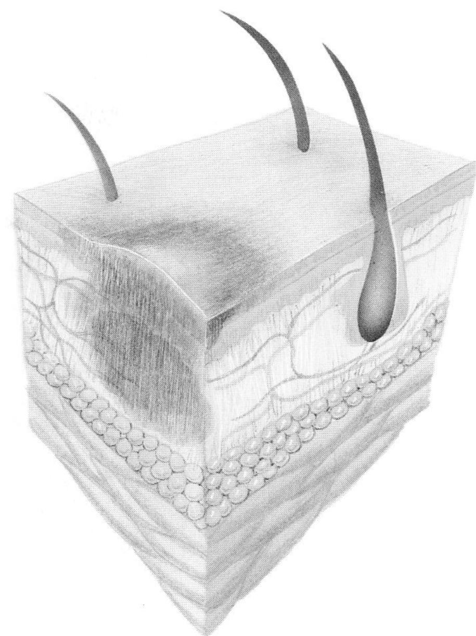

Figure 12-19 An infected wound may become swollen and may have a pus discharge.

ointment if one is available and your organization's protocols allow you to do so.

- Apply a new sterile or clean dressing.
- Hold the dressing in place with a bandage or tape or a Band-Aid® type bandage.

Infection

Since the skin tends to collect microorganisms, even minor injuries involving breaks in the skin can become infected unless properly cared for.

Preventing Infection

Injuries causing breaks in the skin carry great risk of infection. The best initial defense against infection is to cleanse the area thoroughly. For minor wounds, that is, those that are small and do not bleed severely, wash the area with soap and water. Most soaps are effective in removing harmful bacteria. Do not use alcohol because it can damage tissues. Wounds that require medical attention because of more extensive tissue damage or bleeding need not be washed immediately. These wounds will be cleaned thoroughly in the medical facility as a routine part of the care. It is more important for you to control bleeding.

Signs of Infection

Sometimes even the best care for a soft tissue injury is not enough to prevent infection. When a wound becomes infected, the area around the wound becomes swollen and red. The area may feel warm or throb with pain. Some wounds have a pus discharge (Fig. 12-19). Red streaks may develop that progress from the wound toward the heart. More serious infections may cause a person to develop a fever and feel ill. Serious infections require a physician's care.

◆ BURNS

Burns are another type of soft tissue injury, caused primarily by heat. Burns can also occur when the body is exposed to certain chemicals, electricity, or solar or other forms of radiation.

When burns occur, they first affect the top layer of skin, the epidermis. If the burn progresses, the dermis, the second layer, can also

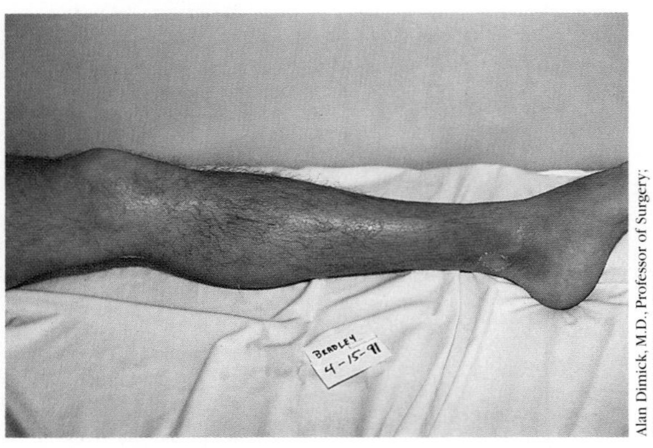

Alan Dimick, M.D., Professor of Surgery; Director UAB Burn Center

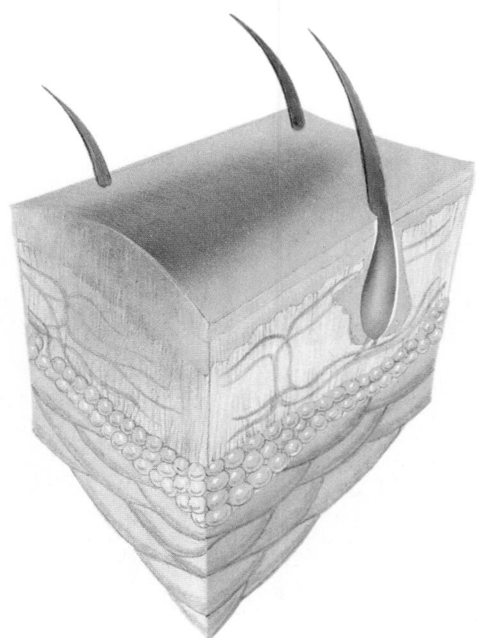

Figure 12-20 A Superficial Burn

be affected. Deep burns can damage underlying tissues. Burns that break the skin can cause infection, fluid loss, and loss of temperature control. Burns can also damage the respiratory system and the eyes.

The severity of a burn depends on the—

- Temperature of the source of the burn.
- Length of exposure to the source.
- Location of the burn.
- Size of the burn.
- Victim's age and medical condition.

In general, people under age 5 and over age 60 have thinner skin and often burn more severely. People with chronic medical problems also tend to have more severe burns, especially if they are not well-nourished, have heart or kidney problems, or are exposed to the burn source for a prolonged period because they are unable to escape.

Types of Burns

Burns are classified by their source, such as heat, chemicals, electricity, or radiation. They are also classified by depth. The deeper the burn, the more severe it is. Generally, three depth classifications are used: superficial (first degree), partial-thickness (second degree), and full-thickness (third degree).

Superficial Burns (First Degree)

A ***superficial burn*** involves only the top layer of skin, the epidermis (Fig. 12-20). The skin is red and dry, and the burn is usually painful. The area may swell. Most sunburns are superficial burns. Superficial burns generally heal in 5 to 6 days without permanent scarring.

Partial-Thickness Burns (Second Degree)

A ***partial-thickness burn*** involves both the epidermis and the dermis (Fig. 12-21). These injuries are also red and have blisters that may open and weep clear fluid, making the skin appear wet. The burned skin may look blotched. These burns are usually painful, and the area often swells. The body loses fluid and the burn is susceptible to infection. Although the burn usually heals in 3 or 4 weeks, extensive partial-thickness burns can be serious, requiring

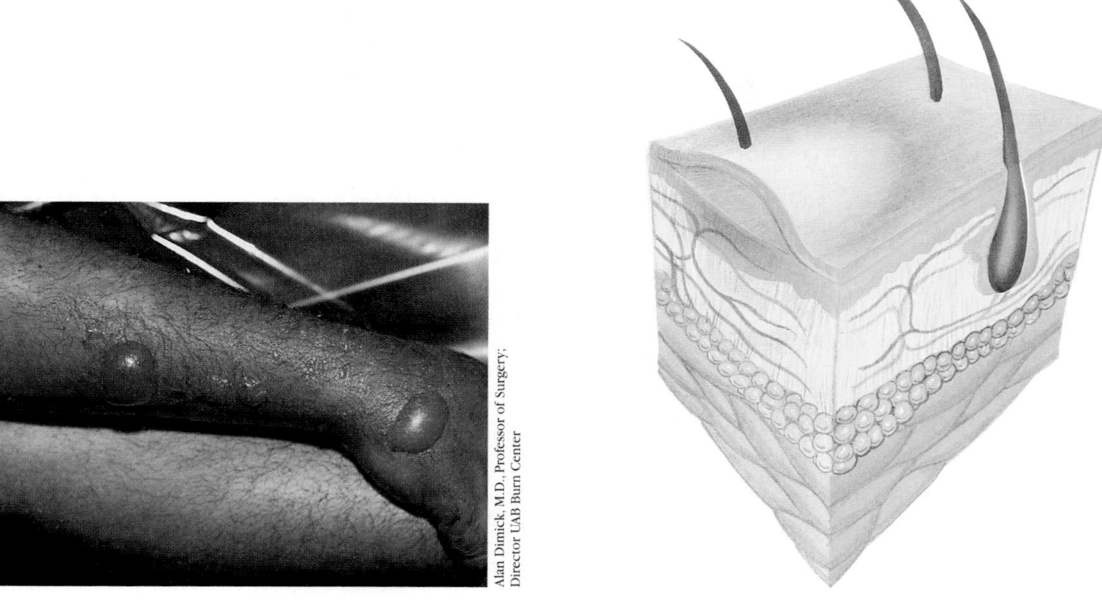

Figure 12-21 A Partial-Thickness Burn

more advanced medical care. Scarring may occur from partial-thickness burns.

Full-Thickness Burns (Third Degree)

A ***full-thickness burn*** destroys both layers of skin, as well as any or all of the underlying structures — fat, muscles, bones, and nerves (Fig. 12-22). These burns may look brown or charred (black), with the tissues underneath sometimes appearing white. They can be either extremely painful or relatively painless if the burn destroys nerve endings in the skin.

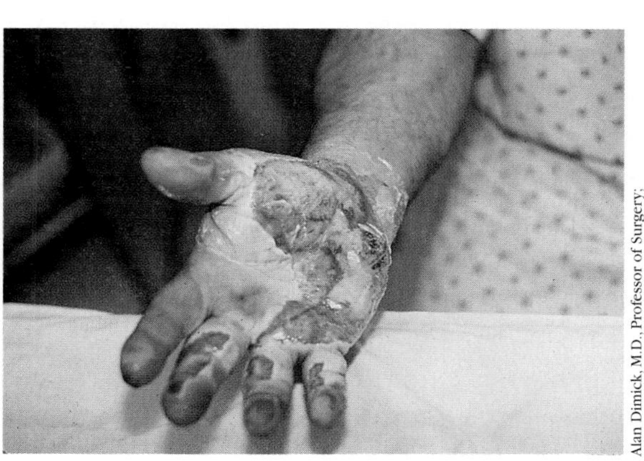

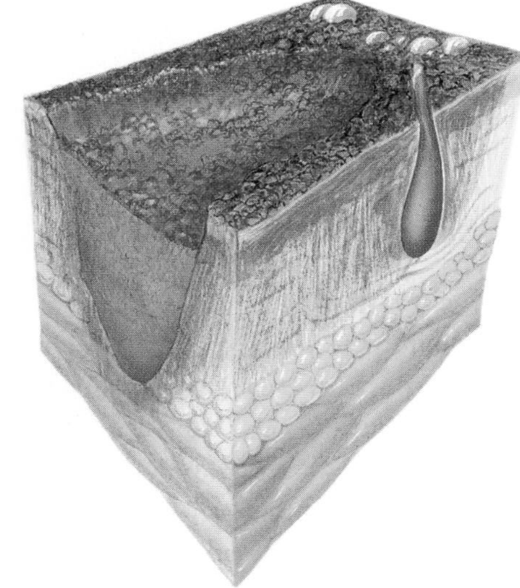

Figure 12-22 A Full-Thickness Burn

Full-thickness burns are often surrounded by painful partial-thickness burns.

Full-thickness burns can be life threatening. Because the burns are open, the body loses fluid and shock is likely to occur. These burns also make the body highly prone to infection. Scarring occurs and may be severe. Many burn sites eventually require skin grafts.

Identifying Critical Burns

It is important that you be able to identify a critical burn. A ***critical burn*** requires the immediate attention of more advanced medical personnel. Critical burns are potentially life threatening, disfiguring, or disabling. Knowing whether you should summon more advanced medical personnel for a burn injury can sometimes be difficult. It is not always easy or possible to assess the severity of a burn immediately after injury. Even superficial burns to large areas of the body or to certain body parts can be critical. You cannot judge severity by the pain the victim feels because nerve endings may have been destroyed. Call for more advanced medical personnel immediately for assistance in caring for the following burns:

- Burns causing breathing difficulty or signs of burns around the mouth and nose
- Burns covering more than one body part
- Burns to the head, neck, hands, feet, or genitals
- Any partial-thickness or full-thickness burn to a child or an elderly person
- Burns resulting from chemicals, explosions, or electricity

Expect that burns caused by flames or hot grease will require medical attention, especially if the victim is under 5 or over 60 years of age. Hot grease is slow to cool and difficult to remove from the skin. Burns that involve hot liquid or flames contacting clothing will also be serious, since the clothing prolongs the heat contact with the skin. Some synthetic fabrics melt and stick to the body. The melted fabrics may take longer to cool than the soft tissues. Although these burns may appear minor at first, they can continue to worsen for a short time.

Estimating the Extent of Burns

When communicating with more advanced medical personnel about a burned victim, you may be asked how much of the body is burned. The Rule of Nines is a common method for estimating what percentage of the body is affected by burns (Fig. 12-23).

In an adult, the head equals 9 percent of the total body surface. Each arm also equals 9 percent of the body. Each leg equals 18 percent. So does the front or back of the trunk. For example, if the front of the trunk (18 percent) and one entire arm (9 percent) is burned, you would estimate that 27 percent of the body's surface area has been burned.

If you do not remember the Rule of Nines, simply communicate how the burn occurred, the body parts involved, and the approximate type of burn. For example, "The victim was injured when an overheated car radiator exploded. The victim has partial-thickness burns on her face, neck, chest, and arms."

Care for Thermal (Heat) Burns

As you approach the victim, decide if the scene is safe. Look for fire, smoke, downed electrical wires, and warning signs for chemicals or radiation. If the scene is unsafe and you have not been trained to manage the situation, summon other specially trained personnel.

If the scene is safe, approach the victim cautiously. If the source of heat is still in contact with the victim, take steps to remove and extinguish it. Doing so may require you to smother the flames or extinguish them with water or to remove smoldering clothing. If the burn is caused by hot tar, cool the area with water but do not attempt to remove the tar.

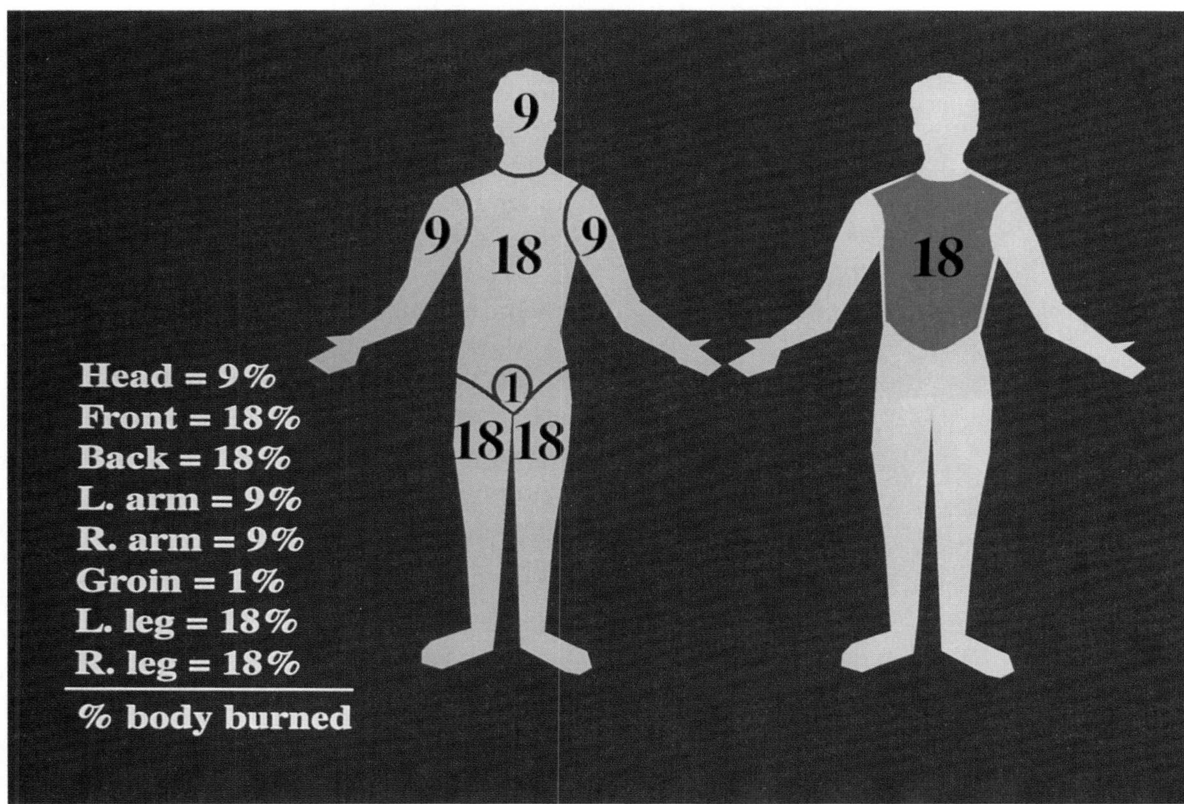

Figure 12-23 The Rule of Nines is one method to help determine how much of the body is burned.

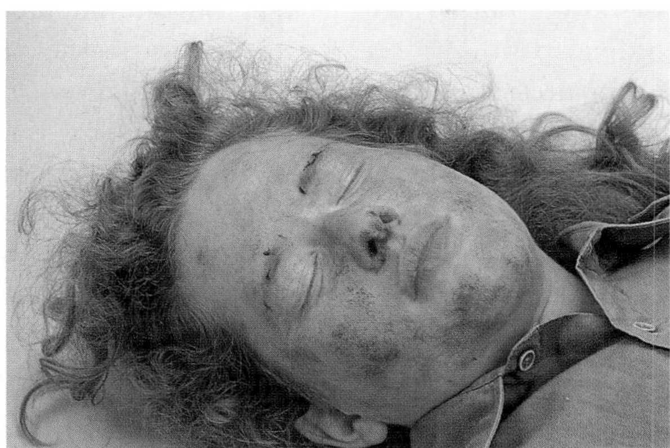

Figure 12-24 Burns or soot on the face may signal that air passages or lungs have been burned.

Do an initial assessment. Pay close attention to the victim's airway. Note soot or burns around the mouth or nose or the rest of the face, which may signal that air passages or lungs have been burned (Fig. 12-24). If you suspect a burned airway or burned lungs, continually monitor breathing and call for advanced medical personnel immediately. Air passages may swell, impairing or stopping breathing. Oxygen should be administered if it is available and you are trained to use it.

As you do a physical examination, look for additional signs of burn injuries. Look also for other injuries, especially if there was an explosion or electric shock.

If thermal burns are present, follow these three basic care steps:

- Cool the burned area.
- Cover the burned area.
- Minimize shock.

Cool the Burned Area

Even after the source of heat has been removed, soft tissue will continue to burn for

A

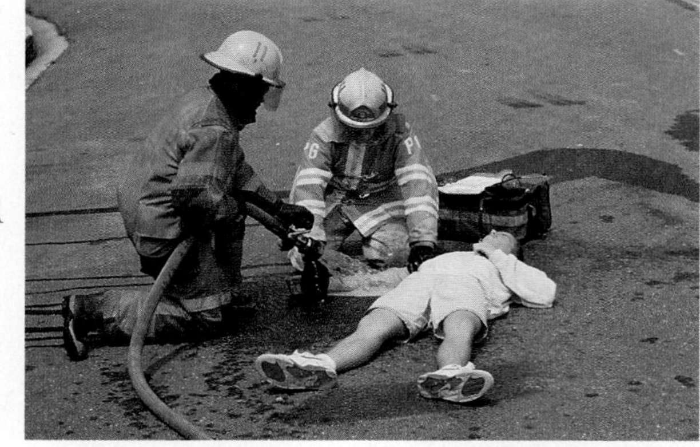

B

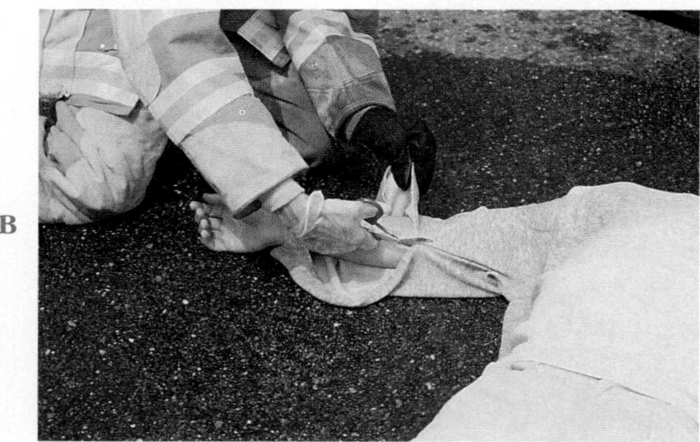

C

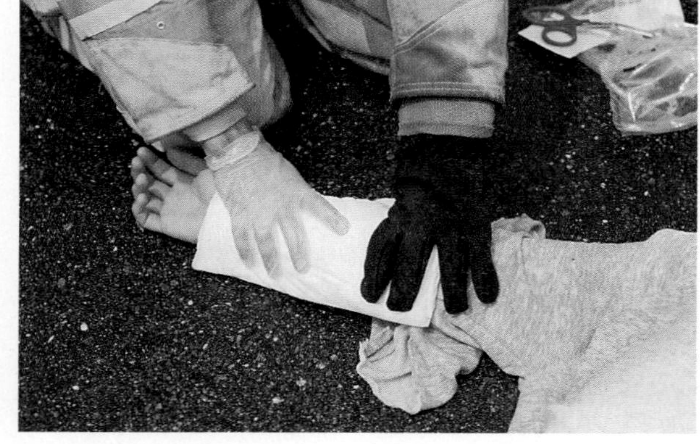

Figure 12-25 **A**, Large amounts of cool water are essential to cool burned areas. **B**, Remove any clothing covering the burned area. **C**, Cover the burned area.

minutes afterwards, causing more damage. Therefore it is essential to cool any burned areas immediately with large amounts of cool water (Fig. 12-25, *A*). Do not use ice or ice water on other than small superficial burns. Ice or ice water can cause critical body heat loss and may also make the burn deeper. Instead, flush or immerse the area using whatever resources are available — a tub, shower, or garden hose is often handy. You can apply soaked towels, sheets, or other wet cloths to a burned face or other area that cannot be immersed. Be sure to keep these compresses cool by adding more cool water, otherwise, they will quickly absorb the heat from the skin's surface.

Allow adequate time for the burned area to cool. If pain continues or if the edges of the burned area are still warm to the touch when the area is removed from the water, continue cooling. When the burn is cool, remove any remaining clothing from the area by carefully removing or cutting material away (Fig. 12-25, *B*). Do not try to remove any clothing that is sticking to skin. Remove any jewelry if doing so will not further injure the victim.

In some areas, you may be provided more specific directions for when and how to cool burns. Follow your local protocols.

Cover the Burned Area

Burns often expose sensitive nerve endings. Cover the burned area to keep out air and help reduce pain (Fig. 12-25, *C*). Use dry, sterile or clean dressings, and loosely bandage them in place. Dressings do not have to be sterile but they must be clean. The bandage should not put pressure on the burn surface. If the burn covers a large area of the body, cover it with clean, dry sheets or other cloth.

Covering the burn helps prevent infection. *Do not put ointments, butter, oil, or other commercial or home remedies on any burn that will receive medical attention.* Oils and ointments seal in heat and do not relieve pain. Other home remedies can contaminate open skin areas, causing infection. Do not break blisters. Intact skin helps prevent infection.

For small superficial burns or small burns with open blisters that are not sufficiently severe or extensive to require medical attention, care for the burned area as an open wound.

Wash the area with soap and water. Cover the burn with a dressing and bandage. Apply an antibiotic ointment if one is available and your protocols permit you to do so. Tell the victim to watch for signs of infection.

Minimize Shock

Full-thickness burns and large partial-thickness burns can cause shock as a result of pain and loss of body fluids. Lay the victim down unless he or she is having difficulty breathing. Elevate burned areas above the level of the heart, if possible. Burn victims have a tendency to chill. Help the victim maintain normal body temperature by protecting him or her from drafts. Administer oxygen if it is available, it is safe to do so and you are trained to use it.

Special Situations

Burns can also be caused by chemicals, electricity, and radiation. These burns require specific care.

Chemical Burns

Chemical burns are common in industrial settings but also occur in the home. Cleaning solutions, such as household bleach, oven or drain cleaners, toilet bowl cleaner, paint strippers, and lawn or garden chemicals, are common sources of caustic chemicals that can eat away or destroy tissue. Caustic chemicals cause **chemical burns**. Typically, burn injuries result from chemicals that are strong acids or alkalis. These substances can quickly injure the skin. As with heat burns, the stronger the chemical and the longer the contact, the more severe the burn. The chemical will continue to burn as long as it is on the skin. You must remove the chemical from the skin as quickly as possible and then call for more advanced medical personnel immediately. If you suspect a chemical burn, also check to see whether the eyes are burned.

If the substance is a liquid, flush the burn continuously with large amounts of cool, running water (Fig. 12-26). Always brush dry or powdered chemicals off with a gloved hand or a cloth, if possible. If not, try to flush them off with water. In some cases, a continuous flow of water will remove a dry substance before the water can activate it. Continue flushing until more advanced medical personnel arrive. Have the victim remove contaminated clothing and jewelry, if possible. Take steps to minimize shock.

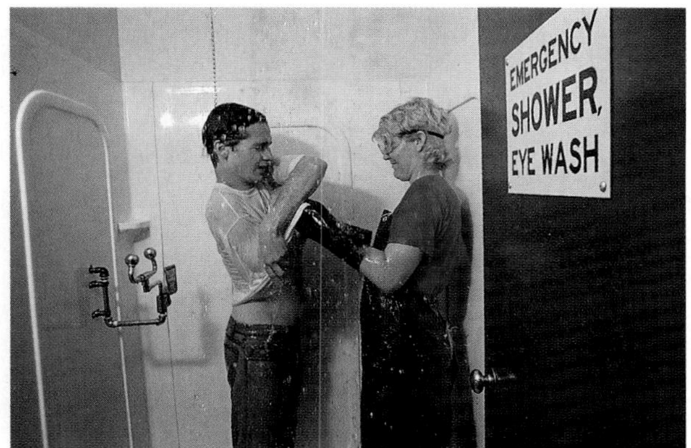

Figure 12-26 Flush a chemical burn with cool running water.

Chemical burns to the eyes can be exceptionally traumatic. If an eye is burned by a chemical, flush the affected eye until more advanced medical personnel arrive or for at least 20 minutes (Fig. 12-27). Flush the affected eye from the nose outward and downward to prevent washing the chemical into the unaffected eye.

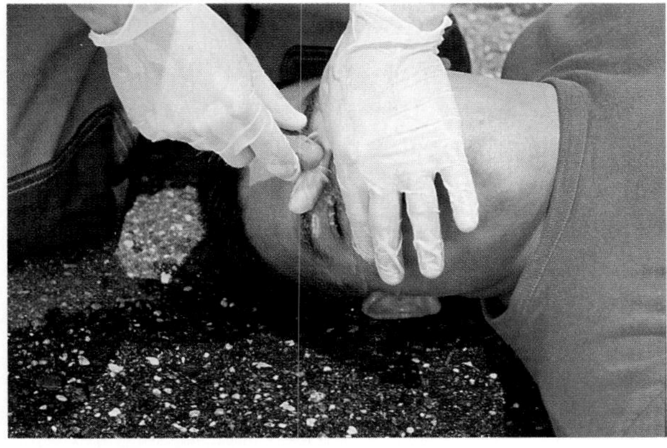

Figure 12-27 Continuously flush an eye that has been burned by a chemical with cool water.

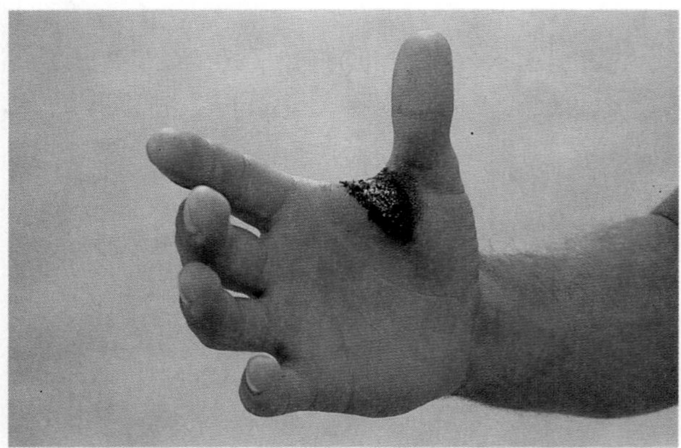

Figure 12-28 An electrical burn may severely damage underlying tissues.

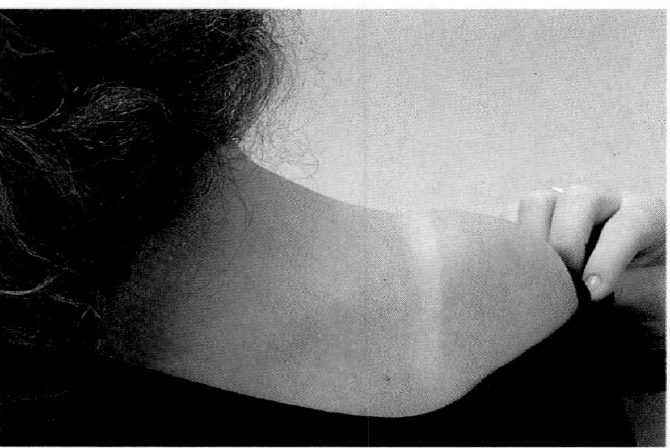

Figure 12-29 Solar radiation burns can be painful.

Electrical Burns

The human body is a good conductor of electricity. When someone comes in contact with an electrical source, such as a power line, a malfunctioning household appliance, or lightning, he or she conducts the electricity through the body. Body parts resist electrical current; some body parts, such as the bones, resist the electrical current more strongly than others. Resistance produces heat, which can cause **electrical burns** along the flow of the current (Fig. 12-28). The severity of an electrical burn depends on the type and amount of contact, the current's path through the body, and how long the contact lasted. Electrical burns are often deep. Although these wounds may look superficial, the tissues beneath may be severely damaged. Some electrical burns will be marked by entry and exit wounds indicating where the current has passed through the body.

In the physical exam, look for two burn sites. Cover any burn injuries with a dry, sterile or clean dressing, and give care to minimize shock. Do not cool the burn(s) with water. Also look for painful, swollen, and deformed extremities because the resistance to the electrical current can cause severe muscle contractions, which may produce injuries.

With a victim of lightning, look and care for life-threatening conditions, such as respiratory or cardiac arrest. The victim may also have fractures, including spinal fracture, so do not move him or her. Caring for any immediate life-threatening conditions takes priority over caring for burns.

Radiation Burns

Both the solar radiation of the sun and other types of radiation can cause **radiation burns**. Solar burns are similar to heat burns. Usually they are mild but can be painful (Fig. 12-29). They may blister, involving more than one layer of skin. Care for sunburn as you would any other burn. Cool the burn and protect the burned area from further damage by keeping it out of the sun.

People are rarely exposed to other types of radiation unless working in special settings, such as certain medical, industrial, or research sites. If you work in such settings, you will be informed and will be required to take precautions to prevent overexposure.

Infant and Child Considerations

Burned infants and children need extra care because they have greater body-surface area relative to their total size than an adult. This greater surface area leads to greater loss of fluid and heat. When burned, infants and children are at extra risk for shock, airway difficulties, and hypothermia. With these victims,

Striking Distance

In medieval times, people believed that ringing church bells would dissipate lightning during thunderstorms. It was an unfortunate superstition for the bell ringers. Over 33 years, lightning struck 386 church steeples and 103 bell ringers died.[1]

Church bell ringers have dropped off the list of people most likely to be struck during a thunderstorm, but lightning strikes remain extremely dangerous. Lightning causes more deaths annually in the United States than any other weather hazard, including blizzards, hurricanes, floods, tornadoes, earthquakes, and volcanic eruptions. The National Weather Service estimates that lightning kills nearly 100 people annually and injures about 300 others. Lightning occurs when particles of water, ice, and air moving inside storm clouds lose electrons. Eventually, the cloud becomes divided into layers of positive and negative particles. Most electrical currents run between the layers inside the cloud. However, occasionally, the negative charge flashes toward the ground, which has a positive charge. An electrical current snakes back and forth between the ground and the cloud many times in the seconds that we see a flash crackle down from the sky. Anything tall — a tower, a tree, or a person — becomes a path for the electrical current.

Traveling at speeds up to 300 miles per second, a lightning strike can hurl a person through the air, burn his or her clothes off, and sometimes cause the heart to stop beating. The most severe lightning strikes carry up to 50 million volts of electricity, enough to keep 13,000 homes running. Lightning can "flash" over a person's body, or, in its more dangerous path, it can travel through blood vessels and nerves to reach the ground.

Besides burns, lightning can also cause neurologic damage, fractures, and loss of hearing or eyesight. The victim sometimes acts confused and amnesic and may describe the episode as getting hit on the head or hearing an explosion.

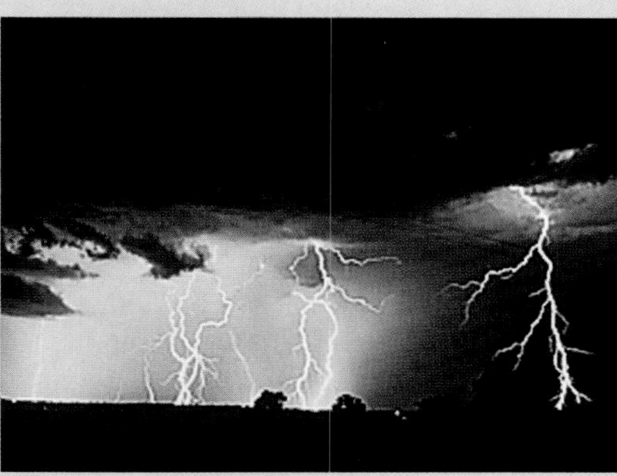

National Oceanic and Atmospheric Administration (NOAA)

Use common sense around thunderstorms. If you see a storm approaching in the distance, do not wait until you are drenched to seek shelter. If a thunderstorm threatens, the National Weather Service advises you to —

- Go inside a large building or home.
- Get inside a car and roll up the windows.
- Stop swimming or boating as soon as you see or hear a storm. Water conducts electricity.
- Stay away from the telephone, except in an emergency.
- Stay away from telephone poles and tall trees if you are caught outside.
- Stay off hilltops; try to crouch down in a ravine or valley.
- Stay away from farm equipment and small metal vehicles such as motorcycles, bicycles, and golf carts.
- Avoid wire fences, clotheslines, metal pipes and rails, and other conductors.
- Stay several yards apart if you are in a group.

References

1. Kessler E: *The thunderstorm in human affairs,* Norman, Oklahoma, 1983, University of Oklahoma.
2. Randall T: 50 million volts may crash through a lightning victim, *The Chicago Tribune,* Section 2D, August 13, 1989.

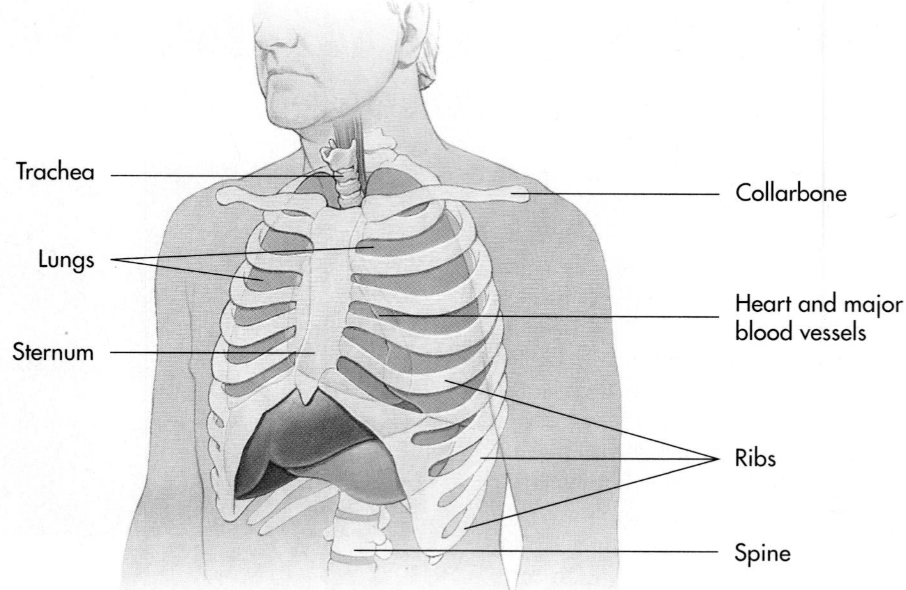

Figure 12-30 The rib cage surrounds and protects several vital organs.

maintain body heat and never douse burns with cold water or ice. Cool water, however, may be used initially to cool the burned area.

With burned children, also be aware of the possibility of child abuse, discussed in Chapter 18. Any suspicions of abuse must be documented and reported to authorities.

◆ CHEST INJURIES

Chest injuries are the second leading cause of trauma deaths each year in the United States. About 35 percent of the deaths from motor vehicle crashes involve chest injuries. Crushing forces, falls, and sports mishaps can also lead to such injuries.

The ***chest*** is the upper part of the trunk, containing the heart, major blood vessels, and lungs. The chest is formed by 12 pairs of ribs, 10 of which attach to the ***sternum*** (breastbone) in front and to the spine in back. The other two pairs attach only to the spine in the back and are sometimes called "floating" ribs. The ***rib cage*** is the cage of bones formed by the 12 pairs of ribs, the sternum, and the spine. It protects vital organs, such as the heart, major blood vessels, and the lungs (Fig. 12-30). Also in the chest are the esophagus, the trachea, and the muscles that assist respiration.

Chest wounds are either open or closed. Open chest wounds occur when an object, such as a knife or a bullet, penetrates the chest wall. Fractured ribs may break through the skin to cause an open chest injury. A chest wound is closed if the skin is not broken. Closed chest wounds are generally caused by a blunt object, such as a steering wheel.

Signs and Symptoms of Chest Injury

You should know the signs and symptoms of serious chest injury. These may occur with both open and closed wounds. They include —

- Difficulty breathing.
- Pain at the site of the injury that increases with deep breathing or movement.

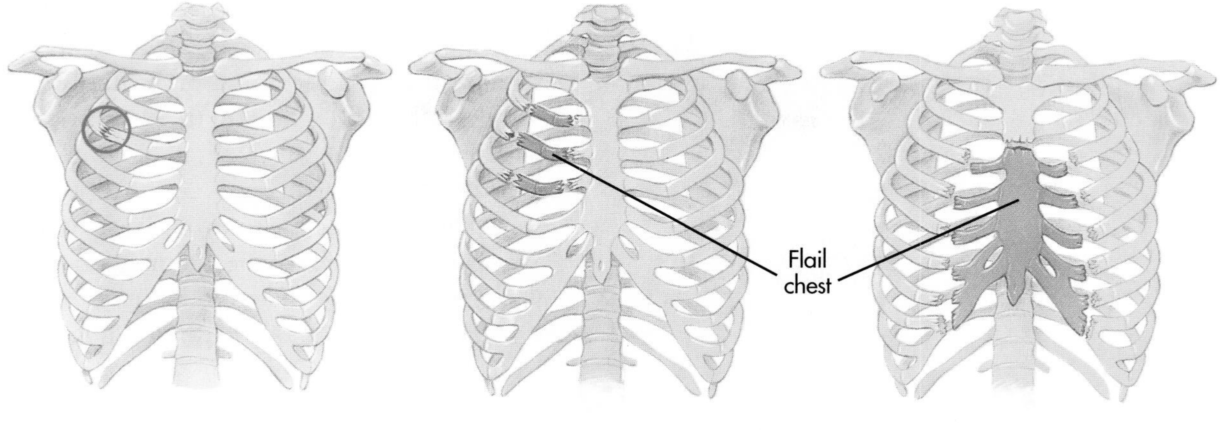

Figure 12-31 Forceful blows to the chest can fracture the ribs.

- Obvious deformity, such as that caused by a fracture.
- Flushed, pale, ashen, or bluish discoloration of the skin.
- Coughing up blood.

Specific Types of Chest Injuries

Certain chest injuries may be life threatening, and others merely cause discomfort. You should be able to recognize severe injuries and summon advanced help.

Rib Fractures

Rib fractures are usually caused by a forceful blow to the chest (Fig. 12-31). Although painful, a simple rib fracture is rarely life threatening. A victim with a fractured rib often breathes shallowly because normal or deep breathing is painful. The victim will usually attempt to ease the pain by leaning toward the side of the fracture and pressing a hand or arm over the injured area.

Serious rib fractures can be life threatening. In severe blows or crushing injuries, multiple ribs can fracture in multiple places. These fractures can produce a loose section of ribs that does not move normally with the rest of the chest during breathing. Usually, the loose section will move in the opposite direction from the rest of the chest. This injury is called a **flail chest**. When a flail chest involves the breastbone (sternum), the breastbone is separated from the rest of the ribs.

If you suspect a fractured rib(s), have the victim rest in a position that will make breathing easier. Binding the victim's arm to the chest on the injured side will help support the injured area and make breathing more comfortable. You can use an object, such as a pillow or rolled blanket, to help support and immobilize the injured area (Fig. 12-32). Serious fractures often cause severe bleeding and difficulty breathing; shock is likely to develop. Administer oxygen if it is available and you are trained to use it, and continue to monitor the vital signs.

Puncture Injuries

Puncture wounds to the chest range from minor to life threatening. Stab and gunshot wounds are examples of puncture injuries. A forceful puncture may penetrate the rib cage and allow air to enter the chest through the wound (Fig. 12-33). This prevents the lungs from functioning normally. The penetrating object can injure any structure within the chest, including the lungs, heart, or major arteries or veins.

Puncture wounds cause varying degrees of

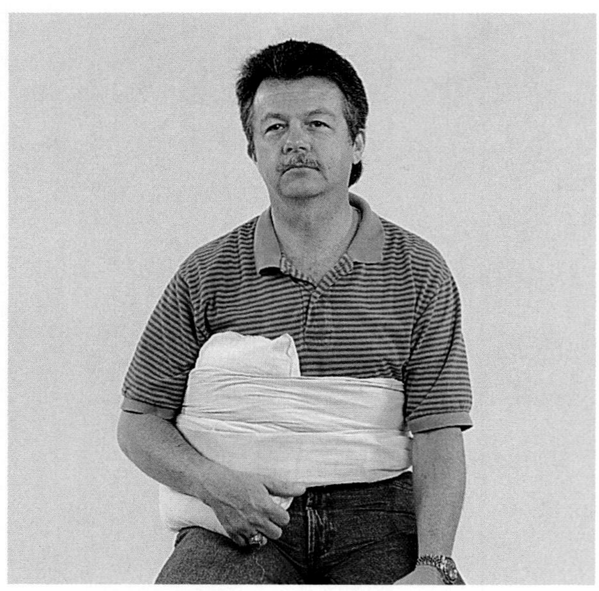

Figure 12-32 For fractured ribs, support and immobilize the injured area.

internal or external bleeding. If the injury penetrates the rib cage, air can pass freely in and out of the chest cavity and the victim cannot breathe normally. With each breath the victim takes, you may hear a sucking sound coming from the wound. This is the primary sign of a penetrating chest injury called a **sucking chest wound.**

Without proper care, the victim's condition will worsen quickly. The affected lung or lungs will fail to function, and breathing will become more difficult. Your main concern is the breathing problem. To care for a sucking chest wound, cover the wound with an **occlusive dressing**—one that does not allow air to pass through it. A plastic bag, a plastic or latex glove, or a piece of plastic wrap or aluminum foil folded several times and placed over the wound can be substituted if a sterile occlusive

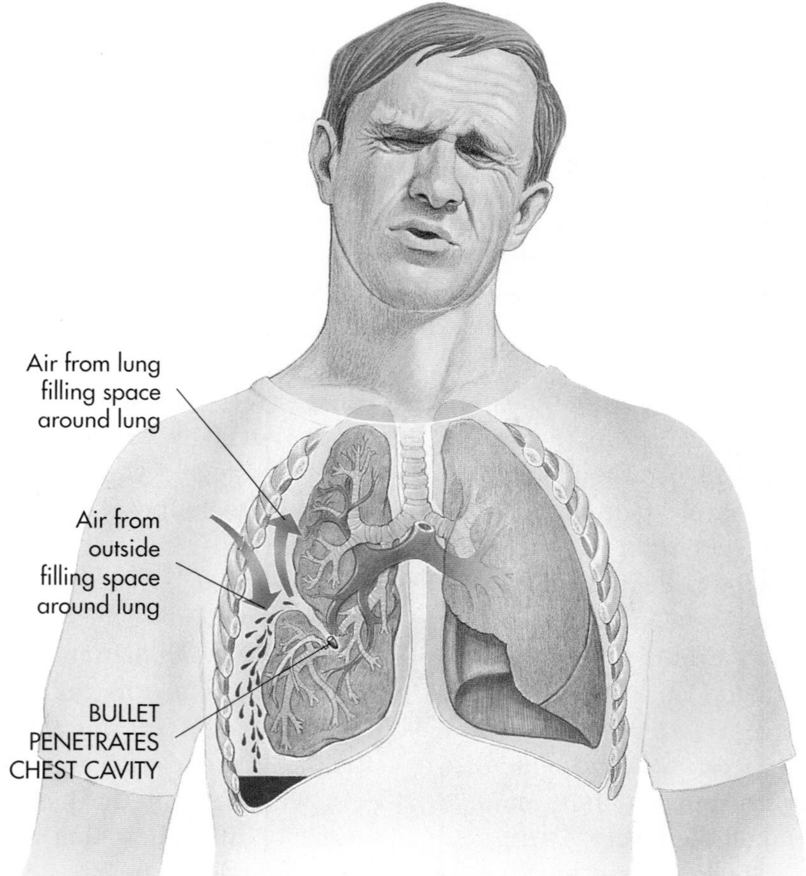

Figure 12-33 A puncture wound that penetrates the lung or the chest cavity surrounding the lung allows air to go in and out of the cavity.

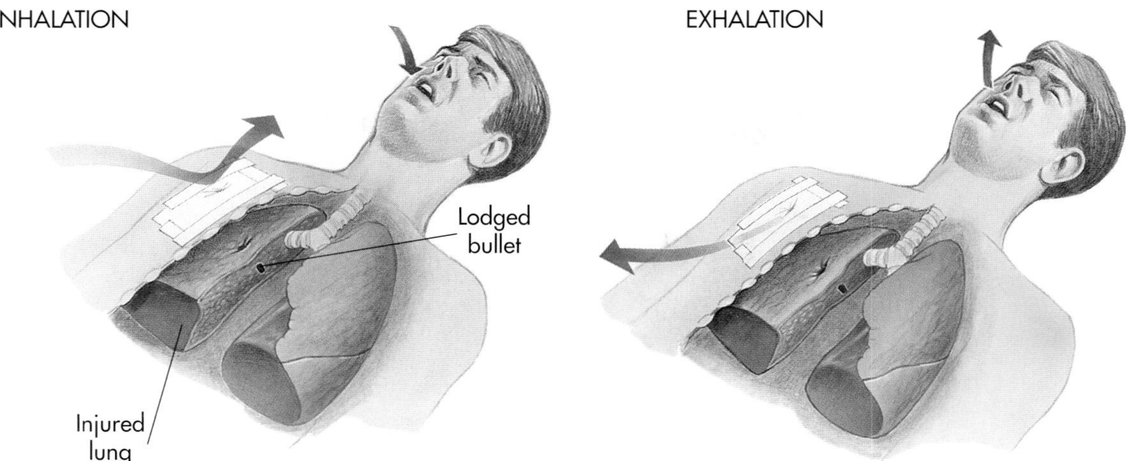

Figure 12-34 A special dressing with one loose side keeps air from entering the wound during inhalation and allows air to escape during exhalation. This helps keep the injured lung from collapsing.

dressing is not available. Tape the dressing in place, except for one side that remains loose (Fig. 12-34). Taping the dressing this way keeps air from entering the wound during inhalation but allows it to escape during exhalation. If none of these materials is available, use a folded cloth or, as a last resort, your gloved hand. Administer oxygen if it is available, and take steps to minimize shock.

◆ INJURIES TO THE ABDOMEN

The **abdomen** is the area immediately under the chest and above the pelvis. It is easily injured because it is not surrounded by bones, although it is protected at the back by the spine. The upper abdomen is only partially protected in front by the lower ribs. The muscles of the back and abdomen also help protect the internal organs, many of which are vital (Fig. 12-35). Certain organs are easily injured or tend to bleed profusely when injured, such as the liver, spleen, and stomach.

The **liver** is rich in blood. Located in the upper right quadrant of the abdomen, this organ is protected somewhat by the lower ribs. However, it is delicate and can be torn by blows from blunt objects or penetrated by a fractured rib. The resulting bleeding can be severe and quickly be fatal. A liver, when injured, can also leak bile into the abdomen, which can cause severe infection.

The **spleen** is located in the upper left quadrant of the abdomen behind the stomach and is protected somewhat by the lower left ribs. Like the liver, this organ is easily damaged. The spleen may rupture when the abdomen is struck forcefully by a blunt object. Since the spleen stores blood, an injury can cause a severe loss of blood in a short time and can be life threatening.

The **stomach** is one of the main digestive organs. The upper part of the stomach changes shape depending on its contents, the stage of digestion, and the size and strength of the stomach muscles. The stomach is lined with many blood vessels and nerves. It can bleed severely when injured, and food contents may empty into the abdomen and possibly cause infection.

Signs and Symptoms of Abdominal Injury

The signs and symptoms of serious abdominal injury include—

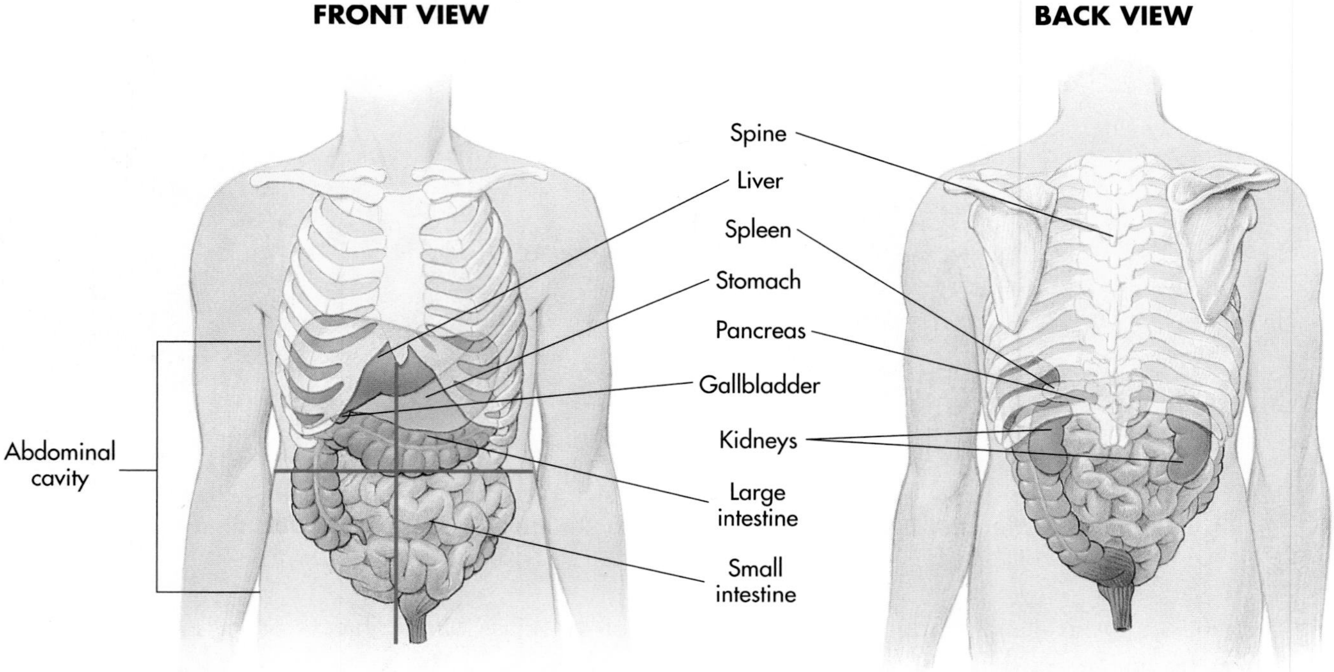

FRONT VIEW   BACK VIEW

Spine
Liver
Spleen
Stomach
Pancreas
Gallbladder
Kidneys
Large intestine
Small intestine
Abdominal cavity

Figure 12-35 Unlike the organs of the chest or pelvis, organs in the abdominal cavity are relatively unprotected.

- Severe pain.
- Bruising.
- External bleeding.
- Nausea and vomiting (sometimes vomit containing blood).
- Pale or ashen, moist skin.
- Weakness.
- Thirst.
- Pain, tenderness, or a tight feeling in the abdomen.
- Organs possibly protruding from the abdomen.

Care for Abdominal Injuries

Like a chest injury, an injury to the abdomen is either open or closed. Even with a closed wound, the rupture of an organ can cause serious internal bleeding that can quickly result in shock. Injuries to the abdomen can be extremely painful. Serious reactions can occur if organs leak blood or other contents into the abdominal cavity.

With a severe open injury, abdominal organs sometimes protrude through the wound (Fig. 12-36, *A*). To care for an open wound in the abdomen, follow these steps (Fig. 12-36, *B-D*):

- Summon more advanced medical personnel.
- Carefully position the victim on the back.
- *Do not* apply direct pressure.
- *Do not* push the organs back in.
- Remove clothing from around the wound.
- Apply moist, sterile or clean dressings loosely over the wound. (Warm tap water can be used.)
- Cover the dressings loosely with plastic wrap if it is available.
- Cover the dressings lightly with a folded towel to maintain warmth.
- Keep the victim from getting chilled or overheated.
- Administer oxygen if it is available.

To care for a closed abdominal injury —

- Carefully position the victim on the back.
- Do not apply direct pressure.
- Bend the victim's knees slightly. Doing so allows the muscles of the abdomen to relax.

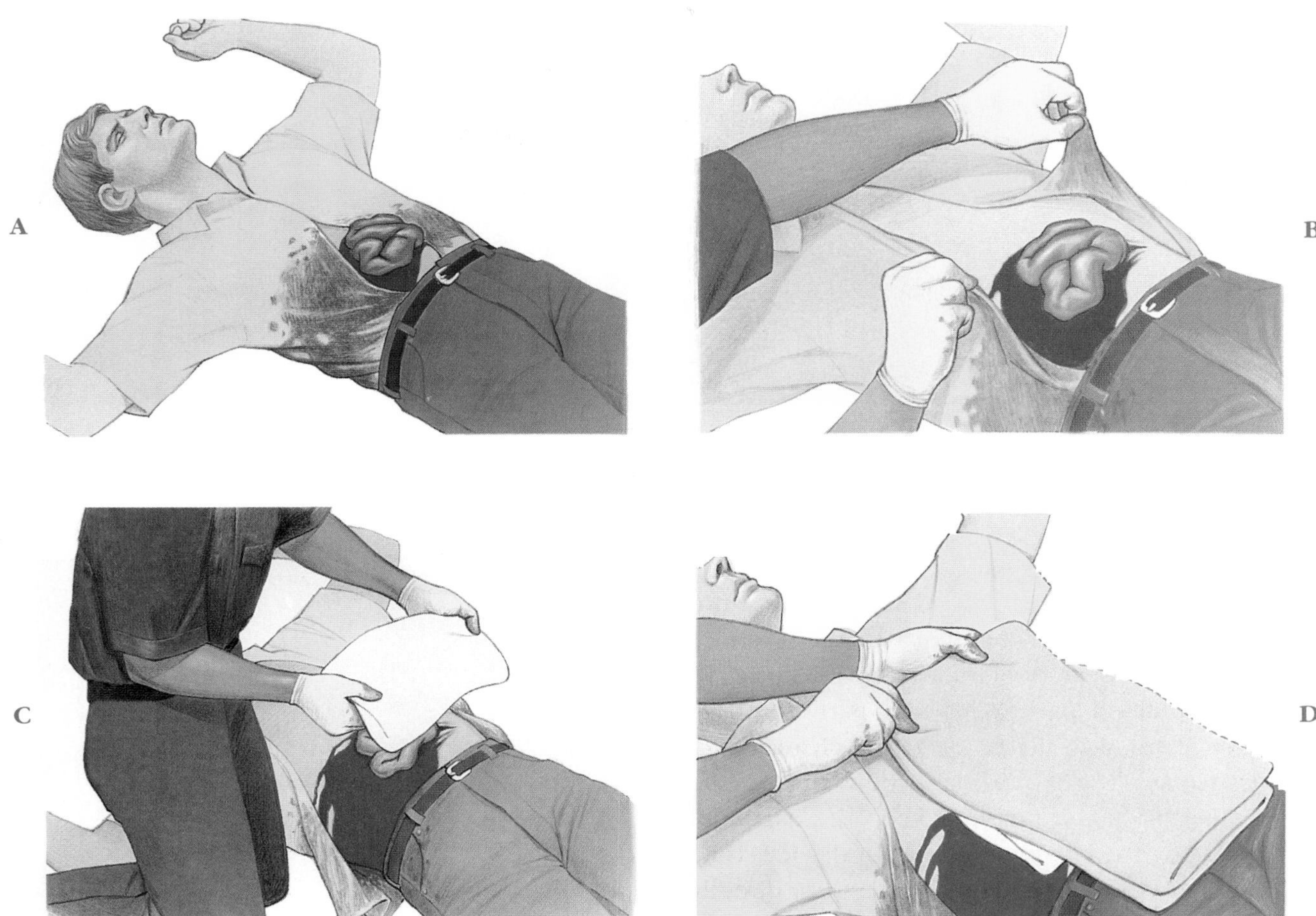

Figure 12-36 **A**, Severe injuries to the abdominal cavity can result in protruding organs. **B**, Carefully remove clothing from around the wound. **C**, Apply a large, moist sterile or clean dressing over the wound and cover it with plastic wrap. **D**, Place a folded towel or other cloth over the dressing to maintain warmth.

Place rolled-up blankets or pillows under the victim's knees. If moving the victim's legs causes pain or you suspect spinal injury, leave the legs straight.

- Administer oxygen if it is available and you are trained to use it.
- Take steps to minimize shock.
- Summon more advanced medical personnel.

Embedded Objects

Do not remove objects lodged in the eye, ear, or nose. An object through the cheek may be removed because it may cause airway damage by lacerating tissues and bleeding down the throat. An embedded object may also be removed if it will interfere with chest compressions. Stabilize an object that is not being removed with bulky dressing (Fig. 12-37, *A*). Control bleeding by bandaging the dressings in place around the object (Fig. 12-37, *B*) and transport the patient.

Amputations

Amputation, the complete severing of a body part, involves the extremities and other body

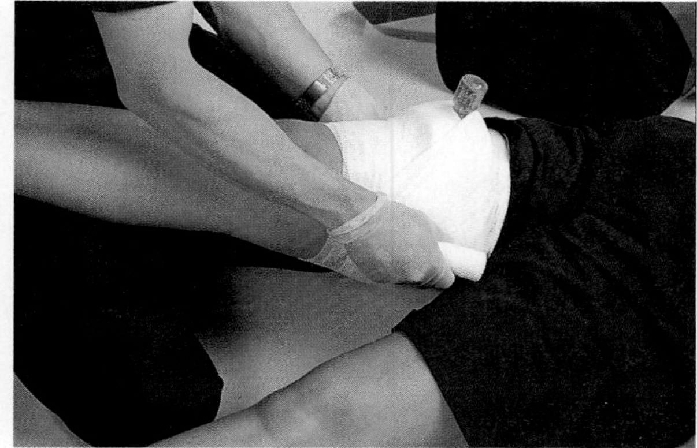

Figure 12-37 **A**, Use bulky dressings to support an embedded object. **B**, Use bandages over the dressing to control bleeding.

parts. The injury may bleed massively or not very much. While tending to the victim's needs, assign searchers to retrieve and preserve the amputated part. Wrap the part in sterile gauze, if any is available, or in any clean material, such as a washcloth. Place the wrapped part in a plastic bag. If possible, keep the part cool by placing the bag on ice (but not dry ice) (Fig. 12-38). Be careful to keep the ice from directly contacting the part so that the part does not freeze. Make sure the part accompanies the victim to the hospital.

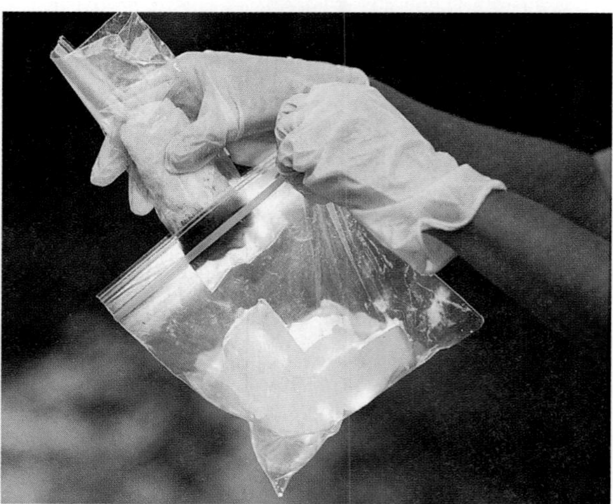

Figure 12-38 Wrap a severed body part in sterile gauze, put it in a plastic bag, and put the bag on ice.

◆ SUMMARY

Caring for wounds is not difficult. You need only follow the basic guidelines to control bleeding and minimize the risk of infection. Remember that with minor wounds your primary concern is to cleanse the wound to prevent infection. With major wounds, you should control the bleeding quickly using direct pressure and elevation and summon more advanced medical personnel. Dressings and bandages, when correctly applied, help control bleeding, reduce pain, and can minimize the danger of infection.

Burn injuries damage the layers of the skin and sometimes the internal structures. Heat, chemicals, electricity, and radiation all cause burns. When caring for a burn victim, always first ensure your personal safety. When the scene is safe, approach the victim and do an initial assessment and a physical examination if necessary.

Once the victim has been removed from the burn source, follow the steps of burn care:

- Cool the burned area with water to minimize additional tissue destruction.
- Keep air away from the burned area by cov-

ering it with dry, sterile dressings, clean sheets, or other cloth.

- Keep the victim from getting chilled or overheated to minimize shock.
- Summon more advanced medical personnel for any critical burn.

In addition, always check for inhalation injury if the person has a heat or chemical burn involving the face. With electrical burns, check carefully for other problems, such as difficulty breathing, cardiac problems, and painful, swollen deformed areas.

In Chapter 13, you will learn how to provide care for injuries involving muscles and bones.

Use the activities in Unit 12 of the workbook to help you review the material in this chapter.

You Are the Responder

It is a hot, muggy day in May. The forecast of rain has not seemed to dampen the spirits of the four beachgoers headed for the coast. After a week of all-night studying and grueling exams, the soon-to-be graduates are anxious to join their friends.

As they approach the bridge, Joe, the driver, decides he can no longer ignore the car's continually climbing temperature gauge. He pulls over to the side of the road, explaining that at the end of the term, he had to decide between a new radiator or beach week. After a few minutes, Joe argues that he can safely open the radiator, since the fluid has had time to cool down.

Despite his friends' objections, Joe takes off his t-shirt and wraps it around the radiator cap. Slowly he releases the cap, a quarter turn at a time. Suddenly, on the last turn, the cap blows off, and scalding fluid and steam burst out of the radiator, burning his chest and arms. As he spins away from the steam, his back is also burned. You happen to be driving by and stop to find out if there is a problem. How do you respond?

ENRICHMENT

◆ INJURIES

Since the end of World War II, 6 million people in the United States have died of injuries, a rate of approximately 400 a day. Injuries claim thousands of lives each year. Approximately 18 million people suffered a disabling injury in 1994.

Injury is a leading cause of death in people aged 1 to 37 years, surpassing major disease groups (cancer, heart disease, stroke) as a cause of death in this age group. Injury is the leading cause of people contacting physicians and the most common cause of hospitalization among people under 45 years old.

Statistics indicate that most people will have a significant injury at some time in their life. Some, because of their professions, are more likely to be injured than others. For example, the International Association of Fire Fighters reports that in 1994, 4 of every 10 fire fighters were injured in the line of duty. Seventy one percent of these were injured at the scene of an emergency incident. Researchers predict that few people will escape the experience of a fatal or permanently disabling injury happening to a relative, co-worker, or friend. In any 10-minute period, it is estimated that 2 people will be killed and about 350 will suffer a disabling injury. The cost of unintentional injury in 1994 was over $440 billion. In 1994, the lost quality of life from injuries was valued at an additional $798.3 billion.

How Injuries Occur

The body has a natural resistance to injury. However, when certain external forms of energy produce forces that the body cannot tolerate, injuries occur. Mechanical forms of energy and the energy from heat, electricity, chemicals, and radiation can damage body tissues and disrupt normal body function. Superficial injuries include minor wounds or burns. Deep injuries include wounds caused by penetrating objects.

Some tissues, such as the soft tissues of the skin, have less resistance and are at greater risk of injury if exposed to trauma than the deeper, stronger tissues of muscle and bone. Some organs, such as the brain, heart, and lungs, are better protected by bones than other organs, such as those in the abdominal cavity. Understanding the forces that cause injury and the kinds of injury that each force can cause will help you recognize certain injuries a victim may have.

Mechanical Energy

Direct, indirect, twisting, and contracting forces are produced by mechanical energy. A direct force is the force of an object striking the body and causing injury at the point of impact. Direct forces can be either blunt or penetrating. For example, a fist striking the chin can break the jaw, or penetrating objects, such as bullets and knives, can injure structures beneath the skin. Direct force can cause internal and external bleeding, head and spine injuries, fractures, and other problems, such as crushing injuries.

An indirect force travels through the body when a blunt object strikes the body and causes injury to a body part away from the point of impact. For example, a fall on an outstretched hand may result in an injury to the arm, shoulder, or collarbone.

In twisting, one part of the body remains stationary while another part of the body turns. A sudden or severe twisting action can force body parts beyond their normal range of motion, causing injury to bones, tendons, ligaments, and muscles. For example, if a ski and its binding keep the lower leg in one position while the body falls in another, the knee may be forced beyond its normal range of motion. Twisting injuries are not always this complex. They more often occur as a result of simple actions such as stepping off a curb or turning to reach for an out-of-the-way object.

Sudden or powerful muscle contractions often result in injuries to muscles and tendons. These injuries commonly occur in sports activities, such as throwing a ball far or hard without warming up or sprinting when out of shape. However, our daily routines also require sudden and powerful muscle contractions, for example, when we suddenly turn to catch a heavy object, such as a falling child. Although it happens rarely, sudden, powerful muscle contractions can even pull a piece of bone away from the point at which it is normally attached.

Figure 12-39 shows how these forces can result in injuries. These four forces, products of mechanical energy, cause the majority of all injuries. Soft tissue injuries and injuries to muscle and bone are most often the result. Soft tissue injuries outnumber musculoskeletal injuries. Combined, they are the major cause of work loss and eligibility for Social Security disability and unemployment compensation in the working age group (16 to 65).

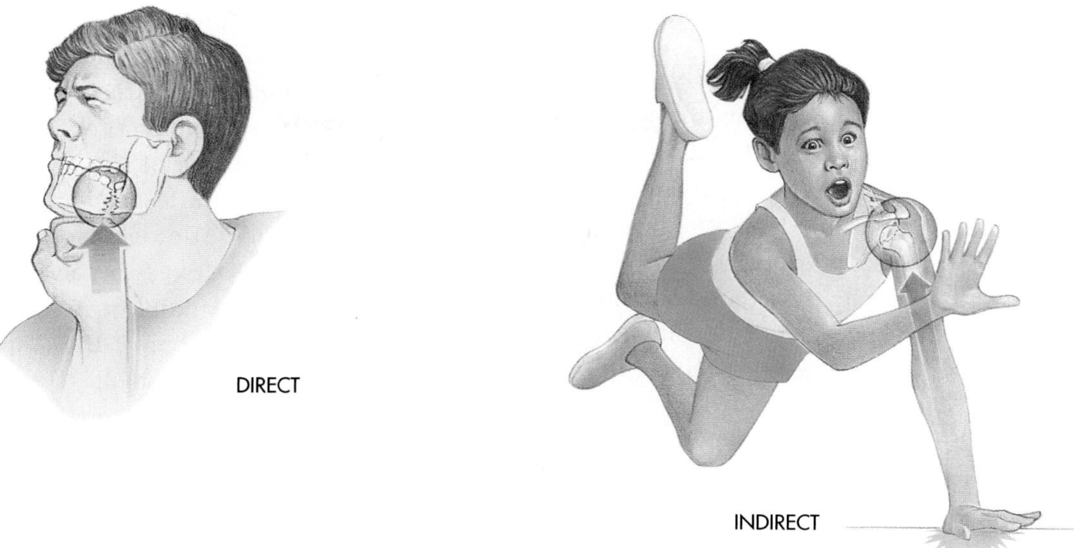

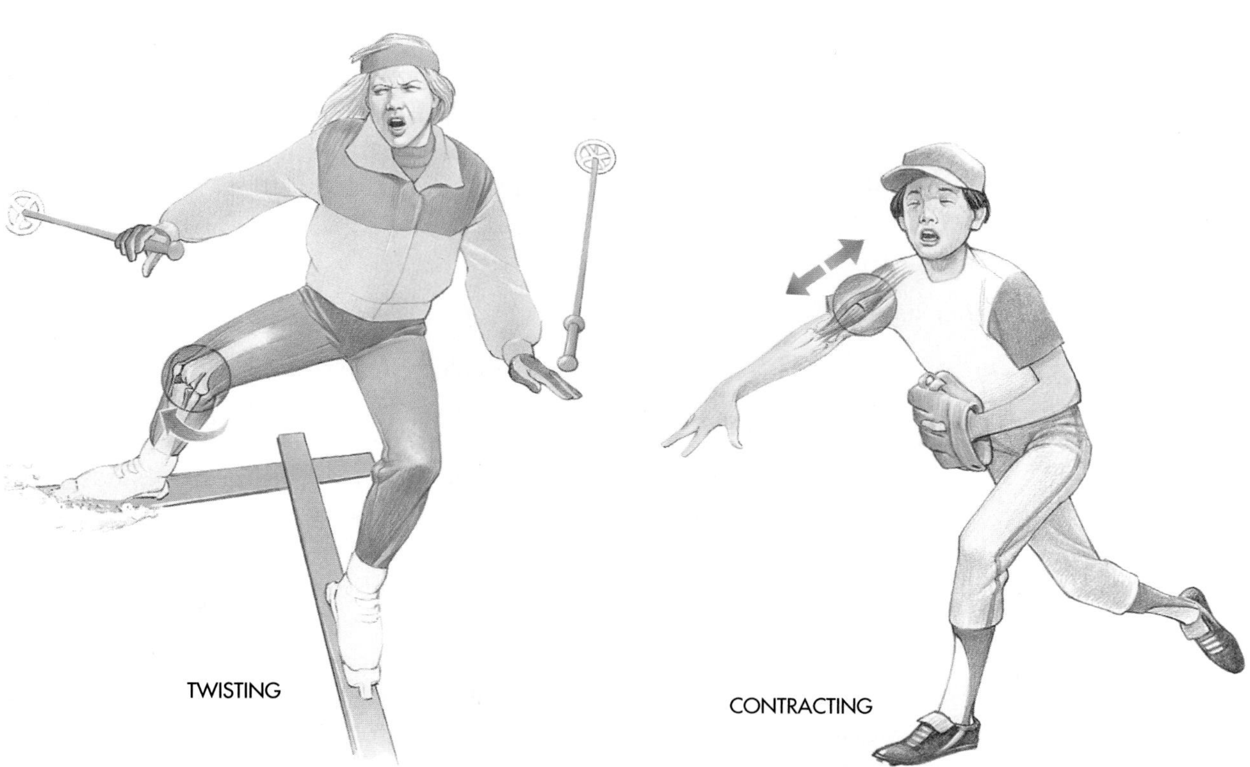

Figure 12-39 Four forces — direct, indirect, twisting, and contracting — cause 76 percent of all injuries.

Burns

In 1994, approximately 4000 people died from fires and burns, making burns the fifth leading cause of unintentional death. Most of those occurred in the home. Over 1 million burn injuries a year require medical attention or result in restricted activity. About one third of these are treated at hospital emergency departments, and over 90,000 people are hospitalized for an average of 12 days. The most common causes of nonfatal burns are scalds from hot liquids or foods and contact with hot surfaces. Fires cause 66 percent of all deaths from burns. Hot liquids cause 27 percent and electricity only 1 percent of burn deaths.

Factors Affecting Injury

A number of factors affect the likelihood of injury — among them age, gender, geographic location, economic status, and alcohol use and abuse. The type and frequency of injuries can also be affected by fads and seasonal activities. As certain activities, such as skateboarding and in-line skating, gain and lose popularity or as activities, such as softball or snow skiing, change with the seasons, the injury statistics reflect these changes.

Injury statistics consistently show that —

- Injury rates are higher among people under age 45.
- The highest rate of deaths from injury occur to the elderly and people aged 15 to 24.
- Males are at greater risk than females for any type of injury.
- Men are 2.5 times more likely to suffer a fatal injury than women.
- Three of four deaths and over half of the injuries suffered by workers in 1989 occurred off the job.

Many factors influence injury statistics. Whether people live in a rural or an urban area, whether a home is built of wood or brick, the type of heat used in the home, and the climate — all affect the degree of risk. Death rates from injury are typically higher in rural areas. The death rate from injuries is twice as high in low-income as in high-income areas.

The use and abuse of alcohol is a significant factor in many injuries and fatalities, even in young teenagers. The deaths of almost half of all fatally injured drivers involve alcohol, as do the deaths of many adult passengers and pedestrians. Over 40 percent of the deaths of 15- to 19-year-olds are the result of motor vehicle crashes. About half of these fatalities involve alcohol. It is estimated that an average of one alcohol-related fatality occurs every 22 minutes.

Alcohol use also contributes to other injuries. It is estimated that a significant number of victims who die as a result of falls, drownings, fires, assaults, and suicides have high blood alcohol concentrations. In one study of emergency department patients, alcohol was in the blood of 30 percent of the patients injured while driving or walking on the road, in 22 percent injured at home, in 16 percent injured on the job, and in 56 percent injured in fights and assaults. Figure 12-40 shows the leading causes of death from injuries in 1993. These figures represent the most current national statistics compiled by the National Safety Council.

Injury Prevention

Many people believe that injuries just happen — their targets are unfortunate victims of circumstance. However, overwhelming evidence exists showing that injury, like disease, does not occur at random. Rather, many injuries are predictable, preventable events resulting from the interaction of people and hazards, whether at home, at work, or during recreation.

Preventing injuries is everyone's responsibility. As a first responder, injury prevention may be part of your job. As an athletic trainer, you are responsible for preventing athletic injuries. As an emergency team member, you may be responsible for ensuring that safety codes and

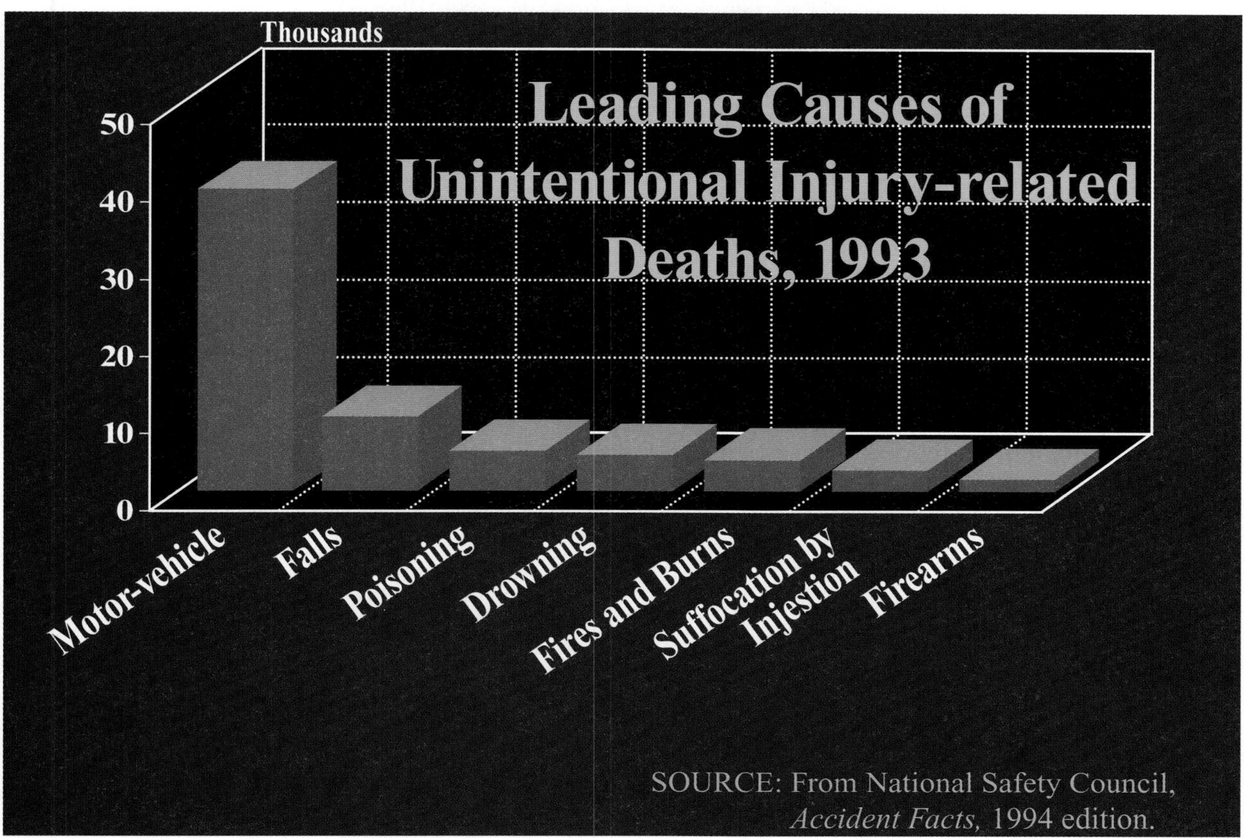

Figure 12-40 Leading Causes of Unintentional Injury-Related Deaths, 1994

regulations are met. A fire fighter or police officer who supervises or instructs others may be responsible for their safety. In any event, all first responders should take all precautions to ensure personal safety and to be role models of safe behavior.

Insurance Institute for Highway Safety

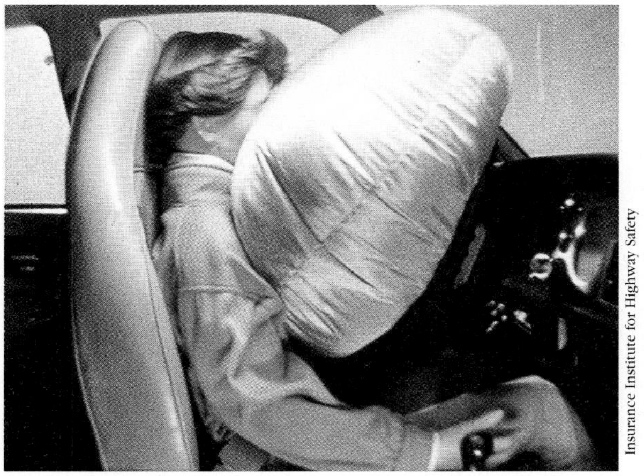

Figure 12-41 Airbags provide automatic protection.

There are three general strategies for preventing injuries:

- Persuade people to alter risky behavior.
- Require behavior change by law and regulation.
- Provide automatic protection through product and environmental design.

Laws and regulations that require people to conform to safety measures, such as wearing safety belts when driving and protective clothing when on the job, are only moderately effective. The most successful injury-prevention strategy is the built-in protection of product design. For instance, automatic protection, such as airbags in motor vehicles, does not allow people to make choices (Fig. 12-41).

Typically, people who engage in risky behaviors are the hardest to influence, regardless of whether safer behaviors are required. For example, despite the overwhelming evidence of alcohol-related injuries and fatalities, people still drink when driving and when operating equipment.

Many people view laws or regulations that require certain behaviors as an infringement of their rights — even though these laws and regulations are intended to protect them from injury. Product designs are equally difficult to influence because of manufacturers' reluctance to bear the costs of design changes. For instance, the evidence favoring safety belts and airbags was largely irrefutable some time ago. However, it took over 20 years of debate before a federal regulation was enacted requiring automobile manufacturers to install automatic restraints in all 1990 model cars.

The American Trauma Society contends that if existing information about prevention were applied, the injury rate could be reduced by 50 percent. Everyone has a personal responsibility to promote safety, both in his or her life, as well as in the lives of others. Taking the following three steps could significantly reduce your risk of injury and the risk of others:

- *Know your injury risk.* Take the time to complete the Healthy Lifestyles Awareness Inventory in Appendix B if you have not already done so.
- *Take measures that can make a difference.* Change to behaviors that decrease your risk of injury and the risk of others, both on the job and off.
- *Think safety.* Be alert for and avoid potentially harmful conditions or activities that increase your injury risk or that of co-workers. Take precautions, such as wearing appropriate protective clothing — helmets, outer garments, and effective barriers — to prevent disease transmission and buckling up when driving or riding in motor vehicles. Let your state and congressional representatives know that you support legislation that ensures a safer environment for us all.

You Are the Responder

1. You are dispatched to the scene of a house fire. You assist three fire victims to exit from the burning structure. One elderly gentleman has burns on his arms and chest. Another man has soot on his face, mouth, and nostrils and appears to be having problems breathing. The child does not appear to be burned anywhere. What care would you provide for these victims?
2. If the child was experiencing difficulty breathing, how would your care change?

Care for a Major Open Wound (Forearm)

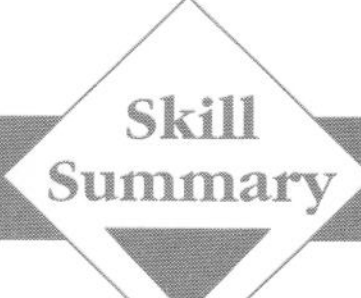

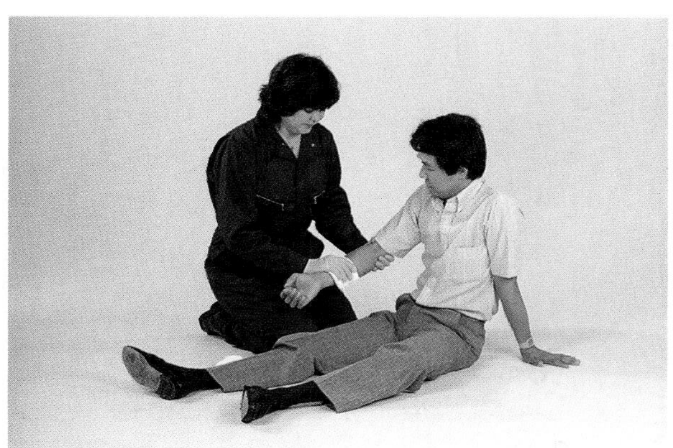

1. Apply direct pressure.

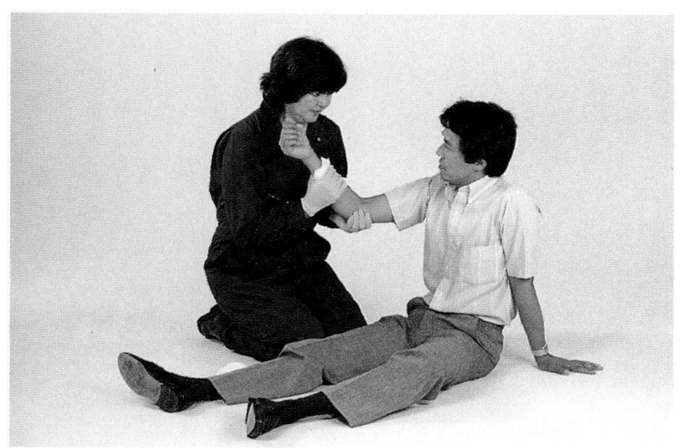

2. Elevate body part.

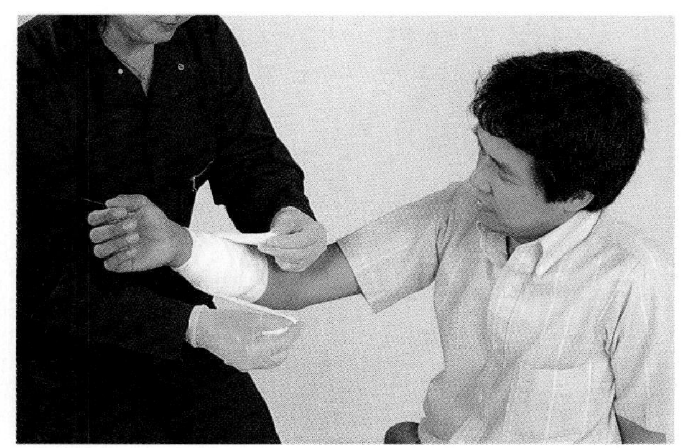

3. Apply pressure bandage.

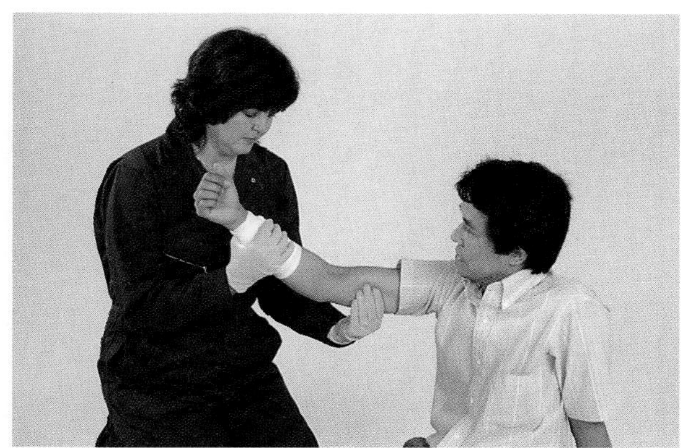

4. Use pressure point if necessary.

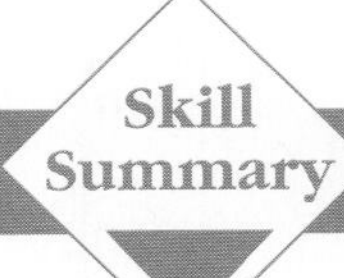

Care for a Major Open Wound (Leg)

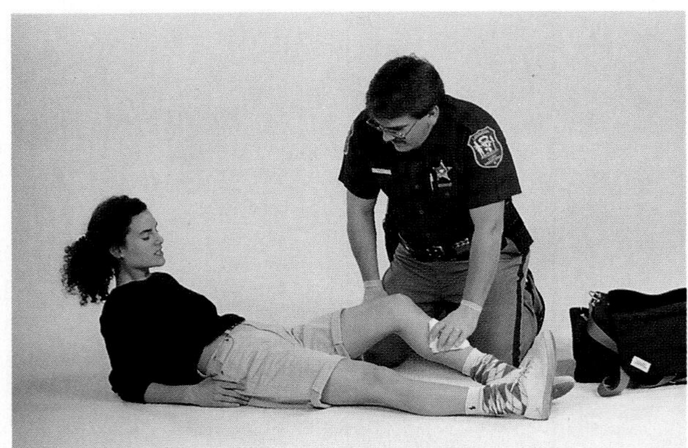

1. Apply direct pressure.

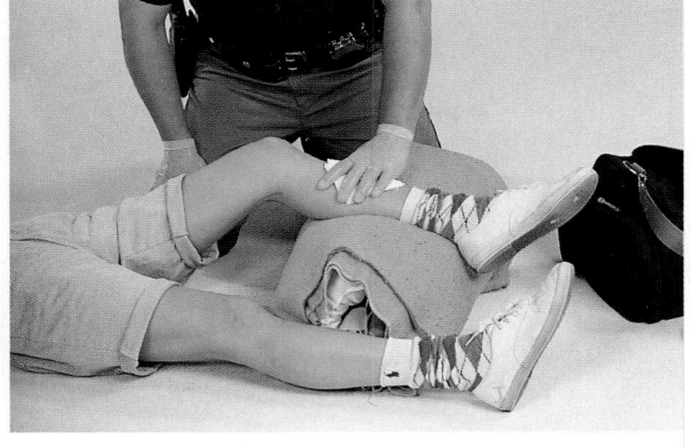

2. Elevate body part.

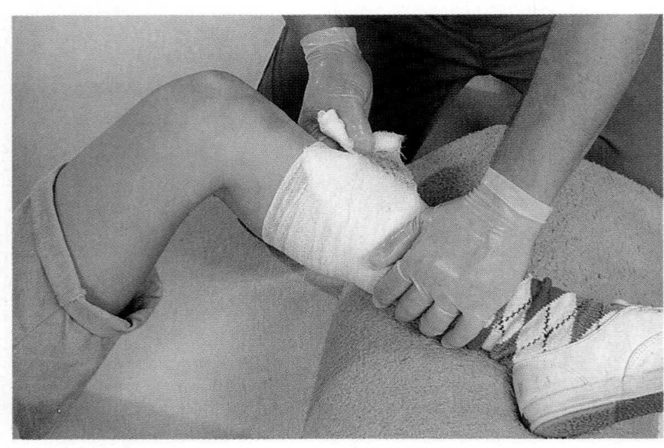

3. Apply pressure bandage.

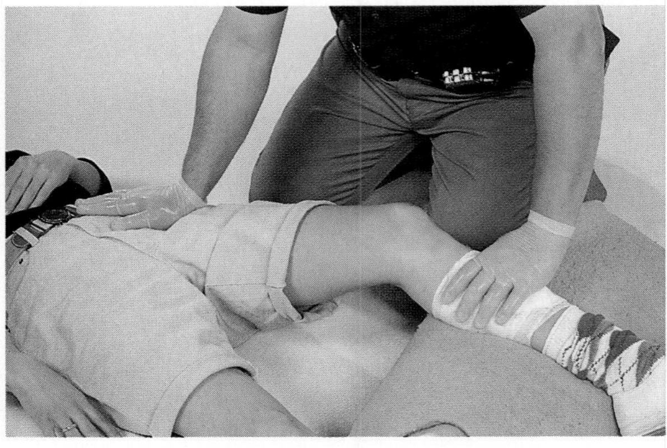

4. Use pressure point if necessary.

Care for a Wound With Embedded Object

Skill Summary

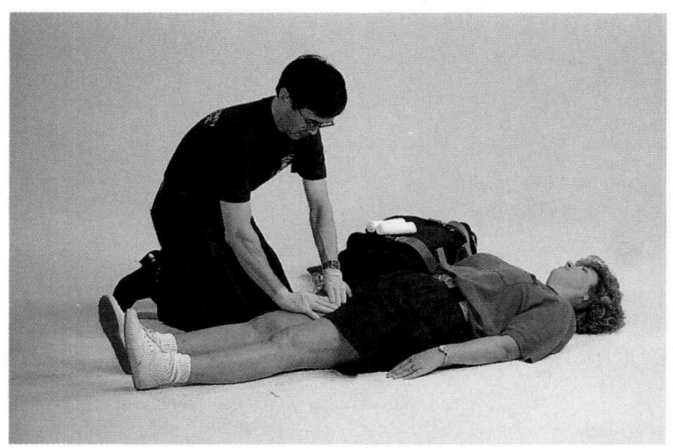

1. Apply direct pressure around object.

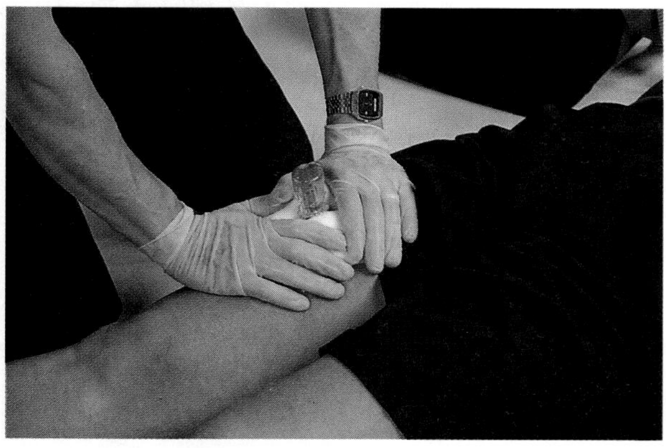

2. Use bulky dressings to support object.

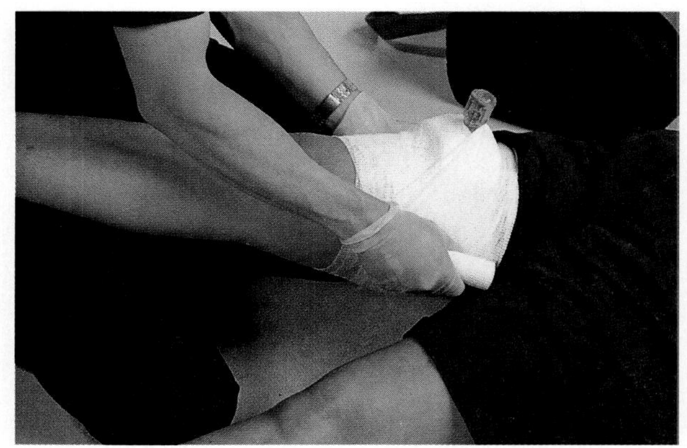

3. Apply pressure bandage.

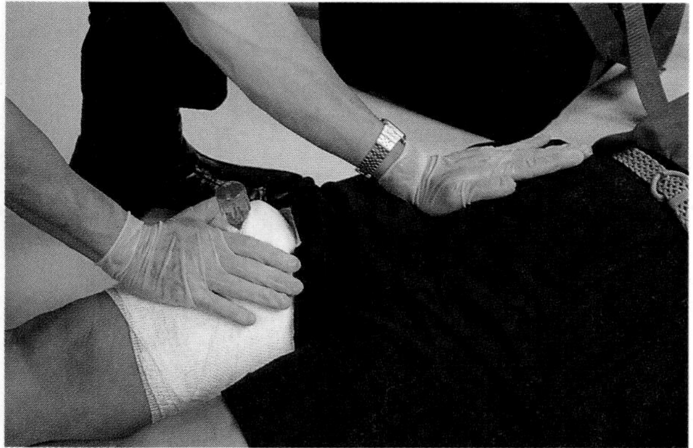

4. Use pressure point if necessary.

Muscle and Bone Injuries

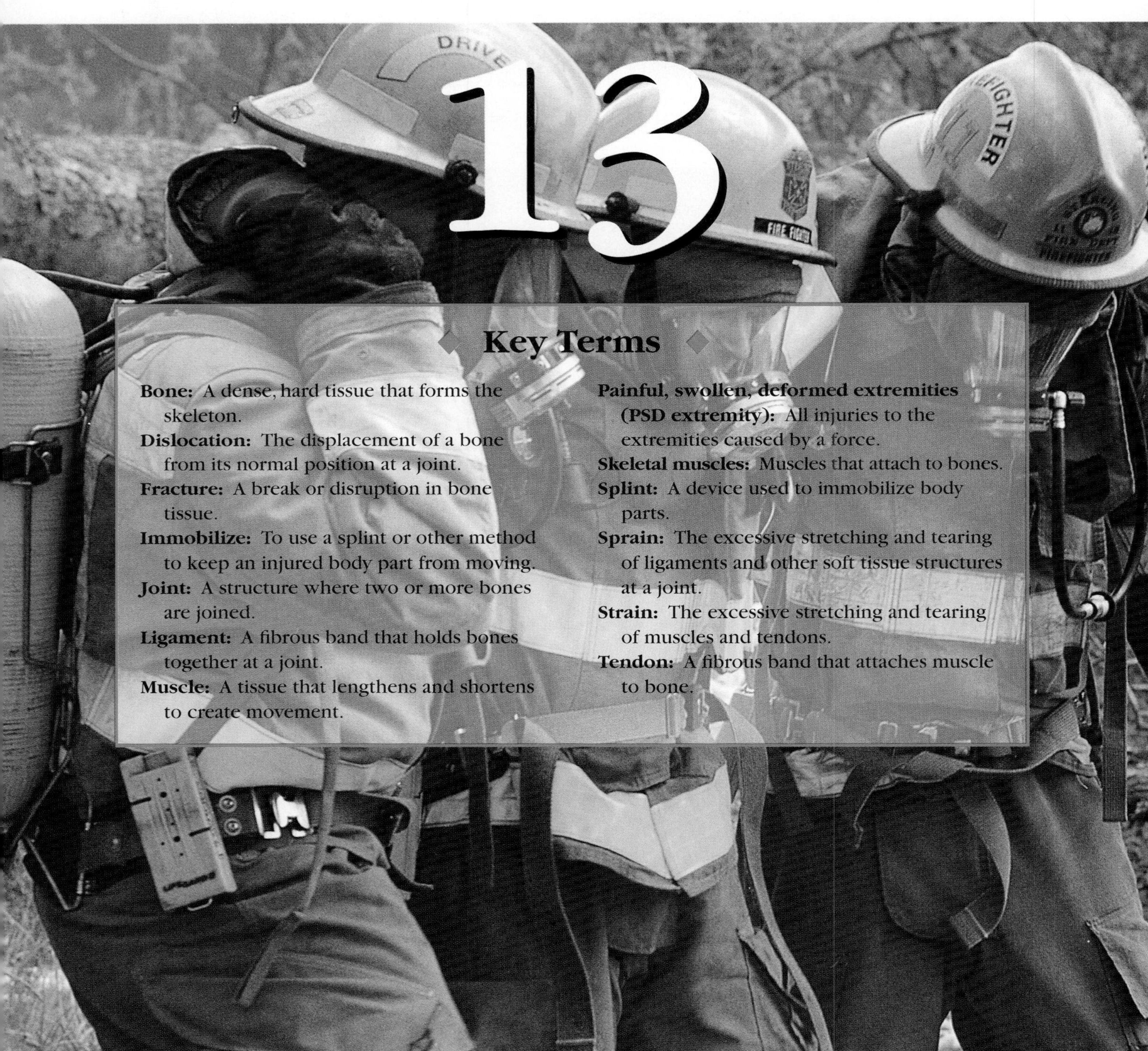

13

Key Terms

Bone: A dense, hard tissue that forms the skeleton.

Dislocation: The displacement of a bone from its normal position at a joint.

Fracture: A break or disruption in bone tissue.

Immobilize: To use a splint or other method to keep an injured body part from moving.

Joint: A structure where two or more bones are joined.

Ligament: A fibrous band that holds bones together at a joint.

Muscle: A tissue that lengthens and shortens to create movement.

Painful, swollen, deformed extremities (PSD extremity): All injuries to the extremities caused by a force.

Skeletal muscles: Muscles that attach to bones.

Splint: A device used to immobilize body parts.

Sprain: The excessive stretching and tearing of ligaments and other soft tissue structures at a joint.

Strain: The excessive stretching and tearing of muscles and tendons.

Tendon: A fibrous band that attaches muscle to bone.

◆ Knowledge Objectives ◆

After reading this chapter and completing the class activities, you should be able to—

- Explain the function of the musculoskeletal system.
- Distinguish between an open and a closed injury to a painful, swollen, deformed extremity.
- Describe the emergency care for a victim who has a painful, swollen, deformed extremity.
- Identify the main structures of the musculoskeletal system.
- List common signs or symptoms of musculoskeletal injuries.
- List signs and symptoms that would cause you to suspect a serious musculoskeletal injury.
- Describe how to care for musculoskeletal injuries.
- List the principles of splinting.
- Identify the types of splints.
- * Explain the use and application of a traction splint.

*Signifies an Enrichment section objective.

◆ Skill Objectives ◆

After reading this chapter and completing the class activities, you should be able to—

- Demonstrate the emergency medical care for a victim who has a painful, swollen, deformed extremity.
- * Demonstrate the application of a traction splint.

*Signifies an Enrichment section objective.

Pete and Kathryn are trying out their new in-line skates. They are alone on a paved, wooded path and Kathryn, the more experienced skater, has rolled on down a slight incline when she hears a thud, followed by Pete screaming. As she skates up the hill, she's thankful they both wore full protective gear.

What can Kathryn expect to find when she reaches Pete, who is clutching his right arm to his chest? Injuries to the musculoskeletal system are common. Millions of people at home, at work, or at play injure their muscles, bones, or joints. No age group is immune. An athlete may fall and bruise the muscles of the thigh, making walking painful. Heavy machinery may fall on a worker and break ribs, making breathing difficult. A person who braces a hand against a dashboard in a car crash may injure the bones at the shoulder, disabling the arm. A person who falls while skiing may twist a leg, tearing the supportive tissues of a knee and making it impossible to stand or move.

◆ INTRODUCTION

Although musculoskeletal injuries are almost always painful, they are rarely life threatening. However, when not recognized and taken care of properly, they can have serious consequences and even result in permanent disability or death. In this chapter, you will learn how to recognize and care for mus-

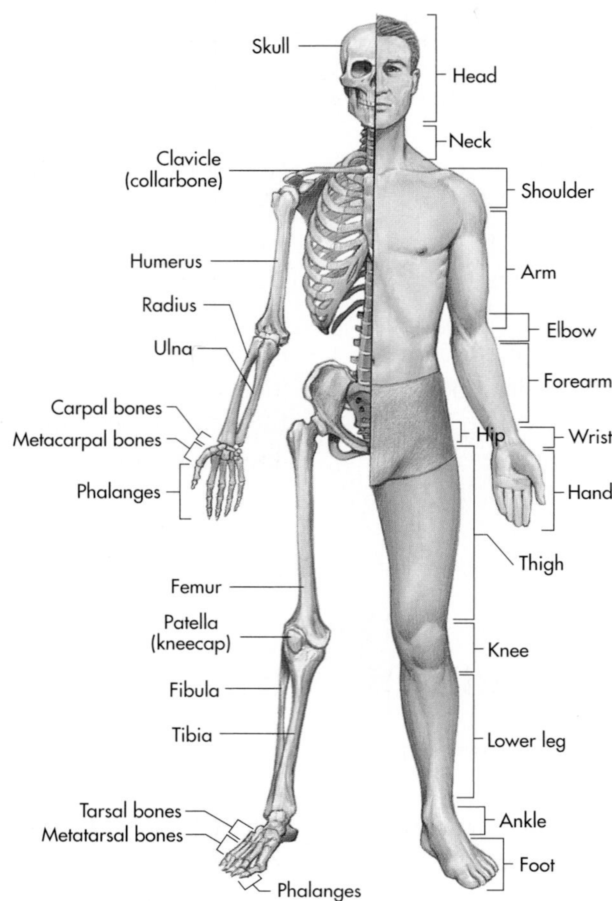

Figure 13-1 Bones that can be seen and felt beneath the skin provide landmarks for locating parts of the body.

culoskeletal injuries. Developing a better understanding of the structure and function of the body's framework will help you assess musculoskeletal injuries and give appropriate care.

The musculoskeletal system is made up of muscles, tendons and ligaments, and bones that form the skeleton. Together, these structures give the body shape, form, and stability. Bones and muscles connect to form various body segments. They work together to provide body movements.

◆ MUSCULOSKELETAL SYSTEM REVIEW

The bony structures that form the skeleton define the parts of the body. For example, the head is defined by the bones that form the skull, and the chest is defined by the bones that form the rib cage. Prominent bones, bones that can be seen or felt beneath the skin, provide landmarks for locating parts of the body (Fig. 13-1). The body has 206 bones.

Muscles are soft tissues. The body has more than 600 muscles (Fig. 13-2). Most are ***skeletal muscles***, which attach to the bones. Skeletal muscles account for most lean body weight (body weight without excess fat).

Unlike the other soft tissues, muscles are able to contract (shorten) and relax (lengthen). All body movements result from skeletal muscles contracting and relaxing. Skeletal muscle actions are under your conscious control. Because you move them voluntarily, skeletal muscles are also called voluntary muscles. Skeletal

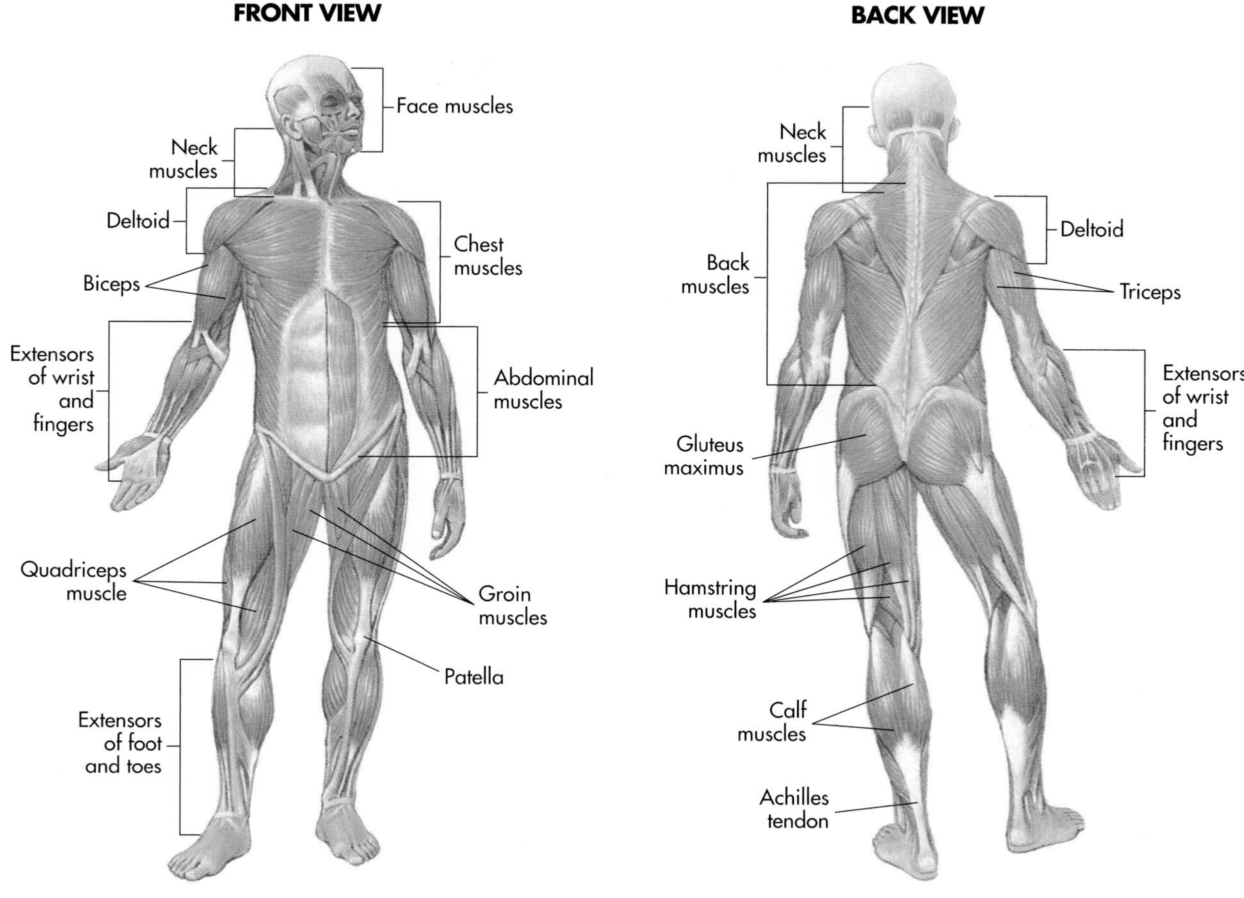

Figure 13-2 Skeletal muscles, muscles that attach to bones, comprise the majority of the body's musculature.

muscles also protect the bones, nerves, and blood vessels.

Most skeletal muscles are anchored to bone at each end by strong, cordlike tissues called ***tendons***. Muscles and their adjoining tendons extend across joints. When the brain sends a command to move, electrical impulses travel through the spinal cord and nerve pathways to the individual muscles and stimulate the muscle fibers to move. When a muscle contracts, the muscle fibers shorten, pulling the ends of the muscle closer together. The muscles pull the bones, causing motion at the joint the muscle crosses.

A ***joint*** is a structure formed by the ends of two or more bones coming together at one place. Most joints allow motion. However, the bone ends at some joints are fused together, which restricts motion. Fused bones, such as the bones of the skull, form solid structures that protect their contents (Fig. 13-3).

Joints are held together by tough, fibrous, connective tissues called ***ligaments***. Ligaments resist joint movement. Joints surrounded by ligaments have restricted movement; joints that have few ligaments move more freely. For instance, the shoulder joint, with few ligaments, allows greater motion than the hip joint, which has more ligaments, although their structure is similar. Joint motion also depends on the bone structure.

Joints that move more freely have less natural support and are therefore more prone to injury. However, all joints have a normal range

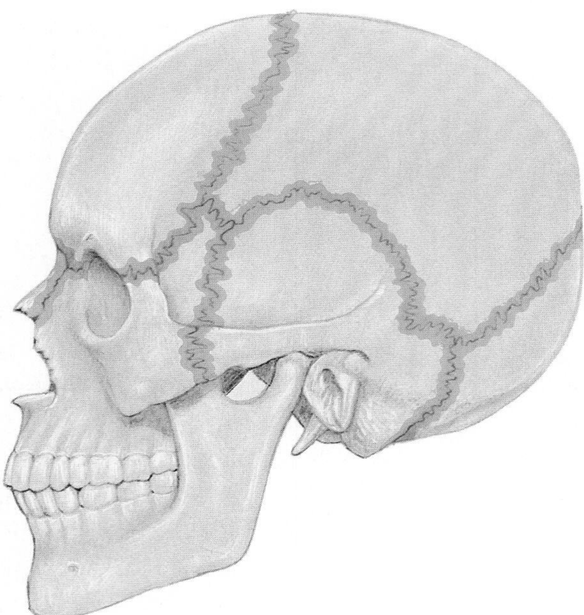

Figure 13-3 Fused bones, such as the bones of the skull, form solid structures that protect their contents.

of movement. When a joint is forced beyond its normal range, ligaments stretch and tear. Stretched and torn ligaments permit too much motion, making the joint unstable. Unstable joints can be disabling, particularly when they are weight-bearing, such as the knee or ankle. Unstable joints are also prone to reinjury and often develop **arthritis,** an inflamed condition of the joints, in later years.

◆ INJURIES TO BONES AND JOINTS

Injuries to bones and joints occur in a variety of ways. They are more commonly caused by forces generated by mechanical forms of energy but can also occur as a result of thermal (heat), chemical, or electrical forms of energy.

Mechanism of Injury

The mechanism of injury, or what caused the injury, is a very important source of clues to what body parts may be injured and how serious the injury may be. The three basic types of mechanisms of injury include —

- Direct force, such as that produced by a fall.
- Indirect force, in which energy is transferred along the length of an extremity and causes damage further along the body part than the point of impact.
- Twisting force, the energy delivered to an extremity that is turned in one direction while the rest of the affected area moves in another direction or remains stationary.

Types of Injuries

Despite the great number of bones in a human body, there are only two basic kinds of injuries to these structures. A **closed** injury leaves the skin unbroken, while an **open** injury causes a break in the continuity of the skin. An open injury is often more serious than a closed injury because of the risks of infection and severe blood loss.

Signs and Symptoms

You identify injuries to the musculoskeletal system during the physical examination. Because these injuries often appear to be similar, it may be difficult for you to determine exactly what type of injury has occurred. As you complete the physical examination, think about how the body normally looks and feels. Compare the injured side to the uninjured side.

Ask how the injury happened. The cause of injury is often enough to make you suspect a serious musculoskeletal injury. As the victim or bystanders explain how the injury occurred, listen for clues, such as a fall from a height or another significant impact to the body that could cause a serious injury. Also ask the victim if any areas are painful.

Then, examine the entire body, beginning with the head. Check each body part. Start with the neck, followed by the shoulders, the chest, and so on. As you perform the physical

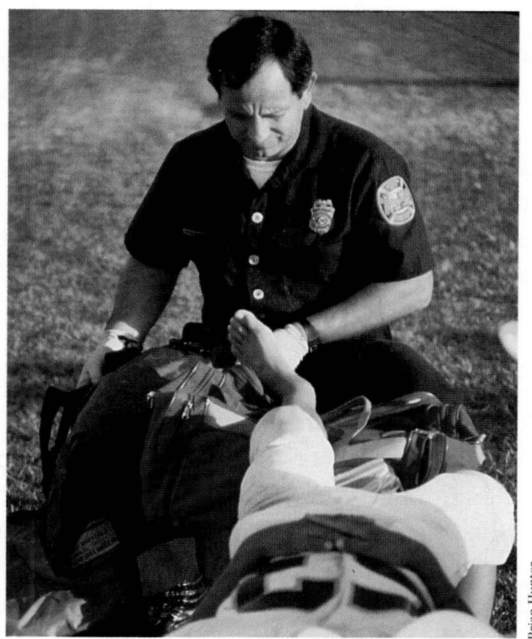

Figure 13-4 Deformity may be obvious when an injured limb is compared to an uninjured limb.

examination, look and listen for clues that may indicate a musculoskeletal injury.

Some common signs and symptoms associated with musculoskeletal injuries are—

- Pain and tenderness.
- Swelling.
- Grating.
- Deformity or **angulation.**
- Bruising (discoloration).
- Exposed bone ends.
- Joint locked into position.
- Inability to use or move an affected part.

Pain, swelling, and discoloration of the skin commonly occur with any significant injury. Irritation to nerve endings that supply the injured area causes pain. Pain is the body's signal that something is wrong. The injured area may be painful to touch and to move. Swelling is caused by bleeding from damaged blood vessels and tissues in the injured area. However, swelling is often deceiving. It may appear rapidly at the site of injury, may develop gradually, or may not appear at all. Swelling by itself, therefore, is not a reliable sign of the severity of an injury or of the structures involved. Bleeding may discolor the skin in surrounding tissues. At first, the skin may only look red. As blood seeps to the skin's surface, the area begins to look bruised.

Deformity is also a sign of significant injury (Fig. 13-4). Abnormal lumps, ridges, depressions, or unusual bends or angles in body parts are types of deformities. Marked deformity is often a sign of fracture or dislocation. Comparing the injured part to an uninjured part may help you detect deformity.

A victim's inability to move or use an injured part may also indicate a significant injury. The victim may tell you he or she is unable to move or that it is simply too painful to move. Moving or using injured parts can disturb tissues, further irritating nerve endings, which causes or increases pain. Often, the muscles of an affected area will **spasm,** or contract abnormally, in an attempt to keep the injured part from moving.

A victim often supports the injury in the most comfortable position. To manage musculoskeletal injuries, try to avoid causing additional pain. Avoid any motion or use of an injured body part that causes pain.

With grating, the ends of broken bones rub and produce a sound that is difficult to describe or reproduce. With exposed bone ends, the pieces of broken bone break through the skin, producing open injuries.

General Care for Bone and Joint Injuries

Remember to use the appropriate protective equipment, such as disposable latex or nitrile gloves, for BSI (body substance isolation). Ensure that the victim is breathing effectively and provide high-flow oxygen if it is available and you are trained to use it. Control major bleeding and life-threatening conditions, and permit the victim to remain in a comfortable

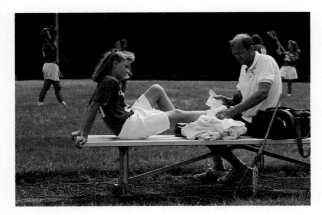

Figure 13-5 General care for all musculoskeletal injuries is similar. Remember rest, ice, and elevation.

position. During your physical examination, summon more advanced medical personnel if —

- The injury involves severe bleeding.
- The injury impairs walking or breathing.
- The injury involves the head, neck, or back.
- You see or suspect multiple injuries.

The general care for all skeletal injuries is similar: rest, ice, and elevation (Fig. 13-5).

Rest

Avoid any movements or activities that cause pain. Help the victim find the most comfortable position. If you suspect head, neck, or back injuries, leave the victim lying flat.

Ice

Apply ice or a cold pack. Cold helps reduce swelling and eases pain and discomfort. Commercial cold packs can be stored in a kit until ready to use, or you can make an ice pack by placing ice in a plastic bag and wrapping it with a towel or cloth. Place a layer of gauze or cloth between the source of cold and the skin to prevent skin damage. Do not apply an ice or cold pack directly over an open fracture because doing so would require you to put pressure on the open fracture site and could cause discomfort to the victim. Instead, place cold packs around the site.

Elevation

Elevating the injured area above the level of the heart helps slow the flow of blood, reducing swelling. Elevation is particularly effective in controlling swelling in extremity injuries. However, never attempt to elevate a seriously injured area of a limb unless it has been adequately immobilized.

◆ IMMOBILIZATION

If you suspect a serious skeletal injury, you must immobilize the injured part before giving additional care, such as applying ice or elevating the injured part. To ***immobilize,*** you use a splint or another method to keep the injured part from moving.

The purposes of immobilizing an injury are to —

- Lessen pain.
- Prevent further damage to soft tissues.
- Reduce the risk of serious bleeding.
- Reduce the possibility of loss of circulation to the injured part.
- Prevent closed ***painful, swollen, deformed extremity*** injuries from becoming open painful, swollen, deformed extremity injuries.

If advanced medical personnel have already been summoned, consider that the ground can temporarily immobilize an injured area effectively. However, if necessary, you can further immobilize an injured part by applying a splint, sling, or bandages to keep the injured body part from moving. A ***splint*** is a device that maintains an injured part in place. To effectively immobilize an injured part, a splint must extend above and below the injury site (Fig. 13-6).

When using a splint, follow these four basic principles:

- Splint only if you can do it without causing more pain and discomfort to the victim.
- Splint an injury in the position you find it.

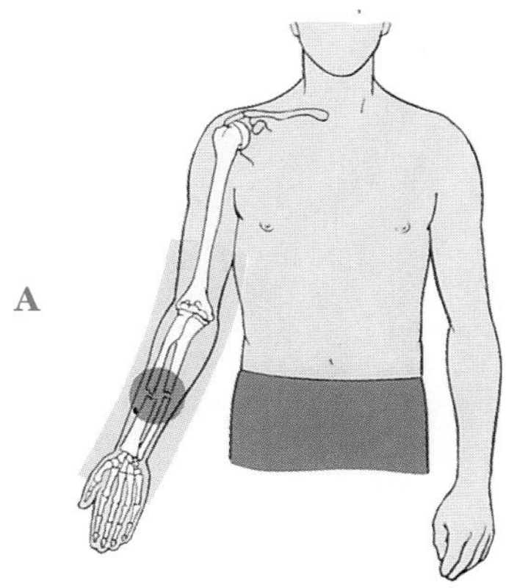

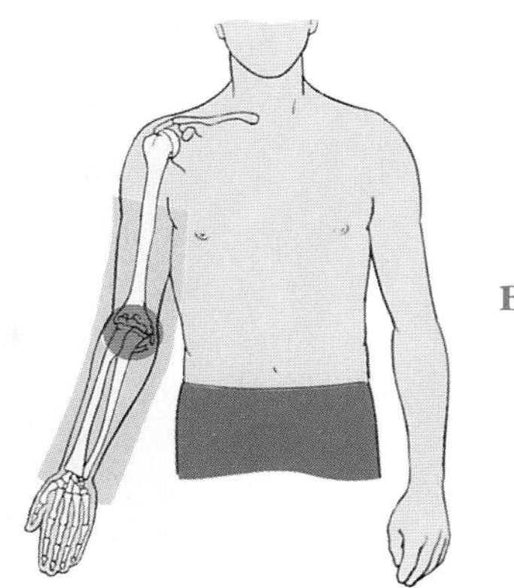

Figure 13-6 **A**, To immobilize a bone, splint the joints above and below the fracture. **B**, To immobilize a joint, a splint must include the bones above and below the injured joint.

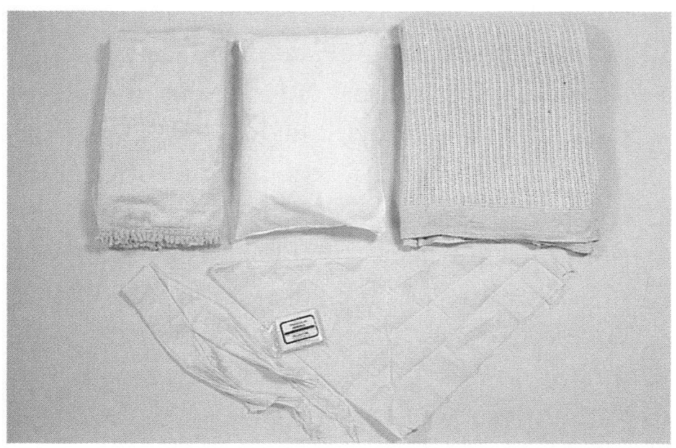

Figure 13-7 Soft splints include folded blankets, towels, pillows, and a sling or cravat.

- Splint the injured area and the joints above and below the injury site.
- Check for proper circulation and sensation before and after splinting.

If splinting a part causes circulation or sensation to become impaired, loosen the splint and wait for advanced medical help to arrive.

Types of Splints

Splints, whether commercially made or improvised, are of four general types—soft, rigid, anatomic, and traction. Soft splints include folded blankets, towels, pillows, and a sling or cravat (Fig. 13-7). A blanket can be used to splint an injured ankle (Fig. 13-8). A **sling**, which can be made from a triangular bandage, is tied to support an arm, wrist, or hand (Fig. 13-9). A **cravat** is a folded triangular bandage used to hold dressings or splints in place.

Rigid splints include boards, metal strips, and folded plastic or cardboard splints (Fig. 13-10). For example, a padded board can be applied to an injured arm (Fig. 13-11). **Anatomic splints** refer to the use of the body as a splint. You may not ordinarily think of the body as a splint, but it works very well and requires no special equipment. For example, an arm can be splinted to the chest. An injured leg can be splinted to the uninjured leg (Fig. 13-12).

As a first responder, you are likely to have commercially made splints immediately available to you. Commercial splints include padded board splints, air splints, specially designed flexible splints, vacuum splints, and traction splints (Fig. 13-13). You should become familiar with the splinting devices you are likely to have before you use them.

Immobilizing Painful, Swollen, Deformed Injuries

Whether using a commercially made splint or improvising from available materials, follow these guidelines when splinting an injured body part:

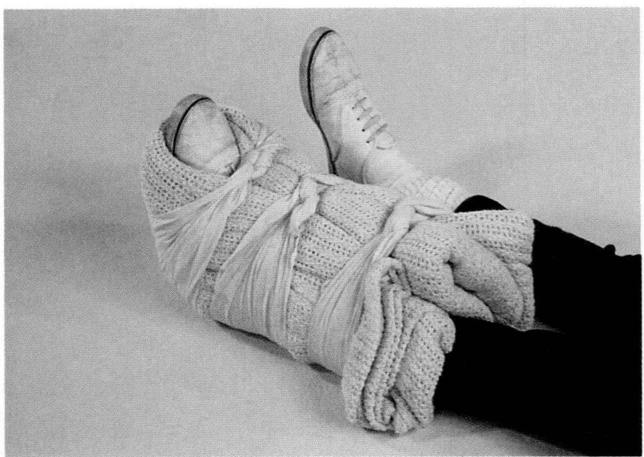

Figure 13-8 A blanket can be used to splint an injured ankle.

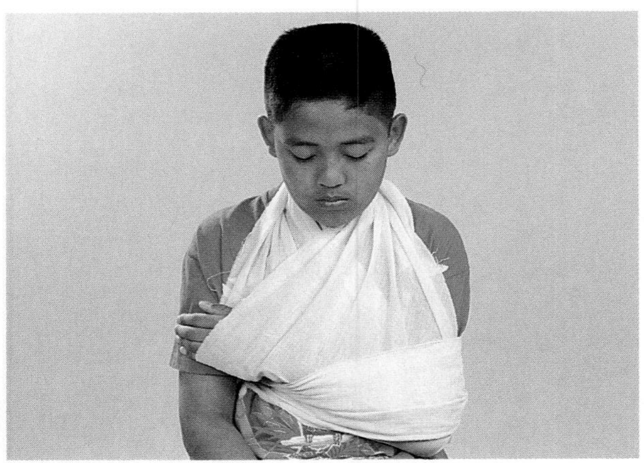

Figure 13-9 A sling supports the arm.

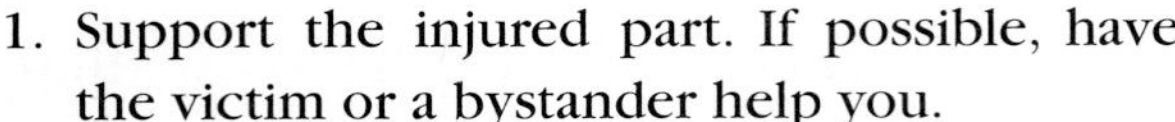

1. Support the injured part. If possible, have the victim or a bystander help you.
2. Cover any open wounds with a dressing and bandage to help control bleeding and prevent infection.
3. If the injury involves an extremity, check for circulation and sensation at a site below (distal to) the injury. Check for a pulse below the injury, feel the hand or foot for warmth, or check for capillary refill in the fingers or toes (infants and children). Ensure that the victim has feeling in the fingers or toes.
4. If using a rigid splint, pad the splint so that it is shaped to the injured part. This padding will help prevent further injury.
5. Secure the splint in place with folded triangular bandages (cravats), roller bandages (gauze), or other wide strips of cloth.
6. Recheck circulation below the injury site to ensure that circulation has not been restricted by applying the splint too tightly. Loosen the splint if the victim complains of numbness or if the fingers or toes turn blue or become cold. It may not be possible to check circulation in a foot, ankle, or leg injury if a sock or shoe is in place or a soft splint is particularly bulky.
7. Elevate the splinted part, if possible.

After the injury has been immobilized, recheck the ABCs and vital signs and take steps to care for shock. Shock is likely to develop as a result of a serious musculoskeletal injury.

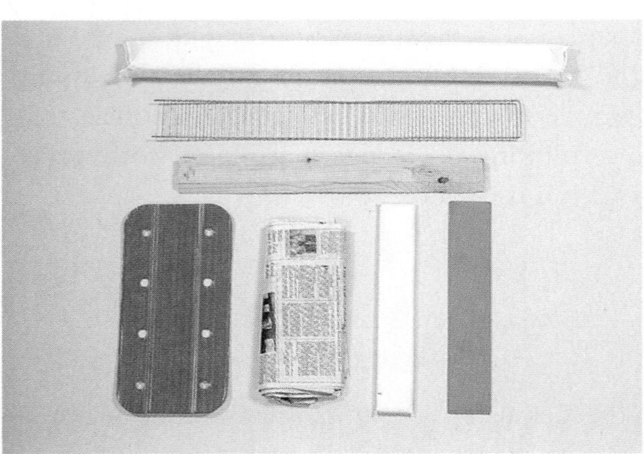

Figure 13-10 Rigid splints include boards, metal strips, and folded cardboard or plastic.

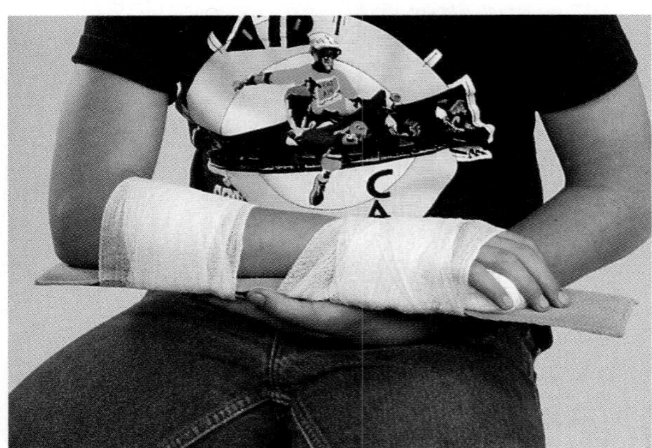

Figure 13-11 A padded rigid splint can be applied to an injured forearm.

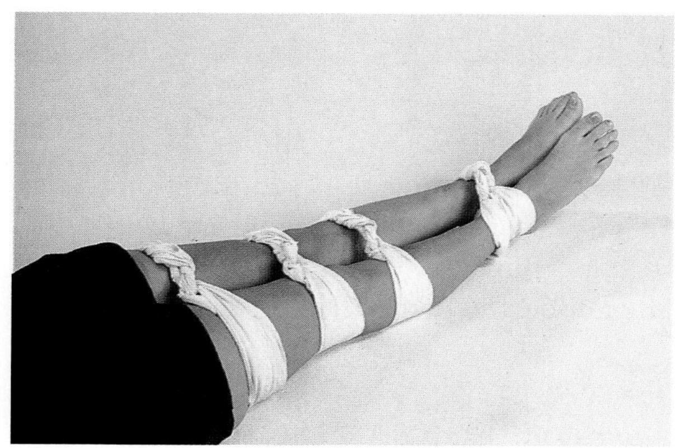

Figure 13-12 An injured leg can be splinted to the uninjured leg.

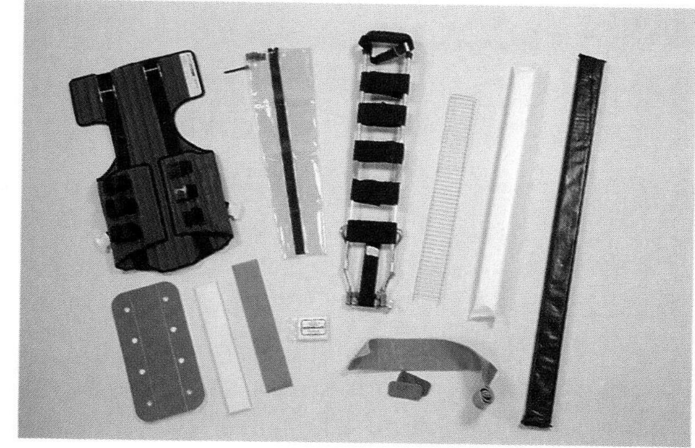

Figure 13-13 Commercial Splints

Help the victim rest in the most comfortable position, apply ice or a cold pack, keep the victim from getting chilled or overheated, and reassure him or her. Determine what additional care is needed and whether to summon more advanced medical personnel if it has not already been done. Continue to monitor the vital signs. Check the victim's level of consciousness, breathing, pulse, skin color and temperature, and blood pressure if you have been trained to do so. Be alert for signs and symptoms of shock or other clues that may indicate the victim's condition is worsening.

Some musculoskeletal injuries are obviously minor. The victim may choose not to get emergency medical care. Others are more serious, requiring more advanced or emergency care. Summon more advanced medical personnel immediately if you suspect an injury involving severe bleeding, injuries to the head, neck, or back, an injury that impairs breathing, or if you see or suspect multiple musculoskeletal injuries. Fractures of large bones can cause severe bleeding and are likely to result in shock.

Some situations may require you to move the victim before an ambulance arrives. If possible, always splint the injury before moving the victim. Follow the general rule: "When in doubt, splint." If you are in a position where you must transport the victim to a medical facility, have someone drive so that you can continue to provide care.

◆ SUMMARY

The musculoskeletal system has four main structures—bones, muscles, tendons, and ligaments. Sometimes it is difficult to tell whether an injury is a fracture, dislocation, sprain, or strain. Since you cannot be sure which of these conditions a victim might have, always care for the injury as if it were serious. If more advanced medical personnel are on the way, do not move the victim. Control any bleeding first. Take steps to minimize shock, and monitor the ABCs and vital signs. If you are going to transport the victim to a medical facility, be sure to first immobilize the injury before moving the victim.

You Are the Responder

1. A basketball players leaps for a rebound. She and another player collide and fall to the ground. What signs and symptoms would you look for that suggest a serious injury?
2. The same player complains for pain in her lower leg and ankle and says that she cannot support her weight. You note a deformity, swelling, and discoloration. Describe how you might provide care for this person.

ENRICHMENT

◆ THE SKELETAL SYSTEM

The **skeleton** is formed by 206 bones of various sizes and shapes (Fig. 13-14). These bones shape the skeleton, giving each body part a unique form. The skeleton protects vital organs and other soft tissues. The skull protects the brain (Fig. 13-15, *A*). The ribs protect the heart and lungs (Fig. 13-15, *B*). The spinal cord is protected by the canal formed by the bones that form the spinal column (Fig. 13-15, *C*).Two or more bones come together to form joints. Ligaments, fibrous bands that hold bones together at joints, give the skeleton stability and, with the muscles, help maintain posture.

Bones

Bones are hard, dense tissues. Their strong, rigid structure helps them withstand stresses that cause injuries. The shape of bones depends on what the bones do and the stresses on them. For instance, the surfaces of bones at

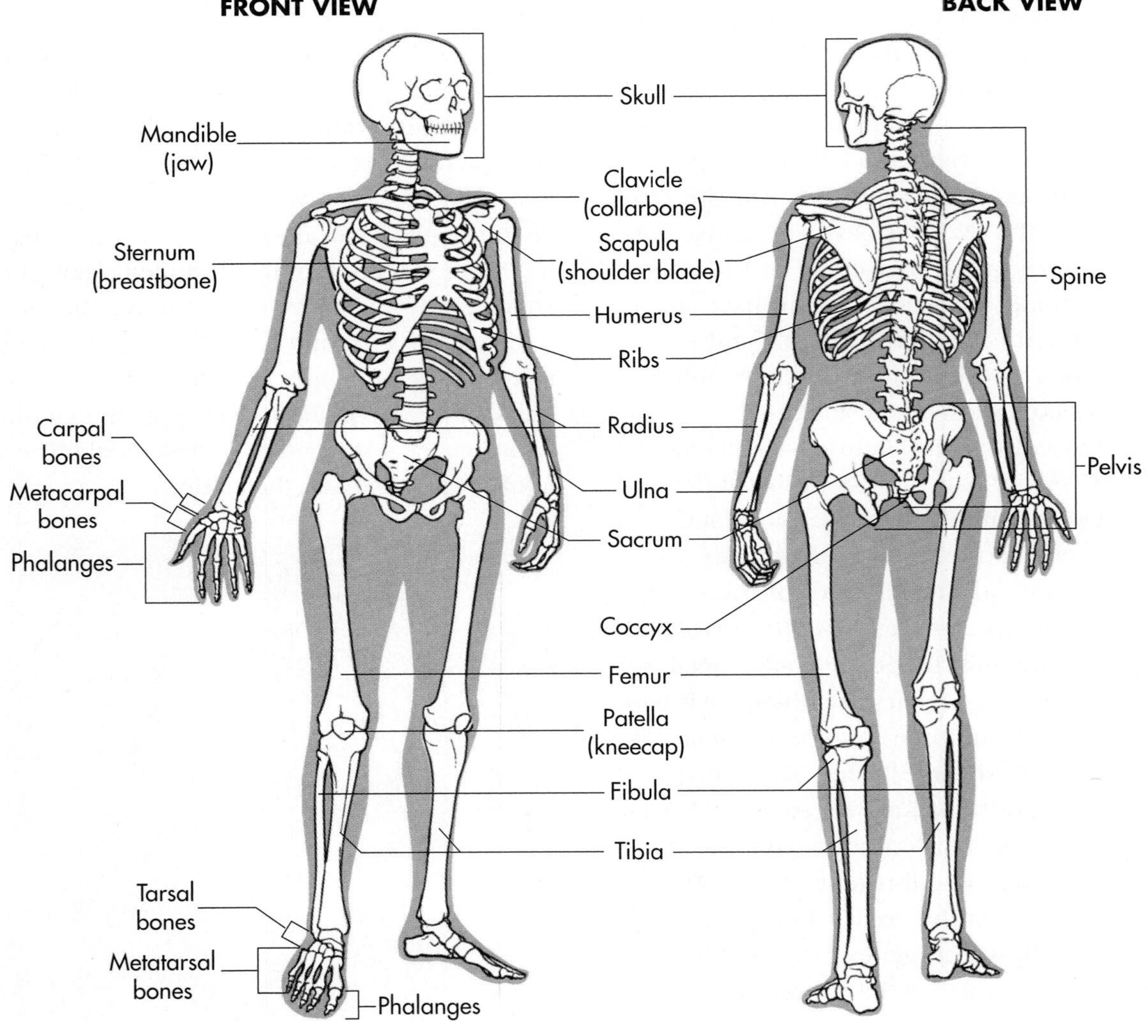

Figure 13-14 The bones of the skeleton give the body its shape and protect vital organs.

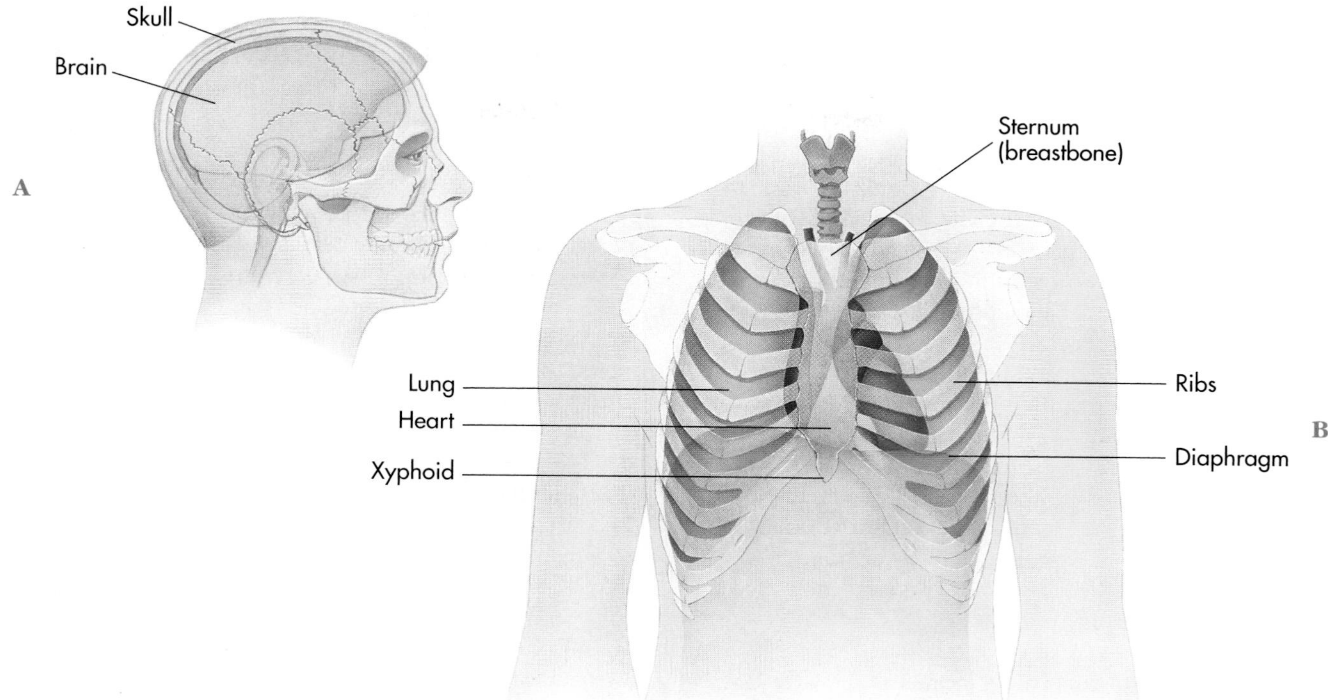

the joints are smooth (Fig. 13-16). Although similar to the bones of the arm, the bones of the leg are much larger and stronger because they carry the body's weight (Fig. 13-17).

Bones have a rich supply of blood and nerves. Some bones store and manufacture red blood cells and supply them to the circulating blood. Bone injuries can bleed and are usually painful. The bleeding can become life threatening if not properly cared for. Bones heal by forming new bone cells. Bone is the only body tissue that can regenerate in this way.

Bones weaken with age. Bones in young children are more flexible than adults' bones, so they are less likely to break. In contrast, elderly people have less dense, brittle bones that are more likely to give way, even under everyday stresses, which can result in significant injuries. For example, the stress created if an elderly person were to pivot with all the body weight on one leg could break the strongest bone in the body, the thigh bone (femur). The gradual, progressive weakening of bone is called **osteoporosis**.

Bones are classified as long, short, flat, or

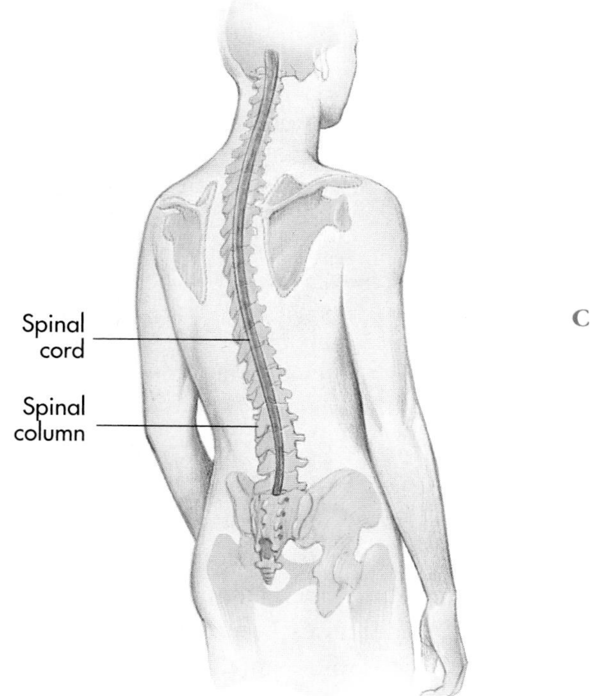

Figure 13-15 **A**, The immovable bones of the skull protect the brain. **B**, The rib cage protects the lungs and heart. **C,** The vertebrae protect the spinal cord.

The Breaking Point

Osteoporosis, a degenerative bone disorder usually discovered after the age of 60, affects 30 percent of people over age 65. It will affect one of four American women and occurs less frequently in men. Fair-skinned women with ancestors from northern Europe, the British Isles, Japan, or China are genetically predisposed to osteoporosis. Inactive people are more susceptible to osteoporosis.

Osteoporosis occurs when there is a decrease in the calcium content of bones. Normally, bones are hard, dense tissues that endure tremendous stresses. Bone-building cells constantly repair damage that occurs as a result of everyday stresses, keeping bones strong. Calcium is a key to bone growth, development, and repair. When the calcium content of bones decreases, bones become frail, less dense, and less able to repair the normal damage they incur.

This loss of density and strength leaves bones more susceptible to fractures. Where once tremendous force was necessary, fractures may now occur with little or no aggravation, especially to hips, vertebrae, and wrists. Spontaneous fractures are those that occur without trauma. The victim may be taking a walk or washing dishes when the fracture occurs. Some hip fractures thought to be caused by falls are actually spontaneous fractures that caused the victim's fall.

Osteoporosis can begin as early as age 30 to 35. The amount of calcium absorbed from the diet naturally declines with age, making calcium intake increasingly important. When calcium in the diet is inadequate, calcium in bones is withdrawn and used by the body to meet its other needs, leaving bones weakened.

Building strong bones before age 35 is the key to preventing osteoporosis. Calcium and exercise are necessary to bone building. The United States Recommended Daily Allowance (U.S. RDA) is currently 800 milligrams of calcium each day for adults. Many physicians recommend 1,000 milligrams for women age 19 and over. Three to four daily servings of low-fat dairy products should provide adequate calcium. Vitamin D is also necessary because it aids in absorption of calcium. Exposure to sunshine enables the body to make vitamin D. Fifteen minutes of sunshine on the hands and face of a young, light-skinned individual are enough to supply the RDA of 5 to 10 micrograms of vitamin D per day. Dark-skinned and elderly people need more sun exposure. People who do not receive adequate sun exposure need to consume vitamin D. The best sources are vitamin-fortified milk and fatty fish such as tuna, salmon, and eel.

Calcium supplements combined with vitamin D are available for those who do not take in adequate calcium. However, before taking a calcium supplement, consult a physician. Many highly advertised calcium supplements are ineffective because they do not dissolve in the body.

Exercise seems to increase bone density and the activity of bone-building cells. Regular exercise may reduce the rate of bone loss by promoting new bone formation and may also stimulate the skeletal system to repair itself. An effective exercise program, such as aerobics, jogging, or walking, involves the weight-bearing muscles of the legs.

irregular (Fig. 13-18). Long bones are longer than they are wide. First responders are not required to learn the medical names for each bone, but some medical names are provided here for reference. Long bones include the bones of the upper arm, the forearm, the thigh, and the lower leg. Short bones are about as wide as they are long. Short bones include the small bones of the hand and feet. Flat bones have a relatively thin, flat shape. Flat bones include the breastbone, the ribs, the shoulder blade (scapula), and some of the bones that form the skull. Bones that do not fit in these three categories are called irregular bones. Irregular bones include the vertebrae and the bones of the face. Bones are weakest at the points where they change shape, and fractures usually occur at these points.

Motion is usually caused by a group of muscles close together pulling at the same time.

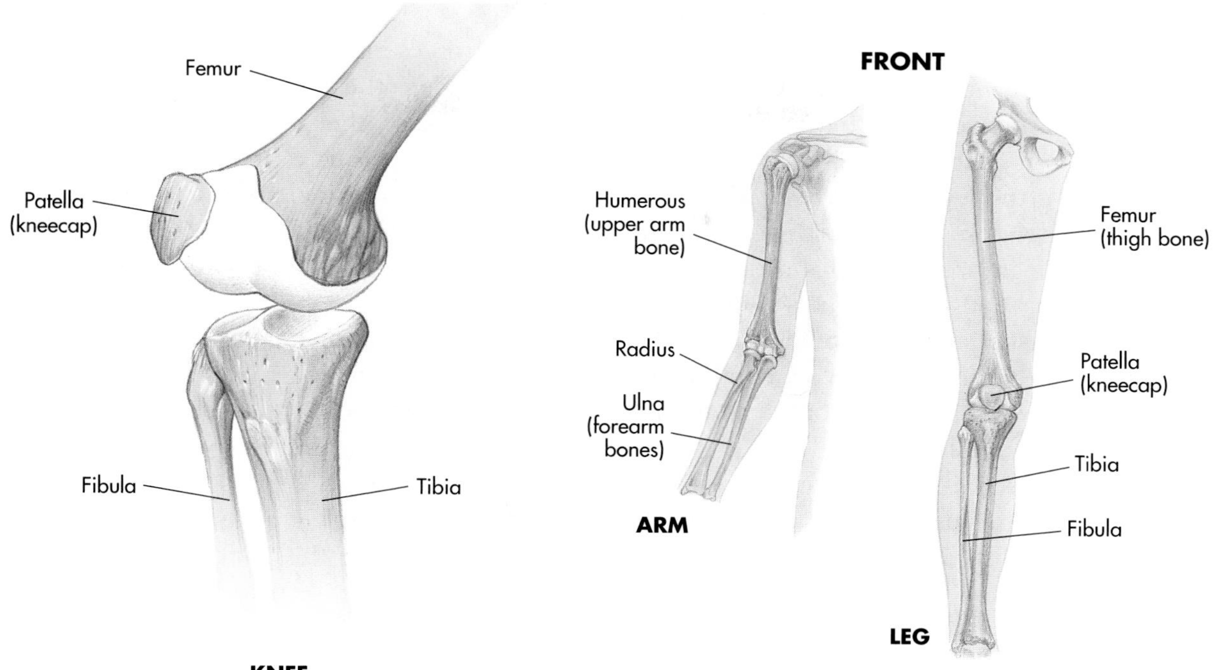

Figure 13-16 Bone surfaces at the joints are smooth.

Figure 13-17 Although similar in shape, the leg bones are larger and stronger than the arm bones because they carry the body's weight.

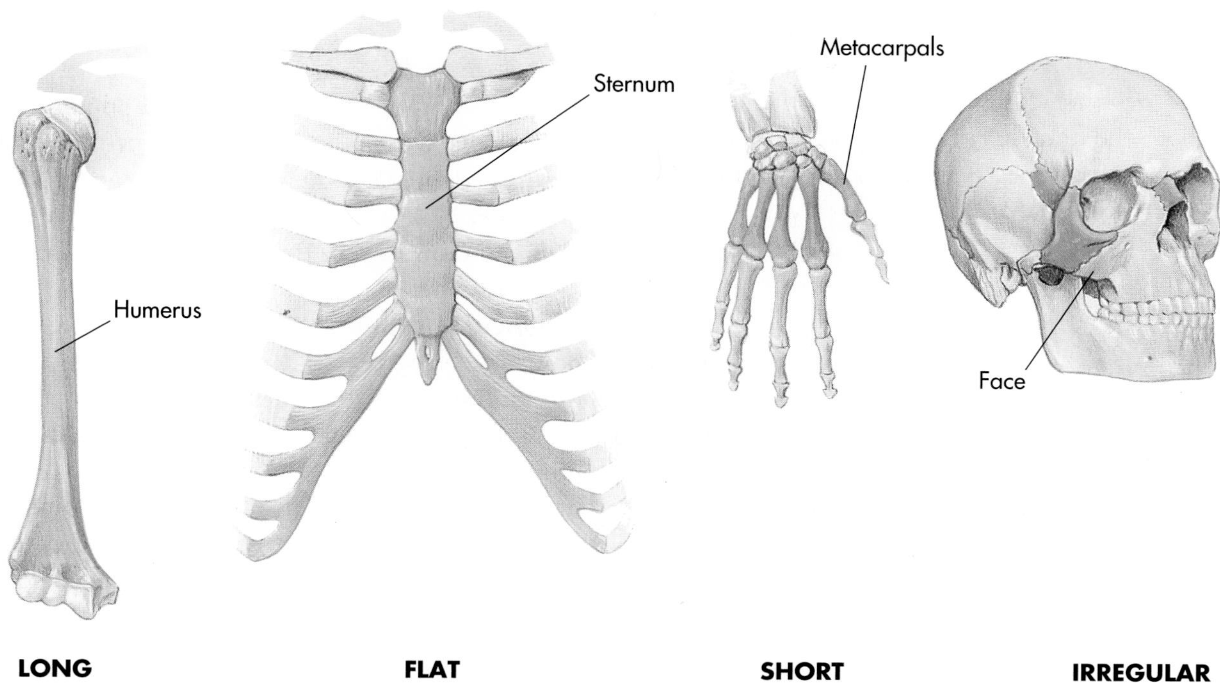

Figure 13-18 Bones vary in shape and size. Bones are weakest at the points where they change shape and usually fracture at these points.

For instance, the hamstring muscles are a group of muscles at the back of the thigh. When the hamstrings contract, the leg bends at the knee. The quadriceps are a group of muscles at the front of the thigh. When the quadriceps contract, the leg straightens at the knee. Generally, when one group of muscles contracts, another group of muscles on the opposite side of the body part relaxes (Fig. 13-19). Even simple tasks, such as bending to pick up an object from the floor, involve a complex series of movements in which different muscle groups contract and relax.

While the general term for musculoskeletal injuries used in this text is "painful, swollen, deformed extremities," a variety of injuries occur.

◆ TYPES OF MUSCULOSKELETAL INJURIES

The four basic types of musculoskeletal injuries are fracture, dislocation, sprain, and strain. Injuries to the musculoskeletal system can be classified according to the body structures that are damaged. Some injuries may involve more than one type of injury. For example, a direct blow to the knee may injure both ligaments and bones. Injuries are also classified by the nature and extent of the damage.

Fracture

A ***fracture*** is a break or disruption in bone tissue. Fractures include chipped or cracked bones, as well as bones that are broken all the way through (Fig. 13-20). Fractures are commonly caused by direct and indirect forces. However, if strong enough, twisting forces and strong muscle contractions can cause a fracture.

Dislocation

A ***dislocation*** is a displacement or separation of a bone from its normal position at a joint (Fig. 13-21). Dislocations are usually caused by severe forces, such as twisting or falls. Some joints, such as the shoulder or fingers, dislocate easily because their bones and ligaments do not provide adequate protection. Others, such as the elbow or the joints of the spine, are well protected and therefore dislocate less easily.

When bone ends are forced far enough beyond their normal position, ligaments stretch and tear. Subsequent dislocations are then more likely to occur. A force violent enough to cause a dislocation can also cause a fracture and can damage nearby nerves and blood vessels.

Dislocations are generally more obvious than fractures because the joint appears deformed (Fig. 13-22). The displaced bone end often causes an abnormal lump, ridge, or depression, sometimes making dislocations easier to identify than other musculoskeletal injuries. Also, an injured person is unable to move a joint that is dislocated because the bones are out of place.

Sprain

A ***sprain*** is the stretching or tearing of ligaments and other tissues at a joint. A sprain usually results when the bones that form a joint are forced beyond their normal range of motion (Fig. 13-23). The more ligaments that are torn, the more severe the injury. The sudden, violent forcing of a joint beyond its limit can completely rupture ligaments and dislocate bones. Severe sprains may also involve a fracture of the bones that form the joint.

Mild sprains, which only stretch ligament fibers, generally heal quickly. The victim may have only a brief period of pain or discomfort and quickly return to activity with little or no soreness. For this reason, people often neglect sprains, and the joint is often reinjured. Severe sprains or sprains that involve a fracture usually cause pain when the joint is moved or used.

Often, a sprain is more disabling than a fracture. When fractures heal, they usually leave the bone as strong as it was before. It is un-

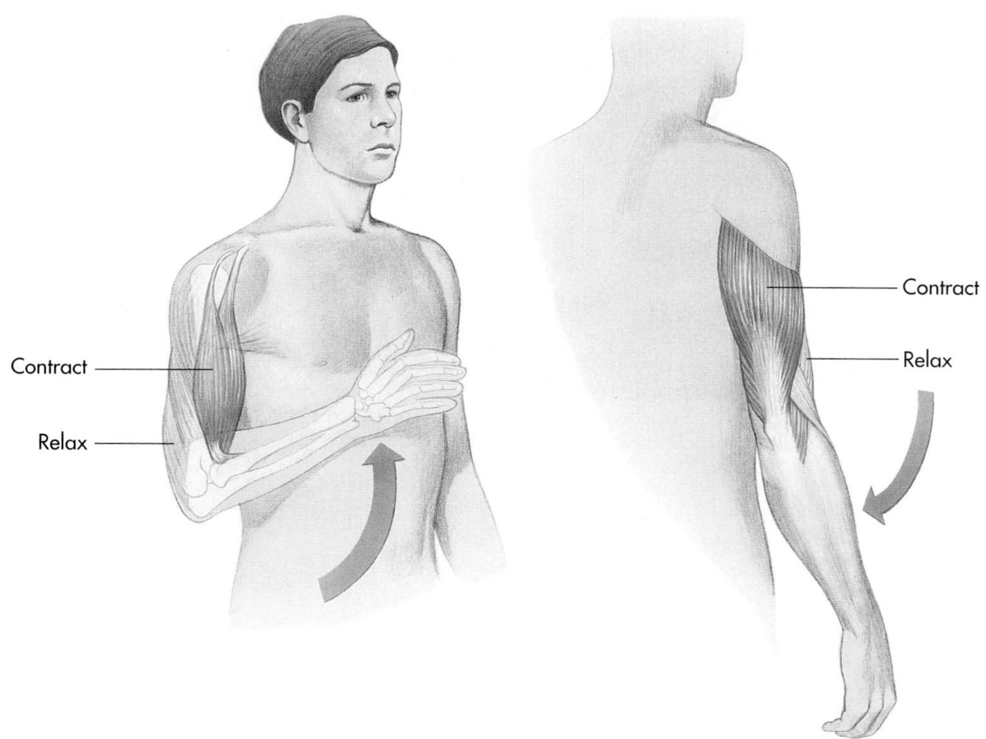

Figure 13-19 Movement occurs when one group of muscles contracts and an opposing group of muscles relaxes.

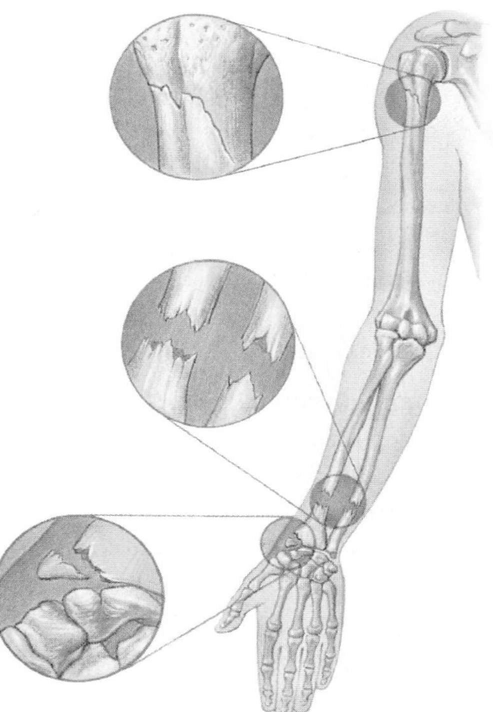

Figure 13-20 Fractures include chipped or cracked bones and bones broken all the way through.

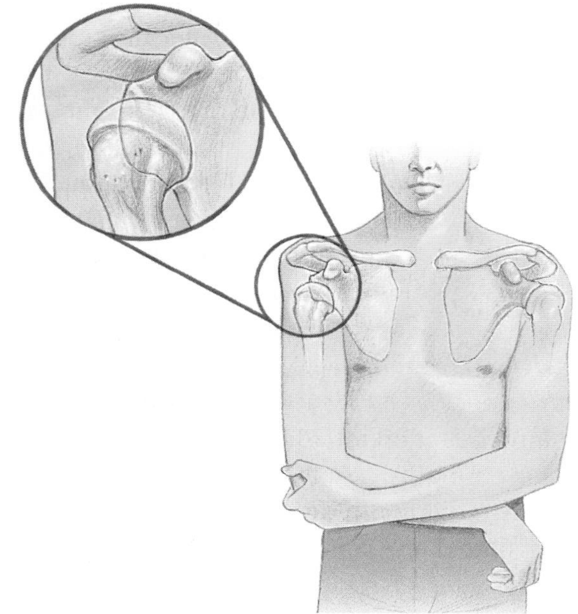

Figure 13-21 A dislocation is a displacement or separation of a bone from its normal position at a joint.

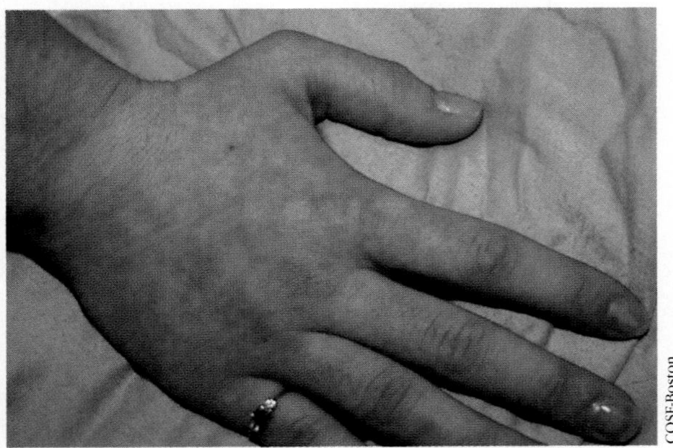

Figure 13-22 A dislocation can cause the joint to appear deformed.

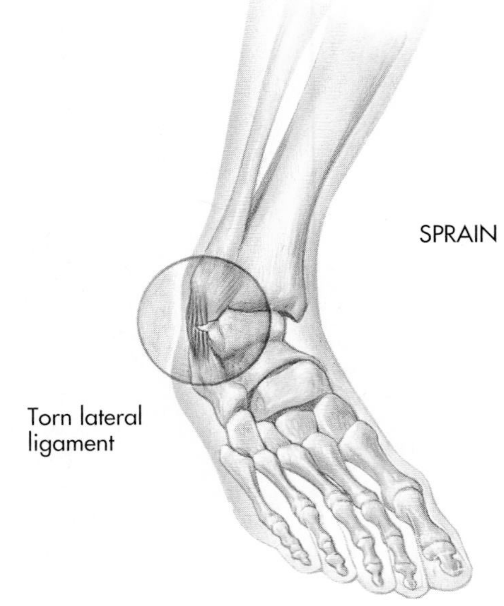

Figure 13-23 A sprain results when bones that form a joint are forced beyond their normal range of motion, causing ligaments to stretch and tear.

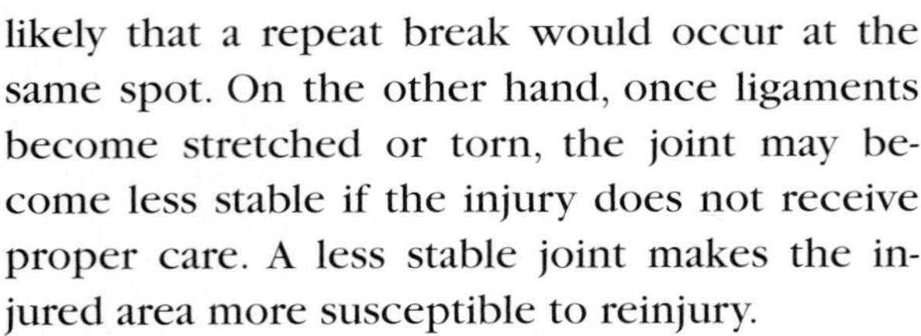
likely that a repeat break would occur at the same spot. On the other hand, once ligaments become stretched or torn, the joint may become less stable if the injury does not receive proper care. A less stable joint makes the injured area more susceptible to reinjury.

Strain

A ***strain*** is the excessive stretching and tearing of muscle or tendon fibers. It is sometimes called a "muscle pull" or "tear." Because tendons are tougher and stronger than muscles, tears usually occur in the muscle or where the muscle attaches to the tendon. Strains often result from overexertion, such as lifting something too heavy or overworking a muscle. They can also result from sudden or uncoordinated movement. Strains commonly involve the muscles in the neck or back, the front or back of the thigh, or the back of the lower leg. Strains of the neck and lower back can be particularly painful and therefore disabling.

Like sprains, strains are often neglected, which commonly leads to reinjury. Strains sometimes reoccur chronically, especially to the muscles of the neck, lower back, and the back of the thigh. Neck and back problems are two of the leading causes of absenteeism from work, accounting for more than $15 billion in workman's compensation claims and lost productivity annually.

◆ CARING FOR SPECIFIC INJURIES TO BONES AND JOINTS

Both the upper and lower extremities have structures that are vulnerable to injury. In general, the care for such injuries is similar.

Upper Extremity Injuries

The **upper extremities** are the arms and hands. The bones of each upper extremity include the **collarbone (clavicle), shoulder blade (scapula),** bones of the upper arm **(humerus)** and **forearm (radius and ulna),** and bones of the hand **(carpals** and **metacarpals)** and fingers **(phalanges).** Figure 13-24 shows the major structures of the upper extremities.

The upper extremities are the most commonly injured area of the body. These injuries occur in many different ways. The most fre-

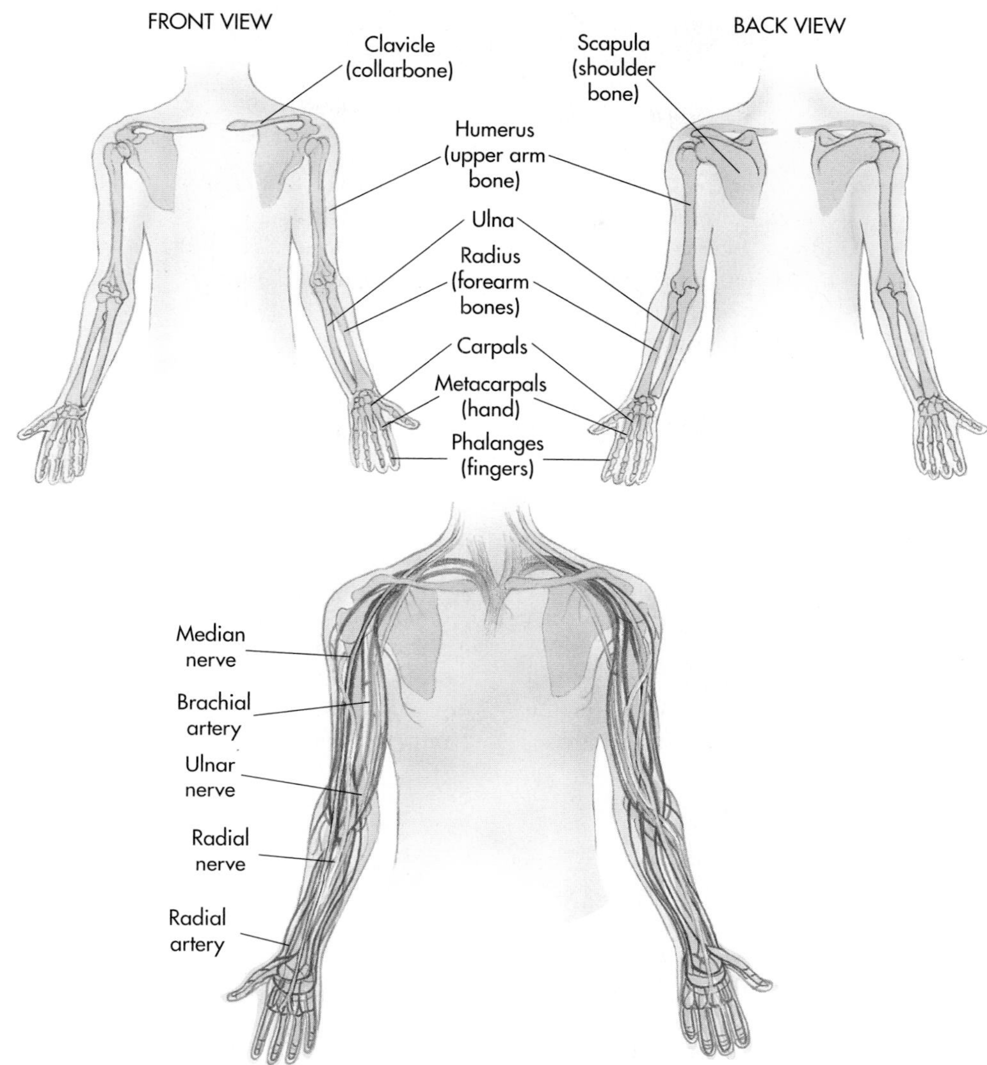

Figure 13-24 The upper extremities include the bones of the arms and hands, nerves, and blood vessels.

quent cause is falling on the hand of an outstretched arm. Since the hands are rarely protected, abrasions occur easily. Because a falling person instinctively tries to break the fall by extending the arms and hands, these areas receive the force of the body's weight. This can cause a serious injury to the hand, forearm, upper arm, or shoulder, such as a severe sprain, fracture, or dislocation (Fig. 13-25).

When caring for serious upper extremity injuries, minimize any movement of the injured part. If an injured person is holding the arm securely against the chest, do not change the position. Holding the arm against the chest is an effective method of immobilization. Instead, allow the person to continue to support the arm in this manner. You can further assist him or her by binding the injured arm to the chest. Doing so eliminates the need for special splinting equipment and still provides an effective method of immobilization.

Injuries to an upper extremity may also damage blood vessels, nerves, and other soft tissues. It is particularly important to ensure that

Sprains and Strains

Spring is the season of flowers, trees, strains, and sprains. Almost as soon as armchair athletes come out of hibernation to become intramural heroes, emergency clinics see an increase in sprained ankles, twisted knees, and strained backs. So what happens when injuries occur? Which do you apply, heat or cold?

The answer is both—first cold, then heat. And it does not matter whether it is a strain or sprain!

How Cold Helps Initially

When a person twists an ankle or strains his or her back, the tissues underneath the skin are injured. Blood and fluids seep out from the torn blood vessels and cause swelling to occur at the site of the injury. Muscles spasm to protect the injured area. This often causes more pain. By keeping the injured area cool, you can help control internal bleeding and reduce pain. Cold causes the broken blood vessels to constrict, limiting the blood and fluid that seep out. Cold reduces pain by numbing the nerve endings, thereby reducing painful muscle spasms.

How Heat Helps Repair the Tissue

A physician will most likely advise applying ice to the injury periodically for up to the first 100 hours or until the swelling goes away. After that, applying heat is appropriate. Heat speeds up chemical reactions needed to repair the tissue. White blood cells move in to rid the body of infections, damaged cells are removed, and other cells begin the repair process. This process enhances proper healing of the injury. If you are unsure whether to use cold or heat on an injured area, always apply cold until you can consult your physician.

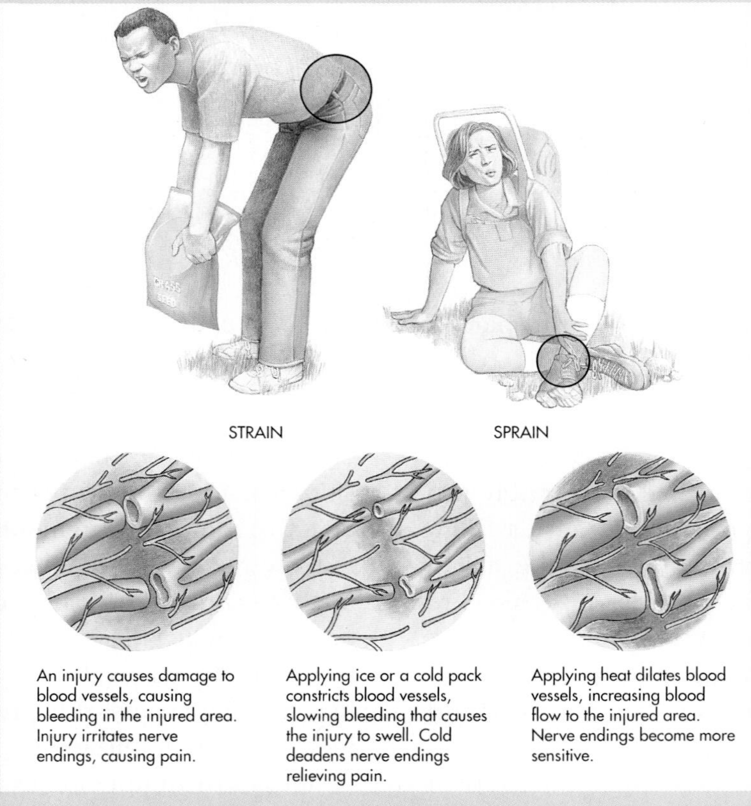

STRAIN
SPRAIN
An injury causes damage to blood vessels, causing bleeding in the injured area. Injury irritates nerve endings, causing pain.
Applying ice or a cold pack constricts blood vessels, slowing bleeding that causes the injury to swell. Cold deadens nerve endings relieving pain.
Applying heat dilates blood vessels, increasing blood flow to the injured area. Nerve endings become more sensitive.

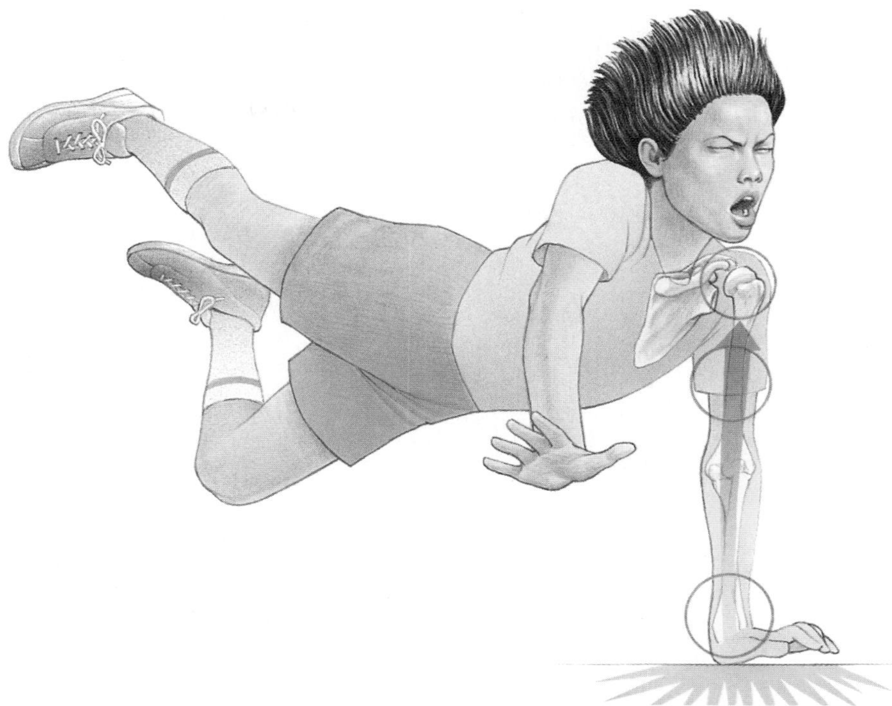

Figure 13-25 A fall can cause a serious injury to the hand, arm, or shoulder.

blood flow and nerve function have not been impaired. Always check for circulation and sensation below the injury site, both before and after splinting. If you suspect that either the blood vessels or the nerves have been damaged, minimize movement of the area and summon more advanced emergency personnel immediately. Sometimes when a splint is applied too tightly, blood flow may be impaired. If this occurs, loosen the splint.

Shoulder Injuries

The shoulder consists of three bones that meet to form the shoulder joint. These bones are the clavicle, scapula, and humerus. The most common shoulder injuries are sprains. However, shoulder injuries may also involve a fracture or dislocation of one or more of these bones.

The most frequently injured bone of the shoulder is the clavicle, or collarbone, more commonly injured in children than adults. Typically, the clavicle is fractured or separates from its original position at its inner or outer end as a result of a fall (Fig. 13-26). A shoulder separation commonly occurs from a fall on the point of the shoulder that forces the outer end of the clavicle to separate fron the joint where it touches the scapula. The victim usually feels pain in the shoulder area, which may radiate down the upper extremity. A person with a clavicle injury usually attempts to ease the pain by holding the forearm against the chest (Fig. 13-27). Since the clavicle lies directly over major blood vessels and nerves to the upper extremity, it is especially important to immobilize a fractured clavicle promptly to prevent injury to these structures.

Scapula fractures are not common. A fracture of the scapula typically results from violent force. The signs and symptoms of a fractured scapula are the same as for any other extremity fracture, although you are less likely to see deformity of the scapula. The most significant signs and symptoms are extreme pain and the inability to move the arm.

Because it takes great force to break the

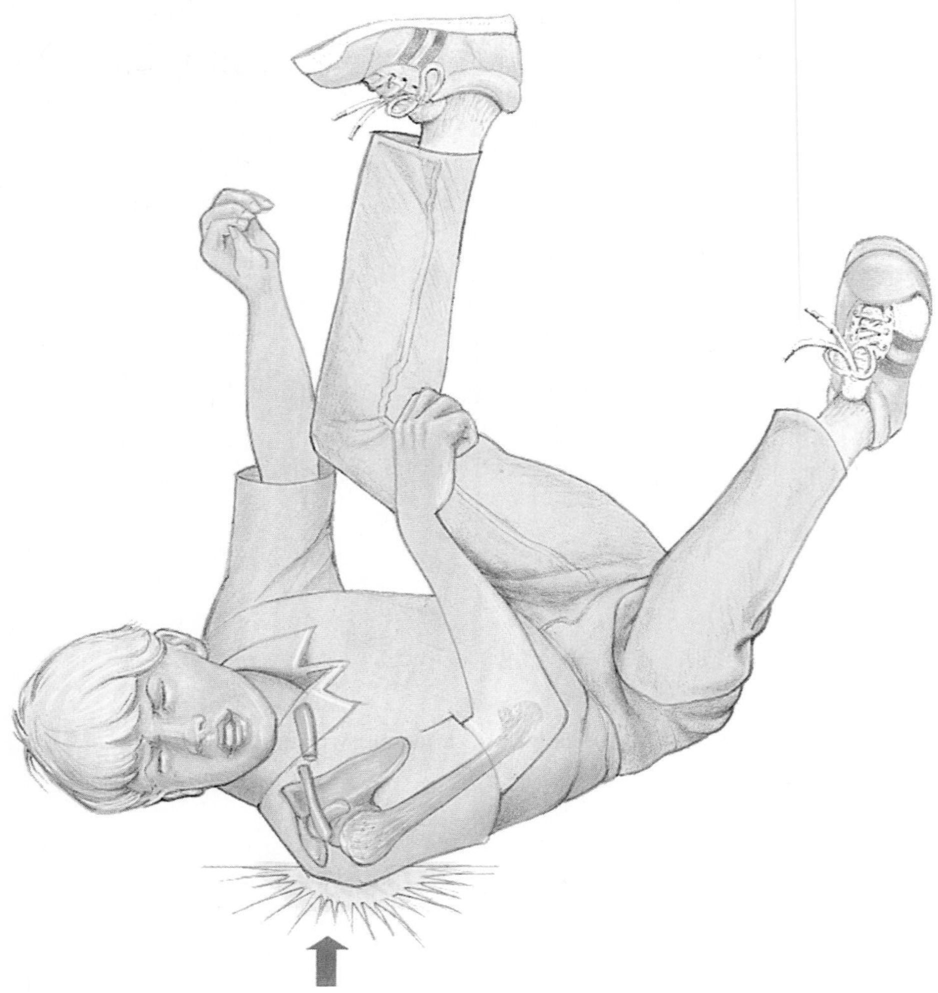

Figure 13-26 A clavicle fracture is commonly caused by a fall.

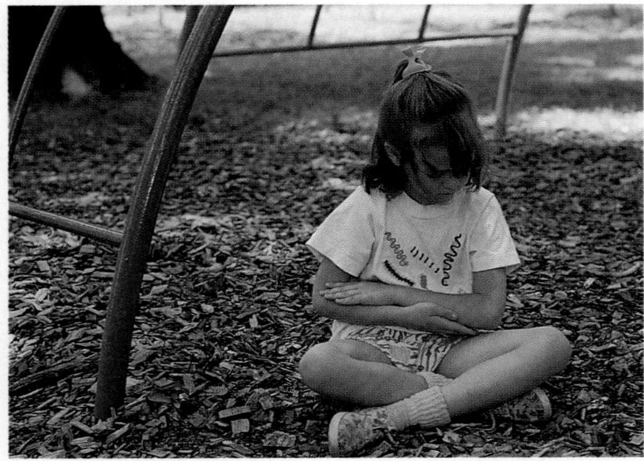

Figure 13-27 Someone with a fractured clavicle will usually support the arm on the injured side.

scapula, you must consider that the force may have been great enough also to injure the ribs or internal organs in the chest. If the chest or its contents are injured, a victim may have difficulty breathing.

A dislocation is another common type of shoulder injury. Like fractures, dislocations often result from falls. This happens frequently in contact sports, such as football and rugby. A player may attempt to break a fall with an outstretched arm or may land on the tip of the shoulder, forcing the arm against the joint formed by the scapula and clavicle. This can result in ligaments tearing, causing the end of the

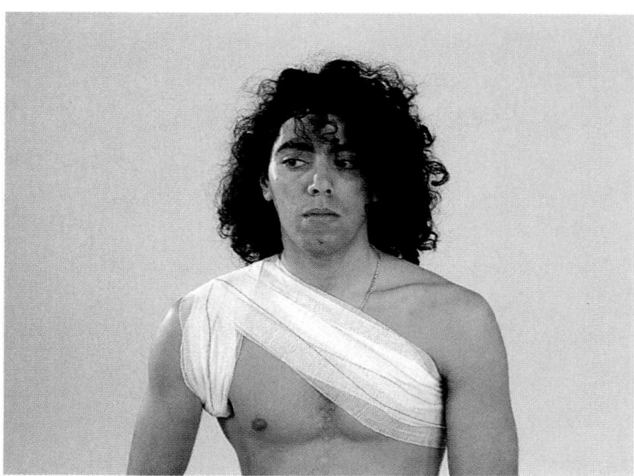

Figure 13-28 Use a figure-eight pattern to apply a pressure bandage to the shoulder.

clavicle to displace. Dislocations also occur at the joint where the humerus meets the socket formed by the scapula. For example, when an arm in a throwing position is hit, it forces the arm to rotate backward. Ligaments tear, causing the upper end of the arm to dislocate from its normal position in the shoulder socket.

Shoulder dislocations are painful and can often be identified by the deformity present. As with other shoulder injuries, the victim often tries to minimize the pain by holding the arm in the most comfortable position.

To care for shoulder injuries, first control any external bleeding with direct pressure. Apply a pressure bandage using a figure-eight pattern (Fig. 13-28). Allow the victim to continue to support the arm in the position in which he or she is holding it (usually the most comfortable position), and splint it in that position if possible. If the victim is holding the arm away from the body, use a pillow, rolled blanket, or similar object to fill the gap between the arm and chest to provide support for the injured area. Check for circulation and sensation in the hand and fingers. Then splint the arm in place. This can be done by merely binding the arm to the chest or by placing the arm in a sling and binding the arm to the chest with a cravat (Fig. 13-29). Recheck for circulation and sensation. Apply cold to the injured area to help minimize pain and reduce swelling. Take steps to minimize shock.

Upper Arm Injuries

The bone of the **upper arm,** the part of the extremity between the shoulder and the elbow, is the humerus. It is the largest bone in the **arm,** the upper extremity from the shoulder to the wrist. This bone can be fractured at any point, although it is usually fractured at the upper end near the shoulder or in the middle

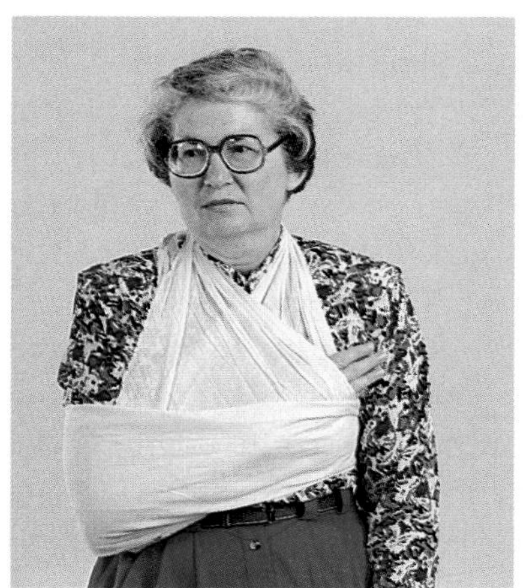

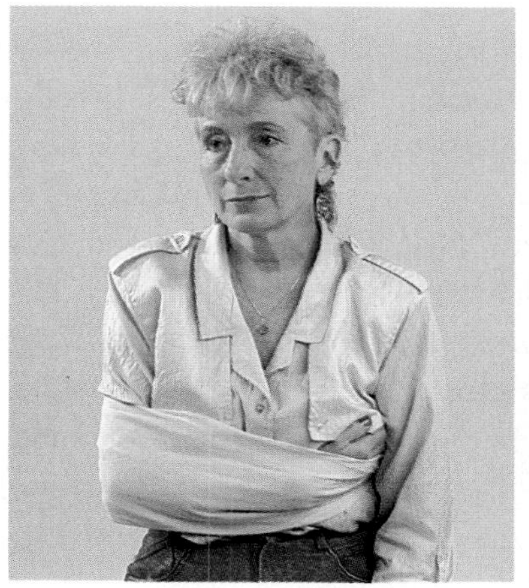

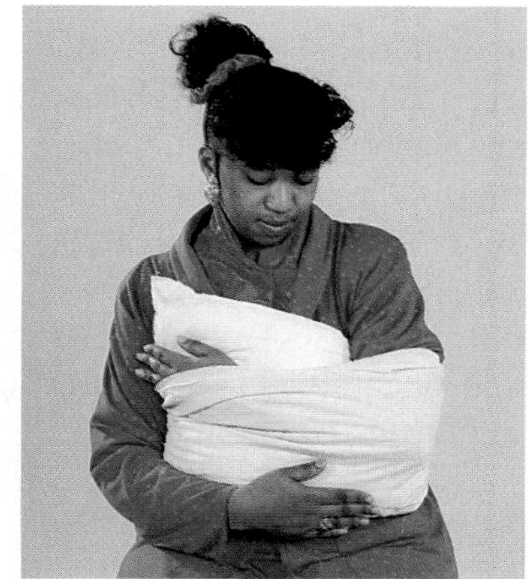

Figure 13-29 Splint the arm against the chest in the position the victim is holding it, using a sling, cravats, and a small pillow or a rolled blanket when necessary.

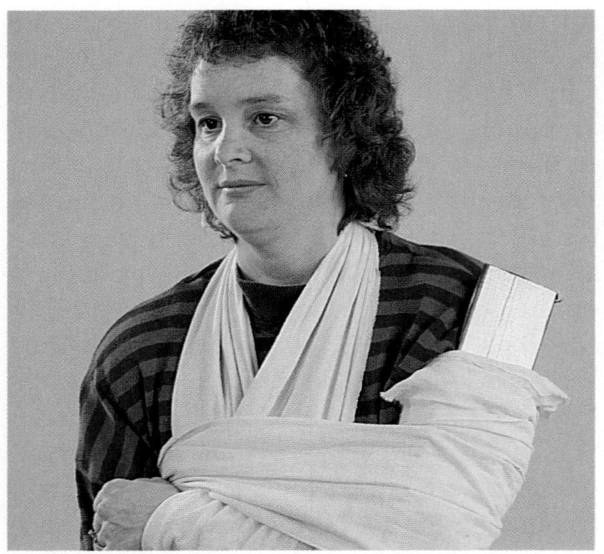

Figure 13-30 A short, padded splint can provide additional support for an injury to the upper arm.

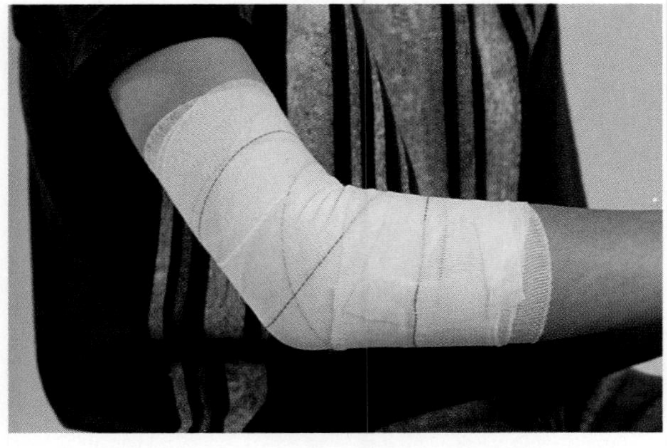

Figure 13-31 Use a figure-eight pattern to apply a pressure bandage to the elbow.

of the bone. The upper end of the humerus often fractures in the elderly and in young children as a result of a fall. Breaks in the middle of the bone occur mostly in young adults. When the humerus is fractured, there is danger of damage to the blood vessels and nerves supplying the entire arm. Most humerus fractures are very painful and prevent the victim from using the arm. A fracture also can cause considerable arm deformity.

To care for a serious upper arm injury, immobilize the upper arm from the shoulder to the elbow. This can be done in the same way as for shoulder injuries. Control any external bleeding with direct pressure. Place the arm in a sling and bind it to the chest with cravats. Apply cold in the best way possible. You can use a short splint, if one is available, to give more support to the upper arm (Fig. 13-30). Always check for circulation and sensation in the hand and fingers before and after immobilizing the injured area.

Elbow Injuries

Like other joints, the elbow can be sprained, fractured, or dislocated. Injuries to the elbow can cause permanent disability, since all the nerves and blood vessels to the forearm and hand go through the elbow. Therefore take elbow injuries seriously. Injuries to a joint like the elbow can be made worse by movement.

If the victim says that he or she cannot move the elbow, do not try to move it. Control any external bleeding with direct pressure and a pressure bandage, using a figure-eight pattern (Fig. 13-31). Check for circulation and sensation. Support the arm and immobilize it from the shoulder to the wrist.

To care for an elbow injury, immobilize the elbow in the position in which you find it. Place the arm in a sling and secure it to the chest, as shown in Figure 13-29. If this is not possible, immobilize the elbow with a splint and two cravats. If the elbow is bent, apply the splint diagonally across the underside of the arm (Fig. 13-32, *A*). The splint should extend several inches beyond both the upper arm and the wrist. If the elbow is straight, apply the splint along the arm. Secure the splint at the wrist and upper arm with cravats or roller bandages (Fig. 13-32, *B*). Recheck for circulation and sensation. Summon more advanced medical personnel. Apply ice or a cold pack and take steps to care for shock.

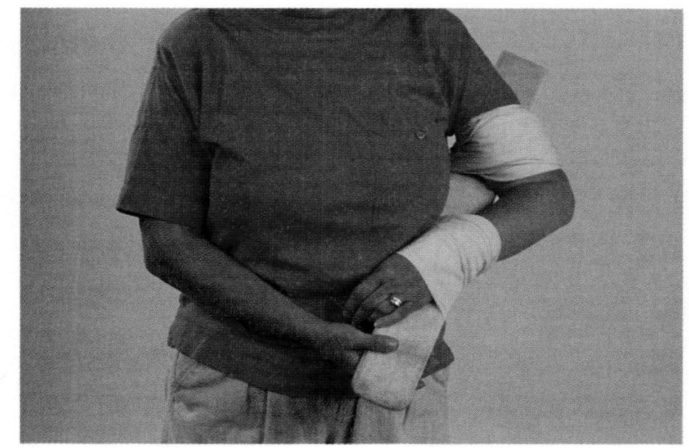

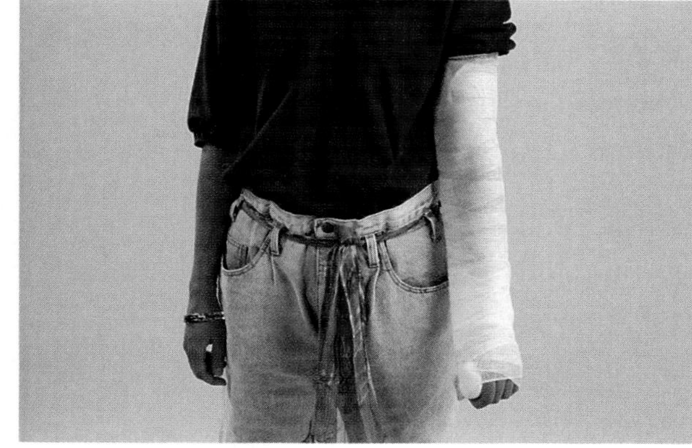

Figure 13-32 **A**, If the elbow is bent, apply a splint diagonally across the underside of the arm. **B**, If the arm is straight, apply a splint along the underside of the arm.

Forearm, Wrist, and Hand Injuries

The **forearm** is the upper extremity from the elbow to the wrist. Fractures of the two forearm bones, the radius and ulna, are more common in children than adults. If a person falls on an outstretched arm, both bones may break, but not always in the same place. With forearm fractures, the arm may look S-shaped (Fig. 13-33). This characteristic shape is why it is sometimes called a "silver-fork" deformity. Because the radial artery and nerve are near these bones, a fracture may cause severe bleeding or a loss of movement in the wrist and hand. The wrist is also a common site of sprains.

Because the hands are used in so many daily activities, they are very susceptible to injury. Most injuries to the hands and fingers involve only minor soft tissue damage. However, a serious injury may damage nerves, blood vessels, and bones. Home, recreational, and industrial mishaps often produce lacerations, avulsions, burns, and fractures of the hands. Because the hand structures are delicate, deep lacerations can cause permanently disabling injuries.

Begin care by controlling any external bleed-

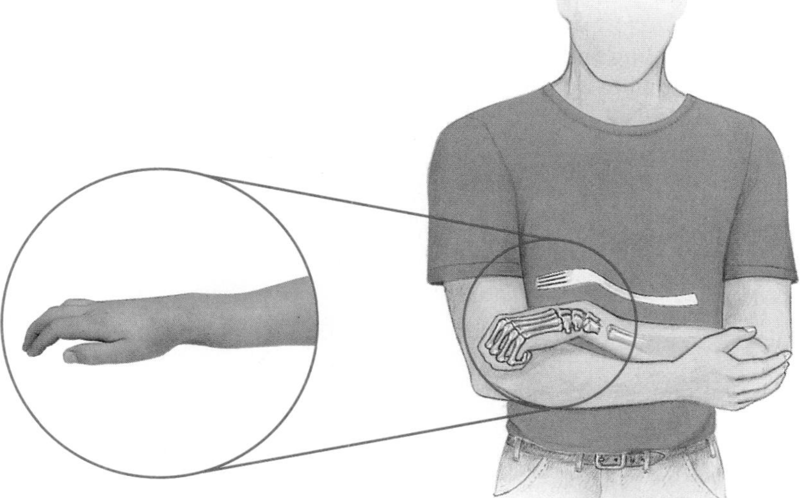

Figure 13-33 Fractures of both forearm bones often have a characteristic S-shaped deformity. This is sometimes called a "silver-fork" deformity.

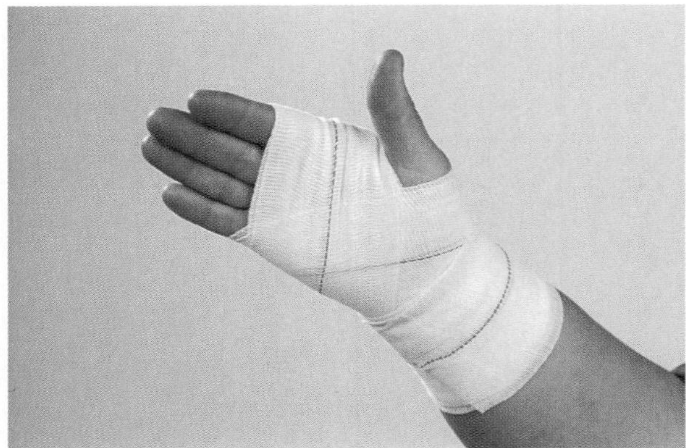

Figure 13-34 A Pressure Bandage for the Palm of the Hand

ing with direct pressure. To bandage the hand, apply a pressure bandage using a figure-eight pattern (Fig. 13-34). Check for circulation and sensation, then care for the injured forearm, wrist, or hand by immobilizing the injured part. When using a rigid splint, support the injured part by placing a splint underneath the forearm. Extend the splint beyond both the hand and elbow. Place a roll of gauze or a similar object in the palm to keep the palm and fingers in a normal position. Then secure the splint with cravats or roller gauze (Fig. 13-35, *A*). Recheck circulation and sensation. Then put the arm in a sling and secure it to the chest (Fig. 13-35, *B*).

You can immobilize hand and finger injuries

A

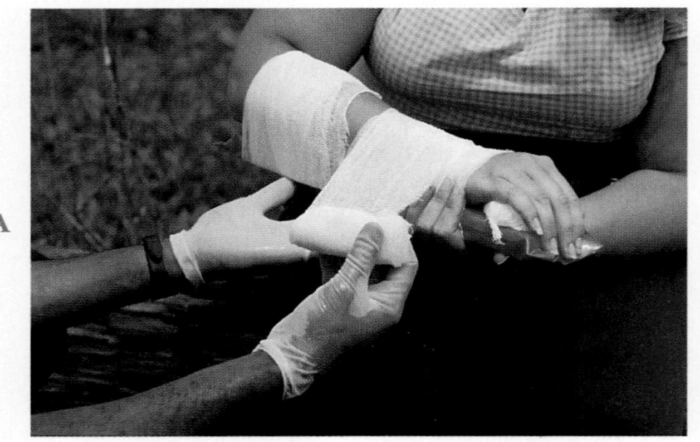

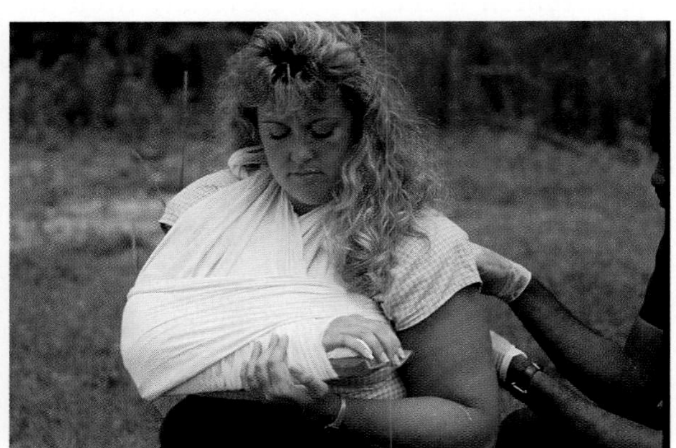

B

Figure 13-35 **A**, If the forearm is fractured, place a splint under the forearm and secure it. **B**, Put the arm in a sling and secure it to the chest with cravats.

A

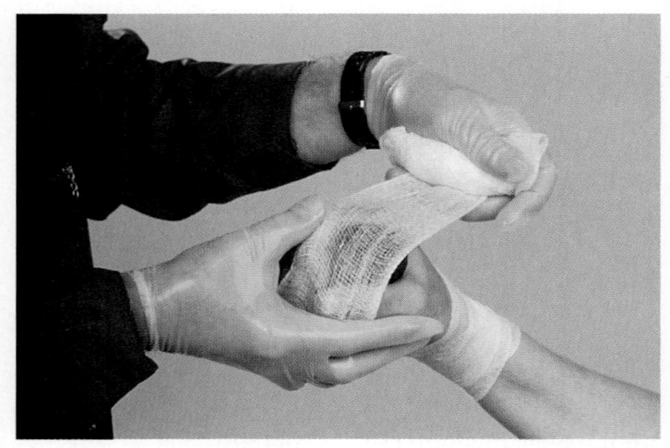

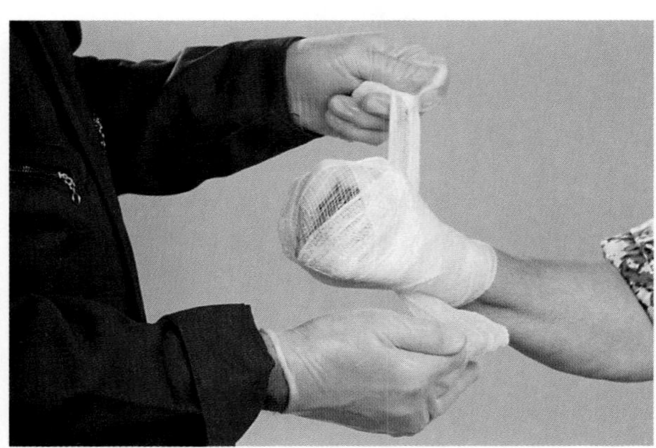

B

Figure 13-36 A soft splint is an effective splint for a **A,** hand or **B,** finger injury.

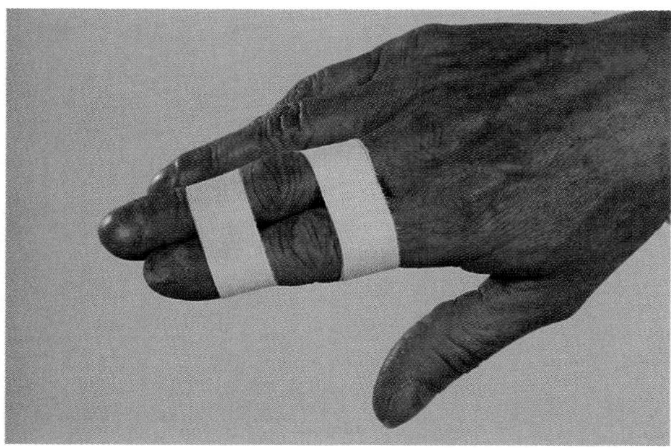

Figure 13-37 An injured finger can be splinted to an adjacent finger.

using a soft splint made of a roll of gauze or rolled up cloth and bandages (Fig. 13-36, *A-B*). You can splint an injured finger to an adjacent finger with tape (Fig. 13-37). *Do not* attempt to put displaced finger or thumb bones back into place. Always apply ice or a cold pack to forearm, wrist, and hand injuries, and elevate the injured area.

Air splints are also an effective way to immobilize the hand and forearm. To avoid cutting off circulation, do not overinflate the splint. When the splint is properly inflated, you should be able to make a slight dent in the surface of the splint with your thumb. A change in temperature or altitude can affect the air in the splint. Moving from a cold area to a warm one or from a lower to a higher elevation can cause the air in the splint to expand, making the splint tighter. Moving from a warm area to a cold one or a higher elevation to a lower can cause the splint to loosen. Continue to check circulation in the limb and proper inflation of the splint. Figure 13-38 shows how to apply an air splint.

Lower Extremity Injuries

Injuries to the **leg,** the entire lower extremity, can involve both soft tissue and musculoskeletal damage. The major bones of the **thigh** (between the pelvis and the knee) and **lower leg** (between the knee and the ankle) are large and strong enough to carry the body's weight. Bones of the leg include the one in the thigh **(femur),** the kneecap **(patella),** the two bones in the lower leg **(tibia and fibula),** the bones of the foot **(tarsals and metatarsals),** and the bones of the toes **(phalanges).** Because of the size and strength of the bones in the thigh and lower leg, a significant amount of force is required to cause a fracture.

The **femoral artery** is the major supplier of blood to the legs and feet. If it is damaged, which may happen with a fracture of the femur, the blood loss can be life threatening.

Figure 13-39 shows the major structures of the lower extremities. Serious injury to the lower extremities can result in their inability to bear weight. Since the victim may be unable to walk, you should summon more advanced medical personnel.

Thigh and Lower Leg Injuries

The femur is the largest bone in the body. Because it bears most of the body's weight, it is most important in walking and running. Thigh injuries range from bruises and torn muscles to severe injuries, such as fractures. The upper end of the femur meets the pelvis at the hip joint (Fig. 13-40). Most femur fractures involve the upper end of the bone. Even though the hip joint itself is not involved, such injuries are often called hip fractures.

A fracture of the femur usually produces a characteristic deformity. When the fracture occurs, the thigh muscles contract. Because the thigh muscles are so strong, they pull the broken bone ends together, causing them to overlap. This may cause the injured leg to be noticeably shorter than the other leg. The injured leg may also be turned inward or outward (Fig. 13-41). Other signs and symptoms of a fractured femur may include severe pain and swelling and inability to move the leg.

A fracture in the lower leg may involve one or both bones. Often both bones are fractured simultaneously. However, a blow to the outside

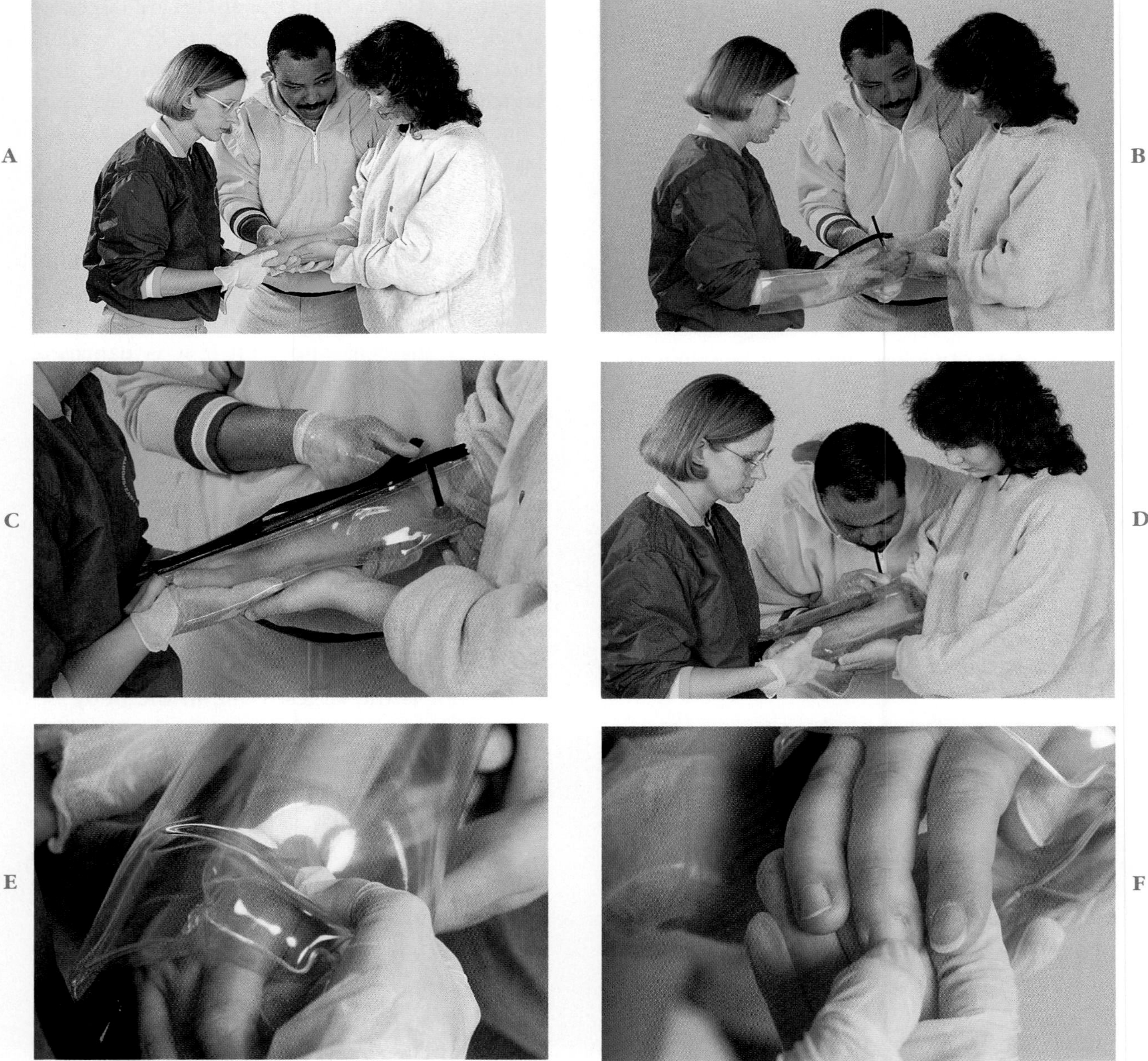

Figure 13-38 To apply an air splint, **A**, support the injured limb. **B**, Slide the closed end of the splint up your arm and grasp the victim's limb. **C**, Position the splint on the injured limb. **D**, Inflate the splint. **E**, Check the splint for proper inflation. **F**, Check circulation and sensation.

of the lower leg can cause an isolated fracture of the smaller bone (fibula). Because these two bones lie just beneath the skin, open fractures are common (Fig. 13-42). Lower leg fractures may cause a severe deformity in which the lower leg is bent at an unusual angle **(angulated).** These injuries are painful and result in an inability to move the leg. However, fractures of the fibula, and some very small fractures of the tibia, may not cause any deformity, and the victim may be able to continue to use the leg.

Initial care for the victim with a serious in-

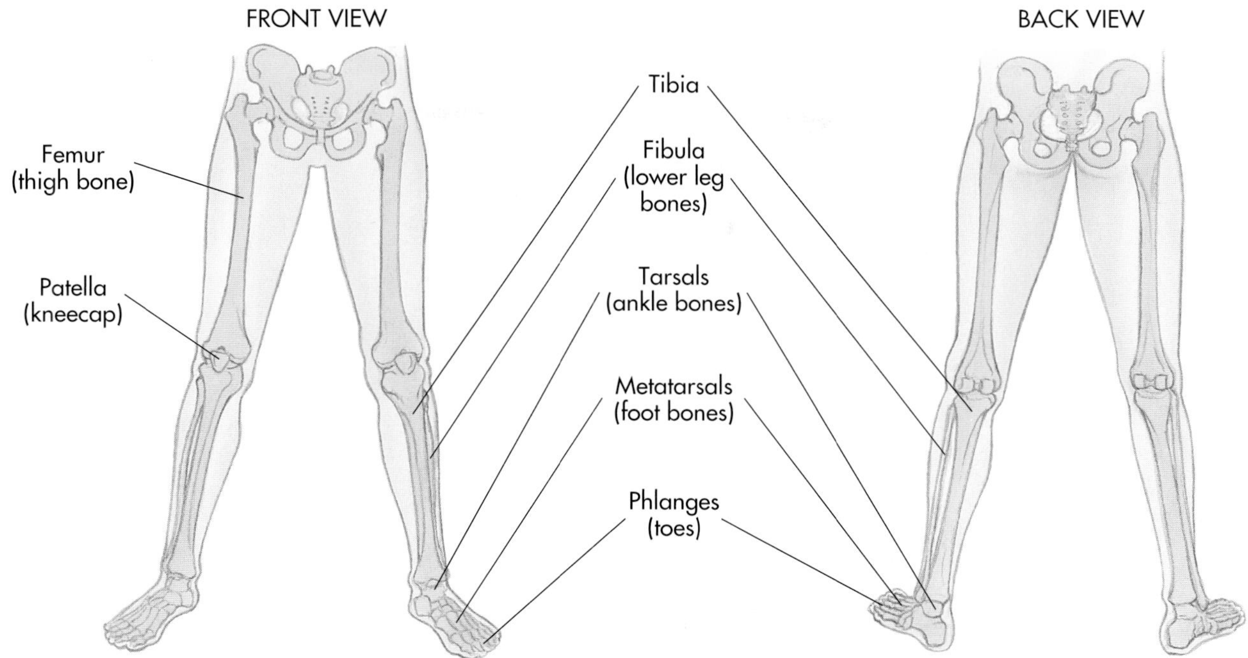

Figure 13-39 The Lower Extremities

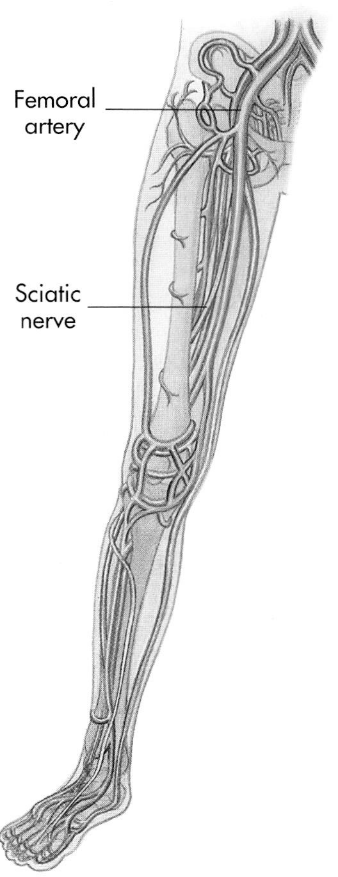

jury to the thigh or lower leg is to stop any external bleeding, immobilize the injured area, and help the victim rest in the most comfortable position. Summon more advanced medical personnel immediately. They are much better prepared to care for and transport a victim with a serious leg injury. The ground can adequately immobilize the legs, if the surface is relatively flat and firm, until more advanced medical personnel arrive.

However, there may be situations, such as moving the victim, in which you will need to splint an injured leg. Securing the injured leg to the uninjured leg with several wide cravats is one simple method. If a pillow or rolled blanket is available, place one between the legs and bind the legs together in several places above and below the site of the injury (Fig. 13-43). If rigid splints are available, apply one long splint to the outside of the injured leg, extending above the hip and beyond the foot. Place a shorter padded one on the inside of the leg, also extending be-

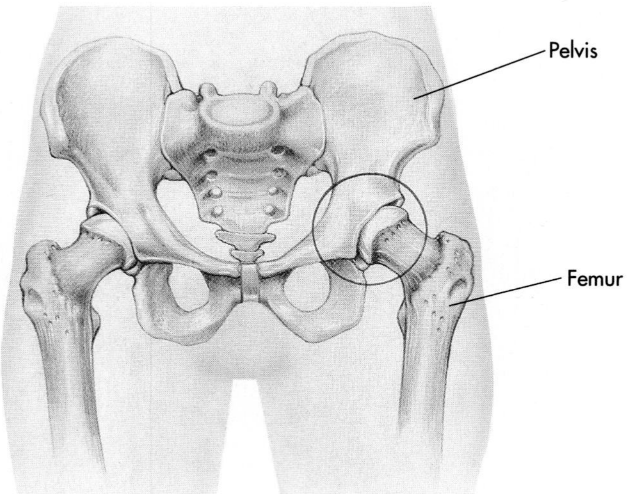

Figure 13-40 The upper end of the femur meets the pelvis at the hip joint.

yond the foot. Secure the splints to the leg with cravats (Fig. 13-44). Other commercial splints, such as air splints or vacuum splints, can also be used if available. Regardless of the type of splint applied, always check and recheck circulation and sensation of the foot. Apply ice or a cold pack to reduce pain and swelling.

A fractured femur can injure the femoral artery, and serious bleeding can result. The likelihood of shock is great. Therefore take steps to minimize shock. Keep the victim lying down and try to keep him or her calm. Keep the victim from getting chilled or overheated, administer oxygen if it is available and you are trained to use it, and make sure that more advanced medical personnel have

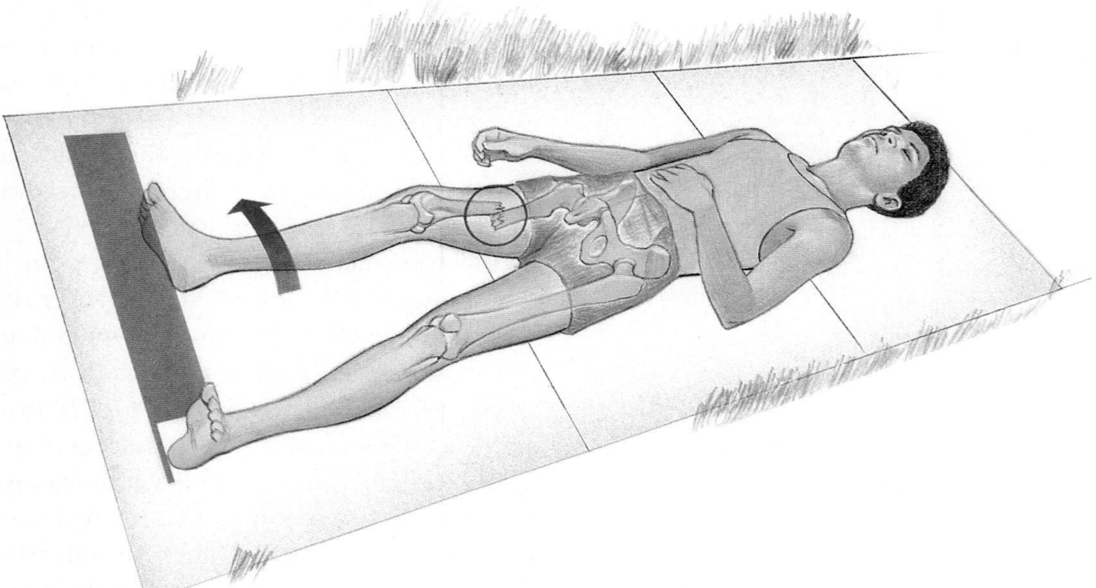

Figure 13-41 A fractured femur often produces a characteristic deformity. The injured leg is shorter than the uninjured leg and may be turned outward.

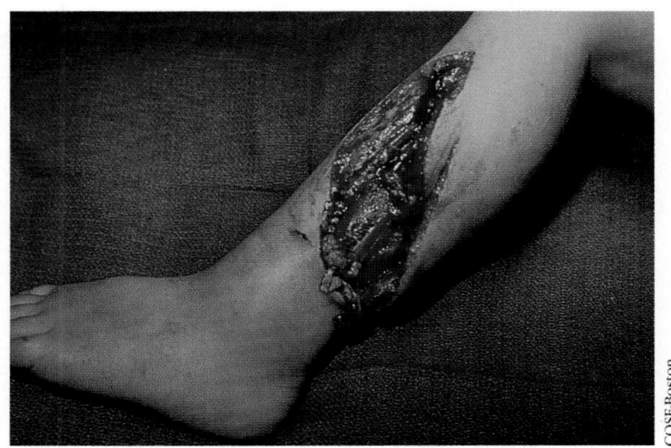

Figure 13-42 Open fractures of the lower leg are common.

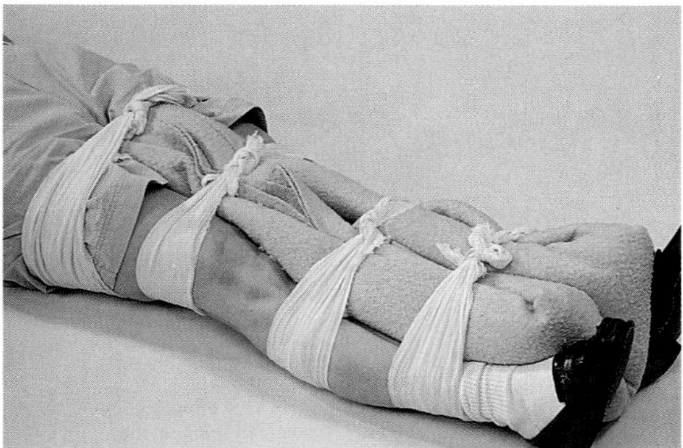

Figure 13-43 To splint an injured leg, secure the injured leg to the uninjured leg with cravats. A pillow or rolled blanket can be placed between the legs.

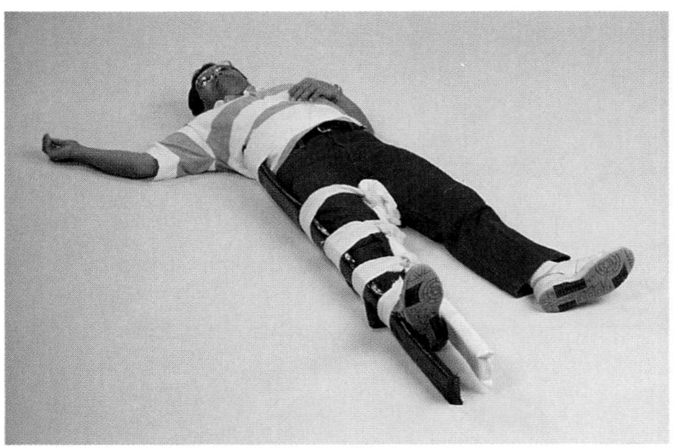

Figure 13-44 Rigid splints can also be used to splint an injured leg.

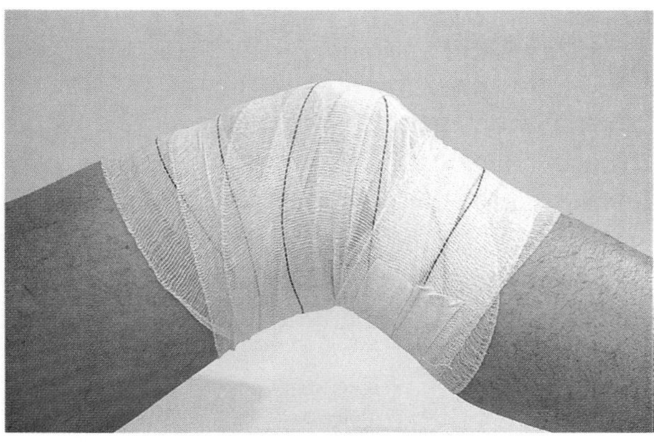

Figure 13-45 A figure-eight pattern is also used to apply a pressure bandage to the knee.

been summoned. Monitor the ABCs and vital signs for changes in the victim's level of consciousness.

Knee Injuries

The knee joint is very vulnerable to injury. The knee includes the lower end of the femur, the upper ends of the tibia and fibula, and the patella (kneecap). The kneecap is a free-floating bone that moves on the lower front surface of the thigh bone. Knee injuries range from cuts and bruises to sprains, fractures, and dislocations. Deep lacerations in the knee area can later cause severe joint infections. Sprains, fractures, and dislocations of the knee are common in athletic activities that involve quick movements or exert unusual force on the knee.

The kneecap is unprotected in that it lies directly beneath the skin. This part of the knee is very vulnerable to bruises and lacerations, as well as dislocations. Violent forces to the front of the knee, such as those caused by hitting the dashboard of a motor vehicle or by falling and landing on bent knees, can fracture the kneecap.

To care for an injured knee, first control any external bleeding. Apply a pressure bandage using a figure-eight pattern (Fig. 13-45). If the knee is bent and cannot be straightened with-

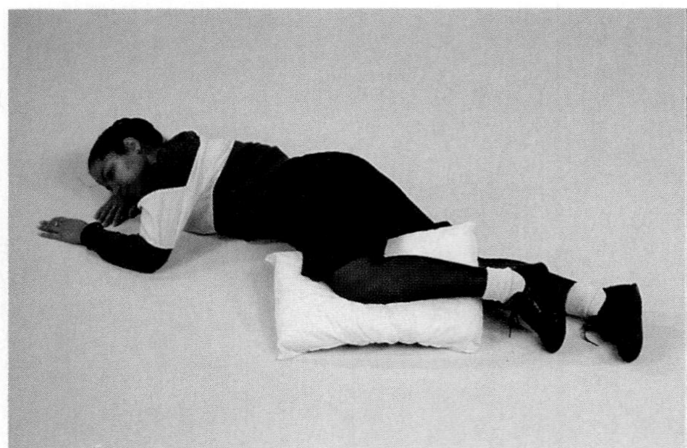

Figure 13-46 Support a knee injury in the bent position if the victim cannot straighten the knee.

out pain, support it in the bent position (Fig. 13-46). If the knee is straight or can be straightened without pain, splint the leg as you would for an injury of the thigh or lower leg or apply a long rigid splint to the leg. Other commercial splints can also be used if available. Apply ice or a cold pack. Help the victim to rest in a comfortable position. Summon more advanced medical personnel.

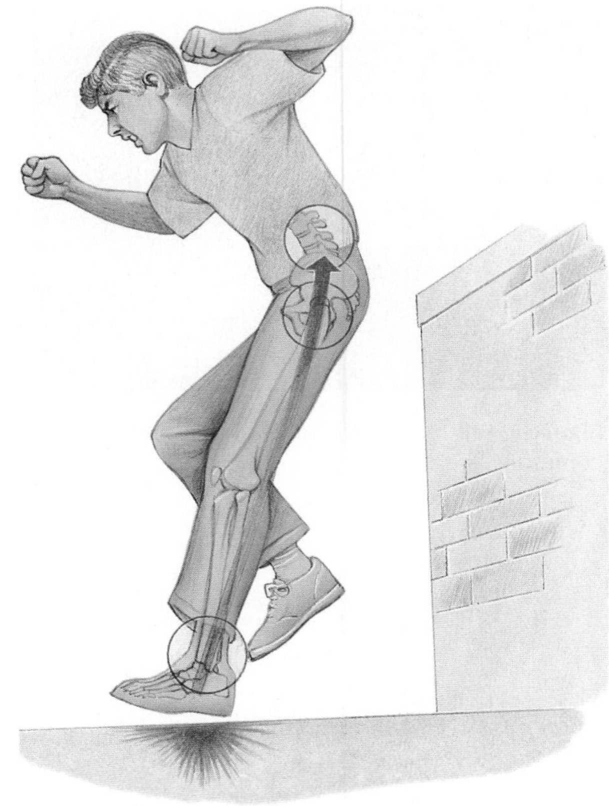

Figure 13-47 In a jump or fall from a height, the impact can be transmitted up the legs, causing injuries to the thighs, hips, or spine.

Ankle and Foot Injuries

Ankle and foot injuries are commonly caused by twisting forces. Injuries range from minor sprains with little swelling and pain that heal with a few days' rest to fractures and dislocations. As with other joint injuries, you cannot always distinguish between minor and severe injuries. You should initially care for all ankle and foot injuries as if they are serious. As with other lower extremity injuries, if the ankle or foot is painful to move, if it cannot bear weight, or if the foot or ankle is swollen, a physician should evaluate the injury. Foot injuries may also involve the toes. Although these injuries are painful, they are rarely serious.

Fractures of the feet and ankles can occur when a person forcefully lands on the heel. With any great force, such as falling from a height and landing on the feet, fractures are possible. The force of the impact may also be transmitted up the legs. This can result in an injury elsewhere in the body, such as the thigh, pelvis, or spine (Fig. 13-47).

Care for ankle and foot injuries by controlling external bleeding and immobilizing the ankle and foot in the best way possible. Some commercial splints are specifically designed for this area. One common splint for the ankle is an air splint (Fig. 13-48). If you must improvise, you can use a soft splint, such as a pillow or folded blanket. Secure the splint to the injured area with two or three cravats or a roller bandage (Fig. 13-49). Once it is splinted, elevate the injured ankle or foot to help reduce the swelling. Apply ice or a cold pack. Suspect that any victim who has fallen or jumped from a

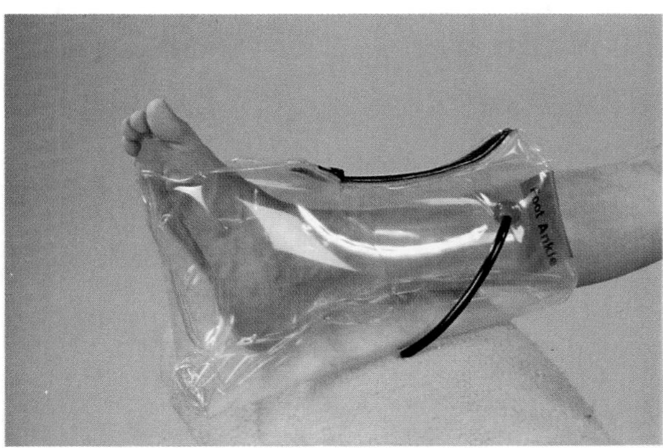

Figure 13-48 An air splint can be used to immobilize an injured foot or ankle.

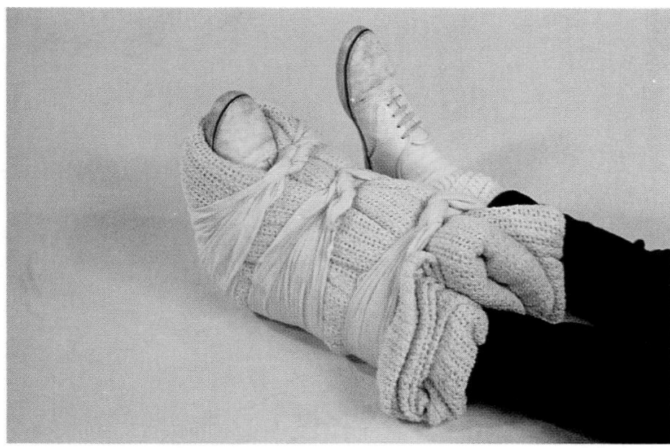

Figure 13-49 An injured ankle can be immobilized with a pillow or folded blanket secured with two or three cravats.

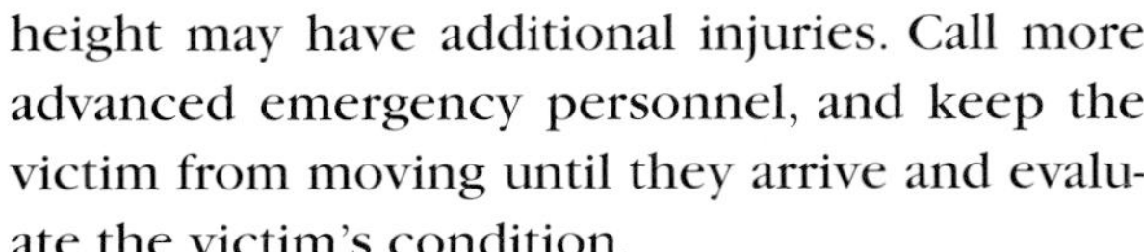
height may have additional injuries. Call more advanced emergency personnel, and keep the victim from moving until they arrive and evaluate the victim's condition.

◆ TRACTION SPLINT

A **traction splint** is a special type of splinting device used primarily to immobilize fractures of the thigh (femur). One end attaches to the hip and the other to the ankle. When traction is engaged, a constant, steady pull is applied against opposite ends of the leg, holding the fractured bone ends in a near-normal position (Fig. 13-50). Because each different commercial brand of traction splint has its own unique method of application, rescuers must be thoroughly familiar with and proficient in the technique of applying the brand of splint being used. It requires two well-trained rescuers working together. Because applying a traction splint requires a special device and two trained rescuers, it is not a device you are likely to use. However, you may be asked to assist more advanced medical personnel in applying a traction splint.

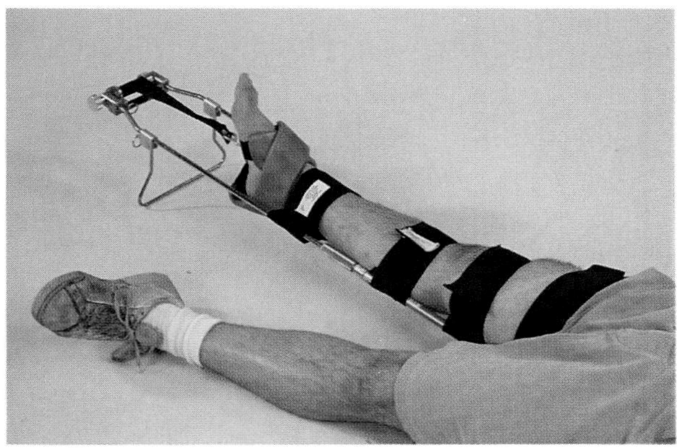

Figure 13-50 A traction splint is primarily used to immobilize fractures of the femur.

Use the activities in Unit 13 of the workbook to help you review the material in this chapter.

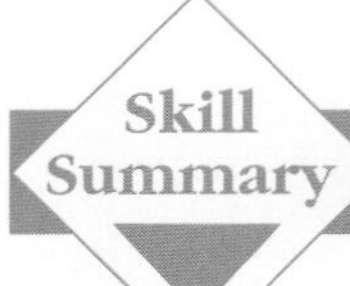

Applying a Rigid Splint

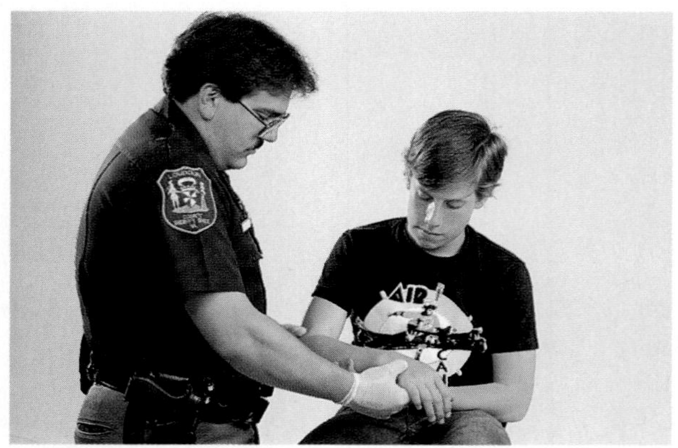

1. Support injured area.

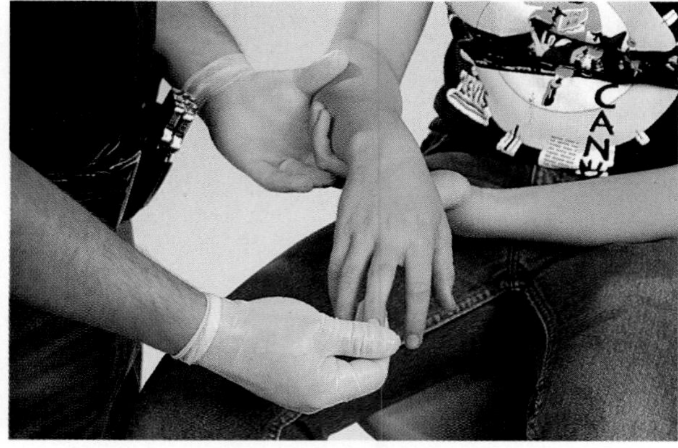

2. Check circulation and sensation below the injured area.

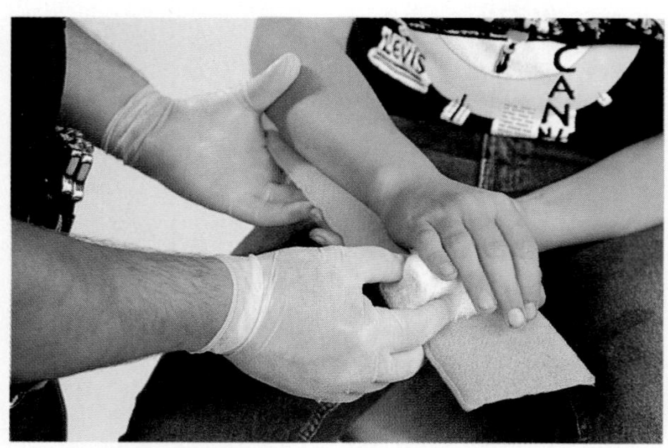

3. Position splint.

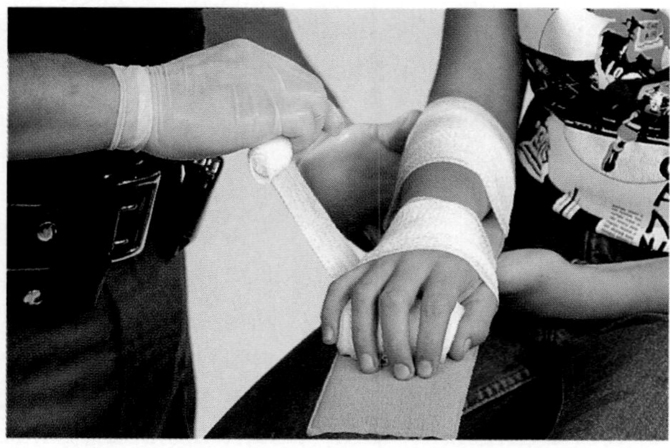

4. Secure splint.

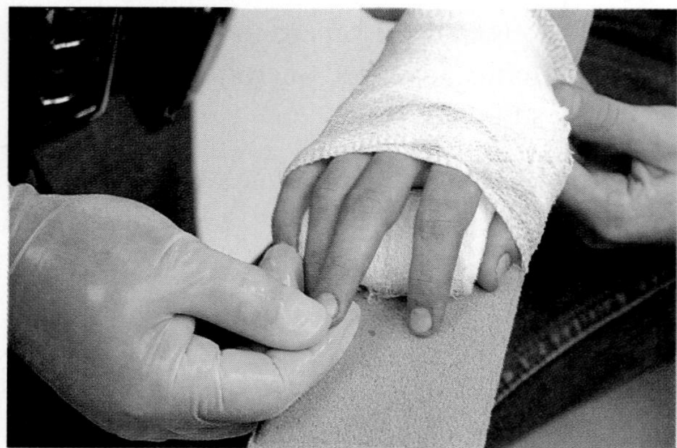

5. Recheck circulation and sensation.

Applying a Sling and Binder

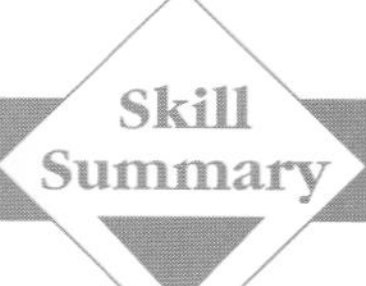

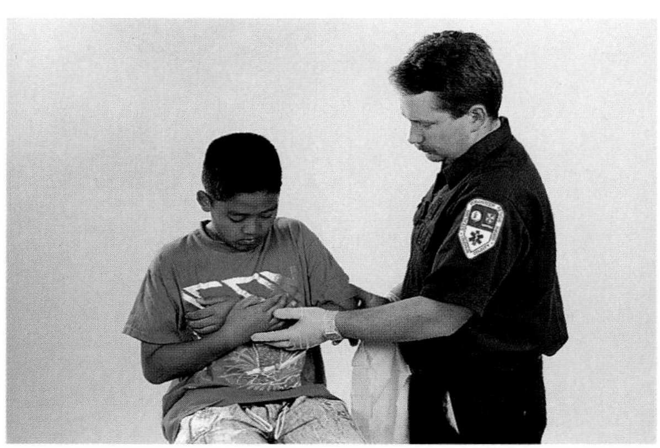

1. Support injured area.

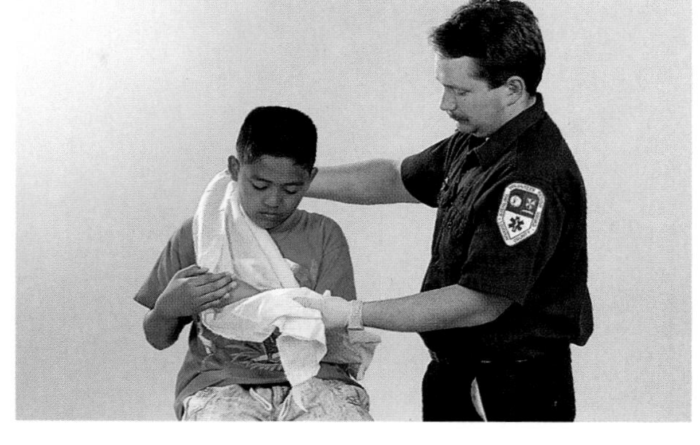

2. Position triangular bandage.

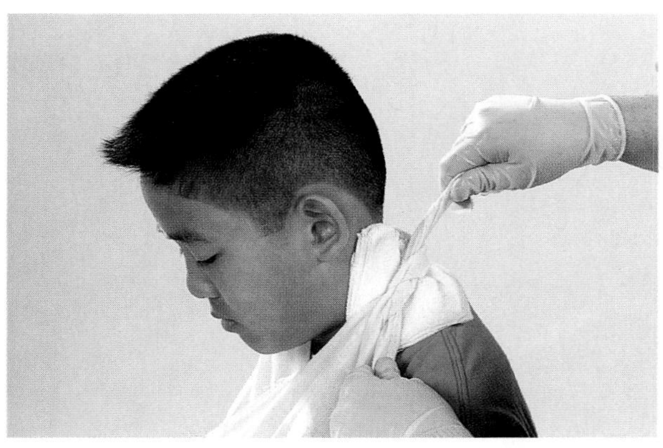

3. Tie ends.

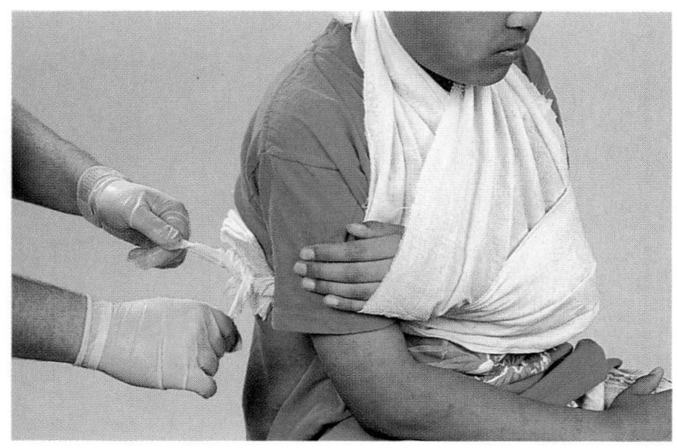

4. Secure arm to chest.

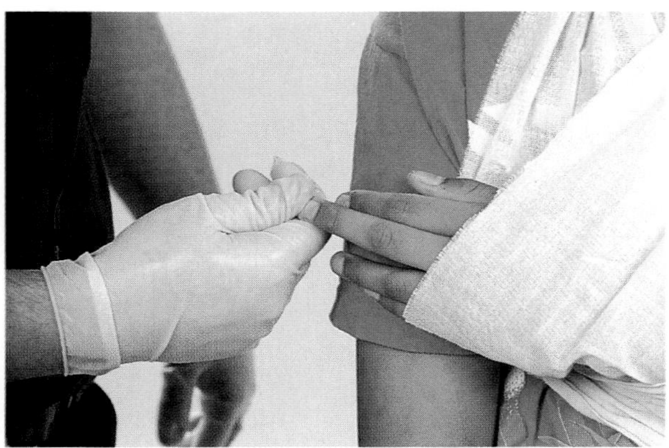

5. Recheck circulation and sensation.

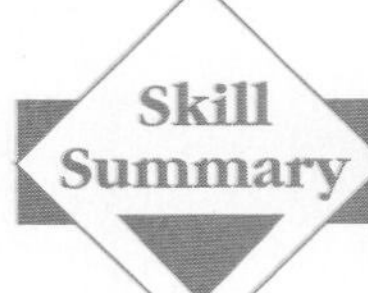

Applying an Anatomic Splint

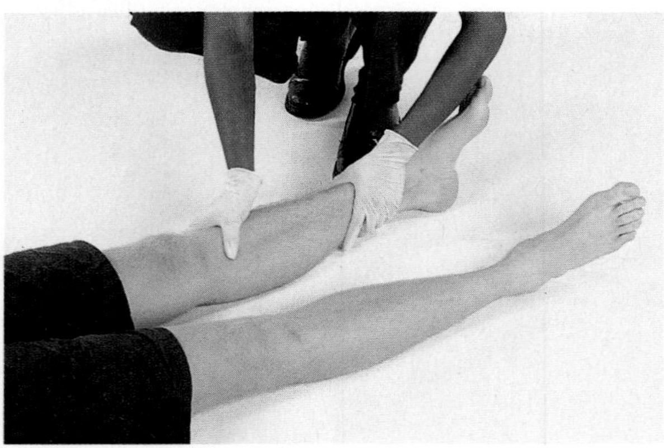

1. Support injured area.

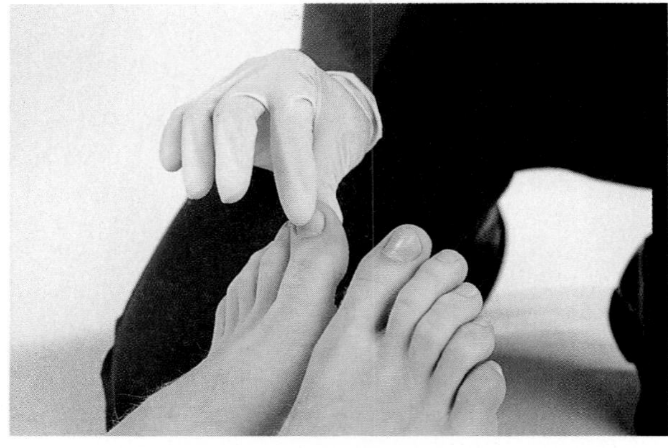

2. Check circulation and sensation below injured area.

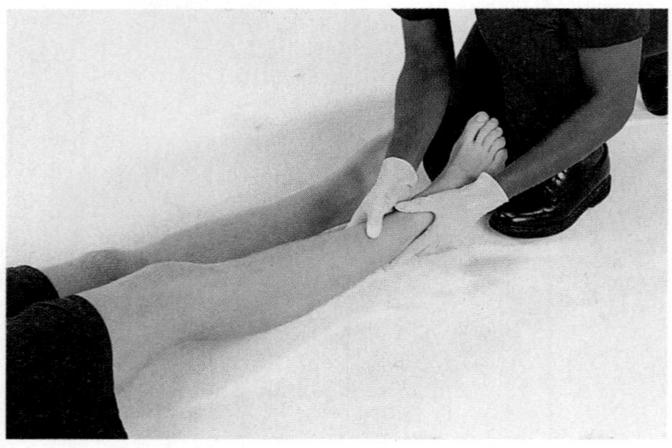

3. Move uninjured limb next to injured limb.

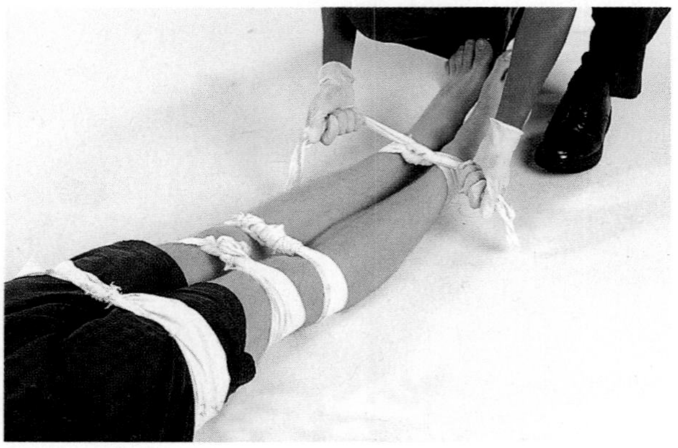

4. Secure injured limb to uninjured limb.

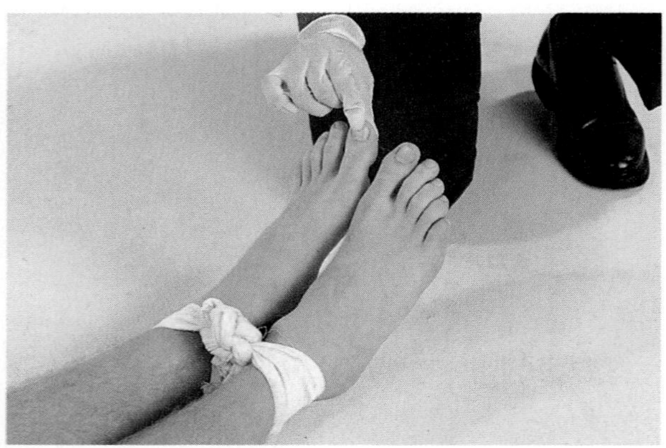

5. Recheck circulation and sensation.

Applying a Soft Splint

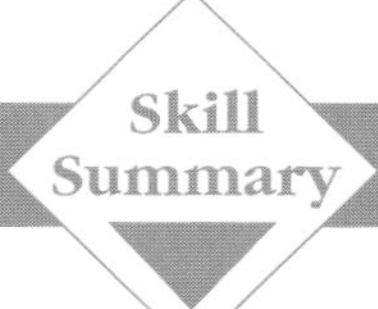

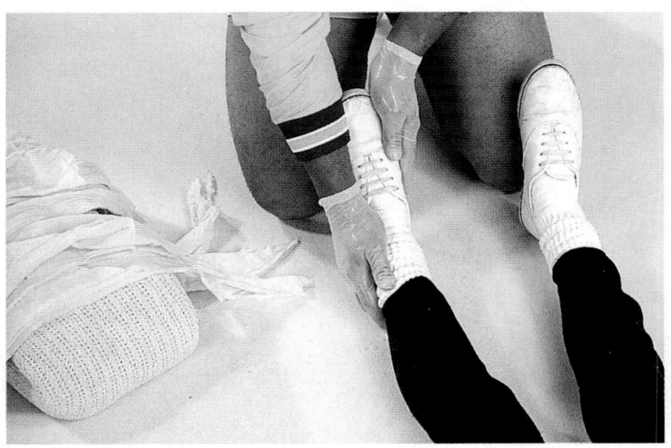

1. Support injured area.

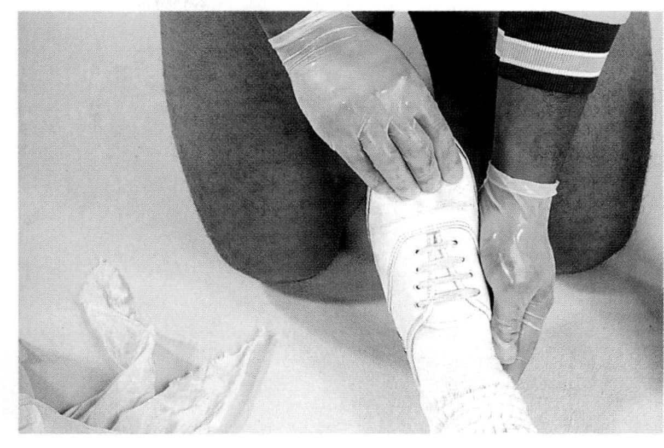

2. Check circulation and sensation below injured area.*

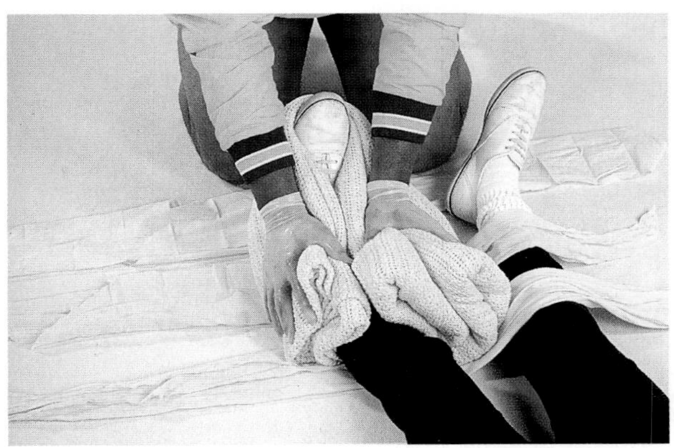

3. Position splint.

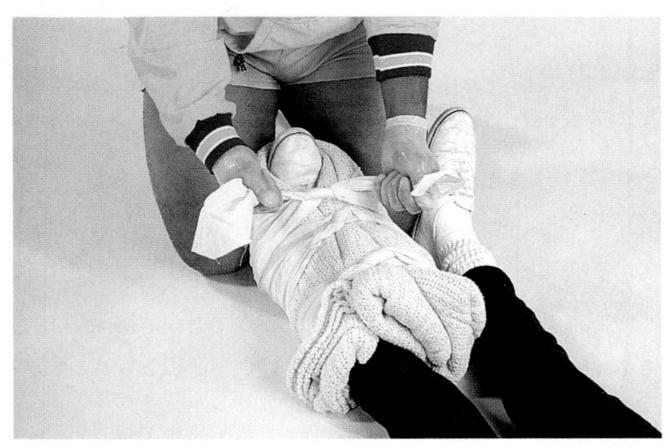

4. Secure splint.

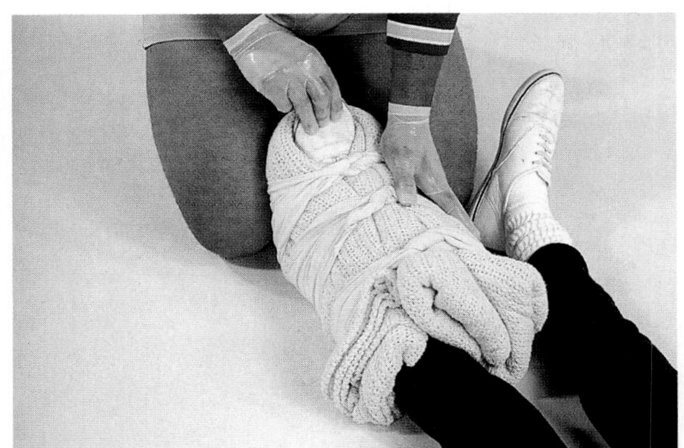

5. Recheck circulation and sensation.*

* It may not be possible to check circulation in an injured foot, ankle, or leg if a sock or a shoe is in place. Also, a recheck may not be possible if the soft splint is particularly bulky.

Injuries to the Head, Neck, and Back

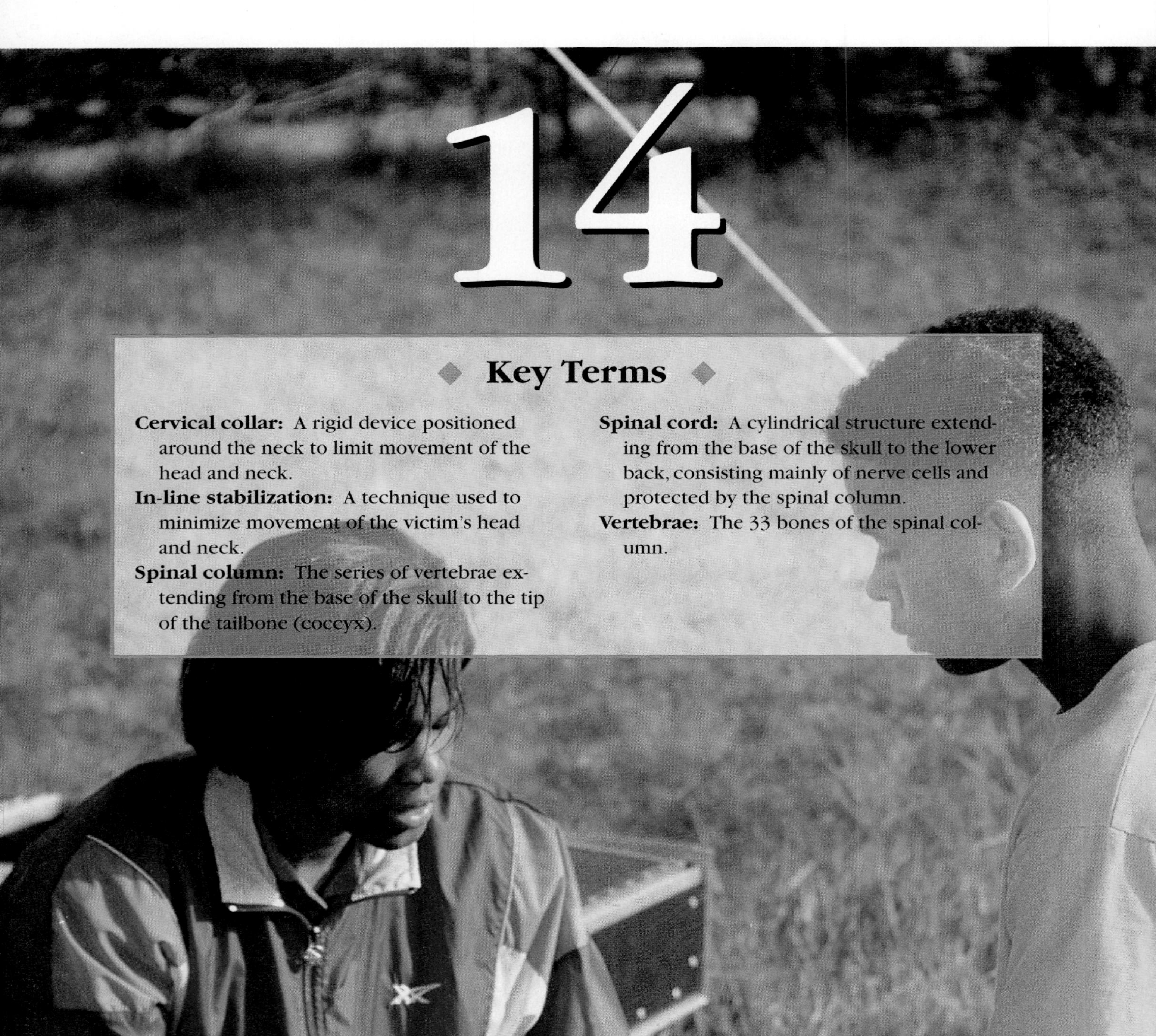

14

Key Terms

Cervical collar: A rigid device positioned around the neck to limit movement of the head and neck.

In-line stabilization: A technique used to minimize movement of the victim's head and neck.

Spinal column: The series of vertebrae extending from the base of the skull to the tip of the tailbone (coccyx).

Spinal cord: A cylindrical structure extending from the base of the skull to the lower back, consisting mainly of nerve cells and protected by the spinal column.

Vertebrae: The 33 bones of the spinal column.

◆ Knowledge Objectives ◆

After reading this chapter and completing the class activities, you should be able to —

- Relate the mechanism of injury to potential injuries of the head, neck, and back.
- List the signs and symptoms of head, neck and back injury.
- Describe the general care for head, neck, and back injuries.
- Describe the care for specific head injuries.
- Describe the method of determining if a responsive patient may have a back injury.
- Explain the importance of minimizing movement of a victim with a possible head, neck, or back injury.
- *Discuss various ways of preventing head, neck, and back injuries.

* Specifies an Enrichment section objective.

◆ Attitude Objectives ◆

After reading this chapter and completing the class activities, you should be able to —

- Understand the long-term consequences of a head, neck, or back injury.

◆ Skill Objectives ◆

After reading this chapter and completing the class activities, you should be able to —

- Perform the proper care for specific head injuries.
- Demonstrate how to open the airway of a victim with suspected head, neck, or back injury.
- Demonstrate how to evaluate a responsive victim with a suspected head, neck, or back injury.
- Demonstrate in-line stabilization of the head and neck.
- *Demonstrate the proper techniques for immobilizing a victim with a possible neck or back injury.

* Specifies an Enrichment section objective.

It's spring break at the beach. High school and college students are having fun in the sun. The weather is great, the water refreshing. The day is perfect for a game of touch football on the beach.

Later in the day, the tide comes in and the game becomes more aggressive. Players lunge into the surf to catch passes and runners. As the game is about to end, the quarterback throws a long pass. The receiver has the

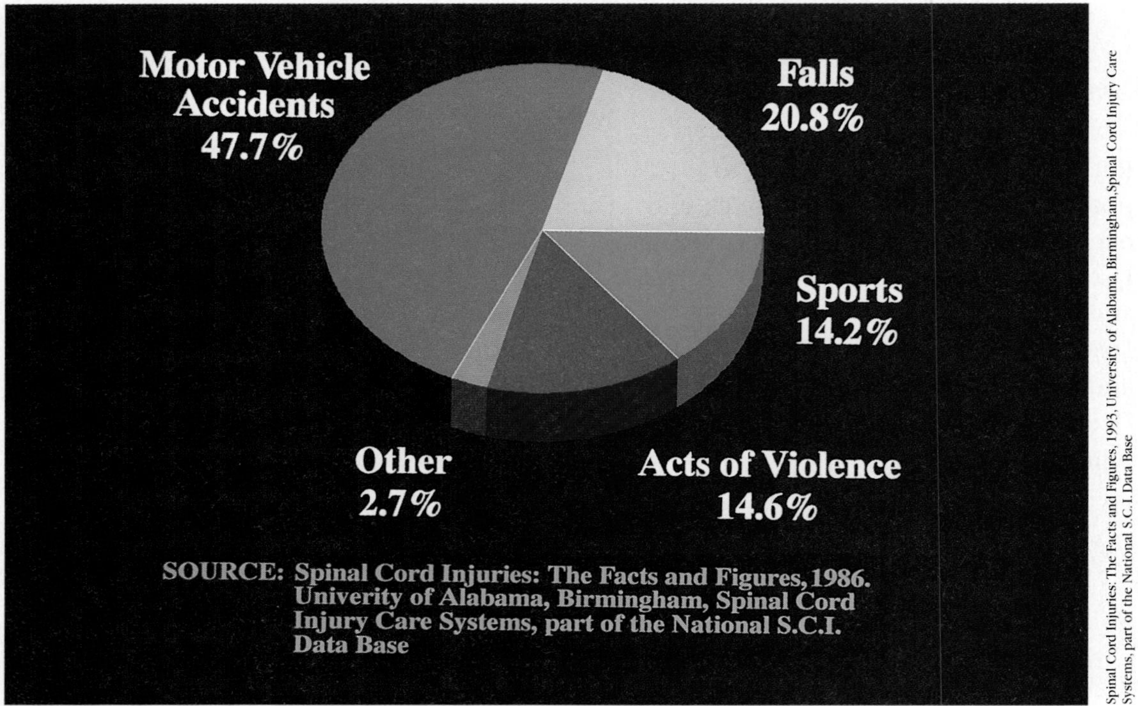

Spinal Cord Injuries: The Facts and Figures, 1993, University of Alabama, Birmingham, Spinal Cord Injury Care Systems, part of the National S.C.I. Data Base

Figure 14-1 Sports-related injuries account for 13 percent of all spinal injuries.

chance to score the winning touchdown, or the defender can intercept the pass to guarantee victory. They both run into the surf and dive headfirst at the ball. As they strike the water, a wave crashes over them, forcing them under water and into a sandbar. Both players strike their heads on the sandy bottom. The result? Both are pulled from the surf by their friends and by lifeguards summoned to the scene. One player is lucky and escapes with only a concussion. The other, not so lucky, suffers a broken neck and is paralyzed for life.

◆ INTRODUCTION

Although injuries to the head, neck, and back account for only a small percentage of all injuries, they cause more than half the fatalities. Each year, nearly 2 million Americans suffer a head, neck, or back injury serious enough to require medical care. Most of these victims are males between the ages of 15 and 30. Motor vehicle collisions account for about half of all head, neck, and back injuries. Other causes include falls, sports and recreational activities, and violent acts, such as assault (Fig. 14-1).

Besides those who die each year in America as a result of head and spine injury, nearly 80,000 victims become permanently disabled. Today there are hundreds of thousands of permanently disabled victims of head, neck, or back injuries in the United States. These survivors have a wide range of physical and mental impairments, including paralysis, speech and memory problems, and behavioral disorders.

Fortunately, prompt, appropriate care can help minimize the damage from most head, neck, and back injuries. In this chapter, you will learn how to recognize when a head, neck, or back injury may be serious. You will also learn how to provide the appropriate care to minimize injuries to the head, neck, and back.

◆ RECOGNIZING SERIOUS HEAD, NECK, AND BACK INJURIES

Injuries to the head, neck, or back can damage both bone and soft tissue, including brain tissue and the spinal cord. It is usually difficult to determine the extent of damage in head, neck, and back injuries. In most cases, the only way to assess the damage is by having a physician examination and X-ray films or a **CAT scan** taken in an emergency department or hospital X-ray department. Since you have no way of knowing exactly how severe an injury is, *always* provide initial care as if the injury is serious.

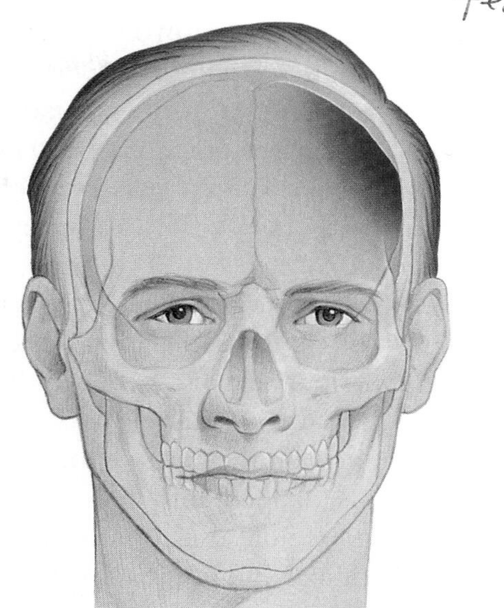

Figure 14-2 Injuries to the head can rupture blood vessels in the brain. Pressure builds within the skull as blood accumulates, causing brain injury.

The Head

The head contains the brain, special sense organs, the mouth and nose, and related structures. It is formed by the skull and the face. The four flat bones of the skull are fused together to form a hollow shell. This hollow shell, the cranial cavity, contains the brain. The face is on the front of the skull. The bones of the face include the bones of the cheek, forehead, nose, and jaw.

Injuries to the head can affect the brain. The brain can be bruised or lacerated when extreme force causes it to move in the skull, stretching and tearing tissue or bumping against the skull. Extreme force, or trauma, can fracture the thick bones of the skull. The major concern with skull fractures is brain damage. Blood from a ruptured vessel in the brain can accumulate in the skull (Fig. 14-2). Bleeding in the skull can occur rapidly or slowly over a period of days. This bleeding will affect the brain, causing changes in consciousness, vision, balance and coordination, and sometimes numbness or weakness of an arm or leg. An altered level of consciousness is often the first and most important sign of a serious head injury.

The Neck

The neck, which contains the larynx and part of the trachea, also contains major blood vessels, muscles and tendons, and the cervical bones of the spine. Any injury to the neck must be considered serious. The neck can be injured by crushing or penetrating forces and by sharp-edged objects that can lacerate tissues and blood vessels or by forces that cause the neck to stretch or bend too far. Injuries to muscles, bones, and nerves can result in severe pain and headaches.

The Back

The back is made up of soft tissue, bones, cartilage, nerves, muscles, tendons, and ligaments. It supports the skull, shoulder bones, ribs, and pelvis and protects the spinal cord and other vital organs. One part of the back that is susceptible to severe injury is the spine.

The **spine** is a strong, flexible column of vertebrae, extending from the base of the skull to the tip of the tailbone, that supports the head and the trunk and encases and protects the spinal cord. The spine is also called the ***spinal***

column or **vertebral column.** The spine consists of small bones, ***vertebrae,*** with circular openings. The vertebrae are separated from each other by cushions of cartilage called **disks** (Fig. 14-3, *A*). This **cartilage** acts as a shock absorber when a person walks, runs, or jumps. The ***spinal cord,*** a cylindrical structure consisting mainly of nerve cells and extending from the base of the skull to the lower back, runs through the hollow part of the vertebrae. Nerve branches extend to various parts of the body through openings on the sides of the vertebrae.

The spine is divided into five regions: the cervical (neck) region, the thoracic (midback) region, the lumbar (lower back) region, the sacrum (lower back, part of the pelvic region), and the coccyx (tailbone), the small triangular bone at the lower end of the spinal column (Fig.14-3, *B*). Injuries to the spinal column include fractures and dislocations of the vertebrae, sprained ligaments, and compression or displacement of the disks between the vertebrae.

Injuries to the back can fracture the vertebrae and sprain the ligaments. These injuries may heal without problems. With severe injuries, however, the vertebrae may shift and compress or sever the spinal cord. Doing so can cause temporary or permanent paralysis, even death. The extent of the paralysis depends on which area of the spinal cord is damaged. A person with a back injury may have tenderness in the injured area or pain when trying to move. The victim may have pain even if he or she is not touched in the injured area or does not try to move. The victim may also have numbness or weakness, tingling in the arms or legs, difficulty breathing, or loss of bladder or bowel control. Ability to move or walk does not rule out the possibility of back injury.

Causes of Injury

Consider the cause of the injury to help you determine whether a person has received a head, neck, or back injury. Size up the scene and think about the forces involved in the injury. Strong forces are likely to cause severe injury to the head, neck, and back. For example, a driver whose head breaks a car windshield in a crash may have a serious head, neck, or back injury. A diver who hits his or her head on the bottom of a swimming pool may also have a serious head, neck, or back injury. Evaluate the scene for clues as to whether a head, neck, or back injury has occurred.

Injury Situations

You should consider the possibility of a serious head, neck, or back injury in a number of situations. These include—

- A fall from a height greater than the victim's height.
- Any diving mishap.
- A person found unconscious for unknown reasons.
- Any injury, such as from a car or other vehicle, involving severe blunt force to the head or trunk.
- Any injury, such as a gunshot wound, that penetrates the head or trunk.
- A motor vehicle crash involving a driver or passengers not wearing safety belts or that results in a broken windshield or a deformed steering wheel.
- Any person thrown from a motor vehicle.
- Any injury in which a victim's helmet is broken, including a motorcycle, bicycle, football, or other sports helmet, or an industrial hard hat.
- Any incident involving a lightning strike.
- Any person found unconscious in water 5 feet deep or less.

Signs and Symptoms of Head, Neck, and Back Injuries

You also may notice certain signs and symptoms that indicate a head, neck, or back injury. These signs and symptoms may be obvious

Figure 14-3 **A,** Vertebrae are separated by cushions of cartilage called disks. **B**, The spine is divided into five regions. Traumatic injury to a region of the spine can paralyze specific body areas.

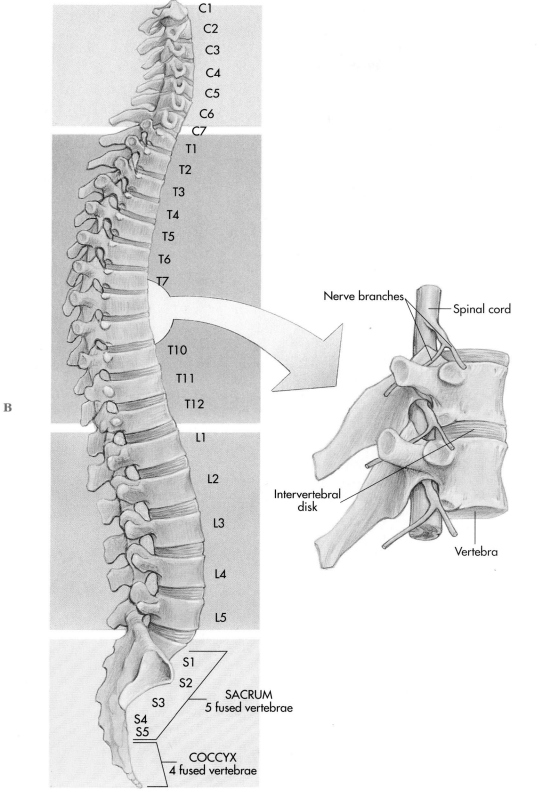

A Call From the Beach

When Liz Linton scanned the surf from one of the lifeguard towers at Newport Beach, she saw a man bobbing awkwardly in the water. As she swam through the surf toward the victim, she felt an uneasy sense of déja vu. As a lifeguard for two summers, Linton had already saved one victim of spinal cord injury from drowning. The memory reminded her of how quickly a serious injury can occur.

As she swam, she marked the victim's position, fearful he would sink before she could reach him. Fortunately, she was able to get to him in time. He told her his head and shoulders had hit the bottom when he dove through a wave. She held him carefully to protect his neck and back from movement and began taking slow steps back to shore. He was partially paralyzed.

The man rescued by Liz Linton was lucky. After many months of rehabilitation, he regained full use of his body. Others are not so lucky. Each year, approximately 1000 people suffer permanent spinal cord damage from diving mishaps. Statisticians describe the typical accident victim with grim accuracy. He is a single, white male between the ages of 15 and 30, an active person who loves sports and the outdoors.

Bill Brooks fits that description. The 29-year-old Davidsonville, Maryland, man was diving through an inner tube into a pool on a Sunday afternoon when his neck hit the tube. As he floated in the water, he remembers being aware of everything, yet powerless to move.

At the hospital, doctors told Brooks he was a "C5" quadriplegic, which described the area of the neck that he had damaged. In college, Brooks had played baseball, and after college, he had taken up slow-pitch softball. In one afternoon, Brooks had lost control of his legs, chest, and arms. He lost the ability to dress himself, feed himself, go to the bathroom by himself, or even hold a softball in his hand.

Months of rehabilitation have improved Brooks's life. Although his right hand remains paralyzed, with his left hand, Brooks can grasp a telephone and control a computer mouse. With the computer mouse, he is learning to design the sprinkler systems he once installed as the foreman for a sprinkler company. Brooks is learning to survive with his injury, but his spinal nerves will never regenerate, so there is little hope that he will ever walk again. Many states and private organizations have begun education and prevention campaigns to reduce the high rate of diving injuries. The American Red Cross offers the following tips to prevent head and back injuries:

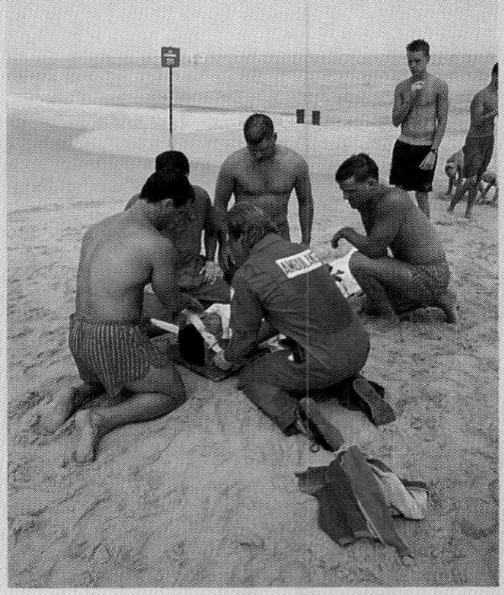

- Check for adequate water depth. When you first enter the water, enter feet first. Even from the edge of a pool or dock, diving into water less than 9 feet deep is potentially dangerous. There is always the possibility of injury if you go straight down and strike the bottom.
- For diving off a 1-meter diving board, the water depth should be a minimum of 11 feet 6 inches. This depth should extend 16 feet in front of the diver. The higher the board, the deeper the water should be. Pools at homes, motels, or hotels often do not have an adequate area for safe diving.
- Never dive into an above-ground pool.
- Starting blocks should be used only by trained swimmers under the supervision of a qualified coach.
- Never drink and dive.
- Never dive in water where you cannot see the bottom. Objects, such as logs or pilings, may be hidden below the surface.
- Running into the water and then diving head-first into the waves is dangerous.
- If you are body surfing, always keep your arms out in front of you to protect your head and neck.

right away or may develop later. These signs and symptoms include—

- Changes in the level of consciousness.
- Pain or pressure in the head, neck, or back.
- Tingling or loss of sensation in the extremities (arms and legs).
- Partial or complete loss of movement of any body part.
- Unusual bumps or depressions on the head, neck, or back.
- Blood or other fluids draining from the ears or nose.
- Profuse external bleeding of the head, neck, or back.
- Seizures.
- Impaired breathing as a result of injury.
- Impaired vision as a result of injury.
- Nausea or vomiting.
- Persistent headache.
- Loss of balance.
- Bruising of the head, especially around the eyes and behind the ears.
- Combative or aggressive behavior.

These signs and symptoms alone do not always suggest a head, neck, or back injury, but they may when combined with the cause of the injury. Regardless of the situation, always summon more advanced medical personnel when you suspect a head, neck, or back injury.

◆ CARE FOR HEAD, NECK, AND BACK INJURIES

Head, neck, and back injuries can become life-threatening emergencies. A serious injury can cause a victim to stop breathing. Care for serious head, neck, and back injuries also involves keeping the respiratory, circulatory, and nervous systems functioning. Provide the following care while waiting for more advanced medical personnel to arrive:

- Minimize movement of the head, neck, and back.
- Maintain an open airway.
- Control any external bleeding.
- Monitor vital signs.
- Keep the victim from getting chilled or overheated.
- Administer oxygen if it is available and you are trained to do so.

Minimize Movement

Caring for a head, neck, or back injury is similar to caring for any other serious soft tissue or musculoskeletal injury. You should immobilize the injured area and control any bleeding. Because movement of an injured head, neck, or back can irreversibly damage the spinal cord, keep the victim as still as possible until you can obtain more advanced care. To minimize movement of the head and neck, use a technique called ***in-line stabilization.***

With this technique, you place your hands on both sides of the victim's head, gently position it, if necessary, in line with the body, and support it in that position. You can do this in various ways, depending on the condition in which you find the victim (Fig. 14-4). This skill is simple to perform and can impact the victim's outcome. Keeping the head in this anatomically correct position helps prevent further damage to the spinal column. If a second rescuer is available, that person can give care for any other conditions while you keep the head and neck stable.

There are some circumstances in which you would *not* move the victim's head in line with the body. These include—

- When the victim's head is severely angled to one side, unless you can gently do so without encountering physical resistance or causing pain.
- When the victim complains of pain, pressure, or muscle spasms in the neck when you begin to align the head with the body.
- When you feel resistance when attempting to move the head in line with the body.

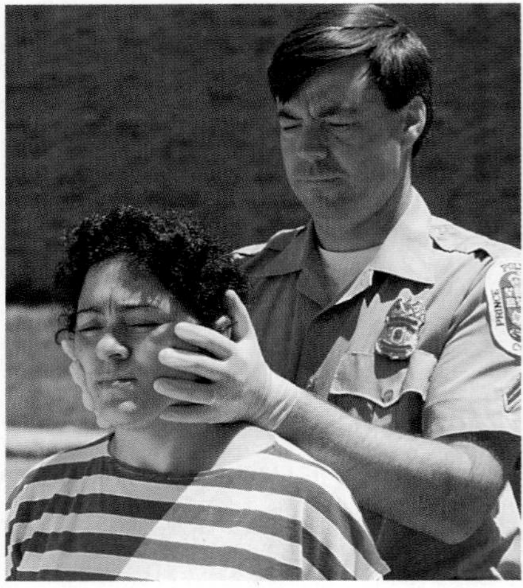

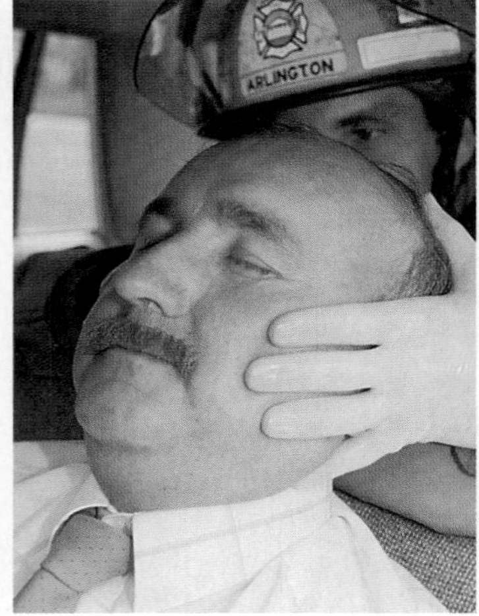

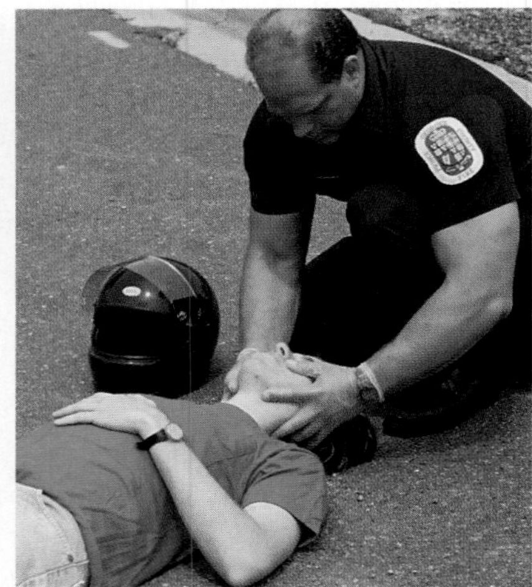

Figure 14-4 Support the victim's head in line with the body using in-line stabilization.

In these circumstances, support the victim's head in the position in which you found it.

After the victim's head is stabilized, as previously described, a rigid ***cervical collar*** should be applied (Fig. 14-5). This collar helps minimize movement of the head and neck and keeps the head in line with the body. Applying a cervical collar requires two rescuers. While one rescuer maintains in-line stabilization, another carefully applies an appropriately sized cervical collar (Fig. 14-6). An appropriately sized collar is one that fits securely, with the victim's chin resting in the proper position and the head maintained in line with the body. Some cervical collars come with specific manufacturer's instructions for proper sizing. Do not apply a cervical collar in a circumstance in which you would not align the head with the body.

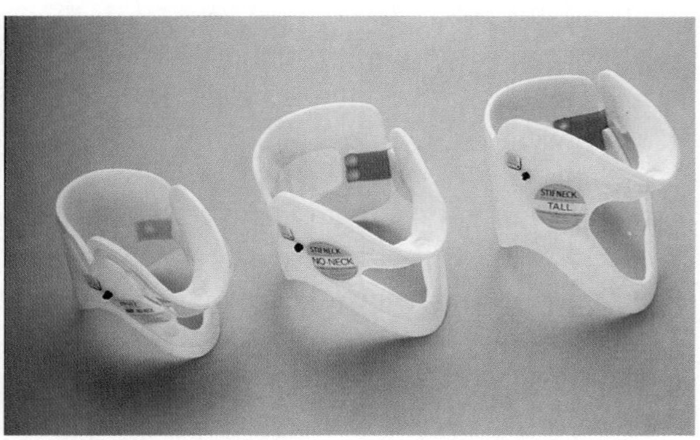

Figure 14-5 There is a variety of rigid cervical collars available.

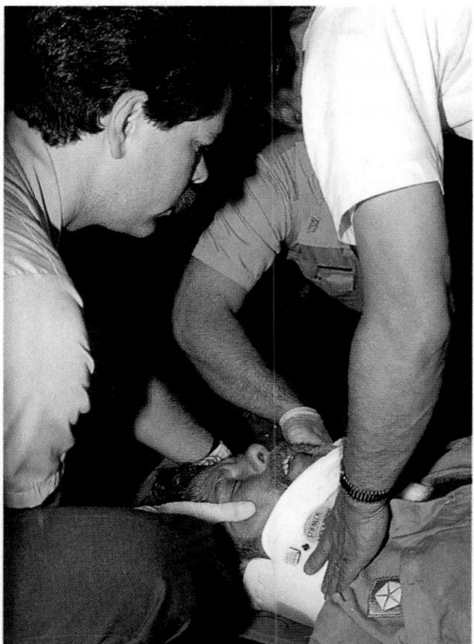

Figure 14-6 Apply a cervical collar that fits securely, with the chin resting in the designated position and the head held in line with the body.

Maintain an Open Airway

A cry of pain, regular chest movement, or the sound of breathing tells you the victim is breathing. If the victim is breathing, maintain in-line stabilization in the position in which you found him or her. If the victim begins to vomit and you have suctioning equipment available, suction the mouth. Otherwise, turn the victim onto one side to keep the airway clear. Turning the victim is more easily done by several people. Ask other rescuers to help roll the victim's body while you maintain in-line stabilization. If the victim is unconscious, attempt to insert an oral or nasal airway to help maintain an open airway. Use the jaw-thrust technique to open the airway to minimize movement of the head and neck. Do not use a nasal airway if you suspect a severe head injury.

Ongoing Assessment

Continue your ongoing assessment and monitor the vital signs. Pay close attention to the victim's level of consciousness and breathing. A serious head injury will often cause changes in the level of consciousness. The victim may give inappropriate responses when asked name, time, place, or what happened or may speak incoherently. The victim may be drowsy, appear to fall asleep, and then suddenly awaken or lose consciousness completely. Breathing may become rapid or irregular. Because injury to the head, neck, or back can paralyze chest nerves and muscles, breathing can stop. If this happens, perform rescue breathing, using the jaw thrust to open the airway. Victims of serious head or back injury need supplemental oxygen. Administer oxygen if it is available and you are trained to do so.

Control External Bleeding

Some head and neck injuries include soft tissue damage. Because there are many blood vessels in the head and two major arteries—the carotid arteries—in the neck, the victim can lose large amounts of blood quickly. If there is external bleeding, control it promptly with dressings, direct pressure, and a pressure bandage while minimizing movement to the head and neck.

Keep the Victim from Getting Chilled or Overheated

A serious injury to the head or back can disrupt the body's normal heating or cooling mechanism. When this mechanism does not function properly, a person is more susceptible to shock. For example, a person suffering a serious head or back injury while outside on a cold day will be more likely to suffer from **hypothermia,** a life-threatening cooling of the body. This is because the normal shivering response to rewarm the body may not work. It is always important to minimize shock by keeping the victim from getting chilled or overheated.

◆ CARE FOR SPECIFIC HEAD INJURIES

The head is easily injured because it lacks the padding of muscle and fat that are in other areas of the body. You can feel bone just beneath the surface of the skin over most of the head, including the chin, cheekbones, and scalp (Fig. 14-7).

Concussion

Any significant force to the head can cause a **concussion,** a temporary impairment of brain function. A concussion usually does not result in permanent physical damage to brain tissue. In most cases, the victim only loses consciousness for an instant and may say that he or she "blacked out" or "saw stars." Sometimes a concussion causes a loss of consciousness for a longer period. At other times, a victim may be confused or have amnesia (memory loss). Anyone who may have a concussion should be examined by a physician. Summon advanced

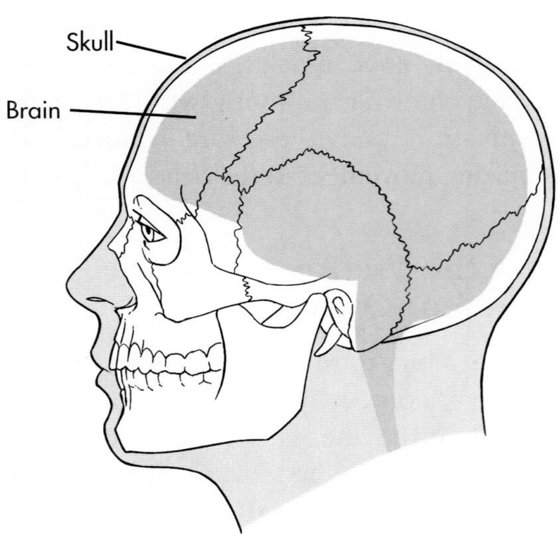

Figure 14-7 The head is easily injured because it lacks the padding of muscle and fat found in other areas of the body.

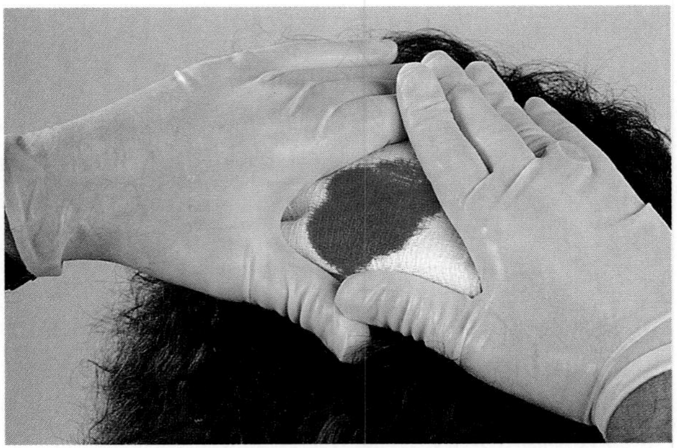

Figure 14-8 To avoid putting pressure on a deep scalp wound, apply pressure around the wound.

medical help if you suspect a person has a concussion.

Scalp Injury

Scalp bleeding can be minor or severe. The bleeding is usually easily controlled with direct pressure. Because the skull may be injured, be careful to press gently at first. If you feel a depression, a spongy area, or bone fragments, do not put direct pressure on the wound. Attempt to control bleeding with pressure on the area around the wound (Fig. 14-8). Examine the injured area carefully because the victim's hair may hide part of the wound. If you are unsure about the extent of a scalp injury, summon more advanced medical personnel. They will be better able to evaluate the injury.

If the victim has only an open wound, control the bleeding with direct pressure. Apply several dressings and hold them in place with your gloved hand (Fig. 14-9, *A*). Secure the dressings with a roller bandage (Fig. 14-9, *B*). Use a pressure bandage if necessary.

A

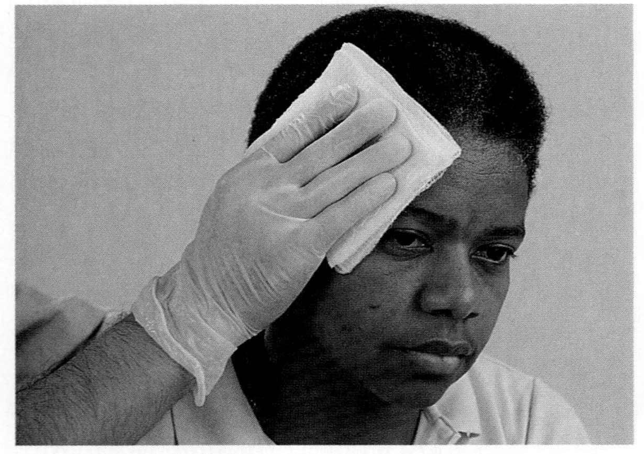

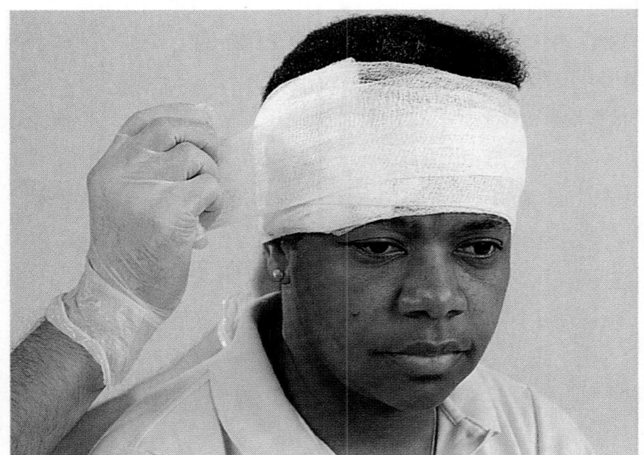

B

Figure 14-9 Apply pressure to control bleeding from a scalp wound. **A**, Hold several dressings against the wound with your hand. **B**, Then secure the dressings with a bandage.

A 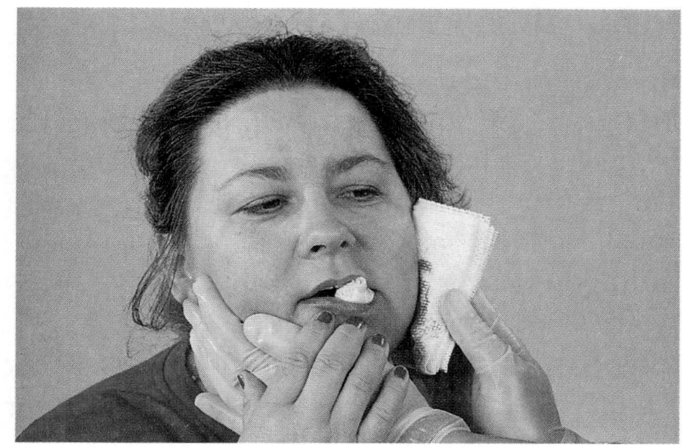

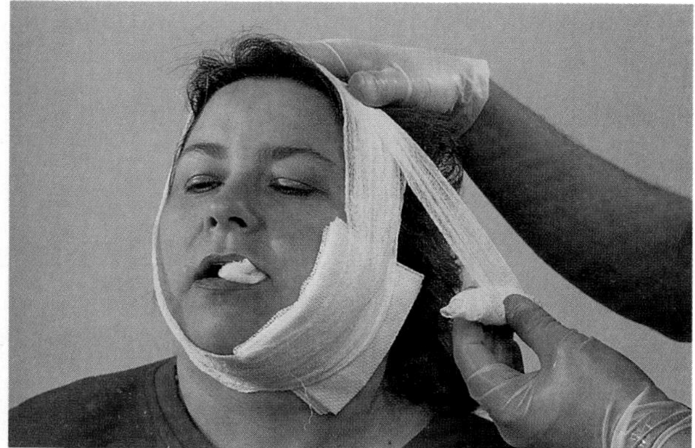 B

Figure 14-10 **A,** Control bleeding inside the cheek by placing a rolled dressing inside the mouth against the wound. Control external bleeding of the cheek using a dressing to apply pressure directly to the wound. **B,** Apply a pressure bandage.

Cheek Injury

Injury to the cheek often involves soft tissue only. Control bleeding from the cheek in the same way as other soft tissue bleeding. The only difference is that you may have to control bleeding on either the outside or the inside of the cheek or in both places. Begin by examining both the outside and inside of the cheek. Bleeding from inside may result from a blow that caused the teeth to cut the inside of the cheek or from a laceration or puncture wound outside. To control bleeding, place several folded dressings inside the mouth, against the cheek. If possible, have the victim hold them in place. If external bleeding is also present, place dressings on the outside of the cheek and apply direct pressure with your gloved hand or a pressure bandage (Fig. 14-10, *A-B*).

If an object passes completely through the cheek and becomes embedded, you may have to remove it to control bleeding and keep the airway open. This circumstance is the only exception to the general rule of not removing embedded objects from the body. An embedded object in the cheek cannot be easily stabilized, makes control of bleeding more difficult, and may become dislodged and obstruct the airway. You can remove the object by pulling it out the same way it entered. If doing this is difficult or is painful to the victim, leave the object in place and stabilize it with bulky dressings and bandages.

If you remove the object, fold or roll several dressings and place them inside the mouth. Be sure not to obstruct the airway. Apply dressings to the outside of the cheek also. The victim may not be able to hold these in place, so you may have to hold them. Bleeding inside the cheek can cause the victim to swallow blood. If the victim swallows enough blood, nausea or vomiting could result, which would complicate the situation. When possible, place the victim in a seated position, leaning slightly forward so that blood will not drain into the throat. As with any situation involving serious bleeding or an embedded object, summon more advanced medical personnel.

Nose Injury

Nose injuries are usually caused by a blow from a blunt object. The result is often a nosebleed. High blood pressure or changes in altitude can also cause nosebleeds. In most cases, you can control the bleeding by having the victim sit with the head slightly forward while

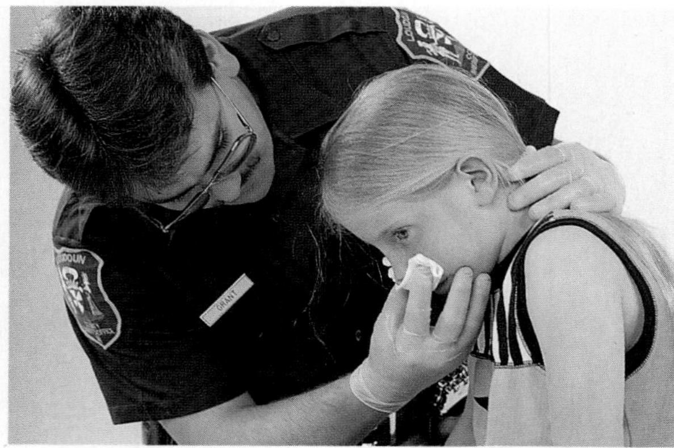

Figure 14-11 To control a nosebleed, have the victim lean forward and pinch the nostrils together for a minimum of 10 minutes.

pinching the nostrils together for a minimum of 10 minutes (Fig. 14-11). Other methods of controlling the bleeding include applying an ice pack to the bridge of the nose or putting pressure on the upper lip just beneath the nose.

Once you have controlled the bleeding, tell the victim to avoid rubbing, blowing, or picking the nose, since this could restart the bleeding. Later, the victim may apply a little petroleum jelly inside the nostril to help keep it moist.

You should summon more advanced medical personnel if the bleeding cannot be controlled, if it stops and then recurs, or if the victim says the bleeding is the result of high blood pressure. If the victim loses consciousness, place the victim on his or her side to allow blood to drain from the nose.

If you think an object is in the nostril, look into the nostril. If you see the object and can easily grasp it with your fingers, then do so. However, do not probe the nostril with your finger. Doing so may push the object farther into the nose and cause bleeding or make it more difficult to remove the object later. If the object cannot be removed easily, the victim should receive medical care.

Eye Injury

Injuries to the eye can involve the eyeball and the bone and the soft tissue surrounding the eye. Blunt objects, like a fist or a baseball, may injure the eye and surrounding area, or a smaller object may penetrate the eyeball. Care for open or closed wounds *around* the eye as you would for any other soft tissue injury.

Injury to the eyeball itself requires different care. Injuries that penetrate the eyeball or cause the eye to be removed from its socket are very serious and can cause blindness. Never put direct pressure on the eyeball. Instead, follow these guidelines when providing care for an eye in which an object has been embedded:

1. Place the victim on his or her back.
2. Do not attempt to remove any object embedded in the eye.
3. Place a sterile dressing around the object (Fig. 14-12, *A*).
4. Stabilize any embedded object in place as best you can. You can do this by placing a paper cup to support the object (Fig. 14-12, *B*).
5. Apply a bandage (Fig. 14-12, *C*).

Foreign bodies that get in the eye, such as dirt, sand, or slivers of wood or metal, are irritating and can cause significant damage. The eye immediately produces tears in an attempt to flush out such objects. Pain is often severe. The victim may have difficulty opening the eye because light further irritates it.

First, try to remove the foreign body by telling the victim to blink several times. Then try gently flushing the eye with water (Fig. 14-13). If the object remains, the victim should receive professional medical attention. Flushing the eye with water is also appropriate if the victim has any chemical in his or her eye. If a chemical is in the eye, the eye should be continuously flushed for at least 15 minutes or until more advanced medical personnel arrive and take over care. Remove, or have the victim remove, contact lenses, since they may trap chemicals against the eyeball.

A

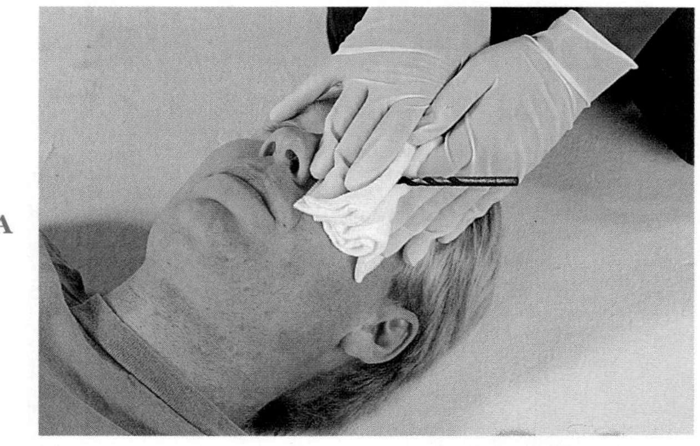

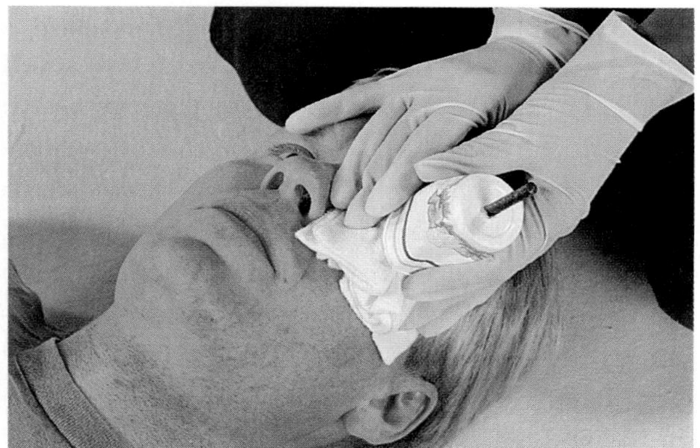

B

C

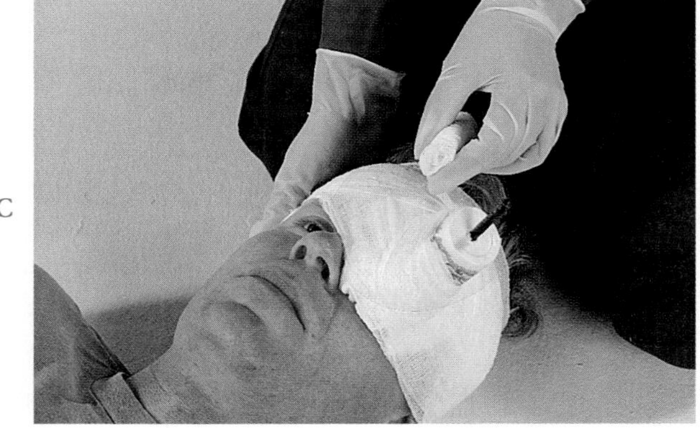

Figure 14-12 **A,** Place sterile dressings around an object impaled in the eye. **B,** Support the object with a paper cup. **C,** Carefully bandage the cup in place.

Ear Injury

Ear injuries are common. Either the soft tissue of the outer ear or the eardrum within the ear may be injured. Open wounds, such as lacerations or abrasions, can result from recreational injuries, such as being struck by a racquetball or falling off a bike. An avulsion of the ear may occur when a pierced earring catches on something and tears the earlobe. You can control bleeding from the soft tissues of the ear by applying direct pressure.

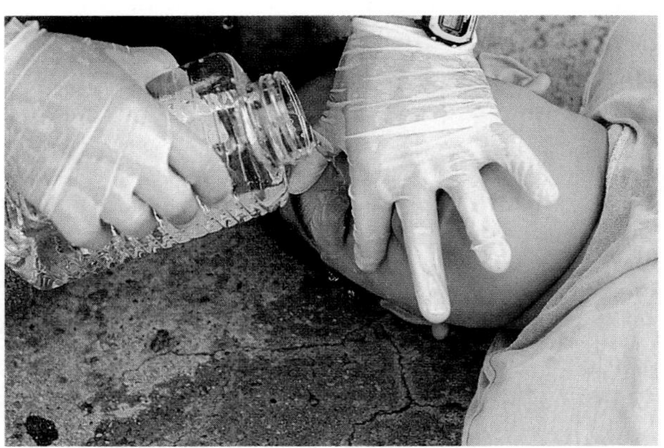

Figure 14-13 If a foreign body is in the eye, flush the eye gently with water.

If the victim has a serious head or back injury, blood or other fluid may be in the ear canal or draining from the ear. *Do not* attempt to stop this drainage with direct pressure. Instead, just cover the ear lightly with a sterile dressing, stabilize the head, neck, and back, and summon more advanced medical personnel.

The ear can also be injured internally. A direct blow to the head may rupture the eardrum. Sudden pressure changes, such as those caused by an explosion or a deep-water dive, can also injure the ear internally. The victim may lose hearing or balance or experience inner ear pain. These injuries require more advanced medical care.

A foreign object, such as dirt, an insect, or a piece of cotton, can easily become lodged in the ear canal. If you can easily see and grasp the object, remove it. Do *not* try to remove any object by using a pin, toothpick, or any sharp item. You could force the object farther back or puncture the eardrum. Sometimes you can remove the object if you pull down on the earlobe, tilt the head to the side, and shake or very gently strike the head on the side. If you cannot easily remove the object, the victim should be seen by a physician.

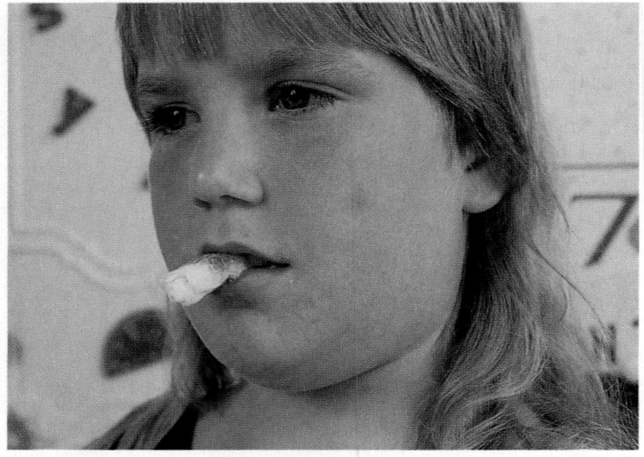

Figure 14-14 If a tooth is knocked out, place a sterile dressing in the space left by the tooth. Tell the victim to bite down.

Mouth, Jaw, and Neck Injury

Your primary concern for any injury to the mouth, jaw, or neck is to ensure an open airway. Injuries in these areas may cause breathing problems if blood or loose teeth obstruct the airway. A swollen or fractured trachea may also obstruct breathing.

If the victim is bleeding from the mouth and you do not suspect a serious head, neck, or back injury, place the victim in a seated position with the head tilted slightly forward. This position will allow any blood to drain from the mouth. If this position is not possible, place the victim on his or her side to allow blood to drain from the mouth.

For injuries that penetrate the lip, place a rolled dressing between the lip and the gum. You can place another dressing on the outer surface of the lip. If the tongue is bleeding, apply a dressing and direct pressure. Applying cold to the lips or tongue can help reduce swelling and ease pain. If the bleeding cannot be controlled, summon more advanced medical personnel.

If the injury knocked out one or more of the victim's teeth, control the bleeding and save any teeth so that they can be reinserted. To control the bleeding, roll a sterile dressing and insert it into the space left by the missing tooth. Have the victim bite down to maintain pressure (Fig. 14-14).

Opinions vary as to how a tooth should be saved. It is best to place the tooth in a cup of milk. If milk is not available, the tooth can be placed in cool water. If the tooth is dirty, first rinse it gently in running water. Hold the tooth by the crown; do not touch the root. Do not scrub the tooth or remove any tissue fragments. Another thought is to place the dislodged tooth or teeth in the injured person's mouth. Doing so is not always the best approach, since a crying child could aspirate the tooth. Also, the tooth could be swallowed with blood or saliva. You also may need to control serious bleeding in the mouth.

If the injury is severe enough for you to summon more advanced medical personnel, give the tooth to them when they arrive. If the injury is not severe, the victim should immediately seek a dentist who can replant the tooth and should get to that dentist within 30 minutes, if possible. Time is a critical factor if the tooth is to be successfully replanted. Ideally, the tooth should be replanted within an hour after the injury.

Injuries serious enough to fracture or dislocate the jaw can also cause other head or back injuries. Be sure to maintain an open airway. Check inside the mouth for bleeding. Control bleeding as you would for other head injuries. Minimize movement of the head and neck. Summon more advanced medical personnel.

Now Smile

Knocked-out teeth no longer spell doom for pearly whites. Most dentists can successfully replant a knocked-out tooth if they can do so quickly and if the tooth is properly cared for.

Replanting a tooth is similar to replanting a tree. On each tooth, tiny root fibers called periodontal fibers attach to the jawbone to hold the tooth in place. Inside the tooth, a canal filled with bundles of blood vessels and nerve ends runs from the tooth into the jawbone and surrounding tissues.

When these fibers and tissues are torn from the socket, it is important that they be replaced within an hour. Generally, the sooner the tooth is replanted, the greater the chance it will survive. The knocked-out tooth must be handled carefully to protect the fragile tissues. Be careful to pick up the tooth by the chewing edge (crown), not the root. Do not rub or handle the root part of the tooth. It is best to preserve the tooth by placing it in a closed container of cool, fresh milk until it reaches the dentist. Milk is not always available at an injury scene; cool water may be substituted.

A dentist or emergency physician will clean the tooth, taking care not to damage the root fibers. The tooth is then placed back into the socket and secured with special splinting devices. The devices keep the tooth stable for 2 to 3 weeks while the fibers reattach to the jawbone. The bundles of blood vessels and nerves grow back within 6 weeks.

REFERENCES

1. Bogert J, DDS, Executive Director, American Academy of Pediatric Dentists: Interview, April 1990.
2. Medford H, DDS: Acute care of an avulsed tooth, *Ann Emerg Med* 11:559, October 1982.

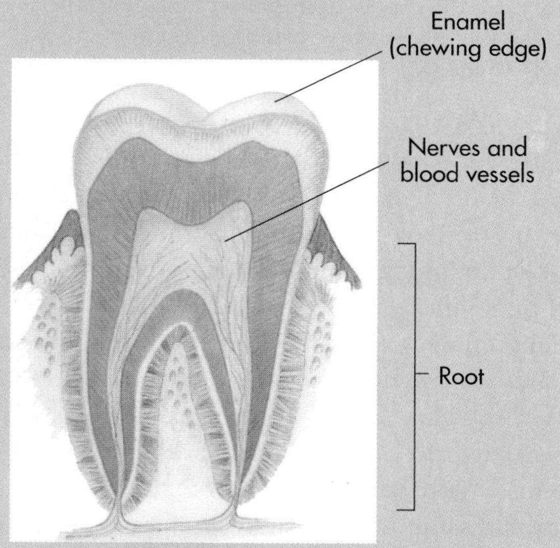

A tooth must be replaced so that periodontal fibers will reattach.

A soft tissue injury of the neck can cause severe bleeding and swelling that may obstruct the airway. Because the back also may be involved, care for a neck injury as you would a possible serious back injury. If the victim struck his or her neck on an object, such as a steering wheel, or was struck hard in the neck by an object, such as a stick, the injury could be devastating. This type of injury can fracture the trachea, causing an airway obstruction that requires immediate advanced medical attention. While waiting for more advanced medical personnel, try to keep the victim from moving and encourage him or her to breathe slowly. Control any external bleeding with direct pressure. Be careful not to apply pressure that constricts both carotid arteries or that interferes with breathing. Apply a pressure bandage so that it does not restrict blood flow (Fig. 14-15).

◆ SUMMARY

In this chapter, you have learned how to recognize and care for serious head, neck, and back injuries and specific injuries to the head and neck. To decide whether an injury is serious, you must consider its cause. Often the cause is

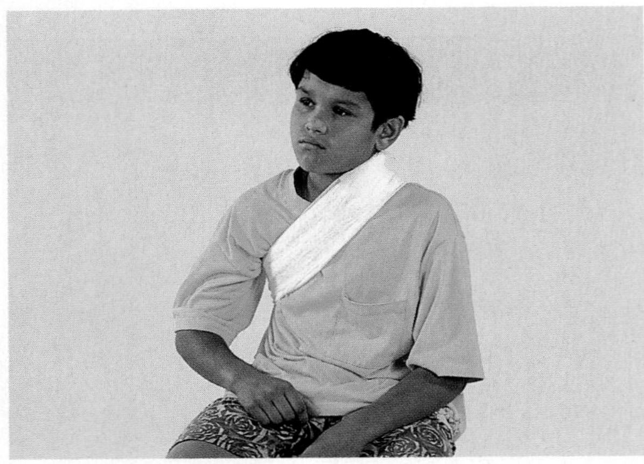

Figure 14-15 Apply a pressure bandage to the neck so that it does not restrict blood flow.

the best indicator of whether an injury to the head, neck, or back should be considered serious. If you have any doubts about the seriousness of an injury, summon more advanced medical personnel.

Like injuries elsewhere on the body, injuries to the head, neck, and back often involve both soft tissues and bone. Control bleeding as necessary, usually with direct pressure on the wound. With scalp injuries, be careful not to apply pressure to a possible skull fracture. With eye injuries, remember not to apply pressure on the eyeball.

If you suspect that the victim may have a serious head, neck, or back injury, minimize movement of the injured area when providing care. Minimizing movement is best accomplished by using in-line stabilization. Administer oxygen if it is available and you are trained to do so. Apply a cervical collar and secure the victim to a backboard if you must move the victim.

Use the activities in Unit 14 of the workbook to help you review the material in this chapter.

You Are the Responder

You respond to an industrial accident involving a person who has fallen from a height of approximately 10 feet. You arrive to find a male victim lying on his side. He is conscious but disoriented. He states he "blacked out" when he struck the ground. He also states that he has a tingling feeling in his legs and feet. Do you consider his injury serious? How would you provide care?

ENRICHMENT

◆ IMMOBILIZING THE VICTIM

Once a cervical collar has been applied and in-line stabilization maintained, the victim's entire body should be immobilized. This can be done using the following equipment:

- Rigid splint, such as a backboard
- Large towel or blanket
- Straps or triangular bandage(s) folded into a cravat(s) or rolls of 4-inch gauze

If you do not have a backboard available, support the victim in the position you found him or her until more advanced medical personnel arrive.

Once a cervical collar is in place, the victim is positioned on a backboard. This is done by "log-rolling" the victim onto the board. This technique keeps the head in line with the body. It requires a minimum of two rescuers: one to support the head and maintain in-line stabilization and another to position the back-

A

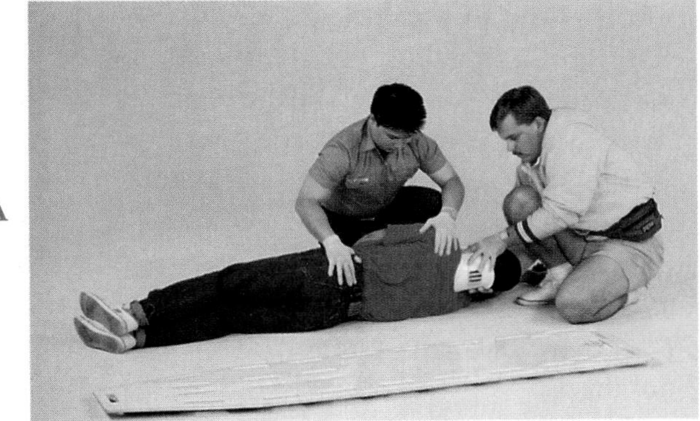

B

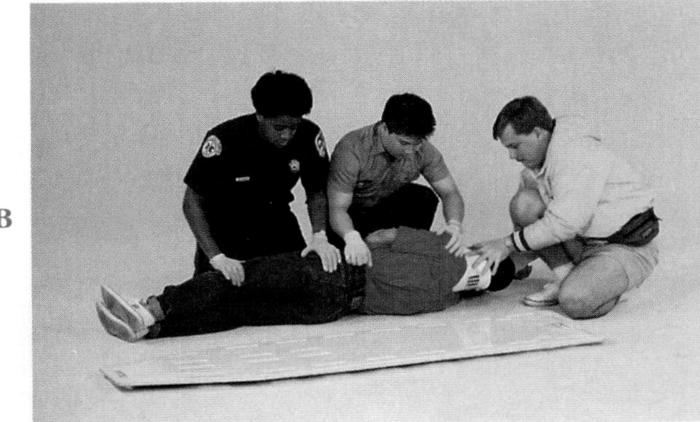

Figure 14-16 **A,** One rescuer maintains in-line stabilization while the second rescuer rolls the victim's body and positions the backboard. **B,** A third rescuer can help log-roll the victim and position the backboard.

board and roll the victim's body (Fig. 14-16, *A*). However, it is highly preferable to have three rescuers available to perform this technique. With three rescuers, one can provide in-line stabilization and the second and third can log-roll the victim and position the backboard (Fig. 14-16, *B*).

Once the victim is on the board, use several straps, cravats, or wide bandages to secure the victim's body to the backboard (Fig. 14-17). There are several ways to apply the straps used to strap the victim onto the board. A common way is to secure the chest by crisscrossing the straps. Regardless of which method is used, the straps should be snug but not so tight as to restrict movement of the chest during breathing. With the remaining straps, secure the victim's hips, thighs, and legs. Secure the hands in front of the body.

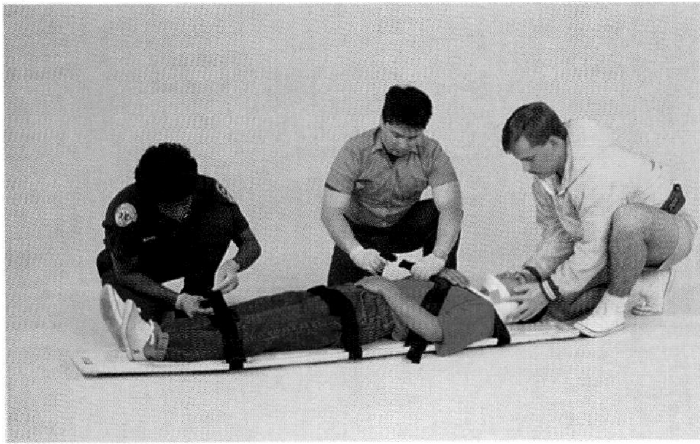

Figure 14-17 Secure the victim to the backboard.

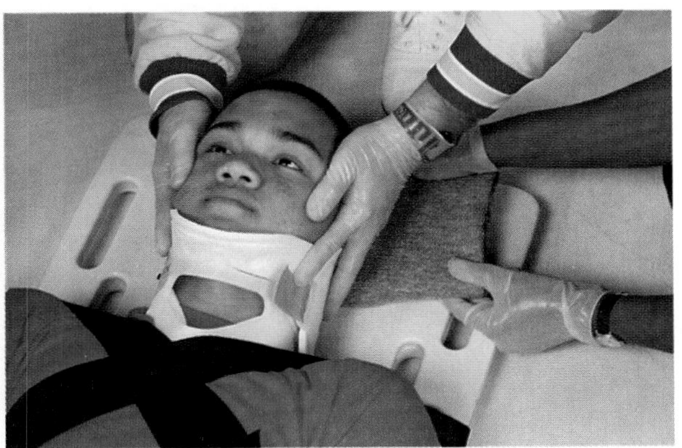

A

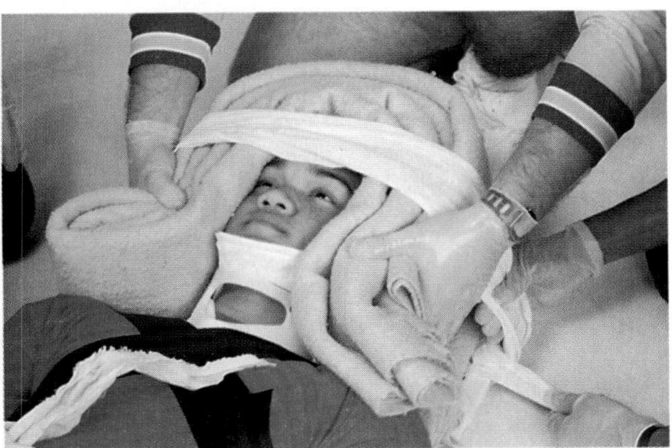

B

Figure 14-18 **A,** You may need to place approximately 1 to $1^1/_2$ inches of padding under the head. **B,** To secure the head, place a rolled blanket around the head and neck, and use a cravat to secure the forehead.

Once the victim's body is secured to the backboard, secure the victim's head. If the victim's head does not appear to be resting in line with the body, you may need to place a small amount of padding, such as a small folded

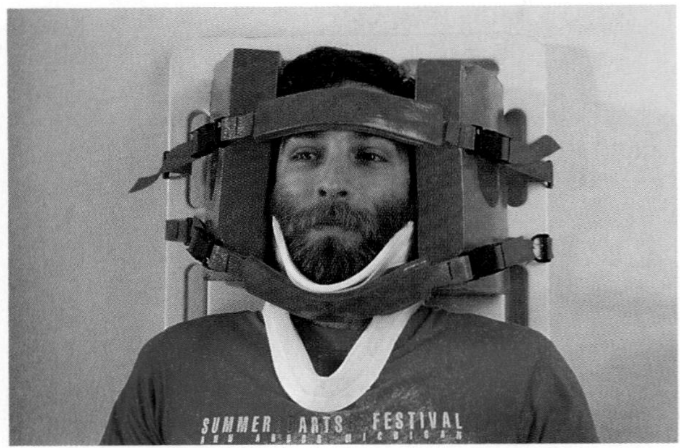

Figure 14-19 A commercial device may be used in place of a blanket and cravat to stabilize the head.

towel, to support the head (Fig: 14-18, *A*). Normally, approximately 1 inch of padding is all that is needed to keep the head in line with the body and at the same time provide comfort for the victim. Next, place a folded or rolled blanket in a horseshoe shape around the victim's head and neck. Use a cravat or tape to secure the forehead (Fig. 14-18, *B*).

You may have a commercially made head-immobilization device available (Fig. 14-19). Many of these devices use Velcro® straps to secure the head. You should follow the manufacturer's directions when using these devices. Sandbags, once traditionally used to secure the victim's head, are no longer recommended. This is because of the force their weight exerts on a vic-

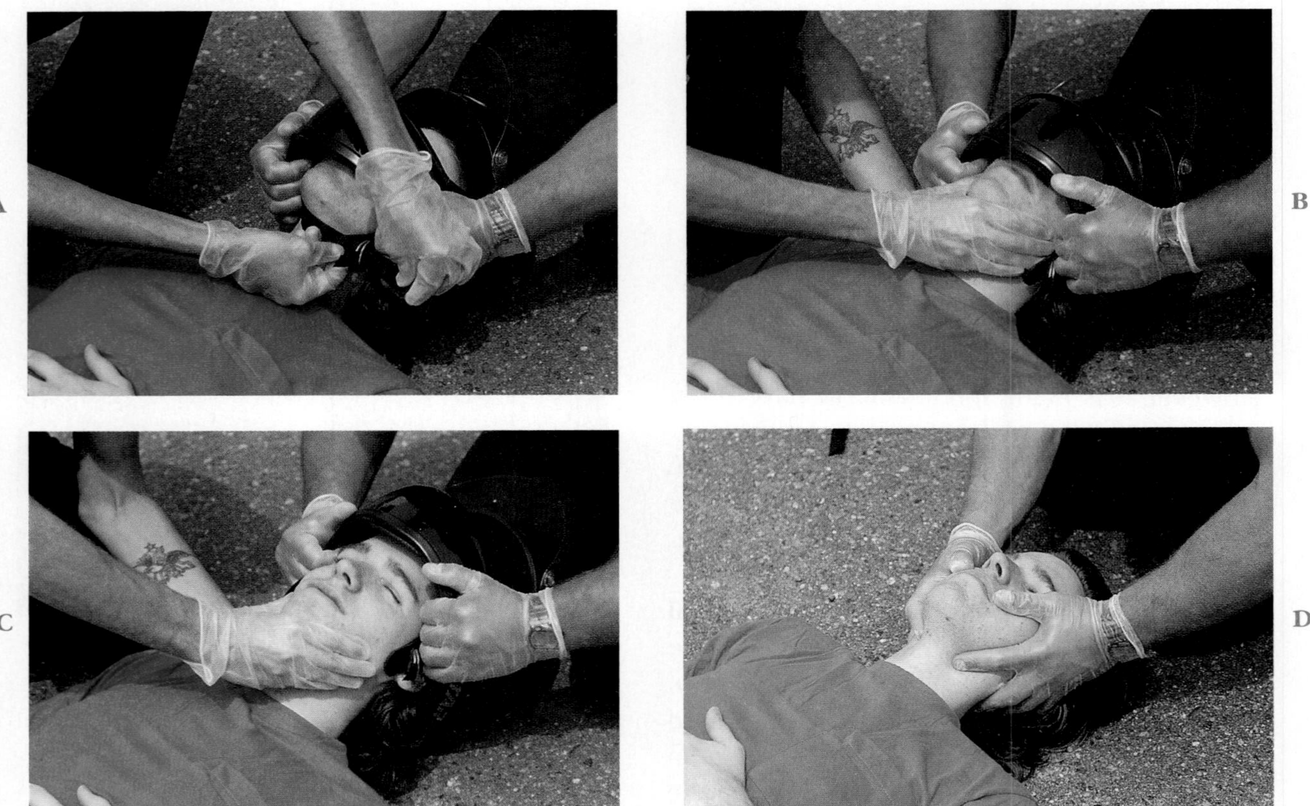

Figure 14-20 To remove a helmet, **A,** the first rescuer removes the chinstrap while the second rescuer holds the head in line with the body. **B,** While the first rescuer supports the head, the second rescuer spreads the sides of the helmet. **C,** The second rescuer slides the helmet off the victim. **D,** Once the helmet is removed, the second rescuer applies in-line stabilization.

tim's neck if the victim must be turned on his or her side to clear the airway while secured to the backboard.

◆ SPECIAL SITUATION—REMOVING A HELMET

There may be a time when someone wearing a helmet, such as a motorcyclist or an athlete, suffers a serious head injury. Since most helmets fit snugly to the head, it is difficult to remove one without moving the head and neck. Fortunately, there is rarely a time when the helmet needs to be removed. If the helmet has a face piece, such as a mask or visor, that interferes with normal breathing, maintaining an open airway, or performing rescue breathing, remove the mask or visor only. Usually, you can remove the face piece by unsnapping, unscrewing, or cutting it.

The only time you should remove a helmet is if it interferes with the care you are providing, such as stabilizing the head in line with the body or performing rescue breathing. In these rare situations, two rescuers should carefully remove the helmet.

To remove a helmet, first remove the chinstrap. Next, as one rescuer supports the head by holding the jaw, a second rescuer spreads the sides of the helmet to clear the ears. While the first rescuer continues to support the head, the second rescuer slides the helmet off, causing as little head movement as possible. The rescuer who removed the helmet then maintains in-line stabilization. Figure 14-20, *A-D,* shows how to remove a helmet.

◆ SPECIAL SITUATION—WATER-RELATED SPINAL INJURY

Along with the risk of drowning, some water activities also involve the risk of spinal injury. Each year in the United States, about 1000 disabling neck and back injuries occur as a result of water activities, such as headfirst entry into shallow water. When the injury damages the spinal cord, severe disability is likely, including permanent paralysis. The person may never be able to move his or her arms or legs again.

Most spinal injuries occur in shallow water. These injuries result from diving into above-ground pools or the shallow end of in-ground pools and striking objects when diving. Unsupervised use of **starting blocks** may also lead to serious injury. Injuries can also result from headfirst entry into the surf at a beach, off a dock at a lake, or from a cliff into a water-filled **quarry.** In this section, you will learn how to recognize a potential spinal injury in the water and what to do to prevent further injury.

Recognizing a Spinal Injury

Usually a spinal injury is caused by hitting the bottom or an object in the water. Your major concern is to keep the person's face out of the water to let him or her breathe and to prevent the person's head and back from moving further. Movement can cause more injury and increase the risk of the person being paralyzed.

If you think the person may have a spinal injury, give care assuming the spine *is* injured. If the person is in the water, your goal is to prevent any further movement of the head or neck and move the person to safety. *Always check first whether a lifeguard or other trained professional is present before touching or moving a person who may have a spinal injury.* This section describes what you can do by yourself or with the assistance of bystanders to care for a victim of spinal injury.

General Guidelines for Care

You can stabilize a person's spine in several ways while the person is still in the water. These methods are described in the next sections. Follow these general guidelines for a per-

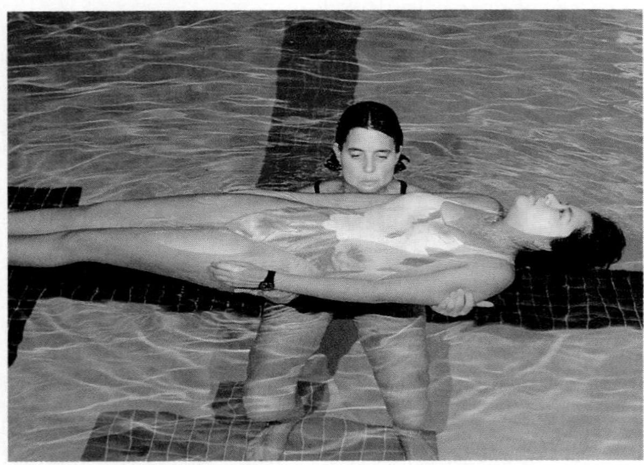

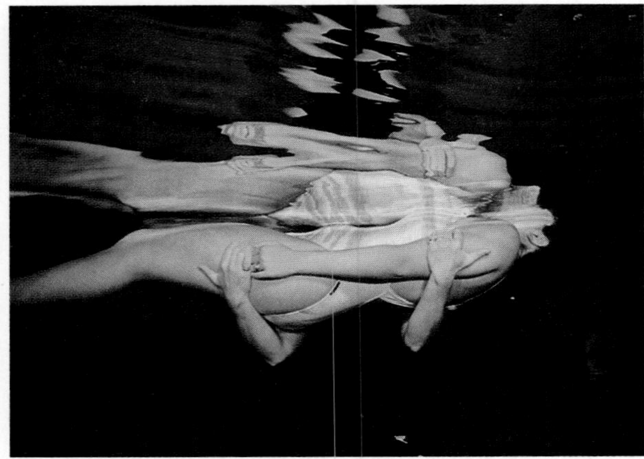

Figure 14-21 The hip/shoulder support helps limit movement of the spine for a victim, while keeping the face clear of water.

son with a suspected spinal injury in shallow water:

1. Be sure someone has called 9-1-1 or the local emergency number. If other people are available, ask someone else in your group or a bystander to help you.
2. Minimize movement of the victim's head, neck, and back. First, try to keep the victim's head in line with the body. Do not pull on the head. Use your hands, arms, or body, depending on which technique you use. The two methods described in the next sections can be used.
3. Position the victim faceup at the surface of the water. You may have to bring a submerged victim to the surface and to a faceup position. Keep the victim's face out of the water to let the victim breathe.
4. Check for consciousness and breathing once you have stabilized the victim's spine. A victim who can talk or is gasping for air is conscious and breathing.
5. Support the victim in the water with his or her head and spine stabilized until help arrives.

In-Line Stabilization Techniques

The following section describes two methods for stabilizing the victim's spine in the water. These methods will enable you to provide care for the victim whether he or she is faceup or facedown.

Hip/shoulder support

This method helps limit movement of the spine. Use it for a victim who is faceup. Support the victim at the hips and shoulders to keep the face out of the water.

1. Approach the victim from the side, and lower yourself to chest depth.
2. Slide one arm under the victim's shoulders and the other under the hip bones. Support the victim's body horizontally, keeping the face clear of the water (Fig. 14-21).
3. Do not lift the victim but support him or her in the water until help arrives.

Head splint

The head splint is used for a person facedown at or near the surface in the water. This victim must be turned faceup to breathe.

1. Approach the victim from the side.
2. Gently move the victim's arms up alongside the head by grasping the victim's arms midway between the shoulder and elbow. Grasp the victim's right arm with your right hand. Grasp the victim's left arm with your left hand.

A

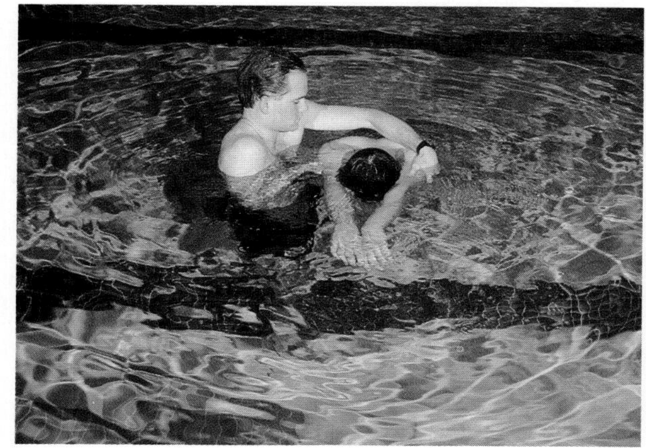

B

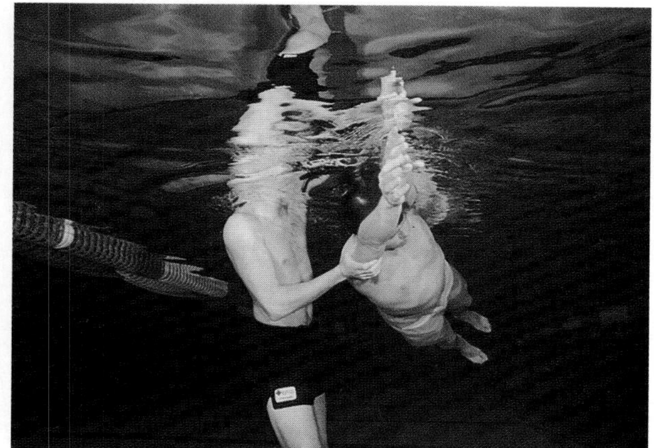

C

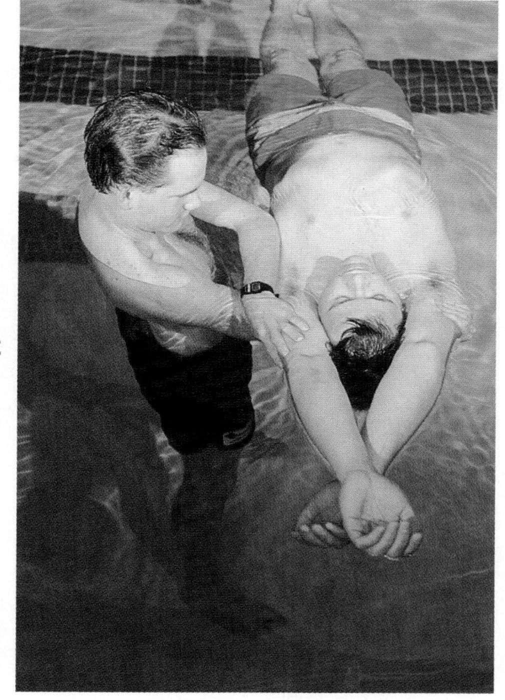

Figure 14-22 When performing the head splint technique, **A,** squeeze the victim's arms against his head, **B,** move the victim slowly forward and rotate the victim toward you until he is faceup, and **C,** position the victim's head in the crook of your arm with the head in line with the body.

3. Squeeze the victim's arms against his or her head. This maneuver helps keep the head in line with the body (Fig. 14-22, *A*).
4. With your body at about shoulder depth in the water, glide the victim slowly forward.
5. Continue moving slowly and rotate the victim toward you until he or she is faceup. This rotation is done by pushing the victim's arm that is closest to you under water, while pulling the victim's other arm across the surface (Fig. 14-22, *B*).
6. Position the victim's head in the crook of your arm with the head in line with the body (Fig. 14-22, *C*).
7. Maintain this position in the water until help arrives.

Immobilization in the Water

In some situations, you may have to remove, or assist lifeguards in removing, a victim who may have a possible head, neck, or back injury from the water. The objective for immobilizing in the water is the same as for immobilizing on the land; however, you need to adjust to the environment you are working in.

After stabilizing the victim's head and neck with one of the two techniques (head splint and hip and shoulder support) described, fully immobilize the victim using a backboard. At least two rescuers are needed to secure a victim to a backboard, but it is easier with help from more rescuers, when they are available. These others can help hold the backboard under the victim, if necessary.

You can place a victim on a backboard and secure a victim to a backboard in different ways. Just be sure that you safely immobilize the spine. Regardless of the strapping method, the victim's body should always be secured to the backboard before the head is secured.

Figure 14-23, *A-J*, shows the steps for immobilization in the water.

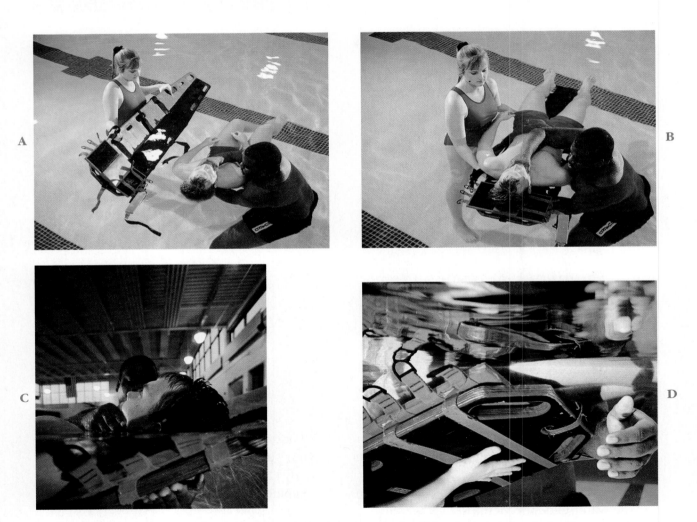

Figure 14-23 **A,** The second lifeguard submerges the backboard next to the victim. **B,** The backboard is positioned under the victim. **C,** The primary lifeguard keeps one hand on the victim's chin and places the other hand under the backboard. **D,** The second lifeguard uses the head and chin support to hold the victim, one hand on the chin, one hand on the board.

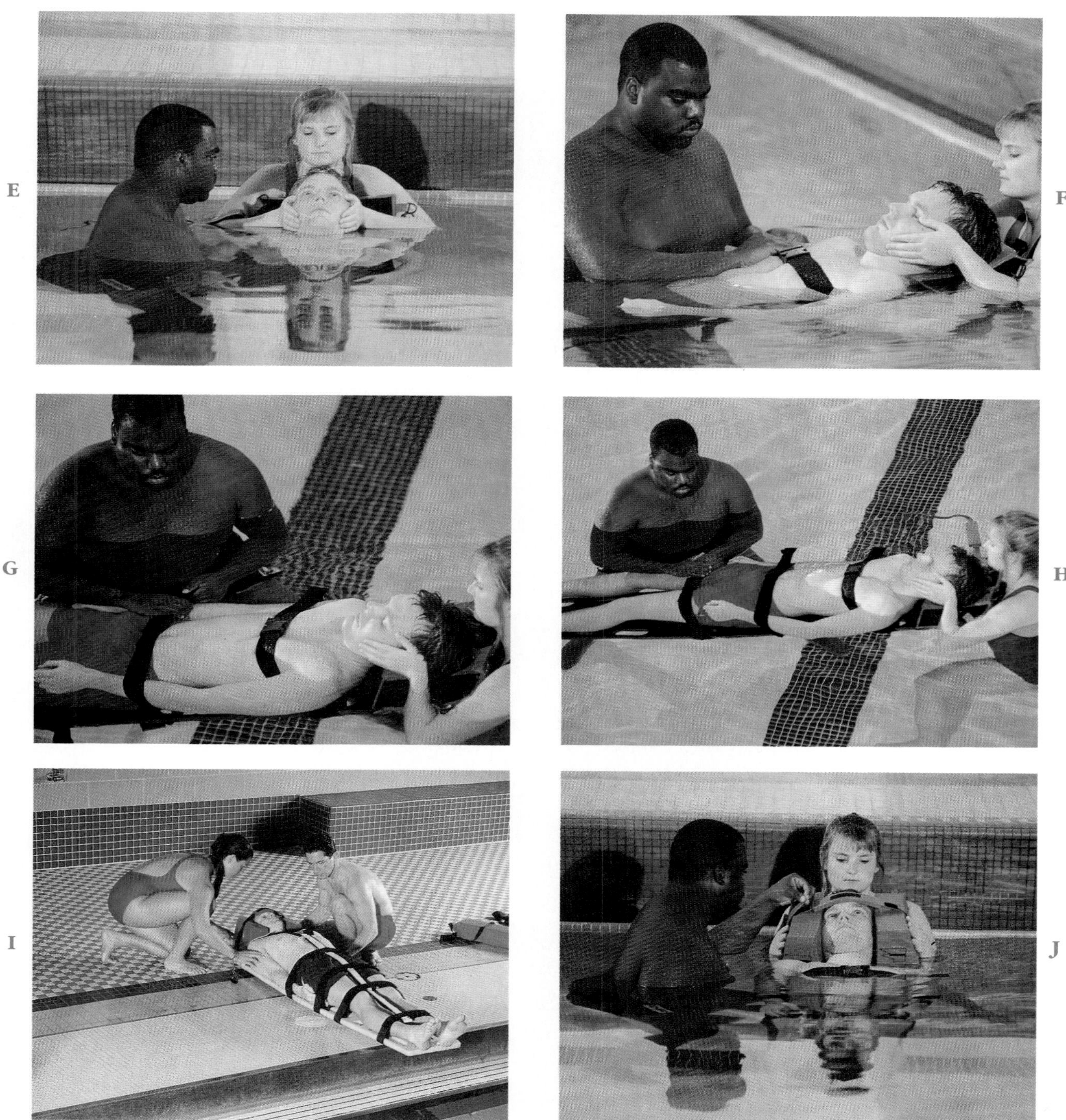

Figure 14-23 (*Continued*) **E,** The second lifeguard supports the board against the chest and shoulders, and squeezes the sides of the backboard with the arms. **F,** Strap under the victim's armpits and across the chest to prevent sliding. **G,** Hip strap securing the hands along the side. **H,** Strap on the thighs. **I,** Spider strap system applied. **J,** The head immobilizer secures the victim's head to the backboard with a strap across the victim's forehead.

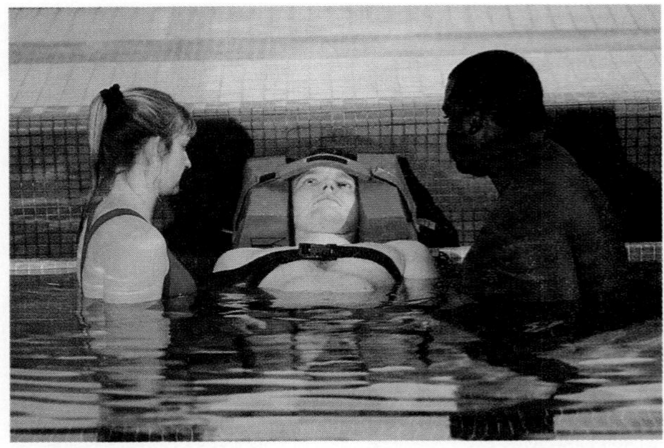

Figure 14-24 Head of backboard placed on the edge of the gutter.

In the American Red Cross Lifeguard Training course, a head immobilizer device is used to secure the head (Fig. 14-24). Be familiar with your area's local protocols for appropriate procedures to follow in cases of head, neck, and back injuries whether they occur on land or in the aquatic environment.

Once the victim is secured on the backboard, remove him or her from the water. Teamwork and communication of the rescuers is of critical importance to ensure the safety of the victim during removal from the water.

Figure 14-25, *A-C,* shows how to remove a victim from the water.

◆ PREVENTING HEAD, NECK, AND BACK INJURIES

Injuries to the head, neck, and back are a major cause of death, disability, and disfigurement. However, many such injuries can be prevented. By using safety practices in all areas of your life, you can help reduce risks to yourself and to others around you.

A

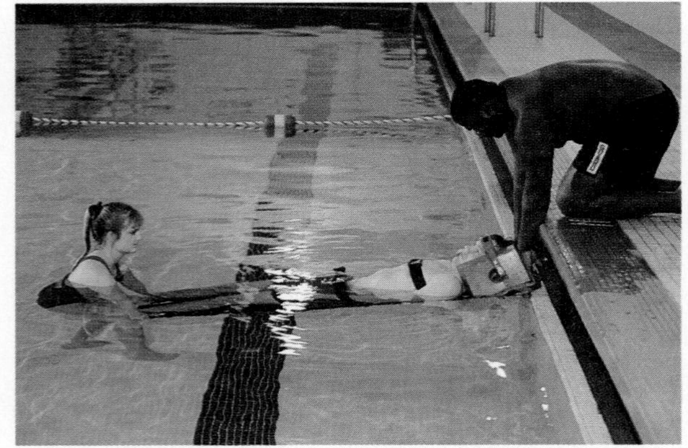

B

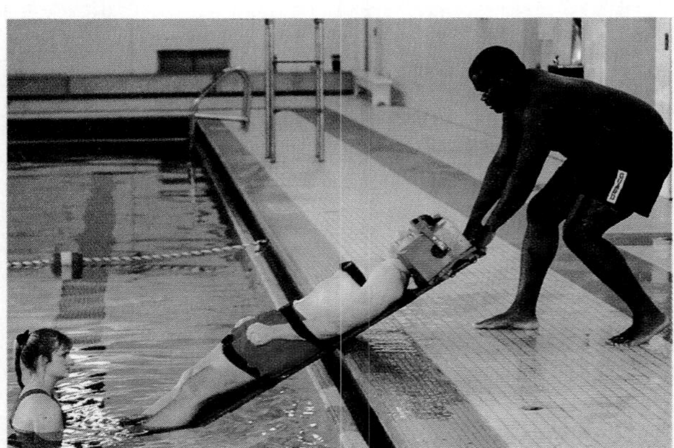

C

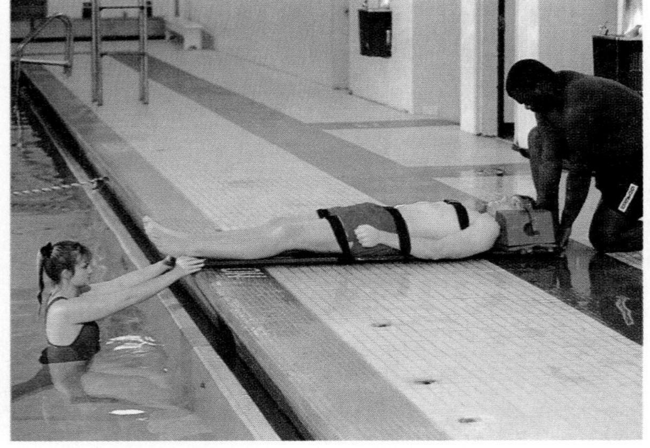

Figure 14-25 **A,** One lifeguard gets out of the pool while the other lifeguard goes to the foot end of the backboard. **B,** The lifeguard on the deck stands up and steps backward, pulling the board. **C,** The backboard is slid onto the deck away from the water.

Safety practices that can help prevent injuries to the head, neck, and back include —

- Wearing safety belts.
- When appropriate, wearing approved helmets, eyewear, face guards, and mouth guards.
- Preventing falls.
- Obeying rules in sports and recreational activities.
- Avoiding inappropriate use of drugs, including alcohol.
- Inspecting work and recreational equipment periodically.
- Thinking and talking about safety.

Wearing Safety Belts

Always wear safety belts, including shoulder restraints, when driving or riding in an automobile. Be sure all passengers also wear them. Airbags, available in some cars, provide additional protection. All small children riding in a car must be in approved safety seats correct for the child's age and weight.

Wearing Helmets and Eyewear

Helmets can prevent many needless injuries to the head, neck, and back. They are designed for different purposes, with varying degrees of protection, and offer protection only for their intended use (Fig. 14-26). For example, the industrial work helmet called a "hard hat" provides adequate protection against falling debris but does not offer the proper protection for riding a motorcycle.

Any open form of transportation, such as a motorcycle, moped, or all-terrain vehicle, exposes the head, neck, and back to injury. Wearing a helmet can help reduce such injuries. The ideal helmet, sometimes called a "full-face helmet," protects the lower face and jaw and has a large clear or tinted face shield. In all cases, the helmet should be the correct size and fit comfortably and securely.

Eyewear can help prevent many needless injuries that result in loss of sight. Any time you operate machinery or perform an activity that may involve flying particles or splashing chemicals, you should wear protective eyewear, such as goggles.

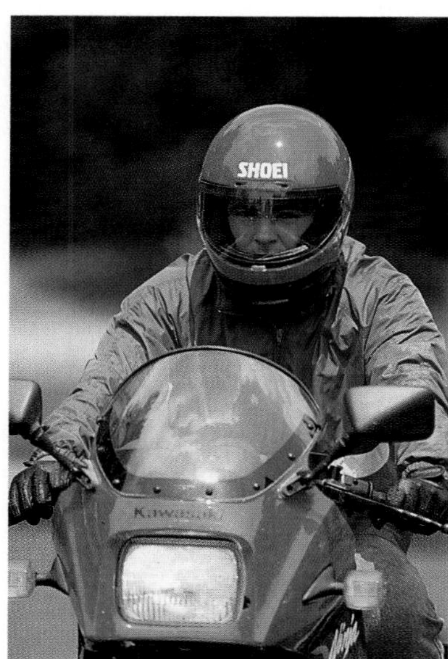

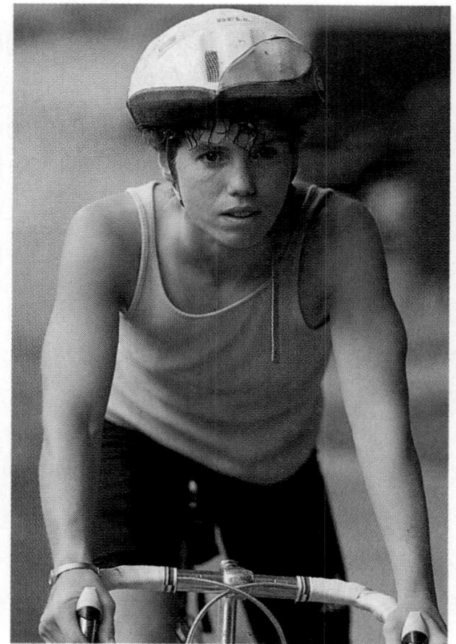
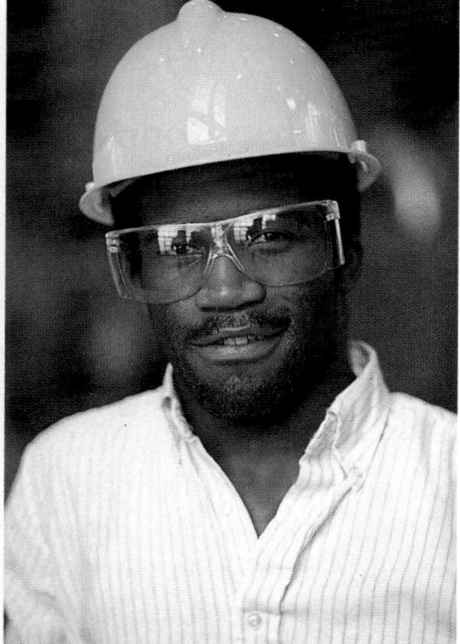

Figure 14-26 Wearing a helmet helps protect against head and spine injuries.

Safeguarding Against Falls

Although most falls occur at home and involve young children and the elderly, falls can and do occur in the workplace. You can take precautions to prevent falls. Floor surfaces should be made of nonslip material. Stairs should have nonslip treads and hand rails. Rugs should be secured to the floor with double-sided tape. If moisture accumulates and causes damp areas on the floor, correct the cause of the problem. Clean up any spills promptly. The bathroom should be safe for all those using it. If necessary, install hand rails by the bathtub and toilet.

Taking Safety Precautions in Sports and Recreation

Participants in sports or recreational activities should know their physical limitations. Proper protective equipment is necessary for any activity in which serious injury may occur. In all sports involving physical contact, participants should wear mouthpieces. Most important, everyone must know and follow the rules. Rules not only make the activity fair, they also help prevent injuries. The coach, athletic trainer, or a more experienced participant may impose additional rules for the safety of newcomers. Never participate in a new activity until you know the rules and risks involved.

Avoiding Inappropriate Drug Use

Alcohol and other drugs used inappropriately cause or contribute to many serious motor vehicle collisions and water-related incidents that involve head and back injuries. Drugs impair judgment and reflexes, causing the body to respond abnormally. Drugs can give the user a feeling of false confidence. Under the influence of a drug, a person may not brake the car quickly enough or may dive into shallow water. Certain prescription and common drugstore medications also have side effects, such as drowsiness, that can make driving or operating machinery dangerous. Follow your physician's directions and the directions and warnings on medication labels. Ask your physician or pharmacist if you have any questions about the safe use of a medication.

Inspecting Equipment

Inspect mechanical equipment, sports equipment, and ladders periodically to ensure good working order. Check for worn or loose parts that could break and cause a mishap. Before climbing a ladder, place its legs on a firm, flat surface and have someone anchor it while you climb.

Thinking and Talking Safety

People too often neglect thinking about safety in their daily lives, yet we are most vulnerable to injury at work, during recreational activities, or while traveling. Take the time to inspect and think about your daily environment. Evaluate your habits. Answer the following five questions:

1. Are there things that you could do in your workplace or home to help prevent injuries to yourself or others?
2. Are you taking unnecessary risks in any activities?
3. Do you follow rules meant for your safety?
4. Do you frequently check the tires on your motor vehicle(s)?
5. Do you ever attempt any activity without being in the physical condition that would allow you to do it without injury?

Talk with others about preventing injuries at work, at home, and in recreation. Everyone needs to know about safety. Seek guidance to help prevent injuries that could permanently affect your life or the lives of others. Discuss safety when using mechanical devices or equipment or when approaching a potentially dangerous scene.

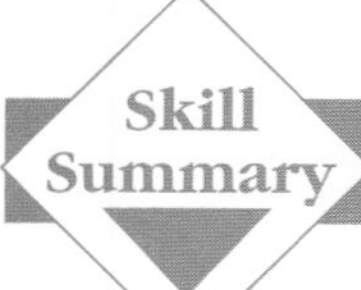

Spinal Immobilization

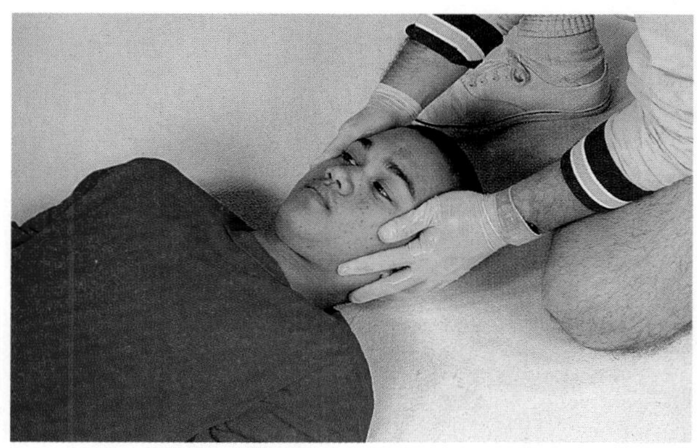

1. Apply in-line stabilization.

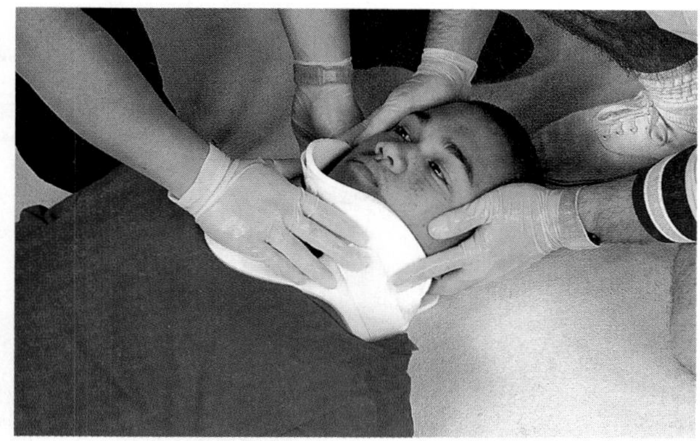

2. Apply cervical collar.

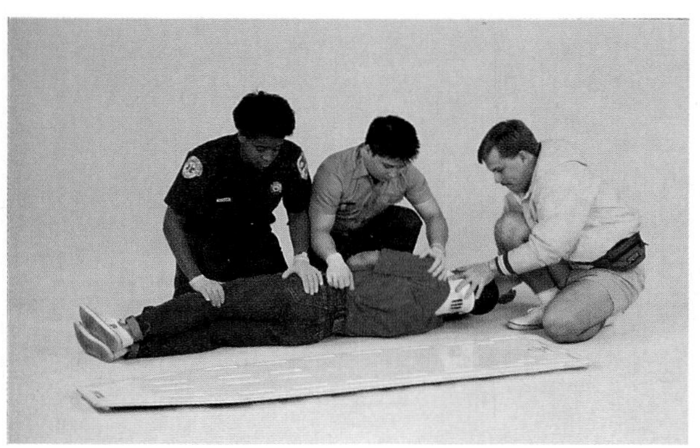

3. Log-roll victim onto backboard.

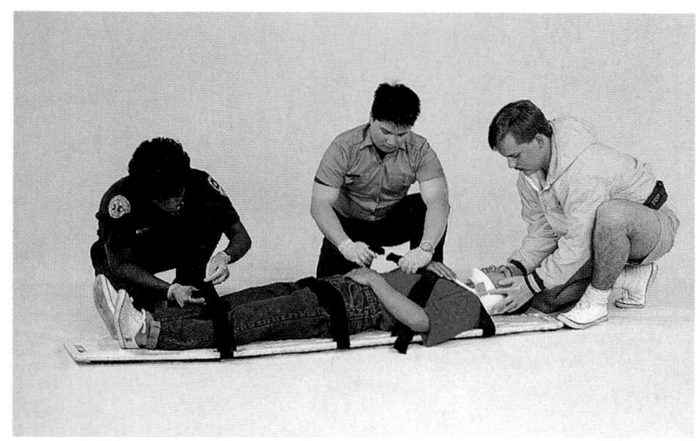

4. Secure victim's body.

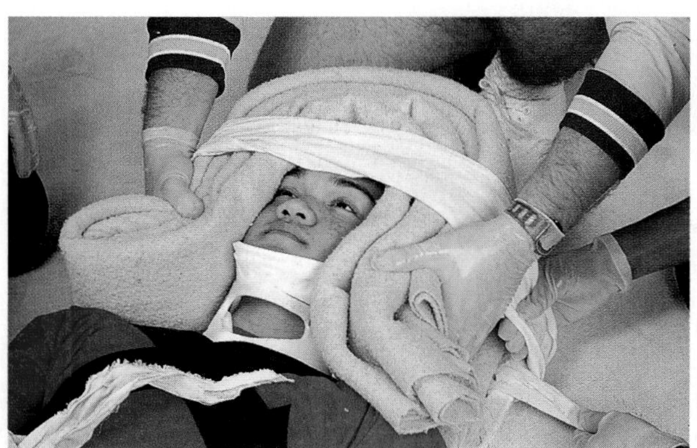

5. Secure victim's head.

Medical and Behavioral Emergencies

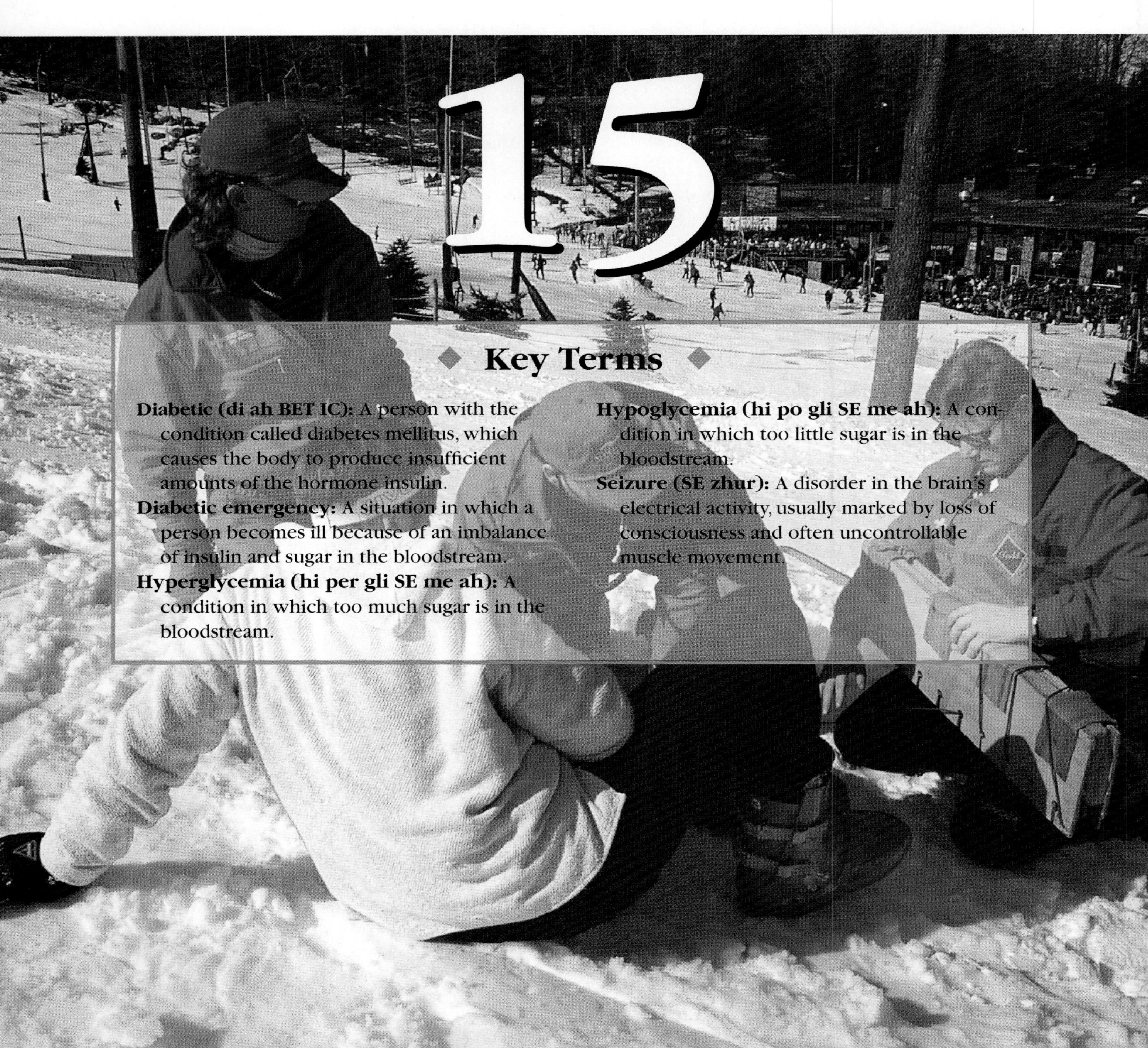

Key Terms

Diabetic (di ah BET IC): A person with the condition called diabetes mellitus, which causes the body to produce insufficient amounts of the hormone insulin.

Diabetic emergency: A situation in which a person becomes ill because of an imbalance of insulin and sugar in the bloodstream.

Hyperglycemia (hi per gli SE me ah): A condition in which too much sugar is in the bloodstream.

Hypoglycemia (hi po gli SE me ah): A condition in which too little sugar is in the bloodstream.

Seizure (SE zhur): A disorder in the brain's electrical activity, usually marked by loss of consciousness and often uncontrollable muscle movement.

◆ Knowledge Objectives ◆

After reading this chapter and completing the class activities, you should be able to —

- Identify a victim who has a general medical complaint.
- Describe the general care for a victim with a general medical complaint.
- Identify the signs and symptoms of altered consciousness and a seizure.
- Describe the care for a victim who has an altered level of consciousness or is experiencing a seizure.
- Identify the signs and symptoms of heat-related illness.
- Describe how to care for a victim who has been exposed to heat.
- Identify the signs and symptoms of cold-related illness.
- Describe how to care for a victim who has been exposed to cold.
- Identify behavior that suggests a person may be experiencing a behavioral emergency.
- Describe how to approach and care for a victim experiencing a behavioral change or psychological crisis.
- *Identify the signs and symptoms of a diabetic emergency and a stroke.
- *Describe the care for a victim who is experiencing a diabetic emergency or stroke.

* Specifies an Enrichment section objective.

◆ Skill Objectives ◆

After reading this chapter and completing the class activities, you should be able to —

- Make appropriate decisions about care when given an example of an emergency in which someone has suddenly become ill.
- Make appropriate decisions about care when given an example of an emergency in which someone is experiencing a behavioral emergency.

You are summoned to assist with an emergency. As you arrive, you notice a woman in her mid 50s, lying motionless on her side on the floor. A man is kneeling helplessly next to her. An empty medicine container, without a label, is on the floor nearby. Saliva is dribbling from the victim's mouth. Her face seems distorted; her mouth droops to one side. She does not respond when you speak to her and tap her on the shoulder. You bend over her and observe that she is breathing rapidly. Her skin is cool and she is sweating heavily.

You ask the man what happened and how long she has been like this. He states he came out of his office and found her sitting on the floor "somewhat conscious" and talking incoherently. Soon, she slumped over and became unconscious. You ask the man if he knows whether the woman has any medical prob-

lems, is taking any medications, or is allergic to anything. The man is uncertain.

Thoughts race through your mind. What causes a loss of consciousness? Heart problems? A stroke? A diabetic problem? A head injury from a fall? Did she have a seizure? Did the man tell everything he knew about the situation?

An ambulance is on the way. You remain calm. You ask the man to find a blanket or a coat to put over the woman's cool body. You make certain her airway is clear. You decide not to move her, but examine her carefully for any clues as to what the problem could be. You want to help the woman more, but because you do not know what the problem is, you are unsure about how to proceed. You feel somewhat helpless. What more should you do?

◆ INTRODUCTION

The dilemma in the preceding scenario is not rare. As a first responder, you could someday face a similar situation involving an unclear medical emergency. Medical emergencies are rarely as clear as easily identifiable problems, such as external bleeding. Therefore you may feel more uncertain about providing care.

When you face an emergency that is unclear, it is normal to feel helpless or indecisive. Yet, like everyone, you still want to help to the best of your ability. Take comfort that giving initial care, even for medical emergencies you do not understand, does not require extensive knowledge. You do not have to "diagnose" or choose among possible problems to be able to provide appropriate care. By following a few basic guidelines for care that you learned in previous chapters, you can provide appropriate care until more advanced medical personnel arrive. Because you know these guidelines for care, you can approach an unclear medical emergency with confidence.

In the scenario, everything that needed to be done was done. Life-threatening conditions were checked for and corrected during the initial assessment. A physical exam and SAMPLE history did not reveal any further information. The victim was kept from getting chilled or overheated, her airway was kept clear, and more advanced medical personnel were summoned.

What if other information had been available, such as a medical alert bracelet indicating the woman was a diabetic or was taking a specific medication? Would that have helped you care for this person? No, even if you had known she was a diabetic or what the medication was, it would not have affected the care you provided. Since she was unconscious, your care would have been the same. Almost all the care you will give a person having a medical emergency is as simple as following a few basic guidelines of care, whether the person is conscious or unconscious.

Behavioral emergencies, like medical emergencies, can also have many causes, and trying to "diagnose" the precise cause is not as important as providing general care. In this chapter, you will learn to recognize signs and symptoms that can indicate medical or behavioral emergencies, as well as the care to provide until more advanced medical personnel arrive.

◆ RESPONDING TO A MEDICAL EMERGENCY

Medical emergencies can develop very rapidly (acute conditions) or gradually and persist for a long time (chronic conditions). Sometimes, there are no warning signs and symptoms to alert you or the victim that something is about to happen. Older people or those with diabetes, for example, may have a heart attack without chest pains. At other times, the victim may feel ill or state that he or she feels that something is wrong. Medical emergencies can result from illness.

Medical emergencies include chronic problems caused by diseases, such as heart and lung disease. They can involve hormone imbalances, such as diabetes. Medical emergencies also can involve illnesses, such as epilepsy, in which an occasional seizure occurs, or allergies, in which exposure to a certain substance causes a severe reaction. Overexposure to heat or cold also can cause serious illness.

Medical emergencies can have a variety of signs and symptoms, including sudden, unexplained altered mental status. A person may complain of feeling lightheaded, dizzy, or weak. He or she may feel nauseated or may vomit. Breathing, pulse, and skin characteristics may change. If a person looks and feels ill, there is a problem.

The assessment and care for these conditions follows the same general guidelines:

- Survey (size up) the scene.
- Conduct your initial assessment to identify and correct any immediately life-threatening conditions.
- Conduct a physical exam and a SAMPLE history to gather additional information, whenever possible.
- Summon more advanced medical personnel.
- Help the victim rest comfortably.
- Keep the victim from getting chilled or overheated.
- Provide reassurance.
- Prevent further harm.
- Administer oxygen if it is available and you are trained to do so.

◆ SPECIFIC MEDICAL CONDITIONS

This section provides information about some specific medical conditions you are likely to encounter, such as altered mental status, seizure, and heat and cold exposure. As you read, you will see that even though each of these medical conditions occurs for a different reason, they have many of the same signs and symptoms.

Altered Mental Status

Altered mental status can result from many causes. These include —

- Fever.
- Infection.
- Poisoning, including substance abuse or misuse.
- High or low blood sugar or insulin reaction.
- Head injury.
- Any condition resulting in decreased blood flow or oxygen to the brain.
- Conditions resulting from mental, emotional, or behavioral disorders.

Signs and Symptoms of Altered Mental Status

Altered mental status is one of the most common medical emergencies. It is often characterized by a sudden or gradual change in a person's level of consciousness, including drowsiness, confusion, and partial or complete loss of consciousness. Sometimes altered mental status is caused by a temporary reduction of blood flow to the brain, such as occurs when blood collects in the legs and lower body. When the brain is suddenly deprived of its normal blood flow, it momentarily shuts down. This condition is called **fainting**.

Fainting can be triggered by an emotional shock, such as the sight of blood. It may be caused by pain, specific medical conditions like heart disease, standing for a long time, or overexertion. Some people, such as pregnant women or the elderly, are more likely to faint when suddenly changing positions, for example, when moving from lying down to standing up. Any time that changes inside the body momentarily reduce the blood flow to the brain, fainting may occur.

Fainting may occur with or without warning. Often, the victim may first feel lightheaded or dizzy. He or she may show signs of shock, such as pale or ashen, cool, moist skin. The victim may feel nauseated and complain of numbness or tingling in the fingers and toes. The victim's breathing and pulse may become faster.

Care for Altered Mental Status

To care for victims with altered mental status, complete an initial assessment and a physical exam and history as needed. Do an ongoing assessment. Make sure the airway is open, and place an unconscious victim in the recovery position. Have suction equipment available if needed. If the victim is conscious or becomes conscious, comfort and reassure him or her. Do not give the victim anything to eat or drink.

Sometimes a person may briefly faint and slowly begin to regain consciousness. Fainting often resolves itself when the victim moves from a standing or sitting position to a lying down position, because normal circulation to the brain then often resumes. The victim usually regains consciousness within a minute.

Fainting itself does not usually harm the victim, but injury may occur from falling. If you suspect head, neck, or back injury, take the necessary precautions when providing care. If you can reach a person who is starting to collapse, lower him or her to the ground or another flat surface and position the person on the back. If possible, elevate the victim's legs 8 to 12 inches (Fig. 15-1). Check the ABCs. Loosen any restrictive clothing, such as a tie or collar. Do not give the victim anything to eat or drink. Eating or drinking can increase the chance of vomiting. Do not splash water on the victim's face. Doing so does little to stimulate the victim, and the victim could aspirate the water. Administer oxygen if it is available and you have been trained to use it.

Although a fainting victim usually recovers quickly, you will not be able to determine whether the fainting is linked to a more serious condition. For this reason, more advanced medical personnel should be summoned.

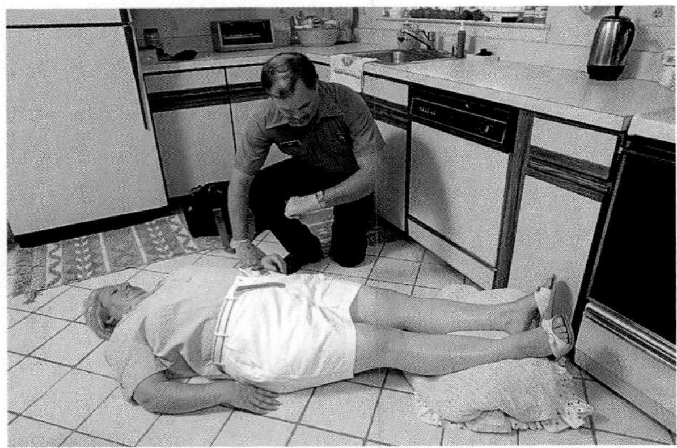

Figure 15-1 To care for fainting, place the victim on his or her back, elevate the feet, and loosen any restrictive clothing, such as a belt, tie, or collar.

Seizures

When the normal functions of the brain are disrupted by injury, disease, fever, infection, or any condition causing a decreased oxygen level, the electrical activity of the brain becomes irregular. This irregularity can cause a loss of body control known as a ***seizure***.

Seizures may be caused by an acute or a chronic condition. The chronic condition is known as **epilepsy**. More than 2 million Americans have epilepsy, and 125,000 new cases are diagnosed annually. Epilepsy is usually controlled with medication. Approximately 70 percent of people who have epilepsy can be expected to enter remission (a lack of signs and symptoms), defined as 5 years without seizures. Most people who are seizure free for 2 to 5 years can be taken off medication. Still, some people with epilepsy, even when on medication, have seizures from time to time. Others may think the condition has gone away and stop taking their medication. These people may then have a seizure again. The most clearly established risk factors for seizures are severe head trauma, central nervous system infections, having a family member who has epilepsy, and stroke.

Signs and Symptoms of Seizures

Before a seizure occurs, the person may experience an aura. An **aura** is an unusual sensation or feeling, such as a visual hallucination; a strange sound, taste, or smell; or an urgent need to get to safety. If the person recognizes the aura, he or she may have time to tell bystanders and sit or lie down before the seizure occurs.

Seizures generally last 1 to 3 minutes and can produce a wide range of signs and symptoms. When a seizure occurs, breathing may become irregular and even stop temporarily. The victim may drool, the eyes may roll upward, and the body may become rigid. The victim may also urinate or defecate. Seizures that cause the victim to experience mild blackouts that others may mistake for daydreaming are commonly known as nonconvulsive seizures because the body remains relatively still during the episode. More severe seizures, known as convulsive seizures, may cause the victim to experience sudden uncontrollable muscular contractions, or convulsions, lasting several minutes.

Infants and young children may be at risk for epilepsy, as well as for seizures brought on by a rapid increase in body temperature. These are called **febrile (heat-induced) seizures** and are most common in children under the age of 5. Additional information on febrile seizures is included in Chapter 18.

Care for Seizures

Although it may be frightening to see someone unexpectedly having a seizure, you can easily help care for the victim. Remember that he or she cannot control the seizure or any convulsions that may occur, so do not try to stop the seizure. Do not attempt to hold or restrain the victim, since doing so could cause musculoskeletal injuries.

Your objectives for care are to protect the victim from injury and keep the airway open. First, move away nearby objects, such as furniture, that might cause injury. Protect the victim's head, and keep the airway clear by rolling the victim onto his or her side (recovery position). Place the victim in the recovery position only if you do not suspect any spinal injury. If fluid, such as saliva or vomit, is in the victim's mouth, this position will help the fluid to drain from the mouth. Apply suction to help clear the airway. If you are unable to open the airway in a victim whose teeth are clenched, consider using a nasal airway, if your organization's protocols allow.

Do not try to place anything between the victim's teeth. People having seizures rarely bite their tongues or cheeks with enough force to cause any significant bleeding. However, some blood may be present, so positioning the victim on his or her side will also help any blood drain out of the mouth.

In many instances, the seizure will be over by the time you arrive to help. The victim will be drowsy and disoriented. Do a physical exam and SAMPLE history, checking to see if he or she was injured during the seizure. Offer comfort and reassurance. The victim will be tired and will want to rest. If the seizure occurred in public, the victim may be embarrassed and self-conscious. Try to provide a measure of privacy for the victim. Ask bystanders not to crowd around. Stay with the victim until he or she is fully conscious and aware of the surroundings.

If the victim is known to have periodic seizures, you do not necessarily need to summon more advanced medical personnel immediately. The victim usually will recover from a seizure in a few minutes. However, more advanced medical personnel should always be called if—

- The seizure lasts more than a few minutes.
- The victim has repeated seizures.
- The victim appears to be injured.
- You are uncertain about the cause of the seizure.
- The victim is pregnant.
- The victim is a known diabetic.
- The victim is an infant or child.
- The seizure takes place in water.
- The victim fails to regain consciousness after the seizure.

Heat and Cold Exposure

The human body is equipped to withstand extremes of temperature. Usually, its mecha-

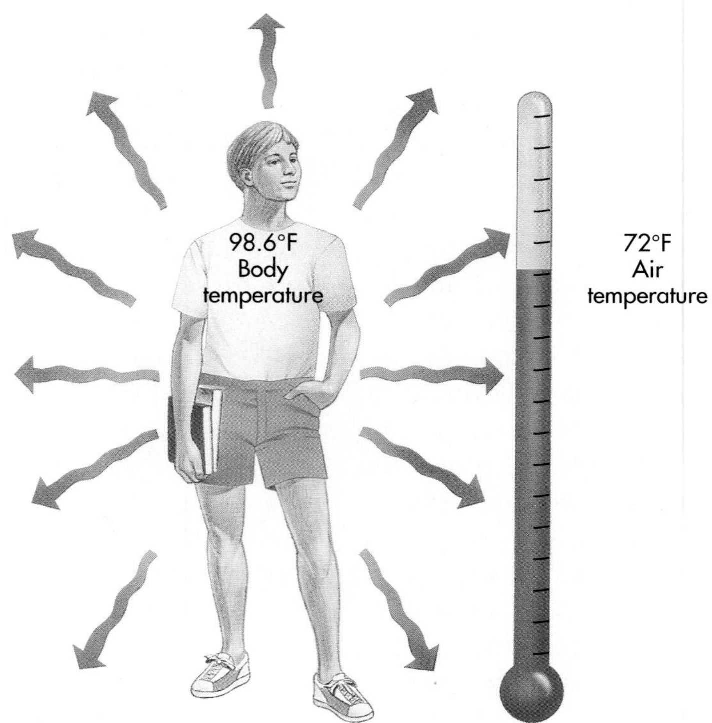

Figure 15-2 Since the body is usually warmer than the surrounding air, it tends to lose heat to the air.

nisms for regulating body temperature work very well. However, when the body is overwhelmed by extremes of heat and cold, illness occurs.

Extreme temperatures can occur anywhere, both indoors and outdoors, but a person can develop a heat- or cold-related illness even if temperatures are not extreme. The effects of humidity, wind, clothing, living and working environment, medications, physical activity, age, and an individual's health are all factors in heat- and cold-related illnesses.

Illnesses caused by exposure to temperature extremes are progressive and can become life threatening. Once the signs and symptoms of a heat- or cold-related illness begin to appear, a victim's condition can rapidly deteriorate, leading to death. If the victim shows any of the signs and symptoms of sudden illness, notice the weather conditions and decide if they suggest the possibility of a heat- or cold-related illness. If so, give the appropriate care. Immediate care can prevent the illness from becoming life threatening. In this chapter, you will learn how extremes of heat and cold affect the body, how to recognize temperature-related emergencies, and how to provide care.

Body temperature must remain constant for the body to work efficiently. Normal body temperature is about 99 degrees F. Body heat is generated primarily through the conversion of food to energy. Heat is also produced by muscle contractions, as in exercise or shivering. Heat always moves from warm areas to cooler ones. Since the body is usually warmer than the surrounding air, it tends to lose heat to the air. The body maintains its temperature by constantly balancing heat loss with heat production (Fig. 15-2). The heat produced in routine activities is usually enough to balance normal heat loss.

When body heat increases, the body removes heat through the skin. Blood vessels near the skin dilate, or widen, to bring more

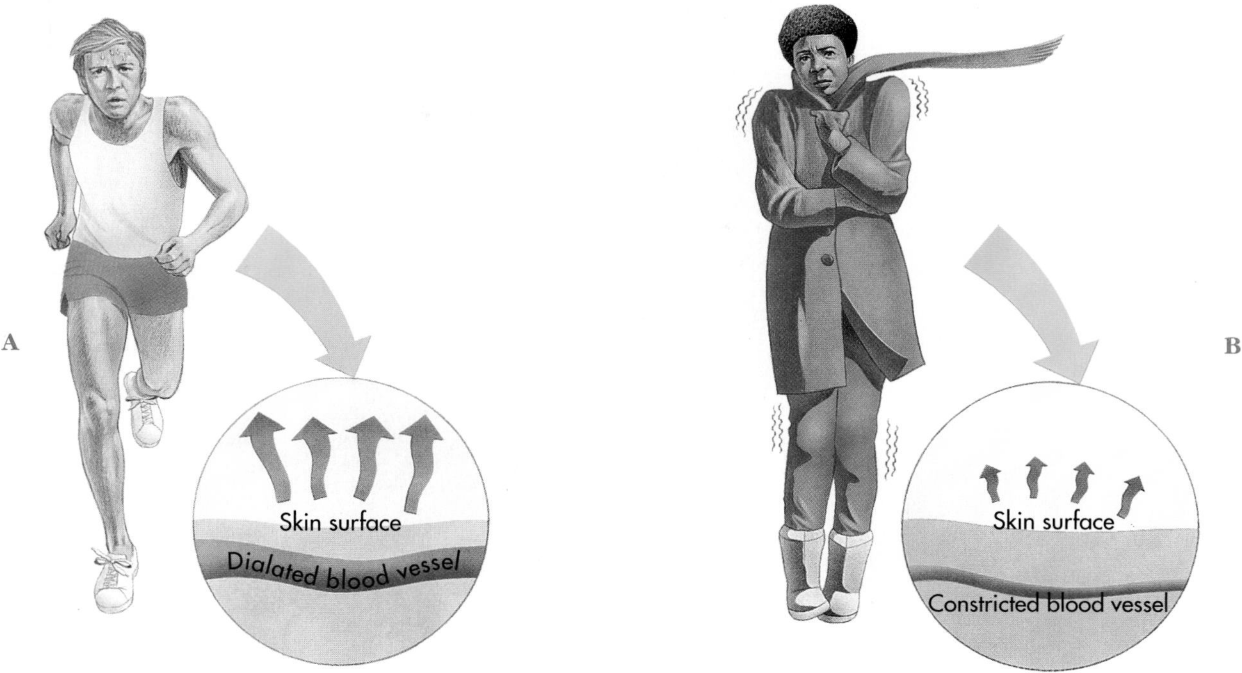

Figure 15-3 **A**, Your body removes heat by dilating the blood vessels near the skin's surface. **B**, The body conserves heat by constricting the blood vessels near the skin.

warm blood to the surface. Heat then escapes and the body cools (Fig. 15-3, *A*).

The body is also cooled by the evaporation of sweat. When the air temperature is very warm, dilation of blood vessels is a less effective means of removing heat. Therefore, sweating increases. But when the humidity is high, sweat does not evaporate as quickly. It stays longer on the skin and has little or no cooling effect.

When the body reacts to cold, blood vessels near the skin constrict, or narrow, which moves warm blood to the center of the body. Thus less heat escapes through the skin, and the body stays warm (Fig. 15-3, *B*). When constriction of blood vessels fails to keep the body warm, shivering results. Shivering produces heat through muscle action.

Three external factors affect how well the body maintains its temperature — air temperature, humidity, and wind. Humidity and wind multiply the effects of heat or cold. Extreme heat or cold accompanied by high humidity hampers the body's ability to effectively maintain its normal temperature (Fig. 15-4). A cold temperature combined with a strong wind rapidly cools exposed body parts. The combination of temperature and wind speed form the "wind chill factor."

Other factors, such as the clothing you wear, how often you take breaks from exposure to extreme temperature, how much water you drink and how often, and how intense your activity is, also affect how well your body manages temperature extremes. These are all factors you can control to prevent heat- or cold-related illnesses.

People at Risk for Heat- or Cold-Related Illnesses

People at risk for heat- or cold-related illnesses include —

- Those who work or exercise strenuously outdoors or in unheated or poorly cooled indoor areas.
- Elderly people.
- Young children.

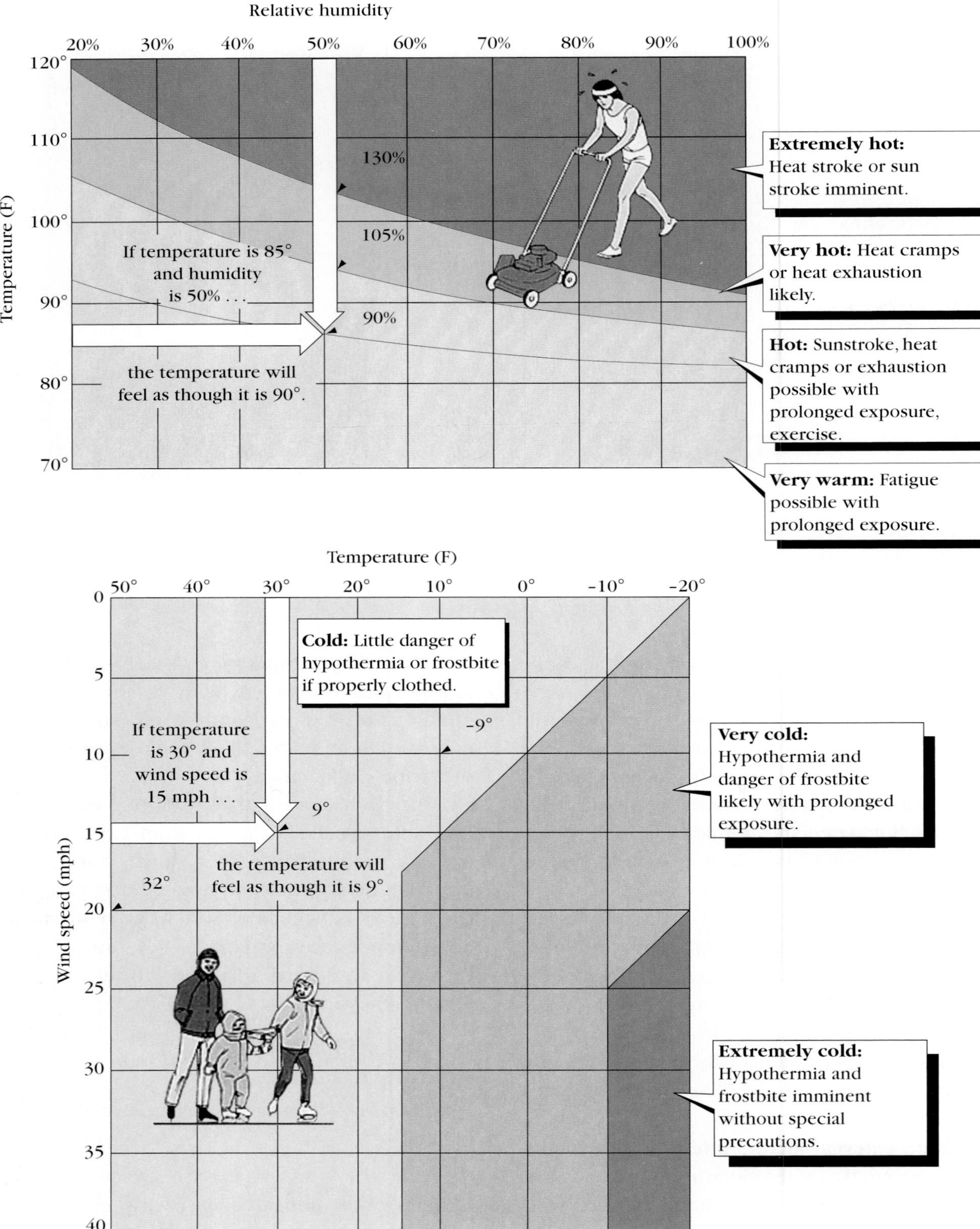

Figure 15-4 Temperature, humidity, and wind are the three main environmental factors affecting body temperature.

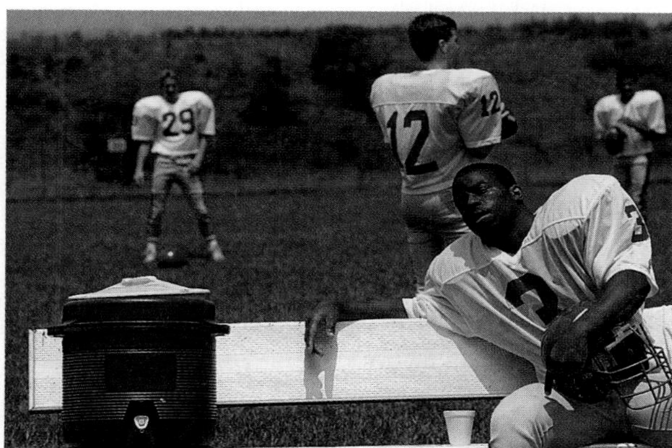

Figure 15-5 In certain situations, it is difficult to escape temperature extremes.

- Those who have had a heat- or cold-related illness in the past.
- Those who have respiratory disease, cardiovascular disease, or other conditions that cause poor circulation.
- Those who use specific drugs or medications, such as alcohol or diuretics (to eliminate water from the body).

Usually people seek relief from an extreme temperature before they begin to feel ill. However, some people do not or cannot easily escape these extremes (Fig. 15-5). People who work or participate in strenuous activity outdoors or in hot, humid indoor conditions often keep working after they develop the first signs or symptoms of illness, which they may not recognize.

Heat- and cold-related illnesses occur more frequently in the elderly, especially those living in poorly ventilated or poorly insulated buildings or in buildings with poor heating or cooling systems. Young children and people with health problems are also at risk because their bodies respond less effectively to temperature extremes.

Heat Exposure

Heat-related emergencies can occur as a result of fluid and electrolytes (salts) loss from heavy sweating. Loss of fluid and electrolytes can begin to produce painful spasms of skeletal muscles, usually in the legs and the abdomen. Body temperature is usually normal, and the skin is moist. Over time, the victim loses fluid through sweating, which decreases the blood volume. Blood flow to the skin increases, reducing blood flow to the vital organs. Because the circulatory system is affected, the person goes into mild shock. At this point, the victim's body temperature will usually be normal or below normal. Other signs and symptoms include —

- Cool, moist, pale or ashen skin. (Skin may be red in the early stage, immediately after exertion.)
- Headache.
- Nausea.
- Dizziness and weakness.
- Exhaustion.

In this stage, heat-related illness can usually be reversed with prompt care. Often the victim feels better when he or she rests in a cool place and drinks cool water.

Signs and symptoms of life-threatening heat-related illness

If the heat-related illness is allowed to progress, the victim's condition will worsen. Body temperature will continue to climb. A victim may vomit and begin to show changes in his or her level of consciousness. Without prompt care, the body systems are overwhelmed by heat and begin to stop functioning. Sweating may stop because body fluid levels are low. When sweating stops, the body cannot cool itself effectively and body temperature rapidly rises. It soon reaches a level at which the brain and other vital organs, such as the heart and kidneys, begin to fail. If the body is not cooled, convulsions, coma, and death will result. This situation is a life-threatening medical emergency. You must recognize the signs and symptoms of this later stage of heat-related illness and provide care immediately. In this late stage, the signs and symptoms include —

- High body temperature (often as high as 106 degrees F).
- Red, hot, dry skin.
- Progressive loss of consciousness.
- Rapid, weak pulse.
- Rapid, shallow breathing.

The victim may at first have a strong, rapid pulse, as the heart works hard to rid the body of heat by dilating blood vessels and sending more blood to the skin. As consciousness deteriorates, the circulatory system begins to fail and the pulse becomes weak and irregular. Without prompt care, the victim will die.

Care for heat exposure

When signs or symptoms of sudden illness develop and you suspect the illness is caused by overexposure to heat, follow these general care steps immediately —

- Check the ABCs.
- Summon more advanced medical personnel.
- Remove the victim from the hot environment.
- Have the victim lie down in a cool or shady area. Elevate the legs slightly, if possible.
- Loosen or remove clothing.
- Apply cool, wet towels or sheets or cold packs to the body.
- Fan the victim to help increase evaporation.
- If you only have ice or cold packs, place them on the victim's wrists and ankles, in each armpit, and in the groin to cool the large blood vessels.
- Give small amounts of cool water to a fully conscious victim.
- *Do not apply rubbing (isopropyl) alcohol.* The alcohol may cause poisoning, either through the skin or through inhalation.
- Monitor vital signs.

A person suffering from the later stage of heat-related illness may experience respiratory or cardiac arrest. Be prepared to do rescue breathing or CPR.

Cold Exposure

Cold-related emergencies can be generalized — commonly called hypothermia — or localized — commonly called frostbite. Frostbite occurs when body tissue exposed to the cold freezes. Hypothermia is a general body cooling that develops when the body can no longer generate sufficient heat to maintain normal body temperature.

Several factors contribute to how well the body maintains its normal temperature. These include —

- Air temperature.
- Humidity.
- Wind.
- Clothing.
- Intensity of the activity.
- The body's ability to adapt to compensate for the cold environment.

Those at greatest risk for problems associated with cold exposure include —

- Young children.
- The elderly.
- Those without adequate clothing, equipment, or training for a cold environment.
- Those with health problems.
- Those using illicit drugs or medications such as diuretics.

Generalized cold exposure (hypothermia)

In hypothermia, the entire body cools when its warming mechanisms fail. The victim will die if not given care. In hypothermia, body temperature drops below 95 degrees F. Most thermometers do not measure below 94 degrees F. As the body temperature cools, the heart begins to beat erratically and eventually stops. Death then occurs.

The signs and symptoms of hypothermia include —

- Cool skin in the core area of the body, as well as the extremities.
- Shivering. This is an early response of the

body to create heat through muscle contractions. Shivering may be absent in later stages.
- Numbness.
- Poor coordination.
- Speech difficulty.
- Rigid muscles.
- Decreasing level of consciousness.

The air temperature does not have to be below freezing for people to develop hypothermia. Elderly people in poorly heated homes, particularly people who receive poor nutrition or who get little exercise, can develop hypothermia at higher temperatures. The homeless and the ill are also at risk. Certain substances, such as alcohol and barbiturates, can also interfere with the body's normal response to cold, causing hypothermia to occur more easily. Medical conditions, such as infection, insulin reaction, stroke, and brain tumor, also make a person more susceptible to the effects of cold. Anyone remaining in cold water or wet clothing for a prolonged time may also easily develop hypothermia.

Localized cold exposure (frostbite)

Frostbite occurs when body tissues freeze. This freezing causes cells to be damaged or destroyed when the fluid in and between the cells freezes and swells. Frostbite usually occurs in exposed areas of the body, depending on the air temperature, length of exposure, and the wind, and in areas with the poorest blood supply, such as the ear lobes, fingertips, and the tip of the nose. It can affect superficial or deep tissues. With superficial frostbite (frostnip), the skin is frozen but the tissues below are not. Superficial frostbite is the most common form. In deep frostbite, both the skin and underlying tissues are frozen. Frostbite can cause the loss of fingers, hands, arms, toes, feet, and legs.

The signs and symptoms of frostbite vary according to whether the injury is superficial or deep. With superficial frostbite, the skin remains soft but blanches (turns very pale) when it is palpated or examined by touch. The victim complains of loss of feeling or sensation. The victim also feels a tingling sensation as the affected area is rewarmed. In deep frostbite, the skin appears white and waxy and feels firm. Swelling and blisters may be present. When rewarmed, the affected area may appear red, with areas of blue and purple.

Care for cold exposure

To care for frostbite, handle the area gently. Never rub an affected area or break any blisters. Rubbing causes further damage because of the sharp ice crystals in the skin. Remove wet clothing and any jewelry from the affected area. Cover the affected area with dry dressings and bandage it loosely. Do not apply direct heat. Do not re-expose the injured area to cold. Additional information on the care for frostbite can be found in the Enrichment section of this chapter.

To care for hypothermia, do an initial assessment and care for any life-threatening problems. Summon more advanced medical personnel. Handle the victim gently and do not bump him or her, especially on the chest. Such a blow could cause cardiac arrest. Remove the victim from the cold environment. Remove any wet clothing and dry the victim. Have the victim stop all activity and rest.

If the victim is on the cold ground, put some insulation under him or her, protecting the back from movement if you suspect neck or back injury. Warm the body gradually by wrapping the victim in blankets or putting on dry clothing. Hot water bottles, heating pads (if the victim is dry), or other heat sources can help rewarm the body. Apply the heat sources only to the trunk, at the armpits and groin. Keep a barrier, such as a blanket, towel, or clothing, between the heat source and the victim to avoid burning him or her. *Do not warm the victim too quickly*, for instance, by immersing in warm water. Rapid rewarming can cause dangerous heart rhythms. If the victim is fully conscious, give him or her hot, nonalcoholic, noncaffeinated liquids.

In cases of severe hypothermia, shivering will cease and the victim may be unconscious. Breathing may have slowed or stopped. The pulse may be slow and irregular. The body may feel stiff as the muscles become rigid. Rescue breathing should be started immediately if the victim is not breathing. Before starting CPR, check the victim's pulse for up to 45 seconds. If you cannot detect a pulse, begin CPR. Summon more advanced medical personnel. Remove any wet clothing. Be prepared to start CPR.

Preventing Heat- or Cold-Related Emergencies

Generally, emergencies caused by overexposure to extreme temperatures are preventable. To prevent heat- or cold-related emergencies from happening to you or anyone you know, follow these guidelines:

- Do not work in the hottest or coldest part of the day, if possible.
- Take frequent breaks to rewarm or cool the body.
- Take breaks to replenish the body with food and fluids.
- Reduce the intensity of the work.
- Wear appropriate clothing for the task and the environment.

Drinking cool or warm fluids helps the body maintain a normal temperature. Do not drink beverages containing caffeine or alcohol. Caffeine and alcohol hinder the body's temperature-regulating mechanism.

Always wear appropriate clothing for the environmental conditions and your activity level. When possible, wear light-colored cotton clothing in the heat. Cotton absorbs perspiration and lets air circulate through the material. This lets heat escape and perspiration evaporate, cooling the body. Light-colored clothing reflects the sun's rays.

When you are in the cold, wear layers of clothing made of tightly woven fibers, such as wool or polypropylene, that trap warm air against your body. Wear a head covering in both heat and cold. A hat protects the head from the sun's rays in the summer and prevents heat from escaping in the winter. Also protect areas of the body, such as the fingers, toes, ears, and nose, from cold exposure by wearing protective coverings. Carry in an emergency kit two extra pairs of socks (one to use as mittens) and two small plastic bags to wear between your shoes and socks in wet areas. Two lawn and leaf-size plastic bags make excellent survival outerwear in situations that require unexpected exposure to cold, wind, and rain.

◆ BEHAVIORAL EMERGENCIES

A person's behavior refers to how he or she acts, which is noticeable to others. A **behavioral emergency** is a situation in which the victim exhibits abnormal behavior that is unacceptable or intolerable. Such is often the case with people who become violent, attempt to take their lives, or believe that people are out to harm them. A behavioral emergency can pose unique problems that you must manage.

Causes of Behavioral Emergencies

Injury, physical or mental illness, and extreme stress are the primary causes of behavioral emergencies. Any condition that reduces the amount of oxygen to the brain, such as head injury, can also result in a significant change in behavior. Too little oxygen could make a normally calm person suddenly become very anxious or even violent. Physical illness as a result of substance abuse, diabetic emergencies, heat or cold exposure, or problems with the nervous system associated with aging, can lead to alterations in behavior.

Mental illness can also cause behavioral emergencies. The exact cause of mental illness is often not known, but it is sometimes the result of a chemical abnormality in the brain. The behavior exhibited by a victim with mental illness can be bizarre and can include excited or depressed behavior. The victim may —

- Be agitated.
- Speak rapidly or incoherently.
- Pace about the room.
- Be subdued or withdrawn.
- Lack the desire to do anything.
- Express feelings of extreme sadness and emptiness.

As you learned in Chapter 2, emotional crises can lead to extreme stress, which affects people in different ways. The impact of the incident and the way the victim copes or fails to cope with the stress can lead to an emotional situation that the victim cannot handle. The victim may react with uncontrollable crying, denial, anger, frustration, or depression.

Recognizing Behavioral Emergencies

The four most common signs and symptoms of behavioral emergencies are —

- Violent behavior towards self or others.
- Psychological disorders causing the victim to lose touch with reality.
- Threatened or attempted suicide.
- Frustration, anger, and depression associated with emotional crisis.

Violent behavior can take many forms, from verbal abuse to punching, kicking, biting, and using weapons. While the violence may not be directed toward you, you could easily become an indirect victim caught in the middle, or these acts may only be targeted to people in positions of authority, like yourself.

A victim's posture and comments can indicate potential violence. Threatening comments and posture, such as clenched fists or assuming a fighting stance, may indicate the victim's intentions (Fig. 15-6).

Mental illness can cause a victim to lose touch with reality. The victim's behavior is often

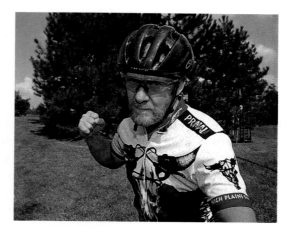

Figure 15-6 A victim's posture, such as clenched fists or assuming a fighting stance, may indicate potential violence.

characterized as irrational, and the victim may have hallucinations. The victim can experience a significant change in mood over a short period of time. The victim may initially appear to be willing to cooperate with you and then suddenly become withdrawn and uncooperative. This victim may also pose a potential or actual threat to himself or herself, as well as to others. Sometimes an individual will attempt to commit suicide. More suicide attempts are made by females than males, but males are more likely to succeed. The most common method of attempting suicide is by drug overdose. However, most actual suicides occur from the use of a firearm, which accounts for more than 50 percent of all deaths from suicide. Any victim who has discussed or attempted suicide in the past is at risk of trying it again, especially if the individual has discussed a definite plan for the suicide attempt.

Caring for Behavioral Emergencies

Your personal safety should always be a concern whenever you encounter a victim with a behavioral emergency. Size up the scene to gather information relevant to safety. Consider the mechanism of injury or illness, and consider the hazards of the scene. Do not enter a dangerous situation until it can be corrected.

This may mean waiting until law enforcement personnel arrive and get the situation under control.

When it is safe to enter, remain cautious as you approach the victim. Just because the scene may appear safe does not necessarily mean that it is. The victim may have a weapon or other objects in his or her possession, or nearby, that could cause injury. Always be prepared for any potential threat. Always keep your eyes on the victim and never turn your back. Always stay between the victim and the exit, if possible.

As you interact with the victim, remember that there are steps that you can take to help calm the victim. Involve other people whom the victim trusts. Avoid unnecessary physical contact. Maintain a comfortable and safe distance from the victim. Your body position can display positive or negative emotions. Get in front of the victim and at his or her level. Maintaining eye contact shows that you are attentive to what the other person has to say. Try to assume a non-threatening posture. A non-threatening posture is one in which you avoid a defensive stance, such as standing rigidly, crossing your arms, standing sideways, or assuming a fighting stance.

When speaking to the victim, speak slowly, clearly, and in a normal tone of voice. Use the victim's name whenever possible. Do not falsely reassure the victim, but let the victim know that everything that can be done to help will be done. Never threaten, challenge, or argue with the victim. Try to comfort the victim, but do not make any effort to "play along" or make statements to support a victim's delusions. Acknowledge that the victim appears upset and that you would like to help. Encourage the victim to discuss whatever is troubling him or her. Always act in a calm, caring manner. In most situations, effective communication techniques can help make your assessment and care easier.

Observe the victim's general appearance and behavior as you talk with him or her. Determine the victim's level of consciousness and activity level. Is the victim active or subdued? How does the victim speak? Explain what you would like to do, including checking his or her vital signs and providing care for any obvious injuries, such as external bleeding. Over time, you may be able to convince the victim that you can be trusted. Before more advanced medical personnel arrive, you may be able to convince the victim of the need for medical care.

A victim with a behavioral emergency needs to be evaluated by professionals trained to handle this type of problem. If the victim refuses to provide consent but you feel that the victim is a threat to himself or herself or others, have law enforcement personnel and more advanced medical personnel intervene. In situations in which the victim is violent or has the potential to become so, the victim may need to be restrained. Restraints, devices that restrict movement, in this case, are for the safety of the victim, as well as others, during transport. Restraints should be used as victim protection in very few circumstances only. As discussed in Chapter 4, restraining a person without justification can give rise to a claim of assault and battery. Before placing a victim in restraints, consider the need for assistance, the type of behavior you have observed or can reasonably anticipate from the victim, the likely consequences of using or not using restraints, and your organization's protocols that govern their use.

Use only **reasonable force** when applying restraints. Reasonable force is the minimal force necessary to keep a victim from injuring both himself or herself and you or others helping to restrain the victim. Applying restraints requires the assistance of rescuers who have been adequately trained in how to apply the restraints used by your agency. Law enforcement personnel are usually available to help you control the victim.

Accurately document the events surrounding your assessment and care of a victim with a behavioral emergency. Proper documentation can help minimize the likelihood of future legal problems. Use attendants of the same sex as the victim whenever possible. Doing so may help minimize accusations of sexual misconduct, commonly alleged by victims with behavioral emergencies.

◆ SUMMARY

Medical emergencies can strike anyone at any time. The signs and symptoms of different emergencies are similar, such as changes in the level of consciousness, confusion, weakness, and ill appearance. Recognizing the general signs and symptoms of medical emergencies will indicate the initial care you should provide. Usually, you will not know the cause of the illness. Altered mental status, diabetic emergencies, seizures, and heat- and cold-related emergencies each have an individual, specific cause. Fortunately, you can provide proper care without knowing the cause. Following the general guidelines of care for any emergency will help prevent the condition from becoming worse. When providing care for sudden illnesses, you should—

- Do no further harm.
- Conduct an initial assessment, physical exam, and SAMPLE history.
- Summon more advanced medical personnel.
- Help the victim rest comfortably.
- Keep the victim from getting chilled or overheated.
- Administer oxygen, if it is available and you are trained to do so.

When responding to a victim with a possible behavioral emergency, begin by assessing the scene for dangers. Do not assess the victim until law enforcement personnel have secured the scene. Approach the victim cautiously, without making any rapid movements. Attempt to determine the victim's problem, gain consent, and provide any care. If the victim's behavior becomes threatening or violent, attempt to calm the victim. If attempts to calm the victim do not work, you may have to leave the scene. In some situations, reasonable force may be needed to restrain the victim for safe transport to a receiving facility. Document the situation carefully to avoid future legal problems.

Use the activities in Unit 15 of the workbook to review the material in this chapter.

You Are the Responder

1. It is a hot afternoon and the swimming pool is crowded. You notice a child acting strangely in the shallow end of the pool. He appears to stagger and then suddenly falls face-down in the water. He is having a seizure. His arms and legs flail wildly about. You rush into the water, support his body, and keep his head above water. The seizure quickly stops and his rigid body goes limp. You remove him from the pool. What care will you provide?
2. On a winter day, you are summoned to check on an elderly woman who has not answered her phone or a neighbor's repeated attempts to get her to come to her door. You go to the house with the neighbor and knock. No one answers. The door is closed but not locked. You enter and realize immediately that inside it is no warmer than outside. A woman bundled in a blanket is huddled close to a space heater. You speak to her and ask how she is. She appears disoriented and responds weakly. She is shivering uncontrollably. What care would you give this woman? Why?

ENRICHMENT

◆ DIABETIC EMERGENCIES

Diabetes mellitus is one of the leading causes of death and disability in the United States today:

- An estimated 14 million Americans currently have diabetes, and more than 600,000 additional cases are diagnosed each year.
- Diabetes contributes to other conditions, such as blindness; kidney, heart, and periodontal (gum) disease; and stroke.

To function normally, body cells need sugar as an energy source. Through the digestive process, the body breaks down food into simple sugars, such as **glucose,** which are absorbed into the bloodstream. However, sugar cannot pass freely from the blood into the body cells. **Insulin**, a hormone produced in the pancreas, is needed for sugar to pass into the cells. Without a proper balance of sugar and insulin in the blood, the cells will starve and the body will not function properly (Fig. 15-7).

There are two major types of diabetes. In Type I, insulin-dependent diabetes, the body produces little or no insulin. Since this type of diabetes tends to develop in childhood, it is commonly called juvenile diabetes. Most people who have Type I diabetes have to inject insulin into their bodies daily. In Type II, non-insulin-dependent diabetes, the body produces insulin, but either the cells do not use the insulin effectively or not enough insulin is produced. Type II diabetes, which is more common than Type I diabetes, is also known as adult-onset diabetes because it usually develops in the adult years. Most people with Type II diabetes can regulate their blood glucose level sufficiently through diet and sometimes oral medications and do not require insulin injections.

Anyone with diabetes must carefully monitor his or her diet and amount of exercise. Insulin-dependent diabetics must also regulate their use of insulin (Fig. 15-8). When diet and exercise are not controlled, either of two problems can occur — too much or too little sugar in the body. This imbalance of sugar and insulin in the blood causes illness.

When the insulin level in the body is too low, the sugar level in the blood is high. This

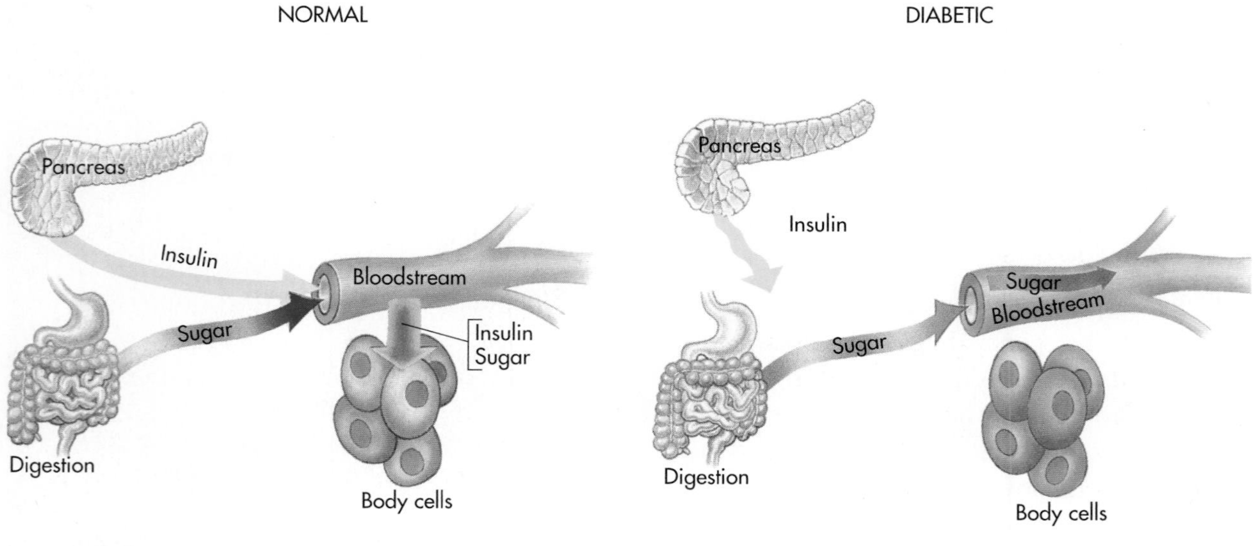

Figure 15-7 The hormone insulin is needed to take sugar from the blood into the body cells.

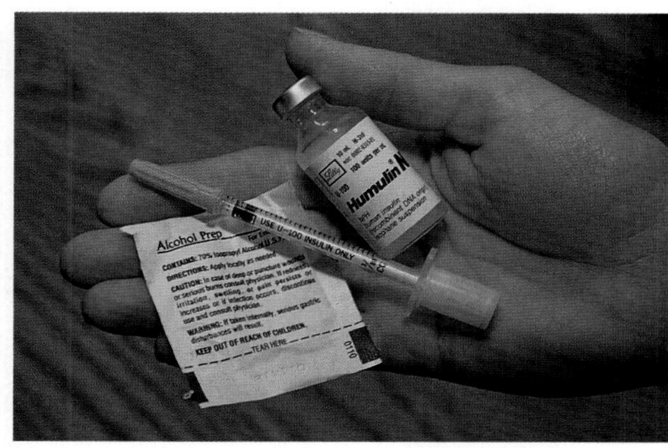

Figure 15-8 Insulin-dependent diabetics inject insulin to regulate the amount in the body.

condition is called ***hyperglycemia*** (Fig. 15-9, *A*). Sugar is present in the blood but cannot be transported from the blood into the cells without insulin. In this condition, body cells become starved for sugar. The body attempts to meet its need for energy by using other stored food and energy sources, such as fats. However, converting fat to energy is less efficient, produces waste products, and increases the acidity level in the blood, causing a condition known as diabetic ketoacidosis. As this occurs, the person becomes ill. He or she may have flushed, hot, dry skin and a sweet breath odor that can be mistaken for the smell of alcohol. The victim may also appear restless or agitated. If this condition is not treated promptly, **diabetic coma,** a life-threatening emergency, can occur.

On the other hand, when the insulin level in the body is too high, the person has a low sugar level. This condition is known as ***hypoglycemia*** (Fig. 15-9, *B*). The blood sugar level can become too low if the ***diabetic***—

- Takes too much insulin.
- Fails to eat adequately.
- Overexercises and burns off sugar faster than normal.
- Experiences great emotional stress.

In this situation, the small amount of sugar is used up rapidly, so not enough sugar is available for the brain to function properly. If left untreated, hypoglycemia from **insulin reaction** can cause brain damage or death.

Many diabetics have blood glucose monitors that can be used to check their blood glucose level at home. Many hypoglycemic and hyperglycemic episodes are now managed at home because of the rapid information these monitors provide.

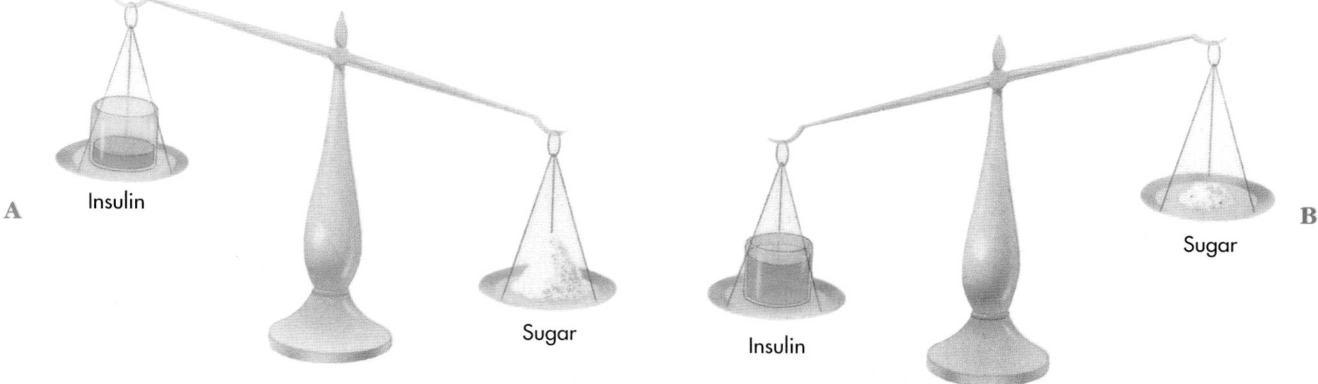

Figure 15-9 **A**, Hyperglycemia occurs when there is insufficient insulin in the body, causing a high level of sugar in the blood. **B**, Hypoglycemia occurs when the insulin level in the body is high, causing a low level of sugar in the blood.

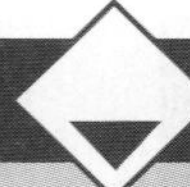

Innovations in the Treatment of Diabetes

Diabetes mellitus is one of the leading causes of death and disability in the United States today. Consider the following facts and figures on diabetes:

- An estimated 14 million Americans currently have diabetes, and more than 600,000 additional cases are diagnosed each year.
- Diabetes contributes to other conditions, such as blindness; kidney, heart, and periodontal gum disease; and stroke.
- Direct costs associated with diabetes were $85 billion in 1992. For the same year, an additional $47 billion in indirect costs was attributed to disability, work loss, and premature mortality.

In an effort to save lives and reduce medical costs, many doctors and researchers have devoted their resources to developing innovative ways to treat diabetes. The following information highlights the technological breakthroughs that have resulted from these endeavors.

New oral medication

Metformin, the first new diabetes medication to be approved in the United States for nearly 30 years, was approved by the Food and Drug Administration in December 1994 and became available by prescription in May 1995. Metformin is an oral medication designed to treat Type II diabetes. Metformin will be sold under the trade name of Glucophage and is estimated to cost about $30 for a month's treatment. Metformin is one of a class of drugs called biguanides. Biguanides improve insulin sensitivity by boosting the effectiveness of insulin already found in the body. Biguanides work by acting on insulin receptors located on the surface of nearly every cell.

Doctors and patients alike are excited about the approval of Metformin because it is affordable, works with the body's natural supply of insulin, can be used in patients who do not respond well to diet and exercise programs, can be prescribed alone or in combination with other diabetes medications, may replace or forestall the need for some insulin injections, and gives patients much better blood sugar control. Metformin is expected to be widely used among those who have Type II diabetes.

Noninvasive glucose monitors

Many patients who have diabetes find it inconvenient or difficult to puncture their fingers several times a day to monitor their blood glucose levels. To overcome resistance to this monitoring process, several companies are attempting to create a noninvasive device that would eliminate the need to puncture the skin.

The most promising device of this kind now in development monitors blood glucose levels by sending a near-infrared laser light beam through a fold in the skin. A patient would put his or her finger or other body part on the monitor, and the blood glucose level would be measured by analyzing the scattering of light passing through the skin.

Doctors and researchers are hopeful that some versions of noninvasive glucose monitors will be ready for review by the FDA in the near future. Once on the market, these monitors are expected to greatly improve the health and quality of life of diabetics.

New insulin analog

Although insulin therapy has come a long way since it was first made commercially available in 1923, present-day therapy still has major shortcomings. Perhaps the greatest difficulty is the inability of insulin injections to accurately mimic the natural concentrations of insulin the body produces in response to diet. When patients inject themselves 30 minutes before a meal, the insulin level peaks between 30 minutes and 2 to 3 hours after the injection and lasts 4 to 6 hours. The result is a risk of high blood glucose levels after a meal and low levels several hours later when food is digested and the insulin is still working.

Scientists are attempting to overcome this problem by creating a faster, short-acting insulin analog. An analog is a drug that resembles another drug in structure and components but pro-

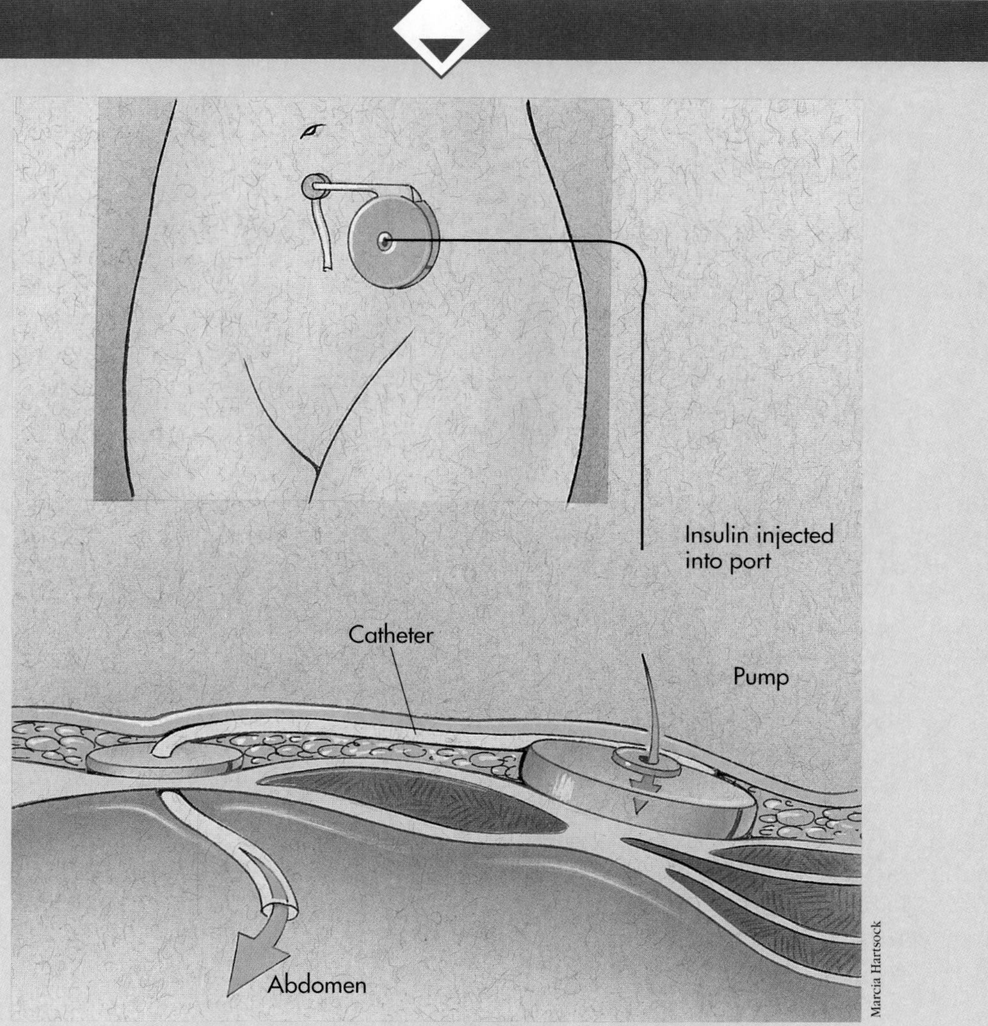

duces different effects. The most promising analog created to date is called Lispro. Lispro works more like natural insulin by going to work quickly, then disappearing rapidly from circulation. Lispro, which can be injected within 5 minutes of eating, peaks in 45 to 50 minutes and stays in the system for about 3 hours. This analog not only provides better glucose control but makes the patient less likely to forget an injection.

Preliminary tests indicate that Lispro is at least as effective as, if not better than, regular insulin. An abstract presented at the June 1994 meeting of the American Diabetes Association concluded that Lispro effectively improved glucose control with fewer insulin reactions than regular insulin. Worldwide testing of Lispro has begun, involving more than 3000 people in 25 countries who have Type I and Type II diabetes. Lispro may be available commercially within the next few years.

Internal programmable pump

Some people who have diabetes wear an external insulin pump, about the size of a beeper, which can be programmed to deliver insulin on demand. Although many patients are pleased with this method of treatment, most of those who have Type I diabetes continue to choose the multiple-injection approach. Dissatisfaction with the external pumps may be from their expense, extensive maintenance, and inconvenience to wear. Now scientists are hoping to spare patients the aggravation of external pumps. On the horizon is a device that will simulate natural insulin delivery through a closed-loop system implanted in the wall of the abdomen, where insulin can be absorbed rapidly.

The closed-loop insulin-delivery machine is so called because the machine would incorporate a sensor to measure plasma or tissue glucose levels continuously, then transfer that information to a pump that would deliver insulin as needed. The pump produces a slight bulge under the skin, much like a pacemaker, but a French study of internal programmable pumps showed excellent results with a minimum of inconvenience. Two American companies are now testing their versions.

Islet cell transplantation

A research team at the Islet Transplantation Center at St. Vincent Medical Center in Los Angeles is perfecting a technique of encapsulating cells from the Islets of Langerhans (pronounced I letz of LAN gur hanz)—the sections of the pancreas responsible for insulin production—and transplanting them into insulin-dependent diabetes patients. In preliminary tests, the transplanted cells appear to function normally, allowing recipients to become insulin independent with normal blood sugar levels.

Experimentation of this kind has been underway for decades. However, the ongoing challenge has been to identify encapsulating substances that prevent or reduce the chances of having the recipient's body reject the cells as foreign material. The most promising encapsulating techniques to date involve the use of a seaweed-derived polymer known as alginate. The encapsulated cells are simply poured into the patient's abdominal cavity through a funnel. Once inside the recipient's abdominal cavity, the encapsulated cells respond to increased levels of glucose just as pancreatic islet cells normally would—by secreting insulin.

Islet transplantation research has been quite successful in recent years. Transplanted cells have been found to function normally in mice for at least a year, and the same procedure is expected to be studied widely in dogs in the near future. To date, the procedure has been attempted in only two humans.

Although these innovations are still being developed and tested, some may not be far from being perfected. Such technologies, once they become widely available, would provide a much greater range of treatment options for both major types of diabetes.

SOURCES

Baum R: "Diabetes treatment: encapsulated cells make insulin in patient," *Chemical and Emergency News* March 21, 1994.

National Diabetes Information Clearinghouse: "Diabetes statistics" September 1994.

Squires S: "New Drug Approved for Type II Diabetics," *Washington Post Health*, May 16, 1995.

Weir GS: "What lies ahead in diabetes care," *Patient Care* February 15, 1995.

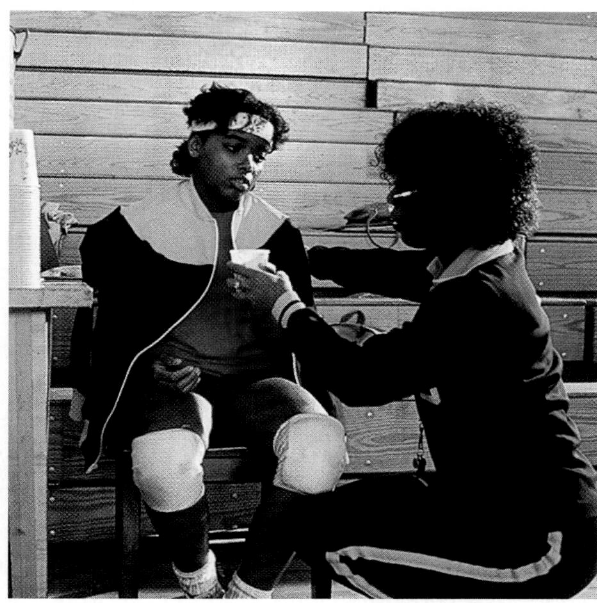

Figure 15-10 If a victim of a diabetic emergency is conscious, give him or her food or fluids containing sugar.

Signs and Symptoms of Diabetic Emergencies

Although hypoglycemia and hyperglycemia are different conditions, their major signs and symptoms are similar. These include—

- Changes in the level of consciousness, including dizziness, drowsiness, and confusion.
- Irregular breathing.
- Abnormal pulse (rapid or weak).
- Feeling and looking ill.
- Abnormal skin characteristics.

It is not important for you to differentiate between insulin reaction and diabetic coma, because the basic care for both conditions is the same.

Care for Diabetic Emergencies

To care for ***diabetic emergencies***, first do an initial assessment and care for any life-threatening conditions. If the victim is conscious, do a physical exam and SAMPLE history, looking for anything visibly wrong. Ask if he or she is a diabetic, and look for a medical alert tag. If the person is a known diabetic and exhibits the signs and symptoms previously stated, then suspect a diabetic emergency.

If the conscious victim can take food or fluids, give him or her sugar (Fig. 15-10). Most candy, fruit juices, and nondiet soft drinks have enough sugar to be effective. Common table sugar, either dry or dissolved in a glass of water, can restore the victim to a normal condition. Commercially available sugar sources also work well. Sometimes, diabetics will be able to tell you what is wrong and will ask for something with sugar in it. If the person's problem is low sugar (hypoglycemia), the sugar you give will help quickly. If the person already has too much sugar (hyperglycemia), the excess sugar will do no further harm.

Unless the person is fully conscious, do not give anything by mouth. Instead, monitor the ABCs, keep the victim from getting chilled or overheated, summon more advanced medical personnel, and administer oxygen if it is available and you are trained to do so. If the victim is conscious but does not feel better within approximately 5 minutes after taking sugar, summon more advanced medical personnel. Oxygen should be administered if it is available and you have proper training.

◆ STROKE

A **stroke**, also called a cerebrovascular accident (CVA), is a disruption of blood flow to a part of the brain, causing permanent damage to brain tissue (Fig. 15-11). Most commonly, a stroke is caused by a blood clot, called a **thrombus** or **embolism**, that forms or lodges in the arteries that supply blood to the brain. Another common cause is bleeding from a ruptured artery in the brain caused by a head injury, high blood pressure, or an aneurysm—a

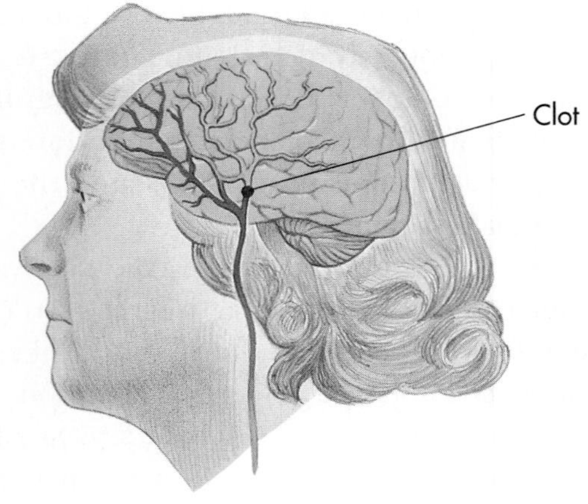

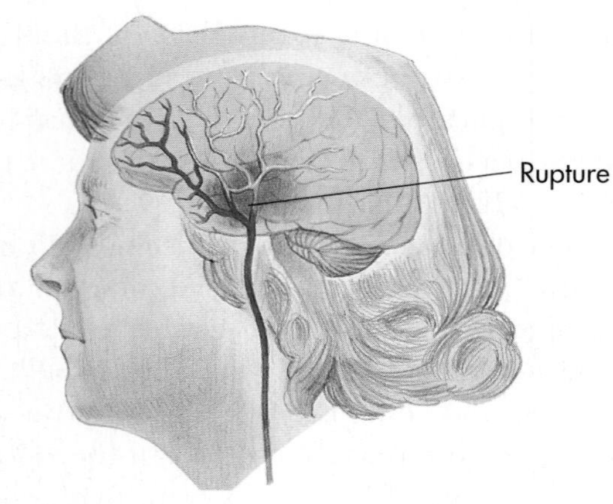

Figure 15-11 A stroke can be caused by a blood clot or bleeding from a ruptured artery in the brain.

weak area in an artery wall that balloons out and can rupture. Fat deposits lining an artery (atherosclerosis) may also cause a stroke. Less commonly, a tumor or swelling from a head injury may cause a stroke by compressing an artery.

A **transient ischemic attack** (TIA), often referred to as a "mini-stroke," is a temporary episode that, like a stroke, is caused by reduced blood flow to a part of the brain. Unlike a stroke, the signs and symptoms of TIA disappear within a few minutes or hours of its onset. Although the indicators of TIA disappear quickly, the person is not out of danger. In fact, someone who experiences a TIA has a nearly 10 times greater chance of having a stroke in the future than someone who has not experienced a TIA.

Signs and Symptoms of Stroke

As with other sudden illnesses, the primary signs and symptoms of stroke or TIA are looking or feeling ill, changes in consciousness, or displaying abnormal behavior. Others include sudden weakness and numbness of the face, arm, or leg. Usually, this occurs only on one side of the body. The victim may have difficulty talking or understanding speech. Vision may be blurred or dimmed; the pupils may be of unequal size. The person may also experience a sudden severe headache, dizziness, confusion, change in mood, or ringing in the ears. The victim may drool, become unconscious, or lose bowel or bladder control.

Care for Stroke

If the victim is unconscious, make sure he or she has an open airway and care for any life-threatening conditions that may occur. If there is fluid or vomit in the victim's mouth, position him or her on one side to allow any fluids to drain out. You may have to use a finger sweep or suction to remove some of the material from the mouth. Summon more advanced medical personnel, stay with the victim, and monitor his or her ABCs. Administer supplemental oxygen if it is available and you are trained to do so. Consider the use of an oral or nasal airway, if necessary and your protocols allow.

If the victim is conscious, do a physical exam and SAMPLE history. A stroke can make the victim fearful and anxious. Offer comfort and reassurance. Often he or she does not understand what has happened. Have the victim rest in a comfortable position. Do not give him or her anything to eat or drink. If the victim is drooling or having difficulty swallowing, place him or her on one side to help drain any fluids or vomit from the mouth.

The Brain Makes a Comeback

Neuroscientists have been mystified for years by the random effects of stroke. For many stroke survivors, talking becomes a tangle of words, a word like "piddlypop" spilling out instead of "hello." One man spoke normally unless he was asked to name fruits and vegetables. Each stroke survivor seemed to have a unique, perplexing set of problems, and doctors found recovery equally unpredictable.

Research into brain function after a stroke has shed new light on the way the brain works. Many strokes are caused when blood flow to the brain is cut off by a blood clot or hemorrhage. The oxygen-deprived brain cells rupture and die. Neuroscientists once believed that the cells died from lack of oxygen. However, their conclusion did not explain why stroke survivors sometimes got worse over a period of several hours.

Researchers have found that when oxygen-deprived brain cells rupture, they release huge quantities of the amino acid glutamate. Glutamate gushes into surviving brain cells and destroys them. Normally, small amounts of glutamate act as transmitters between the cells, but large amounts are damaging to these cells. Researchers believe that if they could inhibit the reaction of glutamate within the cell, they could prevent the most severe brain damage and, perhaps, the death of stroke victims.

Researchers are developing several drugs to try to block the flood of glutamate that occurs after a stroke. They have found that drugs similar to phencyclidine, a potent animal tranquilizer and street drug known as PCP, have proven the most effective. Like PCP, the drugs cause temporary hallucinations. However, doctors say the promising results outweigh the side effects.

Another drug that is now being tested as a possible treatment for the damage caused by stroke is omega-conotoxin. Omega-conotoxin is derived from the venom of the cone snail, which can instantly paralyze a fish and even kill a human. Recent research shows that when Omega-conotoxin is administered after a stroke, it temporarily blocks the channels that deliver the damaging flood of glutamate to the brain cells. When rats were given a synthesized version of Omega-conotoxin, the death of neurons in the brain was slowed down or even halted.

Strokes still present many mysteries, but scientists are learning more about stroke every day. With more than 3 million stroke survivors in the United States today, doctors are hopeful that new drugs may eventually eliminate the long-term effects.

SOURCES

American Heart Association: 1993 *Heart and Stroke Facts Statistics.*

Blakeslee S: "Pervasive Chemical Crucial to the Body Is Indicted as an Agent in Brain Damage," *The New York Times*, November 29, 1988.

Killer snails, healer snails, *Discover* May 1994, p 32.

Preventing Stroke

The risk factors for stroke and TIA are similar to those for heart disease. Some risk factors are beyond your control, such as age; gender; or a family history of stroke, TIA, diabetes, or heart disease.

You can control other risk factors. One of the most important is **hypertension**, or high blood pressure. Hypertension increases your risk of stroke approximately 7 times. High blood pressure puts pressure on arteries and makes them more likely to burst. It also causes atherosclerosis. Even mild hypertension can increase your risk of stroke. You can often control high blood pressure by losing weight, changing your diet, exercising routinely, and managing stress. If those measures are not sufficient, your physician may prescribe medication.

Cigarette smoking is another major risk factor for stroke. Smoking is also linked to heart disease and cancer. It increases blood pressure and makes blood more likely to clot. If you do not smoke, do not start. If you do smoke, seek help to try to stop. No matter how difficult or painful quitting may be, it is well worth it. The benefits of not smoking start as soon as you stop.

Diets that are high in saturated fats and cholesterol increase your chance of stroke by increasing the possibility of fatty materials building up on the walls of your blood vessels. Keep your intake of these foods at a moderate level.

Regular exercise reduces your chances of stroke by increasing blood circulation, which develops more channels for blood flow. These additional channels provide alternate routes for blood if the primary channels become blocked.

◆ RAPID REWARMING OF FROSTBITE

If advanced medical personnel are going to be considerably delayed, causing an extremely long transport time, consider rapid rewarming the localized cold injury (frostbite). Warm the area gently by soaking the affected part in water between 102 degrees F and 104 degrees F. Use a thermometer to check the water, if possible. If not, test the water temperature yourself.

A

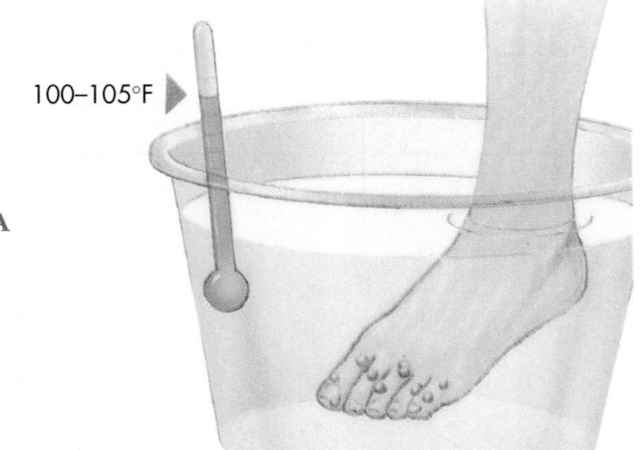

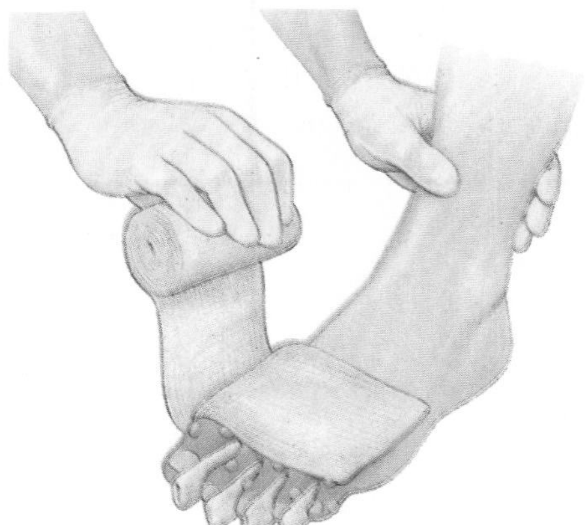

B

Figure 15-12 **A**, Warm the frostbitten area gently by soaking the area in water. Do not allow the frostbitten area to touch the container. **B**, After rewarming, bandage the area with dry, sterile dressing. If fingers or toes are frostbitten, place gauze between them.

If the temperature is uncomfortable to your touch, the water is too warm. Do not let the affected body part touch the bottom or sides of the container (Fig. 15-12, *A*). Keep the frostbitten part in the water until it appears red and feels warm. Bandage the area with a dry, sterile dressing. If fingers or toes are frostbitten, place cotton or gauze between them (Fig. 15-12, *B*). Avoid breaking any blisters. Seek professional medical attention as soon as possible. Do not rewarm if the victim is going to be exposed to cold again. Only rewarm where there is no danger of refreezing, such as in a house or an effective, warm shelter.

Poisoning

16

Key Terms

Absorbed poison: A poison that enters the body through the skin.

Addiction: The compulsive need to use a substance. Stopping use would cause the user to suffer mental, physical, and emotional distress.

Anaphylaxis: A severe allergic reaction in which air passages may swell and obstruct breathing; a form of shock.

Cannabis products: Substances, such as marijuana and hashish, that are derived from the *Cannabis sativa* plant; can produce feelings of elation, distorted perceptions of time and space, and impaired motor coordination and judgment.

Dependency: The desire or need to continually use a substance.

Depressants: Substances that affect the central nervous system to slow physical and mental activity.

Designer drug: A potent and illegal street drug formed from a medicinal substance whose chemical composition has been modified (designed).

Drug: Any substance other than food intended to affect the functions of the body.

Hallucinogens (hah LU si no jenz): Substances that affect mood, sensation, thought, emotion, and self-awareness; alter perceptions of time and space; and produce delusions.

Ingested poison: A poison that is swallowed.

Inhalants: Substance, such as a medication, that a person inhales to counteract or prevent a specific condition; a substance inhaled to produce a mood-altering effect.

Inhaled poison: A poison breathed into the lungs.

Injected poison: A poison that enters the body through a bite, sting, or syringe.

Medication: A drug given to prevent or correct the effects of a disease or condition or otherwise enhance mental or physical welfare.

Narcotics: Powerful depressant substances used to reduce pain.

Overdose: The use of an excessive amount of a substance, resulting in adverse reactions ranging from mania (mental and physical hyperactivity) and hysteria to coma and death.

Poison: Any substance that causes injury, illness, or death when introduced into the body.

Poison control center (PCC): A specialized health center that provides information in poisoning or suspected poisoning emergencies.

Stimulants: Substances that affect the central nervous system to speed up physical and mental activity.

Substance abuse: The deliberate, persistent, excessive use of a substance without regard to health concerns or accepted medical practices.

Substance misuse: The use of a substance for unintended purposes or for intended purposes but in improper amounts or doses.

Tolerance: A condition in which the effects of a substance on the body decrease as a result of continual use.

Withdrawal: The condition of mental and physical discomfort produced when a person stops using or abusing a substance to which he or she is addicted.

◆ Knowledge Objectives ◆

After reading this chapter and completing the class activities, you should be able to—

- List the ways poisons enter the body.
- List signs and symptoms of poisoning.
- Describe the general principles of care for victims of poisoning.
- Describe specific care for victims of ingested, inhaled, injected, and absorbed poisons.
- Identify the categories of commonly abused or misused substances.
- Identify signs and symptoms of possible substance abuse or misuse.
- Describe the general care for someone suspected of misusing or abusing a substance.
- Describe the signs and symptoms of anaphylaxis.
- Describe how to care for a victim of anaphylaxis.

◆ Attitude Objectives ◆

After reading this chapter and completing the class activities, you should be able to—

- Value the important role that poison control centers play in the care of a victim of poisoning.

◆ Skill Objectives ◆

After reading this chapter and completing the class activities, you should be able to —

- Make appropriate decisions about care when given an example of an emergency in which someone may have been poisoned.

◆ INTRODUCTION

Chapter 15 described medical emergencies caused by conditions inside the body. Poisoning can also be a medical emergency, but unlike sudden illnesses, such as fainting and stroke, poisoning results when an external substance enters the body. The substance could be a food that is swallowed, a pesticide absorbed through the skin, or venom that might enter the body through a bite or sting. In this chapter, you will learn how to recognize and care for poisoning.

Between 1 and 2 million poisonings occur each year in the United States. More than 90 percent of all poisonings take place in the home. Unintentional poisonings far outnumber intentional ones, and most unintentional poisonings occur in children under age 5. Although the death rate from poisoning in children under age 5 has dropped in the last 30 years, poisoning fatalities still pose a serious risk. In fact, among adults 18 and older, poisoning fatalities have markedly increased during the same period.

This increase in poisoning fatalities among adults can be linked to two factors: (1) increases in intentional poisonings (suicides) and (2) increases in drug-related poisonings. Although use of illegal street drugs, like cocaine, attracts more attention, the misuse and abuse of prescription medications and alcohol are actually more prevalent. About two thirds of all unintentional poisonings involve drugs and medications. Half of all drug overdoses are caused by prescribed medication that is misused or abused.

◆ HOW POISONS ENTER THE BODY

A ***poison*** is any substance that can cause injury, illness, or death when introduced into the

Common Causes of Poisoning (by age group)

Under 6	6-19	Over 19
Analgesic medications	Analgesic medications	Analgesic medications
Cleaning substances	Bites and stings	Antidepressant drugs
Cosmetics and personal care products	Cleaning substances	Bites and stings
Cough and cold remedies	Cosmetics	Chemicals
Gastrointestinal medications	Cough and cold remedies	Cleaning substances
Plants	Food products/food poisoning	Food products/food poisoning
Topical medications	Plants	Fumes and vapors
Vitamins	Stimulants and street drugs	Insecticides
		Sedatives and hallucinogenic drugs

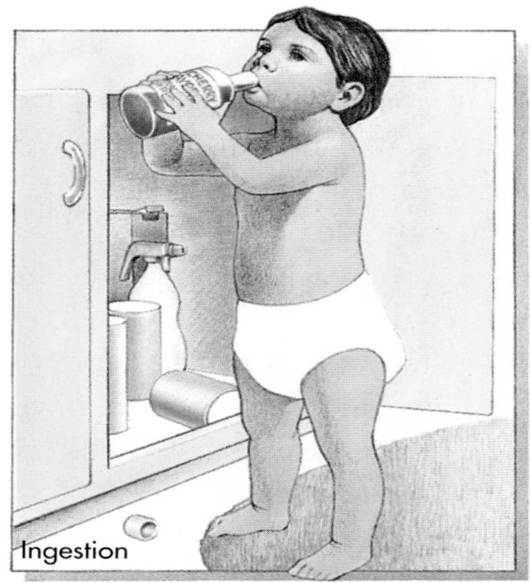

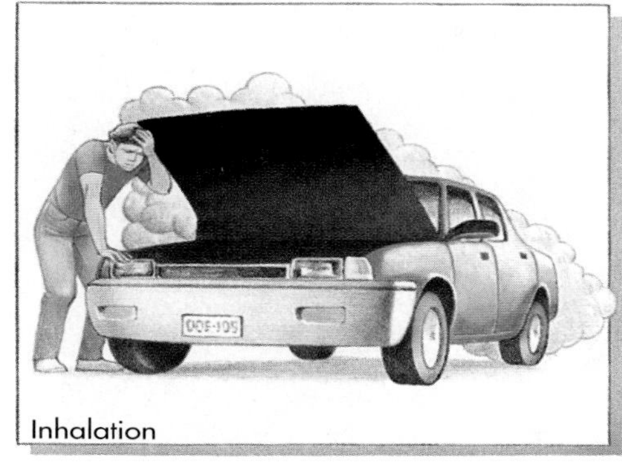

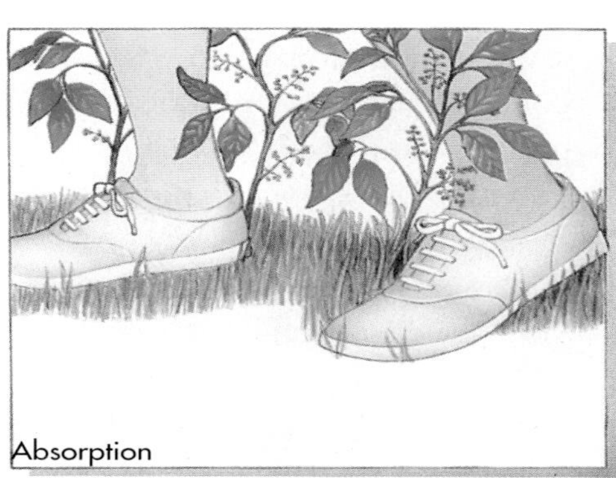

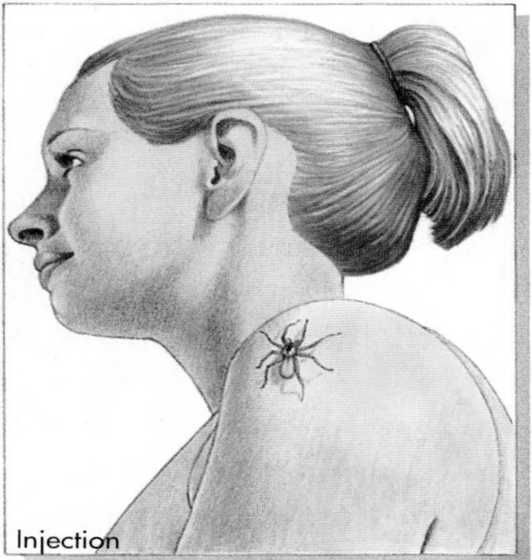

Figure 16-1 A poison can enter the body in four ways: ingestion, inhalation, absorption, and injection.

body in relatively small amounts. Poisons include solids, liquids, **vapors,** gases, and **fumes.** A poison can enter the body in four ways (Fig. 16-1):

- Inhalation
- Ingestion
- Absorption
- Injection

Poisoning by inhalation occurs when a person breathes in toxic substances. ***Inhaled poisons*** include —

- Gases, such as carbon monoxide, from an engine, kerosene heater, or other source of combustion.
- Gases, such as carbon dioxide, that can occur naturally from decomposition.
- Gases, such as nitrous oxide, used for medical purposes.
- Gases, such as chlorine, found in some commercial swimming facilities.
- Vapors from household products, such as glues and paints.
- Vapors from drugs, such as crack cocaine.

Ingestion means swallowing. ***Ingested poisons*** include foods, such as certain mushrooms and shellfish; drugs, such as alcohol; medications, such as aspirin; and household and garden items, such as cleaning products, pesticides, and plants (Fig. 16-2). Many substances not poisonous in small amounts are poisonous in larger amounts. Any medication (prescription or over-the-counter) can be poisonous if it is not taken as prescribed or directed.

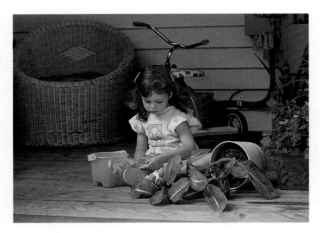

Figure 16-2 Many common household plants are poisonous.

An ***absorbed poison*** enters the body after it comes in contact with the skin. Absorbed poisons include fertilizers and pesticides used in lawn and plant care. While they are not absorbed into the body, the oils in the leaves and other parts of poison ivy, poison oak, and poison sumac plants can cause irritations to people who are allergic to them if they come in contact with the skin. The plants are not actually poisonous. The stinging nettle plant, however, actually injects poison into the skin when you brush up against one.

Injected poisons enter the body through the bites or stings of certain insects, spiders, ticks, marine life, animals, and snakes or as drugs or medications injected with a hypodermic needle.

◆ SIGNS AND SYMPTOMS OF POISONING

The most important thing is to recognize that a poisoning may have occurred. As with other serious emergencies, check the scene and the condition of the victim, then get any possible information from the victim or bystanders. Doing so could help you decide whether the victim has been poisoned.

As you approach the victim, survey the scene to make sure it is safe to enter. Be aware of any unusual odors, flames, smoke, open or spilled containers, an open medicine cabinet, an overturned or damaged plant, or other signals of possible poisoning.

When you reach the victim, check for life-threatening and nonlife-threatening conditions. The victim of poisoning generally looks ill and has signs and symptoms common to other medical emergencies. The signs and symptoms of poisoning include nausea, vomiting, diarrhea, chest or abdominal pain, difficulty breathing, sweating, loss of consciousness, seizures, headache, dizziness, weakness, irregular pupil size, burning or tearing eyes, and abnormal skin color. Other signs of poisoning are burn injuries around the lips or tongue or on the skin. You may also suspect a poisoning based on any information you have from or about the victim. Look also for any **drug paraphernalia,** or devices used to contain or administer drugs, such as syringes, and empty containers at or near the scene.

Common Signs and Symptoms of Poisoning

- Nausea
- Vomiting
- Diarrhea
- Chest or abdominal pain
- Breathing difficulty
- Sweating
- Loss of consciousness
- Seizures
- Burn injuries around the lips or tongue or on the skin
- Headache
- Dizziness
- Weakness
- Irregular pupil size
- Burning or tearing eyes
- Abnormal skin color

If you suspect a poisoning, try to get answers to the following questions:

- What type of poison did the victim ingest, inhale, inject, absorb, or contact?
- How much poison did the victim ingest, inhale, inject, absorb, or contact?
- When did the poisoning take place (approximate time)?

This information will help you provide the most appropriate care.

◆ POISON CONTROL CENTERS

Poison control centers (PCCs) are specialized health-care centers that provide information in cases of poisoning or suspected poisoning emergencies. A network of PCCs exists throughout the United States, as well as abroad. Some PCCs are located in the emergency departments of large hospitals. Medical professionals in PCCs have access to information about virtually all poisonous substances and can tell you how to care for someone who has been poisoned. You should have your local PCC phone number readily available.

PCCs answer over 2 million poisoning calls each year. Since many poisonings can be cared for without the help of EMS professionals, PCCs help prevent overburdening of the EMS system. If the victim is conscious and does not appear seriously ill, your local protocols may have you call your local or regional PCC first. The center will tell you what care to give and whether more advanced medical attention is needed.

If the victim is unconscious or you do not know your PCC number, summon more advanced medical personnel. The dispatcher may link you with the PCC. The dispatcher may also monitor your conversation with the PCC and provide additional information to the responding ambulance crew. In some situations, this saves time by eliminating the need for a second call (Fig. 16-3).

◆ CARE FOR POISONING

The severity of a poisoning depends on the type and amount of the substance; how and where it entered the body; the time elapsed since the poison entered the body; and the victim's size, weight, and age. Some poisons act quickly and produce characteristic signs and symptoms. Others act slowly and cannot be easily identified. Sometimes you will be able to identify the specific poison, sometimes not. The important thing is to follow the general guidelines of care for any poisoning emergency:

- Check the scene to make sure it is safe to approach and to gather clues about what happened.
- Remove the victim from the source of the poison, if necessary and possible.
- Conduct an initial assessment to check for life-threatening conditions.
- If the victim is conscious, perform a physical exam and take a SAMPLE history to get more information.
- Look for any drug or product containers, and take them with you to the telephone. If the victim goes to the hospital, ensure bottles of all possibly ingested poisons or drugs accompany him or her.
- Call your PCC, hospital, or EMS according to your local protocols.
- Give care according to the directions of PCC personnel or hospital staff.
- Do not give the victim anything to drink or eat unless so advised by medical professionals. If the poison is unknown and the victim vomits, save some of the vomit, which the hospital may analyze to identify the poison. Use a clean container to collect the vomit. Look for pieces of plant, pill fragments, or blood in the vomit and report any such findings to the EMTs or emergency department personnel.

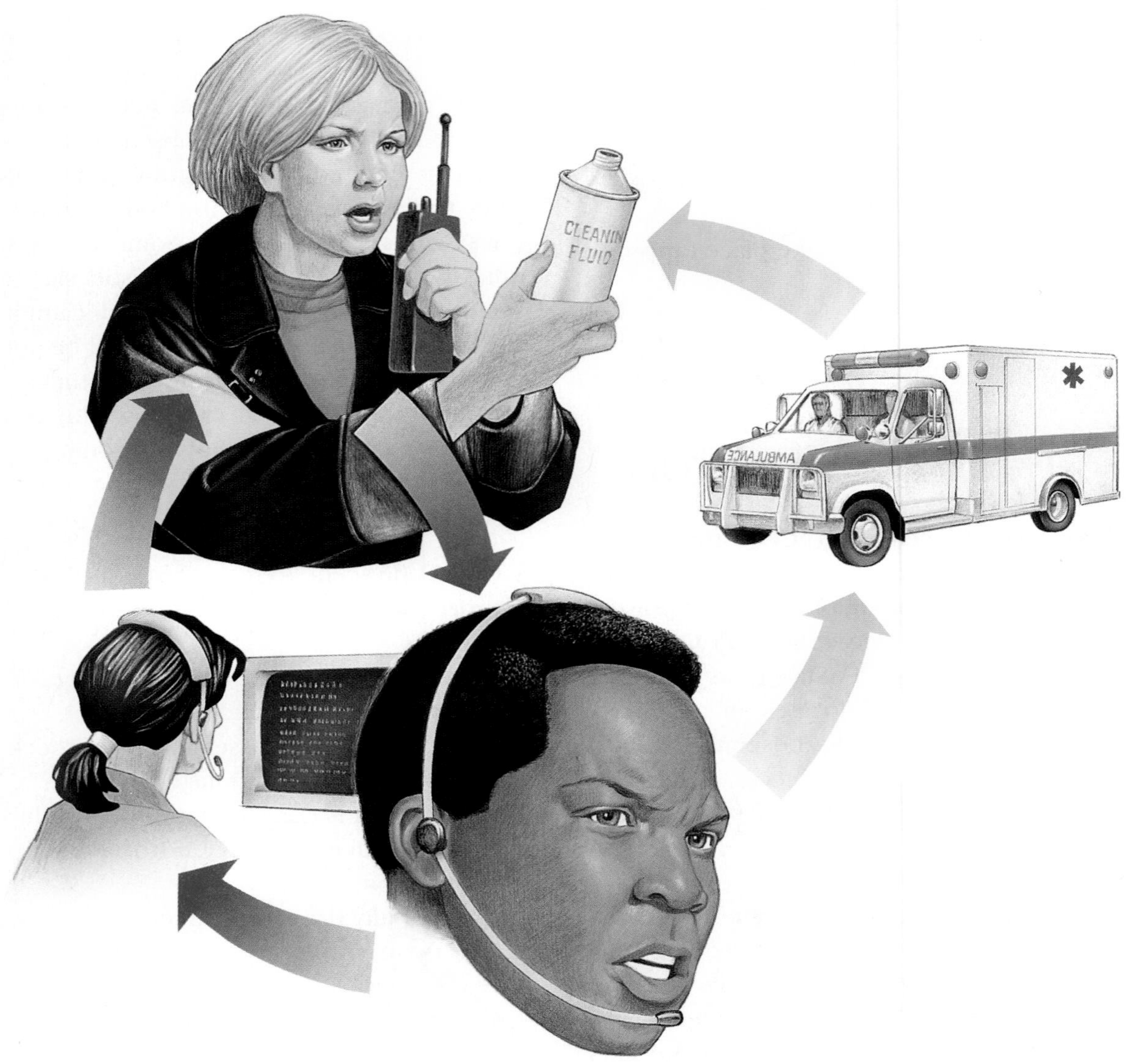

Figure 16-3 A dispatcher can link you with the PCC, monitor your discussion, and provide additional information to the responding ambulance crew.

Inhaled Poisons

When you care for a victim of poisoning, you need to follow precautions to ensure that you do not become poisoned as well. The need for precautions is particularly true with inhaled poisons. **Toxic** fumes, vapors, and gases come from a variety of sources and may or may not have an odor. If you notice clues at the scene of an emergency that might lead you to suspect that toxic fumes are present, such as a strong smell of fuel or a hissing sound like gas escaping from a pipe or valve, you may not be able to reach the victim without risking your safety. Only enter the scene if it is safe to do so.

A commonly inhaled poison is **carbon monoxide (CO).** CO is a colorless, odorless gas that causes more than half of all poisoning deaths in the United States each year. It is present in certain substances, such as car exhaust and tobacco smoke. CO can also be produced

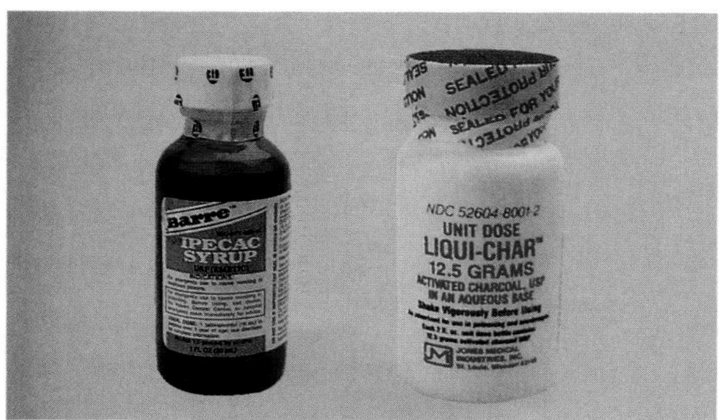

Figure 16-4 Syrup of ipecac and activated charcoal should be part of your emergency supplies.

by fires, defective cooking equipment, defective furnaces, and kerosene heaters. CO is also produced when charcoal is burned indoors. CO is highly lethal and can cause death after only a few minutes of exposure. Nearly 4000 people die each year from CO poisoning, and at least 10,000 others become ill. Carbon monoxide detectors, which work much like smoke detectors, are now available for home use.

A pale, ashen, or bluish skin color, which indicates a lack of oxygen, may signal CO poisoning. For years, people were taught that carbon monoxide poisoning was indicated by a cherry-red color of the skin and lips. However, such redness only occurs after most victims have died.

All victims of inhaled poison need oxygen as soon as possible. First and foremost, remember to check the scene to determine if it is safe for you to help. If you can remove the person from the source of the poison without endangering your life, then do so. You can help a conscious victim by getting him or her to fresh air and summoning more advanced medical personnel. If the victim is unconscious, remove him or her from the environment if it is safe to do so. Summon more advanced medical personnel, and care for any other life-threatening conditions, such as respiratory or cardiac arrest.

Ingested Poisons

In some cases of ingested poisoning, it may be necessary to diminish the effects of the poison by giving activated charcoal. The victim must ingest the **activated charcoal,** a substance that absorbs the poison and helps prevent the patient from absorbing it. Activated charcoal is often supplied in 25-gram bottles (Fig. 16-4). The dose is given based on body weight. Adults usually receive 1 to 2 bottles (25 to 50 grams), and infants and children receive about half the adult dose. Activated charcoal should only be given on the advice of a medical professional.

Some PCCs or local protocols may instruct you to induce vomiting for some types of poisoning. To induce vomiting, you may be asked to give the victim **syrup of ipecac.** Vomiting may prevent the poison from moving from the stomach to the small intestine, where most absorption takes place. *Syrup of ipecac has not been found to be any more effective than activated charcoal. For this reason, inducing vomiting is no longer the preferred treatment. Induce vomiting only if so advised by a medical professional.*

Syrup of ipecac usually comes in a 30-ml bottle (about 2 tablespoons) (see Fig. 16-4). Two tablespoons, followed by a glass of water, is the usual dose for a person over 12 years of age. For children ages 1 to 12, the usual dose is 1 tablespoon followed by half a glass of water. Vomiting usually occurs within 20 minutes. Make sure you read and follow the directions on the syrup of ipecac container.

In some instances, vomiting should not be induced. These instances include when the victim—

- Is unconscious.
- Is having a seizure.
- Is pregnant (in the last trimester, or last 3 months).
- Has ingested a **caustic,** or **corrosive, substance** (such as drain or oven cleaner) or a

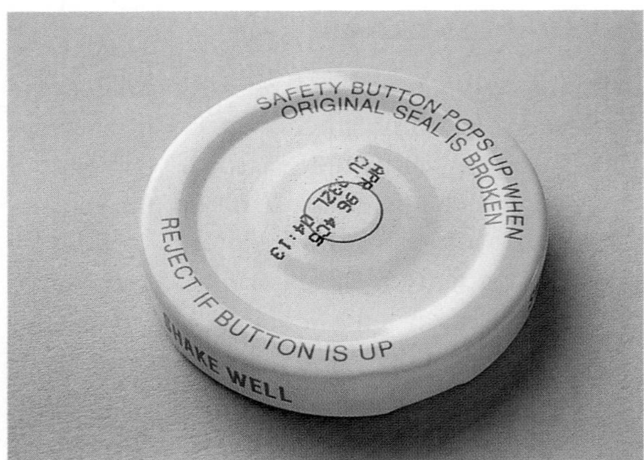

Figure 16-5 Inspect the safety button of the lid before opening canned or bottled food.

petroleum product (such as kerosene or gasoline).

- Is known to have heart disease.

You can dilute some ingested poisons by giving the victim water to drink. Examples of such poisons are caustic, or corrosive, chemicals, such as acids, that eat away or destroy tissues. Vomiting these corrosives could burn the esophagus, throat, and mouth. Diluting the corrosive substance decreases its potential for burning and damaging tissues. Chapter 12 discusses how to care for chemical burns caused by corrosive chemicals.

Foods can be another type of ingested poison. Approximately 33 million Americans are affected by food poisoning each year. Two of the most common categories of food poisoning are bacterial food poisoning and chemical food poisoning (also known as environmental food poisoning). Bacterial food poisoning typically occurs when bacteria grow on food that stands at room temperature after it is cooked or insufficiently cooled. Some bacteria release **toxins,** poisonous substances produced by certain living organisms, into the food. Other bacteria cause illness when ingested. Even when the food is reheated, the toxins may not be destroyed. Foods most responsible for this type of poisoning are ham, tongue, sausage, dried meat, ground meat, fish products, and dairy and dairy-based products. Chemical food poisoning typically occurs when foods containing acid, such as fruit juices or sauerkraut, are stored in containers lined with zinc, cadmium, copper, or in enameled metal pans. Another primary source of chemical poisoning related to food and water is lead, which may be in found pipes that supply water for drinking and cooking.

One of the most common causes of food poisoning is the *Salmonella* bacteria, most often found in poultry and raw eggs. Proper handling and cooking of food and cleaning or kitchen counter surfaces can help prevent *Salmonella* poisoning. The most deadly type of food poisoning is botulism, which is caused by a bacterial toxin that can be produced in home canning of food. The can or lid of canned or bottled food should be inspected before opening to see if it is swollen or if the "safety button" in the center of the lid has popped up (Fig. 16-5). If either has occurred, the food should be thrown away.

The signs and symptoms of food poisoning, which can begin between 1 and 48 hours after eating contaminated food, include nausea, vomiting, abdominal pain, diarrhea, fever, and dehydration. Severe cases of food poisoning can result in shock or death, particularly in children, the elderly, and those with an impaired immune system. Some victims of food poisoning may require antibiotics or antitoxins. Fortunately, most food poisoning can be prevented by proper cooking, refrigeration, and sanitation.

Absorbed Poisons

People can come into contact with poisonous substances that can be absorbed into the body. Pesticides and fertilizers are the most common and most dangerous absorbed poisons. More common poisons can cause an allergic reaction when a person comes in contact with them. Millions of people each year suffer irritating ef-

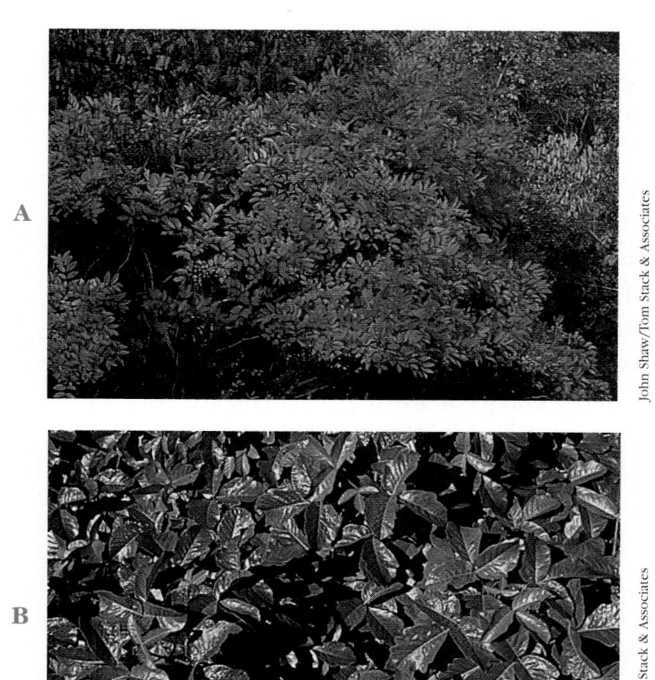

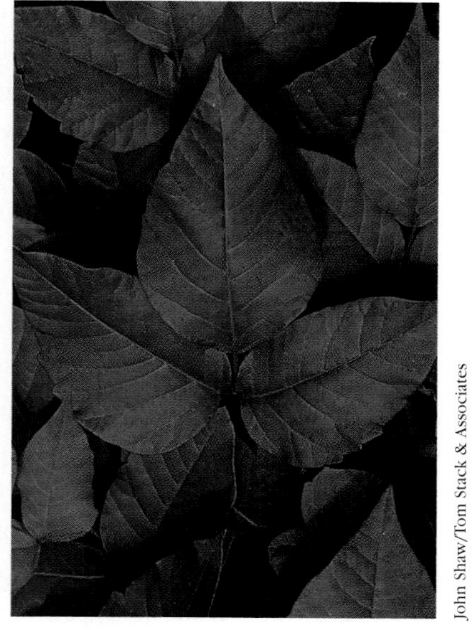

Figure 16-6 Annually, millions of people suffer from contact with plants whose oils irritate the skin: **A**, Poison sumac; **B**, Poison oak; **C**, Poison ivy.

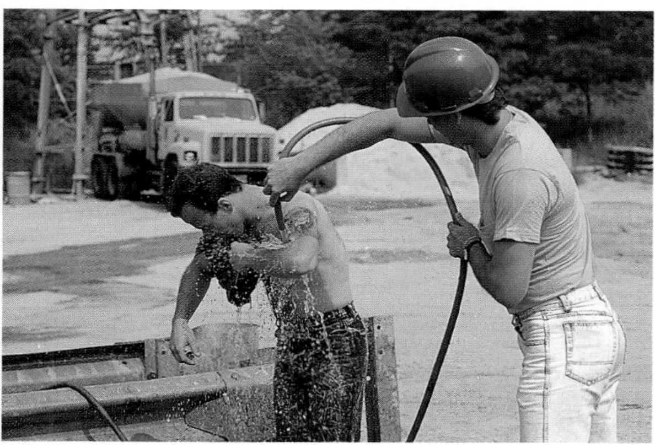

Figure 16-7 Whenever chemical poisons come in contact with the skin, flush the affected area continuously with large amounts of water.

fects after touching or brushing against plants, such as poison ivy, poison oak, and poison sumac (Fig. 16-6, *A-C*). If a rash or weeping lesion (an oozing sore) has developed, advise the victim to see his or her personal physician about possible treatment. Medicated lotions, such as Calamine®, may help soothe the area. **Antihistamines** may also help dry up the lesions and alleviate itching. If the condition worsens and large areas of the body or the face are affected, **anti-inflammatory drugs,** such as **corticosteroid** or other medications, may need to be administered to relieve discomfort.

If poisons, such as dry or wet chemicals, contact the skin, flush the affected area continuously with large amounts of cool running water (Fig. 16-7). Garden hoses and showers suit this purpose well. Before washing the affected area, you may need to have the victim remove his or her jewelry if the jewelry is contaminated or if it constricts circulation as a result of swelling. Summon more advanced medical personnel and continue to flush the affected area until they arrive.

Use your gloved hand or a cloth to brush off dry chemicals. Take care not to get any of the dry chemicals in your eyes or the eyes of the victim or any bystanders. Dry chemicals are activated by contact with water, but if continuous running water is available, it will, in most cases, flush the chemical from the skin before the water can activate it. Running water reduces the threat to you and quickly and easily removes the substance from the victim. Take steps to minimize shock.

Injected Poisons

Insect and animal stings and bites are among the most common sources of injected poisons. This text cannot consider all possible types of stings and bites that could result in poisoning. The following sections describe the care for common stings and bites of insects, spiders, ticks, marine life, snakes, and warm-blooded animals.

Signs and Symptoms of Common Bites and Stings

As with other kinds of poisoning, poisons that are injected through bites and stings may produce various signs and symptoms. Specific signs and symptoms depend on factors such as the type and location of the bite or sting; the amount of poison injected; the time elapsed since the poisoning; and the victim's size, weight, and age. Less severe reactions to bites and stings may trigger signs and symptoms including—

- A bite or sting mark at the point of injection (entry site).
- A stinger, tentacle, or venom sac remaining in or near the entry site.
- Redness at and around the entry site.
- Swelling at and around the entry site.
- Pain or tenderness at and around the entry site.

Care for Specific Bites and Stings

The following sections provide detailed instructions on how to care for specific kinds of bites and stings. Table 16-1 highlights this information.

Insects

Between 1 and 2 million Americans are severely allergic to substances in the venom of bees, wasps, hornets, and yellow jackets. For these people, even one sting can result in a severe allergic reaction known as ***anaphylaxis.*** Such highly allergic reactions account for the nearly 100 reported deaths that occur from insect stings each year. When highly allergic people are stung, they need immediate medical care for anaphylaxis. For most people, insect stings may be painful or uncomfortable but are not life threatening. To give care for an insect sting, first examine the sting site to see if the stinger is in the skin. If it is, remove it to prevent any further poisoning and avoid infection. Scrape the stinger away from the skin with the edge of a tongue depressor or a plastic card, such as a credit card (Fig. 16-8, p. 377). Often the venom sac will still be attached to the stinger. Do not remove the stinger with tweezers, since squeezing the stinger may put pressure on the venom sac and cause further poisoning.

Next, wash the site with soap and water. Cover it to keep it clean. Apply a cold pack to the area to reduce the pain and swelling. Place a layer of gauze or cloth between the source of cold and the skin to prevent skin damage. Observe the victim periodically for signs of an allergic reaction. Be sure to ask the victim if he or she has had any allergic reactions to insect bites or stings.

Ticks

Ticks can contract disease, carry disease, and transmit it to humans. **Rocky Mountain spotted fever (RMSF)** is a serious tick-borne disease. RMSF is caused by the transmission of microscopic parasites from the wood tick or dog tick host to other warm-blooded animals, including humans. The disease gets part of its name from the spotted rash that sometimes appears after a person becomes infected. The rash may first appear on wrists or ankles but spreads rapidly to most other parts of the body. Other signs and symptoms of RMSF include

Table 16-1 Caring for Bites and Stings

Insect bites and stings	Tick bites	Spider bites	Scorpion stings
Signs and symptoms:	**Signs and symptoms:**	**Signs and symptoms:**	**Signs and symptoms:**
Stinger may be present Pain Local swelling Hives or rash Nausea and vomiting Breathing difficulty	Bull's eye, spotted, or black and blue rash around bite or on other body parts Fever and chills Flu-like aches	Bite mark or blister Pain or cramping Nausea and vomitting Difficulties breathing and swallowing Profuse sweating or salivation Irregular heartbeat	Bite mark Local swelling Pain or cramping Nausea and vomitting Difficulty breathing or swallowing Profuse sweating or salivation Irregular heartbeat
Care	**Care**	**Care**	**Care**
Remove stinger; scrape it away with card or knife Wash wound Cover wound Apply a cold pack Watch for signs and symptoms of allergic reactions; take steps to minimize shock if they occur	Remove tick with tweezers Apply antiseptic and antibiotic ointment to wound Watch for signs of infection Get medical attention if necessary	If black widow or brown recluse Call EMS personnel immediately to receive antivenin and have wound cleaned	Wash wound Apply a cold pack Get medical care to receive antivenin Call EMS personnel or local emergency number

Continued

Table 16-1 Caring for Bites and Stings (*continued*)

Snakebites stings	Marine life and wild animal bites	Domestic bites	Human
Signs and symptoms:	**Signs and symptoms:**	**Signs and symptoms:**	**Signs and symptoms:**
Bite mark Severe pain and burning Local swelling and discoloration	Possible marks Pain Local swelling	Bite mark Bleeding Pain	Bite mark Pain
Care	**Care**	**Care**	**Care**
Wash wound Keep bitten part still and lower than the heart Call EMS personnel or local emergency number	If jellyfish — soak area in either vinegar, alcohol, or baking soda paste If stingray — soak area in nonscalding hot water until pain goes away. Clean and bandage wound. Call EMS personnel or local emergency number if necessary	If wound is minor wash wound, control bleeding, apply a dressing, and get medical attention as soon as possible If wound is severe call EMS personnel or local emergency number, control bleeding, and do not wash wound	If wound is minor, wash wound, control bleeding, apply a dressing, and get medical attention as soon as possible. If wound is severe, call EMS personnel or local emergency number, control bleeding, and do not wash wound.

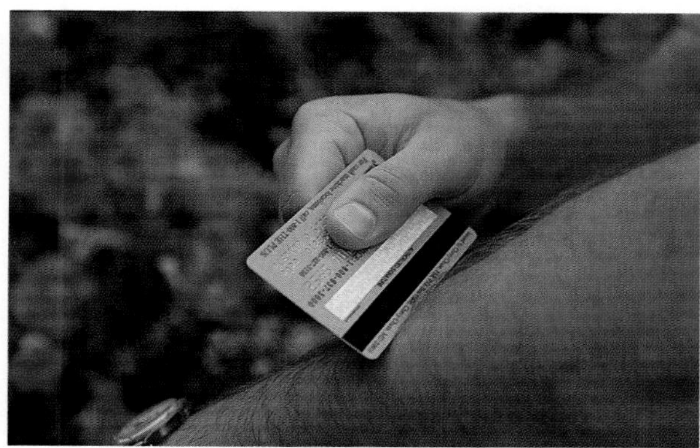

Figure 16-8 If someone is stung and a stinger is present, scrape it away from the skin with a tongue depressor or a plastic card, such as a credit card.

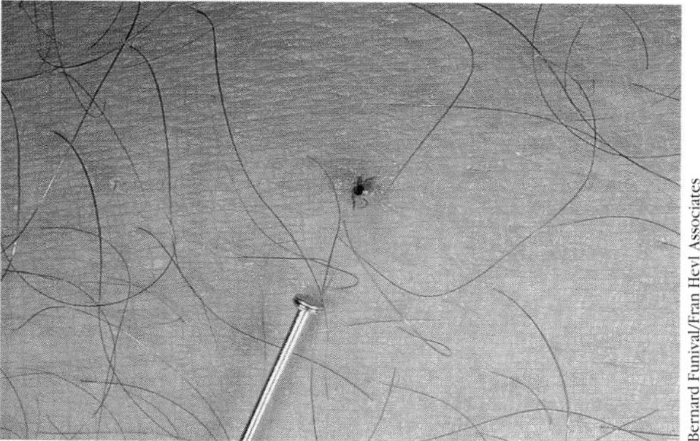

Bernard Funival/Fran Heyl Associates

Figure 16-9 A deer tick can be as small as the head of a pin.

fever and chills, severe headache, and joint and muscle aches.

Early treatment by medical professionals is important because more than 20 percent of untreated patients die from shock or kidney failure. Although the disease was first diagnosed in the western United States, cases of RMSF continue to be reported throughout North and South America today. RMSF is sometimes known by various regional names, such as black fever, mountain fever, tick fever, spotted fever, or pinta fever.

Another disease transmitted by ticks is **Lyme disease**. Lyme disease, or Lyme borreliosis, is an illness that affects a large number of people in the United States. Cases of Lyme disease have been reported in more than 40 states, so everyone should take appropriate precautions to protect against it.

Not all ticks carry Lyme disease. Lyme disease is spread primarily by a type of tick that commonly attaches itself to field mice and deer. It is sometimes called a deer tick. This tick is found around beaches and in wooded and grassy areas. Like all ticks, it attaches itself to any warm-blooded animal that brushes by it, including humans.

Deer ticks are very tiny and difficult to see, especially in the late spring and summer. They are much smaller than the common dog tick or wood tick. They can be as small as a poppy seed, the head of a pin, or the period at the end of this sentence (Fig. 16-9). Even in the adult stage, they are only as large as a grape seed. A deer tick can attach to you without you knowing it is there. Many people who develop Lyme disease do not remember having been bitten.

You can get Lyme disease from the bite of an infected tick at any time of the year. However, the risk is greatest between May and July, when ticks are most active and outdoor activities are at their peak.

The first sign of infection may appear a few days or a few weeks after a tick bite. Typically, a rash starts as a small red area at the site of the bite. It may spread up to 6 to 8 centimeters, or 2 to 3 inches, across (Fig. 16-10). In fair-skinned people, the center of the rash is lighter in color and the outer edges are red and raised, sometimes giving the rash a bull's-eye appearance. In dark-skinned people, the rash area may look black and blue, like a bruise. A rash can appear anywhere on the body, and more than one rash may appear on various body parts. You can even have Lyme disease without developing a rash.

Most other signs and symptoms of Lyme disease are similar to those of RMSF and include fever and chills, headache, weakness or fatigue, and flulike joint and muscle aches. These signs

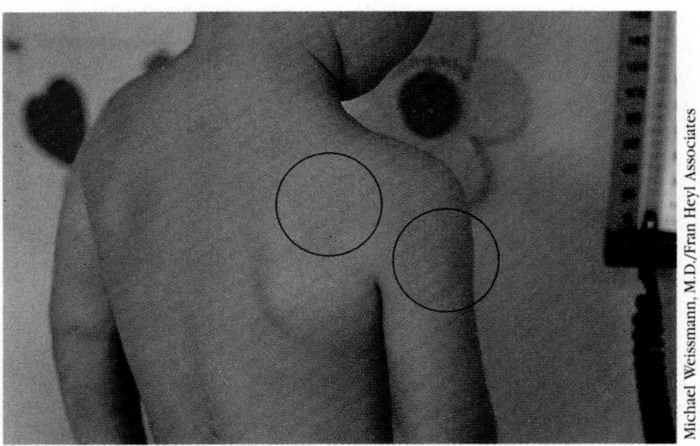

Figure 16-10 A person with Lyme disease may develop a rash.

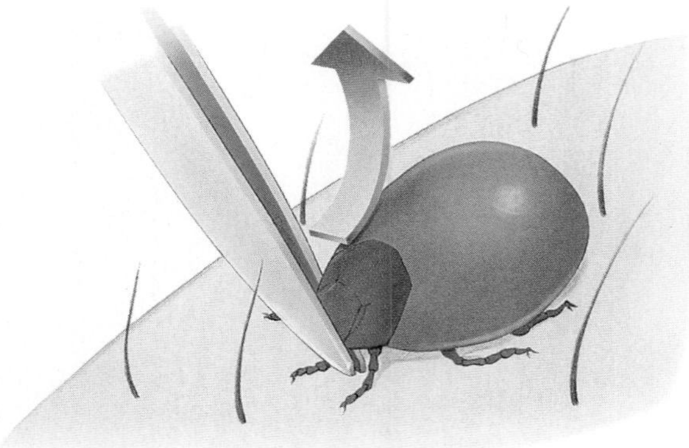
Figure 16-11 Remove a tick by pulling steadily and firmly with fine-tipped tweezers.

and symptoms may develop slowly and may not occur at the same time as a rash. The more severe symptoms of Lyme disease may appear weeks, months, or even years after a tick bite.

Lyme disease can get worse if it is not treated. In its advanced stages, Lyme disease may cause arthritis, numbness, memory loss, problems with vision or hearing, high fever, and stiff neck. Some of these signs and symptoms could indicate brain problems or other nervous system problems. An irregular or rapid heartbeat could indicate heart problems.

If you find an embedded tick, grasp the tick with fine-tipped tweezers as close to the skin as possible, and pull slowly, steadily, and firmly (Fig. 16-11). If you do not have tweezers, use your gloved hand. Do not try to burn a tick off with a hot match or a burning cigarette. Do not use other "home remedies," like coating the tick with petroleum jelly or nail polish or pricking it with a pin. These remedies are not always effective in removing the tick and can cause the victim further harm.

Mouthparts of adult ticks may sometimes remain in the skin, but these will not cause disease. Once the tick is removed, apply an **antiseptic,** such as alcohol, to the site of the bite. If an **antibiotic** ointment is available, apply it to help prevent wound infection as well. Advise the victim to observe the site periodically thereafter. If a rash or flulike symptoms develop, he or she should seek medical help.

A physician will usually prescribe antibiotics to treat Lyme disease and RMSF. Antibiotics work best and most quickly when taken early. Clinical trials are now underway on a Lyme disease vaccine that may be available in the near future. If you suspect that someone may have been infected with Lyme disease or RMSF, summon more advanced medical personnel. Treatment is slower and less effective in advanced stages.

Additional information on Lyme disease and RMSF may be available from your state or local health department. You can also contact the American Lyme Disease Foundation by calling 1-800-876-LYME.

Spiders and scorpions

Few spiders in the United States have venom that causes death. However, the bites of the black widow and brown recluse spiders can make you seriously ill and are occasionally fatal. These spiders live in most parts of the United States. You can identify them by the unique designs on their bodies (Fig. 16-12, *A-B*). The black widow spider is black with a reddish hourglass shape on its underbody. The brown recluse spider is light brown with a darker brown, violin-shaped marking on the top of its body.

Both spiders prefer dark, out-of-the-way places where they are seldom disturbed. Bites usually occur on the hands and arms of people reaching into places, such as wood, rock, and

A

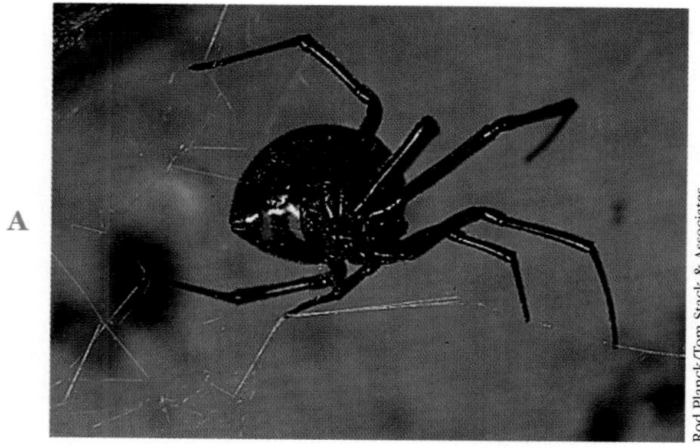

B

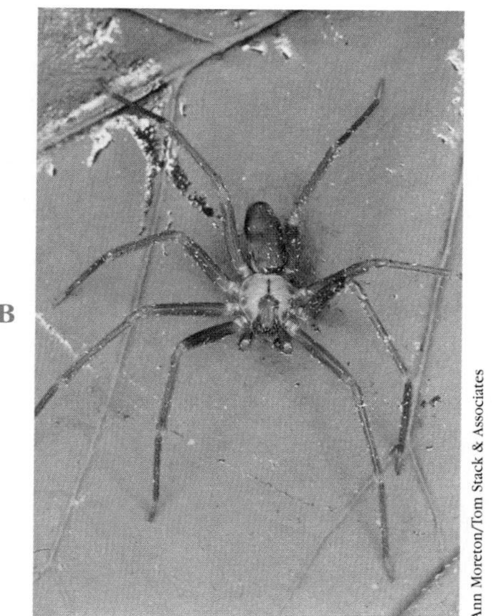

Figure 16-12 **A**, The black widow spider, and **B**, the brown recluse spider have characteristic markings.

brush piles, or rummaging in dark garages and attics. Often, the victim will not know that he or she has been bitten until signs or symptoms develop.

The bite of the black widow spider is the more painful and often the more deadly of the two, especially in very young and elderly victims. Its venom is even deadlier than that of a rattlesnake, although the smaller amount of venom injected by the spider usually produces less of a reaction than that of a snakebite.

The bite of a black widow spider usually causes a sharp pinprick pain followed by a dull pain in the area of the bite. Signs and symptoms of this bite include muscular rigidity in the shoulders, back, and abdomen, as well as restlessness, anxiety, sweating, weakness, and drooping eyelids.

A brown recluse spider bite may produce little or no pain initially, but localized pain develops an hour or more later. A blood-filled blister forms under the surface of the skin, sometimes in a target or bull's eye pattern. The blister increases in size and eventually ruptures, leaving a black scar.

If the victim or you recognize the spider as either a black widow or brown recluse, summon more advanced medical personnel. The victim should be hospitalized. In the hospital, professionals will clean the wound and give medication to reduce the pain and inflammation. An ***antivenin,*** a substance used to counteract the poisonous effects of the venom, is available for black widow bites. Antivenin is used mostly for children and the elderly and is rarely necessary when bites occur in healthy adults.

Scorpions live in dry regions of the southwestern United States and Mexico. They are usually about 3 centimeters, or 1 inch, long, and have 8 legs and a pair of crab-like pincers. At the end of the tail is a stinger, used to inject venom. Scorpions live in cool, damp places, such as basements, junk piles, wood piles, and under the bark of living or fallen trees. They are most active in the evening and at night, which is when most stings occur. Like spiders,

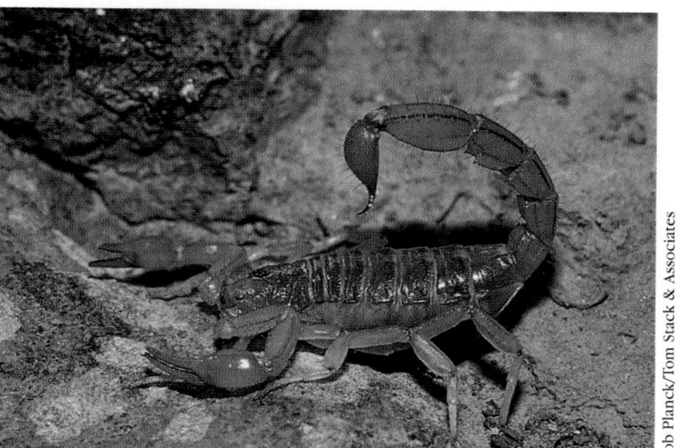

Figure 16-13 The bites of only a few species of scorpions found in the United States can be fatal.

only a few species of scorpions have a potentially fatal sting (Fig. 16-13). In general, scorpions stings are dangerous only if the victim has an allergic reaction. *However, because it is difficult to distinguish the highly poisonous scorpions from the nonpoisonous, all scorpion bites should be treated as a medical emergency.*

Signs and symptoms of spider bites and scorpion stings may include—

- A mark indicating a possible bite or sting.
- Severe pain in the sting or bite area.
- A blister, lesion, or swelling at the entry site.
- Nausea and vomiting.
- Difficulty breathing or swallowing.
- Sweating and salivating profusely.
- Irregular heart rhythms.
- Muscle cramping or abdominal pain.

In the event of a scorpion sting, the victim may need to go to a medical facility. While waiting for more advanced medical personnel, wash the wound and apply a cold pack to the site to reduce swelling. Remember to place a layer of gauze or cloth between the source of cold and the skin to prevent skin damage.

Snakes

Few areas of medicine have provoked more controversy about care for an injury than snakebites. Snakebite care issues, such as whether to use a tourniquet, cut the wound, apply ice, when to apply suction, use electric shocks, or capture the snake, have been discussed at length over the years. All this controversy is rather amazing since, of the 8000 people reported bitten annually in the United States, typically fewer than 12 die. Figure 16-14, *A-D*, shows the four kinds of poisonous snakes found in the United States.

Rattlesnakes account for most snake bites and nearly all deaths from snakebites in the

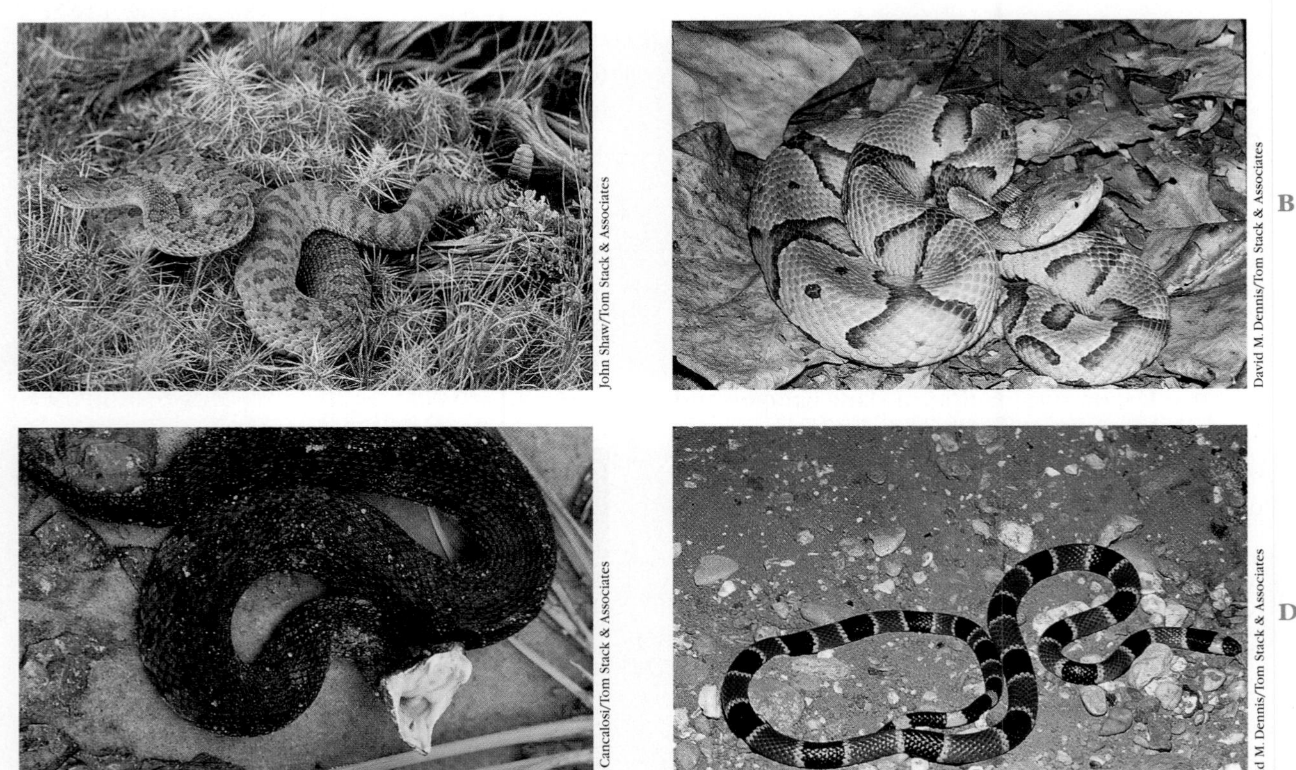

Figure 16-14 There are four kinds of poisonous snakes found in the United States: **A**, Rattlesnake; **B**, Copperhead; **C**, Water moccasin; and **D**, Coral snake.

United States. Most deaths occur because the victim has an allergic reaction, is in poor health, or because too much time passes before the victim receives medical care. Elaborate care is usually unnecessary because, in most cases, the victim can reach professional medical care within 30 minutes. Often care can be reached much faster, since most bites occur near the home, not in the wild.

Signs and symptoms that indicate a poisonous snakebite include—

- One or two distinct puncture wounds, which may or may not bleed. The exception is the bite of the coral snake, which leaves a semicircular mark from the snake's teeth.
- Severe pain and burning at the wound site immediately after or within 4 hours of the incident.
- Swelling and discoloration at the wound site immediately after or within 4 hours of the incident.

Follow these guidelines to care for someone bitten by a snake:

- If you know the snake is poisonous, take the victim to medical care immediately if possible.
- Wash the wound, if possible.
- Immobilize the affected part.
- Keep the affected area lower than the heart, if possible.
- Summon more advanced medical personnel.
- Minimize the victim's movement. If possible, carry a victim who must be transported or have him or her walk slowly.

If you know the victim cannot get advanced care within 30 minutes, consider suctioning the wound using an appropriate snakebite kit. Regardless of what you may have otherwise heard or read—

- *Do not* apply ice. Snake venom, unlike other kinds of venom, gets drawn further into the body as the cold constricts the blood vessels around the wound and the cold causes further tissue destruction.
- *Do not* cut the wound. Cutting the wound can further injure the victim and has not been shown to remove any significant amount of venom.
- *Do not* apply a tourniquet. A tourniquet severely restricts blood flow to the limb, which could result in the loss of the limb.
- *Do not* use electric shock. This technique has not been conclusively shown to affect the poison and can be dangerous. It is inappropriate in the majority of snakebite cases in the United States, since professional help is readily attainable.

Marine life

The stings of some forms of marine life are not only painful but can also make a person ill (Fig. 16-15, *A-D*). The side effects include allergic reactions that can cause breathing and heart problems and paralysis. If the sting occurs in water, move the person to land as soon as possible. Summon more advanced medical personnel if the victim has a history of allergic reactions to marine life stings, is stung on the face or neck, or starts to have difficulty breathing.

If the sting was from a jellyfish, sea anemone, or Portuguese man-of-war, the affected area will need to be soaked in vinegar as soon as possible. Vinegar often works best to offset the toxin and reduce pain. Rubbing alcohol or a baking soda paste may also be used. Do not rub the wound or apply fresh water or ammonia, since these substances will increase pain. Meat tenderizer is no longer recommended, because the active ingredient once used to reduce pain is no longer in most meat tenderizers.

If the sting was from a stingray, sea urchin, or spiny fish, flush the wound with tap water. You can also use ocean water. Immobilize the affected area and soak it in nonscalding hot water (as hot as the person can stand) for about 30 minutes or until the pain goes away. Toxins from these animals are heat sensitive, and dramatic relief of local pain often occurs from one application of hot water. If hot water is not available, packing the area in hot sand may

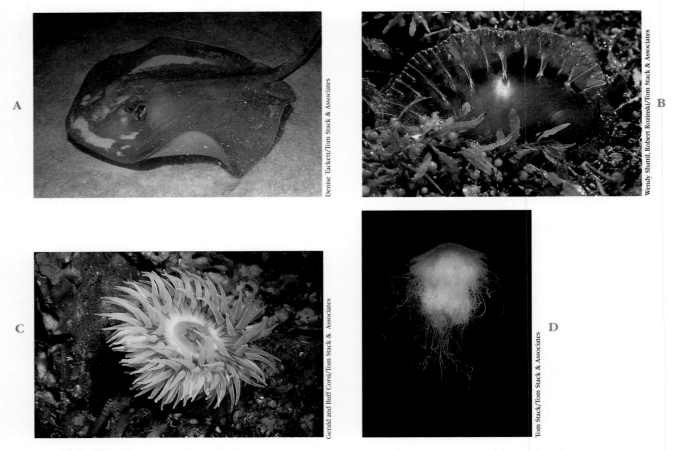

Figure 16-15 The painful sting of some marine animals can cause problems: **A**, Stingray; **B**, Man-of-war; **C**, Sea anemone; and **D**, Jellyfish.

relieve pain if the sand is hot enough. Clean the wound and apply a bandage. Watch for signs of infection, and check with a health-care provider to determine if a tetanus shot is needed.

Domestic and Wild Animals

The bite of a domestic or wild animal carries the risk of infection, as well as soft tissue injury. One of the most serious possible results is rabies. ***Rabies*** is a disease transmitted through the saliva and urine of diseased mammals, such as skunks, bats, raccoons, cats, dogs, cattle, and foxes. Dog bites are the most common of all bites from domestic or wild animals.

Animals with rabies may act in unusual ways. For example, nocturnal animals, such as raccoons, may be active in the daytime. A wild animal that usually tries to avoid humans may not run away when you approach. Rabid animals may salivate, appear partially paralyzed, or act irritable, aggressive, or strangely quiet. To reduce your risk of becoming infected with rabies, do not pet or feed wild or stray animals and do not touch the body of a dead wild animal.

If not treated, rabies is fatal. *Anyone bitten by a wild or domestic animal must get professional medical attention as soon as possible.* To prevent rabies from developing, the victim receives a series of vaccine injections to build up immunity. In the past, caring for rabies meant a lengthy series of painful injections that had many unpleasant side effects. The vaccines used now require fewer and less painful injections and have fewer side effects. The following victims should go to the emergency department or their physician for a tetanus shot:

- Anyone with a wound who has not had a complete series of tetanus shots as a child (or does not remember)
- Anyone with a minor wound who has not had a tetanus shot in the last 10 years
- Anyone with a deep wound, a puncture wound, or a very dirty wound

Tetanus is another potentially fatal infection, one that affects the central nervous system. Tetanus is caused by the transmission of a toxin, which can occur in puncture wounds, such as animal and human bites. The toxin associated with tetanus is one of the most deadly poisons known. More than 50,000 people worldwide die annually from tetanus infection, although fatalities in the United States are few. Wounds to the face, head, and neck are the most likely to be fatal because those areas are close to the brain.

Signs and symptoms of tetanus include irritability, headache, fever, and painful muscular spasms. One of the most common symptoms of tetanus is muscular stiffness in the jaw, which is why tetanus is sometimes known as "lockjaw." It can take anywhere from 3 days to 5 weeks before these signs and symptoms occur. Eventually, if the condition is not treated, every muscle in the body goes into spasms. Care for tetanus includes prompt and thorough cleansing of the wound by a medical professional, followed by a series of immunization injections.

If someone is bitten by a wild or domestic animal, try to get him or her away from the animal without endangering yourself. Do not try to restrain or capture the animal. If the wound is minor, cleanse it, control any bleeding, apply a dressing, and take the victim to a doctor or medical facility. If the wound is bleeding heavily, control the bleeding but do not clean the wound. Seek medical attention immediately. The wound will be properly cleaned at a medical facility.

If possible, try to remember what the animal looks like and the area in which it was last seen. Call 9-1-1 or the local emergency number. The dispatcher will get the proper authorities, such as animal control, to the scene.

Humans

Human bites are quite common. They account for up to 23 percent of all bites cared for by urban physicians. Human bites differ from other bites in that they may be more contaminated with bacteria, tend to occur in higher-risk areas of the body (especially on the hands), and often receive delayed care. At least 42 different species of bacteria have been reported in human saliva, so it is not surprising that serious infection often follows a human bite. *However, according to the Centers for Disease Control and Prevention (CDC), human bites are not considered to carry a risk of transmitting the human immunodeficiency virus (HIV), the virus that causes the acquired immunodeficiency syndrome (AIDS).* Children often inflict and receive human bite wounds.

As with animal bites, it is important to get the victim of a human bite to professional medical care as soon as possible so that antibiotic therapy can be prescribed if necessary. If the wound is not severe, wash it with soap and water, control any bleeding, apply a dressing, and take the victim to a doctor or medical facility. If the bite is severe, control bleeding and call EMS personnel. The wound will be properly cleaned at a medical facility.

◆ ANAPHYLAXIS

Severe allergic reactions to poisons are rare. But when one occurs, it is truly a life-threatening medical emergency. This reaction, called anaphylaxis, is a form of shock. It can be caused by an insect bite or sting or by contact with drugs, medications, foods, and chemicals. Anaphylaxis can result from any of the kinds of poisoning described in this chapter.

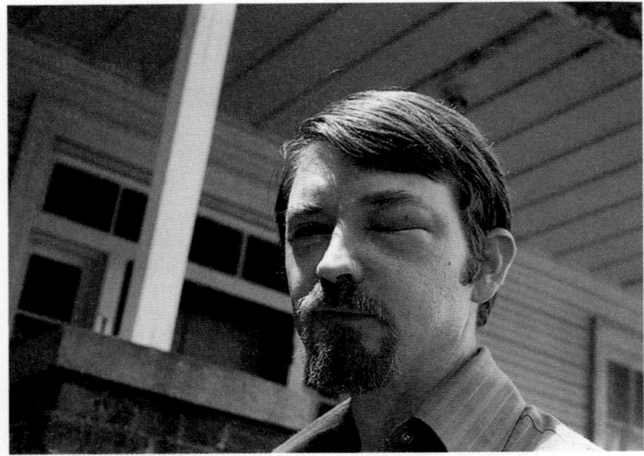

Figure 16-16 In anaphylaxis, the skin or area of the body usually swells and turns red.

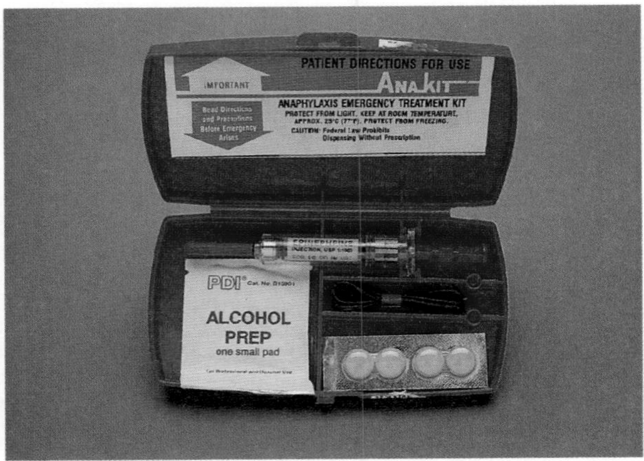

Figure 16-17 Anaphylaxis Kit Contents

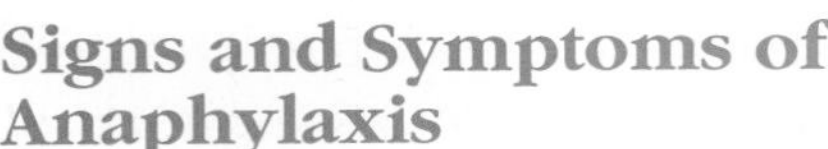

Signs and Symptoms of Anaphylaxis

Anaphylaxis usually occurs suddenly, within seconds or minutes after contact with the substance. The skin or area of the body that came in contact with the substance usually swells and turns red (Fig. 16-16). Other signs and symptoms include hives, itching, rash, weakness, nausea, vomiting, dizziness, and difficulty breathing that includes coughing and wheezing. This breathing difficulty can progress to an obstructed airway as the tongue and throat swell. Death from anaphylaxis usually occurs because the victim's breathing is severely impaired.

Care for Anaphylaxis

If an unusual inflammation or rash is noticeable immediately after contact with a possible source, it could be an allergic reaction. Assess the person's airway and breathing. If the person has any difficulty breathing or complains that his or her throat is closing, summon more advanced medical personnel immediately. Help the victim into the most comfortable position for breathing. Administer oxygen if it is available and you are trained to do so. Monitor the ABCs and try to keep the victim calm.

People who know they are extremely allergic to certain substances usually try to avoid them, although this is sometimes impossible. These people may carry an anaphylaxis kit in case they have a severe allergic reaction. Such kits are available by prescription only (Fig. 16-17). The kit contains a single dose of the drug epinephrine that can be injected into the body to counteract the anaphylactic reaction. Many kits also contain an antihistamine (a substance that reduces the effects of compounds released in allergic reactions).

◆ SUBSTANCE MISUSE AND ABUSE

When you hear the term substance abuse, what thoughts flash through your mind? Narcotics? Cocaine? Marijuana? Because of the publicity they receive, we tend to think of illegal (also known as illicit or controlled) drugs when we hear of substance abuse. In the United States today, however, legal (also called licit or noncontrolled) substances are among those most often misused or abused. Such legal substances include nicotine (found in tobacco products); alcohol (found in beer, wine, and liquor); and over-the-counter medications such as aspirin, sleeping pills, and diet pills.

The term substance abuse refers to a broad range of improperly used medical and nonmedical substances. Substance abuse costs the United States tens of billions of dollars each year in medical care, insurance, and lost productivity. Even more important, however, are the lives lost or permanently impaired each year from injuries or medical emergencies related to substance abuse or misuse.

Effects of Misuse and Abuse

Substance abuse and misuse pose a very serious threat to the health of millions of Americans. According to the Drug Abuse Warning Network (DAWN), drug-related emergency department admissions are at an all-time high. The number of emergency department patients who say that they have used illegal substances has risen dramatically. The greatest increase is in the number of people who admit to using cocaine and crack.

Thousands of Americans die annually as a result of substance abuse. Experts estimate that as many as two thirds of all homicides and serious assaults occurring annually involve alcohol. Other problems directly or indirectly related to substance abuse include dropping out of school, adolescent pregnancy, suicide, involvement in crime, and transmission of the human immunodeficiency virus (HIV), the virus that may lead to, acquired immunodeficiency syndrome (AIDS).

Forms of Substance Misuse and Abuse

Substance misuse is the use of a substance for unintended purposes or for appropriate purposes but in improper amounts or doses. ***Substance abuse*** is the deliberate, persistent, and excessive use of a substance without regard to health concerns or accepted medical practices. Many substances that are abused or misused are not illegal. Other substances are legal only when prescribed by a physician. Some are illegal only for those under age (for example, alcohol). Figure 16-18 shows some commonly misused and abused substances that are legal.

A ***drug*** is any substance, other than food, taken to affect body functions. A drug given therapeutically, to prevent or treat a disease or otherwise enhance mental or physical wellbeing, is a ***medication.*** Any drug can cause ***dependency,*** the desire to continually use the substance. The victim feels that he or she needs the drug to function normally. People with a compulsive need for a substance and who would suffer mental, physical, and emotional distress if they stopped taking it are said to have an ***addiction*** to that substance.

When someone continually uses a substance, its effects on the body decrease—a condition called ***tolerance.*** The person then has to increase the amount and frequency of use to obtain the desired effect.

An ***overdose*** occurs when someone uses an excessive amount of a substance, resulting in adverse reactions ranging from **mania** and hysteria to coma and death. Specific reactions include changes in blood pressure and heartbeat, sweating, vomiting, and liver failure. An overdose may occur unintentionally if a person takes too much medication at one time, for example, when an elderly person forgets that he or she took one dose of a medication and takes an additional dose (Fig. 16-19).

An overdose may be intentional, as in suicide attempts. Sometimes the victim takes a sufficiently high dose of a substance to be certain to cause death. Other times, to gain attention or help, the victim takes enough of a substance to need medical attention but not enough to cause death.

The term ***withdrawal*** describes the condition produced when a person stops using or abusing a substance to which he or she is addicted. Stopping the use of a substance may occur as a deliberate decision or because the person is unable to obtain the specific drug. Withdrawal from certain substances, such as alco-

A B C D

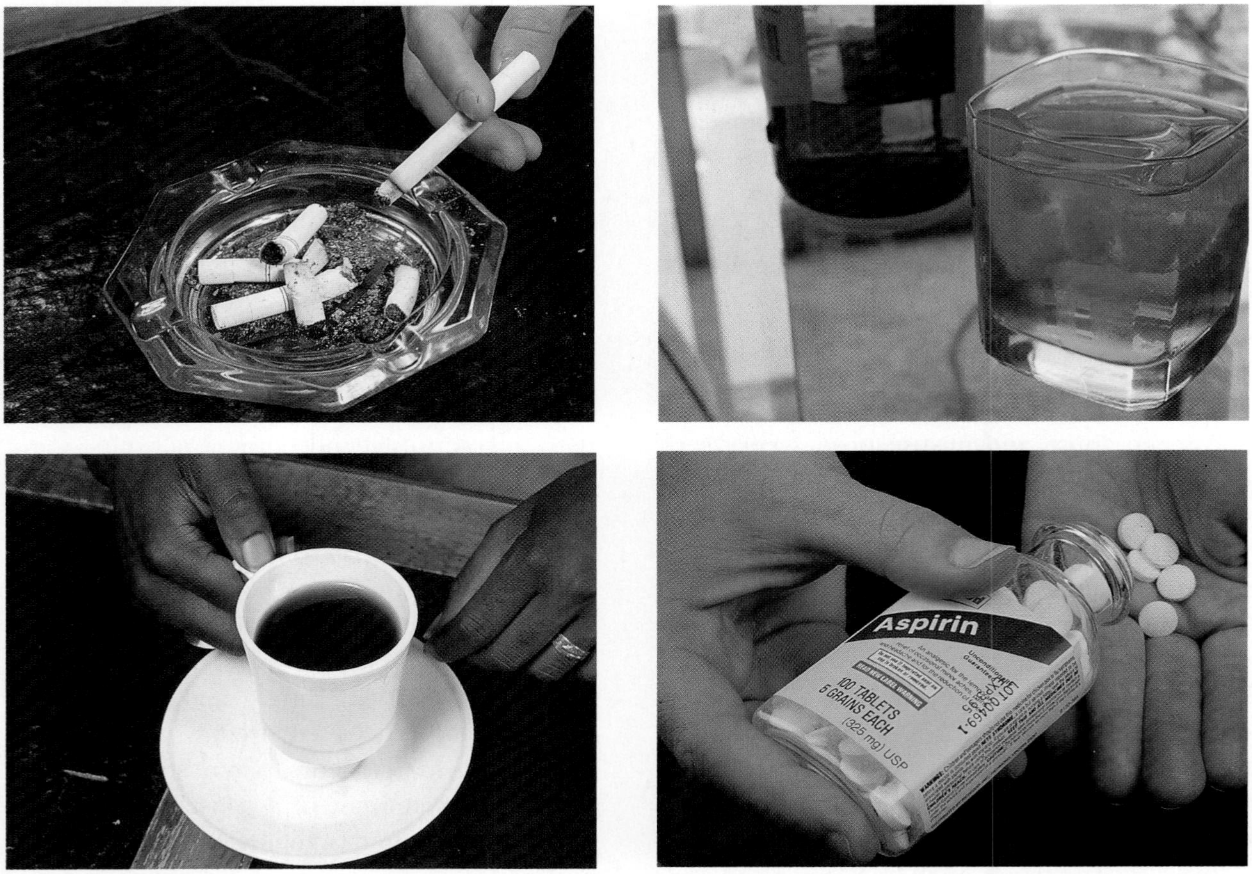

Figure 16-18 Substance abuse and misuse involve a broad range of improperly used medical and nonmedical substances: **A**, Cigarettes, **B**, Alcoholic beverages, **C**, Coffee, and **D**, Aspirin.

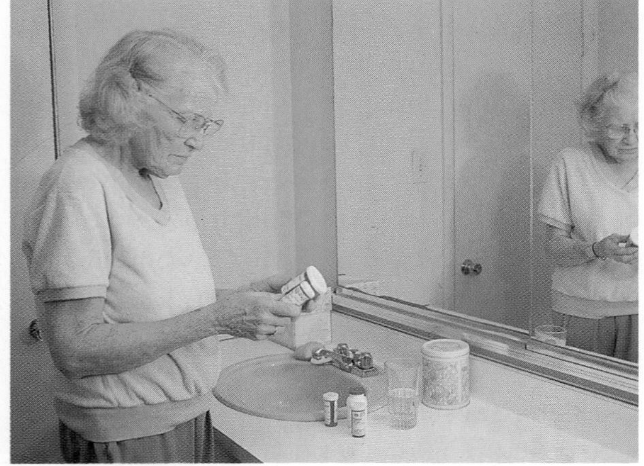

Figure 16-19 Misuse of a medication can occur unintentionally for an elderly person or a person with failing eyesight.

hol, can cause severe mental and physical distress. Because withdrawal may become a serious medical condition, medical professionals often oversee the process.

Misused and Abused Substances

Substances are categorized according to their effects on the body (Table 16-2). The six major categories are stimulants, depressants, hallucinogens, narcotics, inhalants, and cannabis products. The category to which a substance belongs depends mostly on the effects it has on the central nervous system or the way the substance is taken. Some substances depress the nervous system, whereas others speed up

Table 16-2 Commonly Misused and Abused Substances

Category	Substances	Possible effects
Stimulants	Caffeine Cocaine, Crack cocaine Methamphetamines Amphetamines Dextroamphetamines Nicotine Over-the-counter diet aids Asthma treatments	Increase mental and physical activity, produce temporary feelings of alertness, prevent fatigue, suppress appetite.
Hallucinogens	LSD (Lysergic Acid Diethylamide) PCP (Phencyclidine) Mescaline Peyote Psilocybin	Cause changes in mood, sensation, thought, emotion, and self-awareness; alter perceptions of time and space; and may produce profound depression, tension, and anxiety, as well as visual, auditory, or tactile hallucinations.
Depressants	Barbiturates Narcotics Alcohol Antihistamines Sedatives Tranquilizers Over-the-counter sleep aids	Decrease mental and physical activity, alter consciousness, relieve anxiety and pain, promote sleep, depress respiration, relax muscles, and impair coordination and judgment.
Narcotics	Morphine Codeine Heroin Methadone Opium	Relieve pain, may produce stupor or euphoria, may cause coma or death, and are highly addictive.
Inhalants	Medical anesthetics Gasoline and kerosene Glues in organic cements Lighter fluid Aerosol propellants	Alter moods; may produce a partial or complete loss of feeling; may produce effects similar to drunkenness, such as slurred speech, lack of inhibitions, and impaired motor coordination. Can also cause damage to the heart, lungs, brain, and liver.
Cannabis Products	Hashish Marijuana THC (Tetrahydrocannabinol)	Produce feelings of elation, increase appetite, distort perceptions of time and space, and impair motor coordination and judgment. May irritate throat, redden eyes, increase pulse, and cause dizziness.

Continued.

Table 16-2 *(continued)*

Category	Substances	Possible effects
Other	MDMA (Methylenedioxymethamphetamine or ecstasy)	Elevate blood pressure and produce euphoria or erratic mood swings, rapid heartbeat, profuse sweating, agitation, euphoria, and sensory distortions.
	Anabolic steroids	Enhance physical performance, increase muscle mass, and stimulate appetite and weight gain. Chronic use can cause sterility, disruption of normal growth, liver cancer, personality changes, and aggressive behavior.
	Aspirin	Relieve minor pain and reduces fever. Can impair normal blood clotting and cause inflammation of the stomach and small intestine.
	Laxatives	Relieve constipation. Can cause uncontrolled diarrhea and dehydration.
	Decongestant nasal sprays	Relieve congestion and swelling of nasal passages. Chronic use can cause nosebleeds and changes in the lining of the nose, making it difficult to breathe without sprays.

its activity. Some are not easily categorized because they have various effects or may be taken in a variety of ways. Figure 16-20 shows a variety of legal and illegal substances that are commonly misused and abused. A heightened or exaggerated effect may be produced when two or more substances are used at the same time. This is called a **synergistic effect,** which can be deadly.

Stimulants

Stimulants are drugs that affect the central nervous system by increasing physical and mental activity. They produce temporary feelings of alertness and prevent fatigue. They are sometimes used for weight reduction because they also suppress appetite.

Many stimulants are ingested as pills, but some can be absorbed or inhaled. Amphetamine, dextroamphetamine, and methamphetamine are stimulants. Their slang names include uppers, bennies, black beauties, speed, crystal, meth, and crank. One of the more recent and dangerous new stimulants is called "ice." Ice is an extremely addictive smokeable form of methamphetamine.

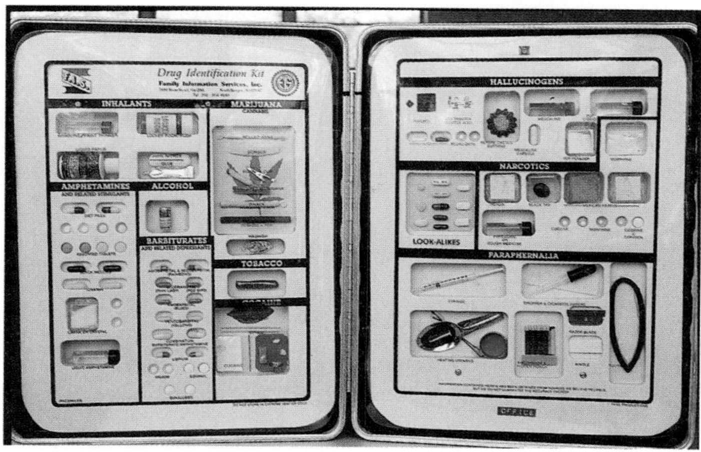

Figure 16-20 Misused and Abused Substances

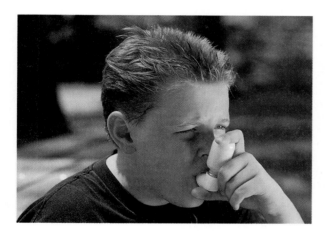

Figure 16-21 Medication used to treat asthma is a common legal stimulant.

Cocaine is one of the most publicized and powerful stimulants. Cocaine can be taken into the body in different ways. The most common way is sniffing it in powder form, known as "snorting." In this method, the drug is absorbed into the blood through capillaries in the nose. Slang names for cocaine include coke, snow, blow, flake, foot, and nose candy. A purer and more potent form of cocaine is crack. Crack is smoked. The vapors that are inhaled into the lungs reach the brain and cause almost immediate effects. Crack is highly addictive. Slang names for crack include rock and freebase rocks.

Interestingly, the most common stimulants in America are legal. Leading the list is caffeine, present in coffee, tea, many kinds of sodas, chocolate, diet pills, and pills used to combat fatigue. The next most common stimulant is nicotine, found in tobacco products. Other stimulants used for medical purposes are asthma medications or decongestants that can be taken by mouth or inhaled (Fig. 16-21).

Hallucinogens

Hallucinogens, also known as psychedelics, are substances that cause changes in mood, sensation, thought, emotion, and self-awareness. They alter one's perception of time and space and produce visual, auditory, and tactile (relating to the sense of touch) delusions.

Among the most widely abused hallucinogens are lysergic acid diethylamide (LSD), called acid; psilocybin, called mushrooms; phencyclidine (PCP), called angel dust; and mescaline, called peyote, buttons, or mesc. These substances are usually ingested, but PCP is also often inhaled.

Hallucinogens often have physical effects similar to stimulants but are classified differently because of the other effects they produce. Hallucinogens sometimes cause what is called a "bad trip." A bad trip can involve in-

A

The George Washington University

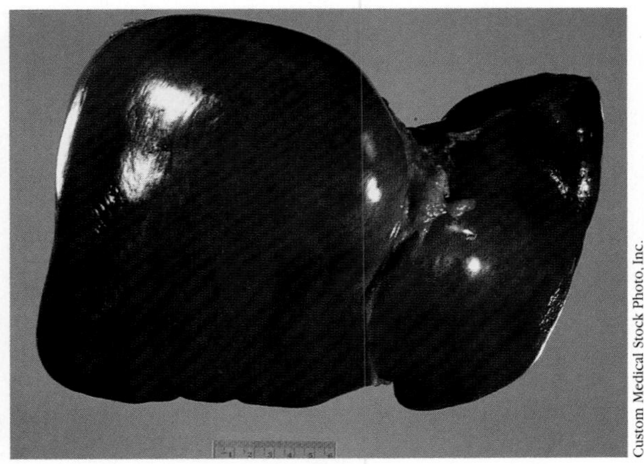

Custom Medical Stock Photo, Inc.

B

Figure 16-22 **A**, Chronic drinking can result in cirrhosis, a disease of the liver. **B**, A healthy liver.

tense fear, panic, paranoid delusions, vivid hallucinations, profound depression, tension, and anxiety. The victim may be irrational and feel threatened by any attempt others make to help.

Depressants

Depressants are substances that affect the central nervous system by decreasing physical and mental activity. Depressants are commonly used for medical purposes. Common depressants are barbiturates, benzodiazepines, narcotics, and alcohol. Most depressants are ingested or injected. Their slang names include downers, rainbows, barbs, goofballs, yellow jackets, purple hearts, nemmies, tooies, reds, Quaaludes, or ludes.

Alcohol is the most widely used and abused substance in the United States. In small amounts, its effects may be fairly mild. In higher doses, its effects can be toxic. Slang names for alcoholic beverages include booze, juice, brew, vino, and hooch.

Alcohol is like other depressants in its effects and risks for overdose. Frequent drinkers may become dependent on the effects of alcohol and increasingly tolerant of those effects. Drinking alcohol in large or frequent amounts causes many unhealthy consequences. Alcohol poisoning can occur when a large amount of alcohol is consumed in a short period of time and can result in unconsciousness and, if untreated, death.

The digestive system may also be irritated by heavy or chronic drinking. Alcohol can cause the esophagus to rupture, or it can injure the stomach lining. Chronic drinking can also affect the brain and cause a lack of coordination, memory loss, and apathy. Other problems include liver disease, such as cirrhosis (Fig. 16-22, *A-B*). In addition, many psychological, family, social, and work problems are related to chronic drinking.

All depressants alter consciousness to some degree. They relieve anxiety, promote sleep, depress respiration, relieve pain, relax muscles, and impair coordination and judgment. Like other substances, the larger the dose or the stronger the substance, the greater its effects.

Narcotics

Narcotics, derived from opium, are drugs used mainly to relieve pain. Narcotics are so powerful and highly addictive that all are illegal without a prescription, and some are not prescribed at all. When taken in large doses, narcotics can produce euphoria, stupor, coma, or death. The most common natural narcotics are morphine and codeine. Most other narcotics, including heroin, are synthetic or semisynthetic.

Inhalants

Substances inhaled to produce mood-altering effects are called ***inhalants.*** Inhalants also depress the central nervous system. In addition, inhalant use can damage the heart, lungs, brain, and liver. Inhalants include medical anesthetics, such as amyl nitrite and nitrous oxide (also known as "laughing gas"), as well as hydrocarbons, known as solvents. Solvents' effects are similar to those of alcohol. People who use solvents may appear to be drunk. Solvents include toluene, found in glues; butane, found in lighter fluids; acetone, found in nail polish removers; fuels, such as gasoline and kerosene; and propellants, found in aerosol sprays.

Cannabis Products

Cannabis products, including marijuana, tetrahydrocannabinol or THC, and hashish, are all derived from the plant *Cannabis sativa.* Slang names for marijuana include pot, grass, weed, reefer, ganja, tea, and dope. Marijuana is the most widely used illicit drug in the United States. It is typically smoked in cigarette form or in a pipe. The effects include feelings of elation, distorted perceptions of time and space, and impaired judgment and motor coordination. Marijuana irritates the throat, reddens the eyes, and causes a rapid pulse, dizziness, and often an increased appetite. Depending on the dose, the person, and many other factors, cannabis products can produce effects similar to those of substances in any of the other major substance categories.

Marijuana, although illegal, has been used for some medicinal purposes. Marijuana or its legal synthetic versions are used as an anti-nausea medication for people who are undergoing chemotherapy for cancer, for treating glaucoma, for treating muscular weakness caused by multiple sclerosis, and to combat the weight loss caused by cancer and AIDS.

Other Substances

Some other substances do not fit neatly into these categories. These substances include designer drugs, steroids, and over-the-counter substances, which can be purchased without a prescription.

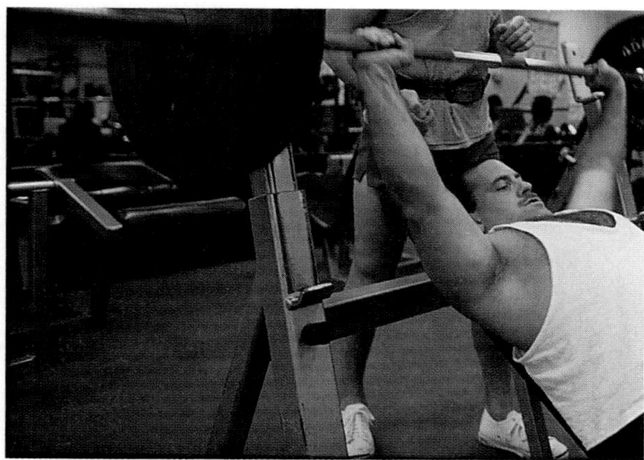

Figure 16-23 Steroids are drugs sometimes used by athletes to enhance performance and increase muscle mass.

Designer drugs

In the early 1980s, the spread of designer drugs was a frightening possibility. Today, it is a reality. ***Designer drugs*** are variations of other substances, such as narcotics and amphetamines. Through simple and inexpensive methods, the molecular structure of substances produced for medicinal purposes can be modified into extremely potent and dangerous street drugs; hence the term "designer drug." When the chemical makeup of a drug is altered, the user can experience a variety of unpredictable and dangerous effects. The modifier may have no knowledge of the effects a new designer drug might produce. One designer drug, a form of the commonly used surgical anesthetic fentanyl, can be made 2000 to 6000 times stronger than its original form.

One of the more commonly used designer drugs is methylenedioxymethamphetamine (MDMA), often called "ecstasy." Although ecstasy is structurally related to stimulants and hallucinogens, its effects are somewhat different from either category. Ecstasy can evoke a euphoric high that makes it popular. Other signs and symptoms of ecstasy use range from

The Incalculable Cost of Alcohol Abuse

The hospital morgue is full: a teenager who drowned while boating, an elderly man who died of a chronic liver disease, and a woman who was shot by her boyfriend. The group seems to share no connection other than that each body lies in the same morgue.

But there is a connection: alcohol.

Public health officials are seeing a growing number of injuries, illnesses, and other social problems in which alcohol plays a role. More than 100,000 people die each year from alcohol-related causes. Currently in the United States, an estimated 10 million adults and 3 million adolescents under the age of 18 are alcoholics. From the child abused by her alcoholic parent to the driver who drinks and causes a six-car pileup, our country feels the influence of alcohol abuse.

Because alcohol impairs judgment and coordination, even a first-time drinker who overindulges can become a death statistic. Each year, alcohol-related motor vehicle crashes result in approximately 17,500 deaths in the United States. In addition, impaired driving is a leading cause of death among persons under 25 years of age. Nearly one third of all drownings and about half of all deaths caused by fire also involve alcohol. Researchers say strength, judgment, stamina, motor skills, speed, and intellect are all factors in injury prevention. Alcohol impairs many of these abilities. Subsequently, alcohol is a major risk factor for nearly every type of injury.

Tragically, drinking alcohol is a risk often taken by young people. In 1988, a 25-year-old Olympic diving champion drove into a group of teenagers at the end of a country road, killing two people and injuring four others. His blood alcohol concentration was 0.20 percent, twice the legal limit. In one night, both his life and the lives of many others were destroyed.

Reckless and violent behavior has been linked to alcohol abuse in study after study. Nearly one half of all homicides, a third of all suicides, and two thirds of all assaults involve alcohol. One of the best predictors of violence is alcohol abuse. Crime and other social problems are also linked to alcohol. Social workers find alcohol abuse a factor in nearly 50 percent of child abuse cases. Prevalence of alcohol abuse among the homeless ranges from 20 percent to 45 percent.

These personal and social consequences create a tremendous economic burden. According to the National Institute on Drug Abuse, the cost of alcohol addiction runs an estimated $118 billion annually. This cost is associated with time missed from work, reduced job productivity, medical bills, support for families, and property damage.

Health-care costs account for $15 to $20 billion of alcohol costs, and research documenting the detrimental health effects of alcohol is growing. Doctors now say that even moderate drinking increases risks of high blood pressure, cirrhosis of the liver, and decreased motor development for children whose mothers drink while pregnant. Prolonged or heavy drinking causes more

the stimulant-like effects of high blood pressure, rapid heartbeat, profuse sweating, and agitation to the hallucinogenic-like effects of paranoia, sensory distortion, and erratic mood swings.

Anabolic steroids

Anabolic steroids are drugs sometimes used by athletes to enhance performance and increase muscle mass (Fig. 16-23). Their medical uses include stimulating weight gain for persons unable to gain weight naturally. They should not be confused with corticosteroids, which are used to counteract the toxic effects of and allergic reactions to plants, such as poison ivy. Chronic use of anabolic steroids can lead to sterility, liver cancer, and personality changes, such as aggressive behavior. Steroid use by younger people may also disrupt normal growth. Slang names for anabolic steroids include androgens, hormones, juice, roids, and vitamins.

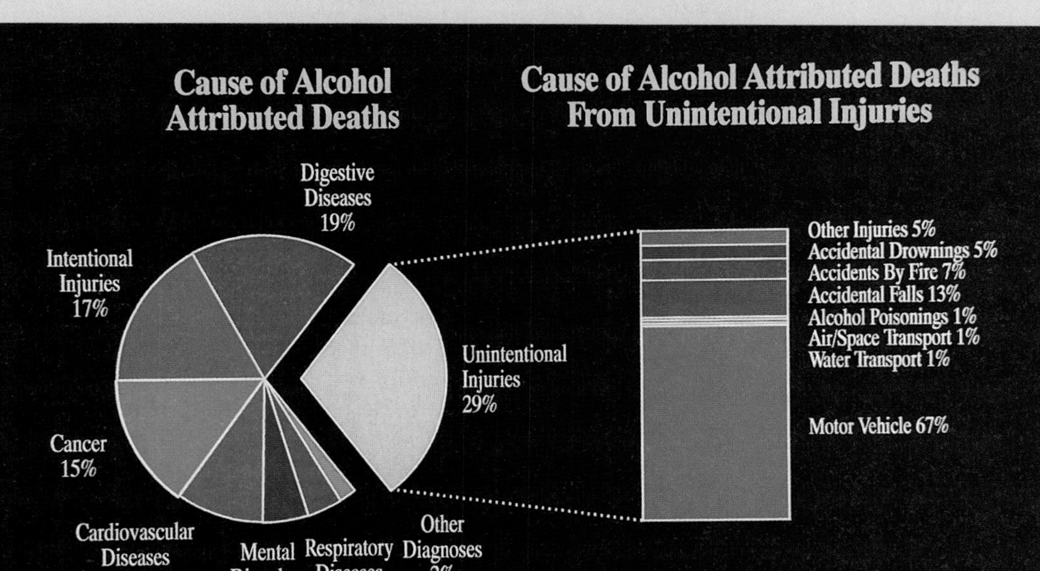

serious long-term effects on your health, including risk of heart attack, many cancers, stroke, gastrointestinal bleeding, kidney failure, and problems of the nervous system, such as tremors and dementia.

Our morgues are filling up with people ravaged by a drug they could and did not control. In terms of economic cost, lives, and productivity, alcohol abuse outdistances cocaine, heroin, and all other drugs. Avoid alcohol or drink moderately so that you will not end up an unfortunate statistic.

SOURCES

Centers for Disease Control: Alcohol-related mortality and years of potential life lost—United States, 1987, *Morbidity and Mortality Weekly Report*, 39(11):173, 1990.

Morbidity and Mortality Weekly Report, December 2, 1994.

Associated Press: *The New York Times*, January 31, 1989, p. 87.

National Clearinghouse for Alcohol and Drug Information. *The Fact is ...OSAP responds to national crisis*, Rockville, MD, Summer 1990, p. 2.

Morbidity and Mortality Weekly Report, March 23, 1990.

Over-the-counter substances

Aspirin, laxatives, and nasal sprays are among the most commonly misused or abused over-the-counter substances. Aspirin is an effective minor pain reliever and fever reducer that is found in a variety of medicines. People use aspirin for many reasons and conditions. In recent years, cardiologists, or heart specialists, have praised the benefits of aspirin for the treatment of heart disease. As useful as aspirin is, misuse can have toxic effects on the body. Typically, aspirin can cause inflammation of the stomach and small intestine that results in bleeding ulcers. Aspirin can also impair normal blood clotting.

Laxatives are used to relieve constipation. They come in a variety of forms and strengths. If used improperly, laxatives can cause uncontrolled diarrhea that may result in **dehydration,** the excessive loss of water from the body

Steroids: Body Meltdown

If you think using steroids is the way to get that sculpted, muscular body typical of bodybuilders and many professional athletes, think again. These drugs may build up bodies on the outside, but they can cause a body meltdown on the inside. Doctors and other public health officials warn of the dangers of steroid abuse and are particularly concerned about the long-term effects of high doses.

Anabolic steroids are synthetic chemicals that mimic the hormone testosterone. Testosterone gives the male his masculine characteristics—deeper voice, beard and mustache, and other sex characteristics. Anabolic steroids have several legitimate, legal uses. They are prescribed by doctors to treat skeletal and growth disorders, certain types of anemia, some kinds of breast cancer, and to offset the negative effects of irradiation and chemotherapy.

Steroids are also used illegally to create proteins and other substances that build muscle tissue, which is why they are popular with some athletes and bodybuilders. In recent years, several professional athletes have made the headlines because of their abuse of steroids. Doctors are now getting a better idea of the devastating effects that illegal steroid use can have on the body. The problem is that some young athletes and bodybuilders are listening to their gym buddies rather than their doctors. Steroids are being used in greater doses than ever before and at earlier ages. Although both young males and females abuse steroids, the abuse of steroids among young males is becoming as prevalent as eating disorders in young females.

Before you listen to another person's opinion of steroids, consider these effects:

- **Stunted growth.** In children, steroids cause the growth plates in the bones to close prematurely. As a teenager, you may have been destined to be six-foot-four, but taking steroids can permanently stunt your growth.
- **Heart disease and stroke.** Steroids cause dangerous changes in cholesterol levels. One study found dramatic drops in the amount of good cholesterol (HDL), which helps remove the fatty deposits on the artery walls, in steroid users. The research also shows dramatic increases in bad cholesterol (LDL), which clogs the arteries and causes heart problems. Your steroid-doped body may look fine on the out-

tissues. The very young and the elderly are particularly susceptible to dehydration.

The abuse of laxatives is frequently associated with attempted weight loss and eating disorders, such as anorexia nervosa or bulimia. **Anorexia nervosa** is a disorder that typically affects young women and is characterized by a long-term refusal to eat food with sufficient nutrients and calories. Anorexics, people with anorexia, typically use laxatives to keep from gaining weight. **Bulimia** is a condition in which victims gorge themselves with food, then purge by vomiting or using laxatives. For this reason, the behavior associated with bulimia is often referred to as "binging and purging." Anorexia nervosa and bulimia have underlying psychological factors that contribute to their onset. The effect of both of these eating disorders is severe malnutrition, which can result in death.

Decongestant nasal sprays can help relieve the congestion of colds or hay fever. If misused, they can cause physical dependency. Using the spray over a long period can cause nosebleeds and changes in the lining of the nose that make it difficult to breathe without the spray.

Signs and Symptoms of Substance Misuse and Abuse

Many of the signs and symptoms of substance misuse and abuse are similar to those of other

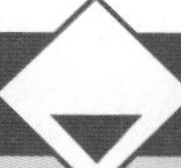

side, but inside, it may look like the body of a man in his fifties whose arteries are so clogged that he needs heart surgery.

- **Aggressive personality and psychological disorders.** Some people who take anabolic steroids become unnaturally aggressive. A few have developed documentable mental disorders. In a *Sports Illustrated* article, a South Carolina football player described his nightmare with steroids. He described pulling a gun on a pizza delivery boy in his dorm and how his family intervened when he began threatening suicide. Many doctors feel the psychiatric effects of steroids may be the most threatening side effect.
- **Lowered white blood cell count.** Taking steroids also affects the number of white blood cells in your body. With fewer white blood cells, your body has fewer antibodies to fight off infections, including cancers and other diseases.
- **Sexual dysfunction and disorders.** Synthetic steroids cause your body to cut off its own natural production of steroids, resulting in shrinking testicles in men. If you are a woman, you may grow facial hair, your breast size may decrease, and your voice may get permanently deeper. In both sexes, steroids may cause sterility and reduce sexual interest.
- **Impaired liver function and liver disease.** Steroids seriously affect the liver's ability to function. They irritate the liver, causing tissue damage and an inability to clear bile. Doctors also have found blood-filled benign tumors in the livers of steroid users.

Steroids pose dangers beyond these physiological side effects. Because steroids are often sold on the black market, they are increasingly sold by drug traffickers who obtain their wares from unsanitary laboratories. Yet another danger comes from the fact that sharing needles to inject steroids increases the increasing of transmission of viruses such as HIV, which causes AIDS, and hepatitis.

SOURCES

Altman L: New breakfast of champions: a recipe for victory or disaster?, *The New York Times,* November 20, 1988.

Chaikin T, and Telander R: The nightmare of steroids, *Sports Illustrated,* 69:18 1988.

USA Today, Vol. 121, No. 2573, February 1993.

National Institute on Drug Abuse. "Anabolic steroids: a threat to body and mind." National Institutes of Health, No. 94-3721, 1991.

medical emergencies. You should not necessarily assume that someone who is stumbling, is disoriented, or has a fruity, alcohol-like odor on the breath is intoxicated by alcohol or other drugs, since he or she may be a victim of a diabetic emergency.

The misuse or abuse of stimulants can have many unhealthy effects on the body that mimic other conditions. For example, a stimulant overdose can cause moist or flushed skin, sweating, chills, nausea, vomiting, fever, headache, dizziness, rapid pulse, rapid breathing, high blood pressure, and chest pain. In some instances, it can cause respiratory distress, disrupt normal heart rhythms, or cause death. The victim may appear very excited, restless, talkative, or irritable or suddenly lose consciousness. Stimulant abuse can lead to addiction and can cause heart attack or stroke.

Specific signs and symptoms of hallucinogen abuse may include sudden mood changes and a flushed face. The victim may claim to see or hear something not present. He or she may be anxious and frightened.

Specific signs and symptoms of depressant abuse may include drowsiness, confusion, slurred speech, slow heart and breathing rates, and poor coordination. A person who abuses alcohol may smell of alcohol. A person who has consumed a great deal of alcohol in a short time may be unconscious or hard to arouse. The person may vomit violently.

Specific signs and symptoms of alcohol withdrawal, a potentially dangerous condition that can be life threatening, include confusion and restlessness, trembling, hallucinations, and seizures. Always call EMS personnel if you suspect a person is suffering from alcohol withdrawal or from any form of substance abuse.

Remember that, as in other medical emergencies, you do not have to diagnose substance misuse or abuse to provide care. However, you may be able to find clues that suggest the nature of the problem. Such clues may help you provide more complete information to more advanced medical personnel so that they can provide prompt and appropriate care. Often these clues will come from the victim, bystanders, or the scene. Look for containers, pill bottles, drug paraphernalia, and signs of other medical problems. If the victim is incoherent or unconscious, try to get information from any bystanders or family members. Since many of the physical signs of substance abuse mimic other conditions, you may not be able to determine that a person has overdosed on a substance. To provide care for the victim, you need only recognize abnormalities in breathing, skin color and moisture, body temperature, and behavior; any of which may indicate a condition requiring professional help.

Care for Substance Misuse and Abuse

Since substance abuse and misuse are forms of poisoning, care follows the same general principles. However, as in other medical emergencies, people who misuse or abuse substances may become aggressive or uncooperative when you try to help. If the person becomes agitated or makes the scene unsafe in any way, retreat until the scene can be secured. *Provide care only if you feel the person is not a danger to you and others.*

Your initial care for substance misuse or abuse does not require that you know the specific substance taken. Follow these general principles as you would for any poisoning:

- Size up the scene to be sure it is safe.
- Perform an initial assessment to check for any life-threatening conditions.
- Summon more advanced medical personnel.
- Perform a physical exam.
- Take a SAMPLE history to try to find out what substance was taken, how much was taken, and when it was taken.
- Calm and reassure the victim.
- Keep the victim from getting chilled or overheated.
- Keep the victim's airway clear.
- Administer oxygen if it is available and you are trained to do so, and the victim is having difficulty breathing.

◆ PREVENTING SUBSTANCE ABUSE

Experts in the field of substance abuse generally agree that prevention efforts are far more cost-effective than treatment. Yet, preventing substance abuse is a complex process that involves many underlying factors. Various approaches, including educating people about substances and their effects on health and attempting to instill fear of penalties, have not by themselves proved particularly effective. It is becoming clearer that, to be effective, prevention efforts must address the various underlying issues of substance abuse and ways to approach it.

The following factors may contribute to substance abuse:

- A lack of parental supervision
- The breakdown of traditional family structure
- A wish to escape unpleasant surroundings and stressful situations
- The widespread availability of substances
- Peer pressure and the basic need to belong

- Low self-esteem, including feelings of guilt or shame
- Media glamorization, especially of alcohol and tobacco, promoting the idea that using substances enhances fun and popularity
- A history of substance abuse in the home or community environments

Recognizing and understanding these factors may help prevent and treat substance abuse.

◆ PREVENTING SUBSTANCE MISUSE

Some poisonings from medicinal substances occur when the victims knowingly increase the dosage beyond what is directed. Medications should be taken only as directed. On the other hand, many poisonings from medicinal substances are not intentional. The following guidelines can help prevent unintentional misuse or overdose—

- Read the product information and use only as directed.
- Ask your doctor or pharmacist about the intended use and side effects of prescription and over-the-counter medication. If you are taking more than one medication, check for possible interaction effects.
- Never use another person's prescribed medications; what is right for one person is seldom right for another.
- Always keep medications in their appropriate, marked containers.
- Discard all out-of-date medications. Time can alter the chemical composition of medications, causing them to be less effective and possibly even toxic.
- Always keep medications out of reach of children.

◆ SUMMARY

Poisonings can occur in four ways: ingestion, inhalation, absorption, and injection. Substance abuse and misuse are types of poisoning that can occur in any of these ways. Substance abuse and misuse can produce a variety of signs and symptoms, most of which are common to other types of poisoning. You do not need to be able to determine the cause of a poisoning to provide appropriate initial care. If you see any of the signs and symptoms of sudden illness, follow the basic guidelines for care for any medical emergency. For suspected poisonings, contact your local or regional poison control center (PCC) or summon more advanced medical personnel. Beyond following the general guidelines for giving care for a suspected poisoning, medical professionals may advise you to provide some specific care, such as neutralizing the poison with activated charcoal.

Six major categories of substances, when abused or misused, can produce a variety of signs and symptoms, some of which are indistinguishable from those of other medical emergencies. Remember, you do not have to know the specific condition to provide care. If you suspect that the victim's condition is caused by substance misuse or abuse, provide care for a poisoning emergency.

Use the activities in Unit 16 of the workbook to review the material in this chapter.

You Are the Responder

You are on your way to work when you see a car on the highway go out of control, narrowly miss hitting other cars, strike a guard rail, and come to a stop, fortunately on the shoulder. You stop, go over to the car, and find the driver coughing, wheezing, and clutching his throat. You notice a red, swollen mark on his left arm, and you see a hornet buzzing on the windshield. What do you do?

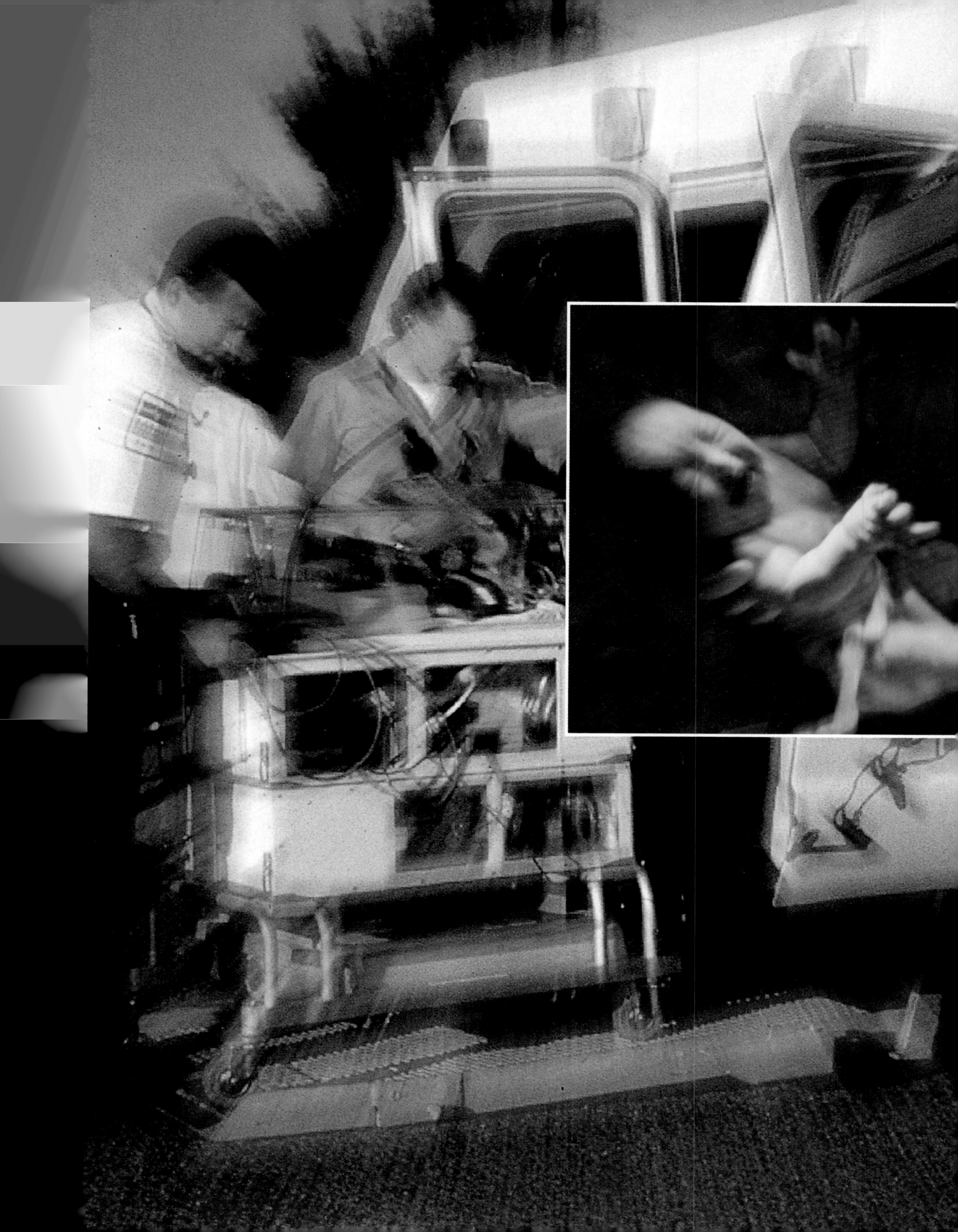

Module Six

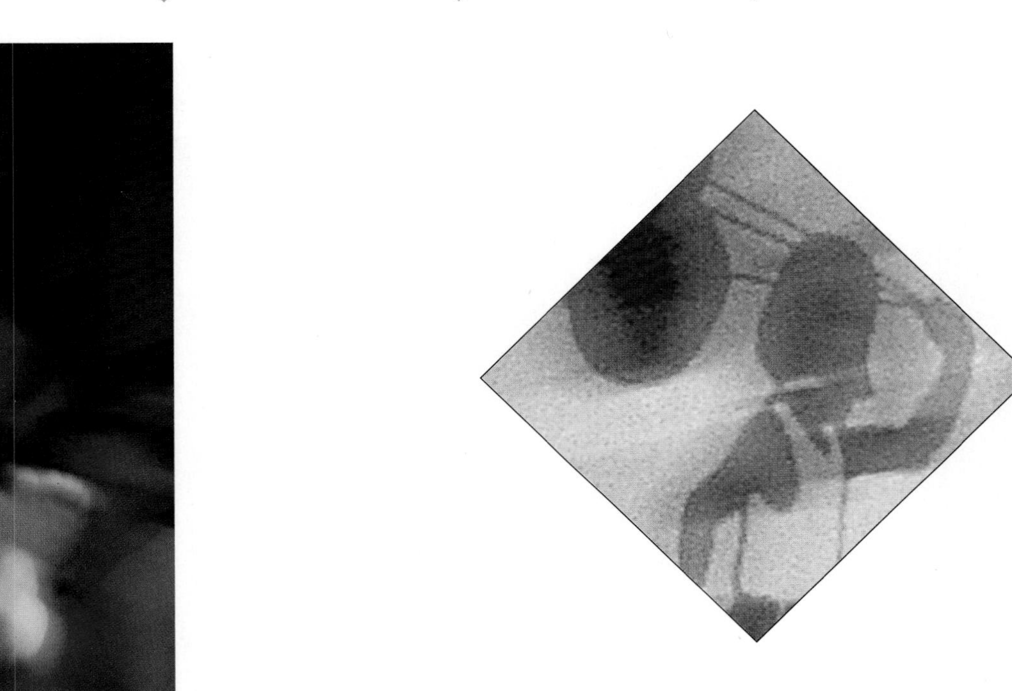

Childbirth and Children

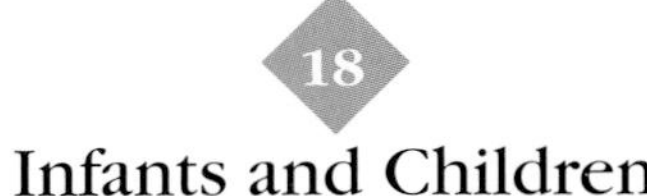

Childbirth

17

Key Terms

Amniotic (am ne OT ik) sac: A fluid-filled sac that encloses, bathes, and protects the developing baby; commonly called the bag of waters.

Birth canal: The passageway from the uterus to the vaginal opening through which a baby passes during birth.

Bloody show: Pink or light red thick discharge from the vagina that occurs during labor. Sometimes this signifies the onset of labor.

*__Breech birth:__ The delivery of a baby feet or buttocks first.

Cervix: The upper part of the birth canal; the opening of the uterus.

Contraction: The rhythmic tightening and relaxing of muscles in the uterus during labor.

Crowning: The time in labor when the baby's head is at the opening of the vagina.

Labor: The birth process; beginning with the contraction of the uterus and dilation of the cervix and ending with the stabilization and recovery of the mother.

Miscarriage (spontaneous abortion): A spontaneous end to pregnancy before the twentieth week, usually because of birth defects in the fetus or placenta.

Placenta (plah SEN tah): An organ attached to the uterus and unborn child through which nutrients are delivered to the baby; expelled after the baby is delivered.

Prolapsed cord: A complication of childbirth in which a loop of umbilical cord protrudes through the vagina before delivery of the baby.

Umbilical cord: A flexible structure that attaches the placenta to the unborn child, allowing for the passage of blood, nutrients, and waste.

Uterus: A pear-shaped organ in a woman's pelvis in which an embryo forms and develops into a baby; also called the womb.

Vagina: *See* **Birth canal.**

◆ Knowledge Objectives ◆

After reading this chapter and completing the class activities, you should be able to—

- Identify the following structures: birth canal, placenta, umbilical cord, amniotic sac.
- Define the following terms: crowning, bloody show, labor, spontaneous abortion.
- State indications of an imminent delivery.
- State the steps in the predelivery preparation of the mother.
- Explain the importance of body substance isolation during childbirth.
- State the steps in assisting with childbirth.
- Describe care of the baby as the head appears.
- Describe the steps in the delivery of the placenta.
- List the steps in the post-delivery emergency medical care of the mother.
- Describe the steps in caring for the newborn.
- * Describe possible complications that may occur during pregnancy and childbirth.
- Describe why it is important to attend to the emotional needs of a person in need of emergency medical care during childbirth.

* Signifies an Enrichment section objective.

◆ Attitude Objectives ◆

After reading this chapter and completing the class activities, you should be able to—

- Acknowledge the need for having a caring attitude toward the mother during childbirth.
- Empathize with the mother during childbirth, as well as with family members and friends of the mother.
- Acknowledge the physical and emotional stress associated with pregnancy and childbirth.

◆ Skill Objectives ◆

After reading this chapter and completing the class activities, you should be able to—

- Demonstrate the steps to assist in a normal head-first delivery.
- Demonstrate the necessary care of the baby as the head appears.
- Demonstrate the post-delivery care of the mother.
- Demonstrate the care of the newborn.

A woman calls 9-1-1 and asks for an ambulance. She says she thinks her baby is coming fast. The response time of the ambulance to reach her rural home is nearly 25 minutes. A police officer nearby hears the call on her radio and decides to help until ambulance personnel arrive.

As she approaches the house, she notices the front door is partially opened. She goes in and finds a woman lying on the floor, in obvious pain. She sees bloody fluid on the floor. When she assesses the woman, she sees the infant's head at the opening of the birth canal. Childbirth is occurring and will not wait for the ambulance crew to arrive. The police officer prepares to help deliver the baby.

◆ INTRODUCTION

Someday you may be faced with a similar situation, requiring that you assist with childbirth. If you have never seen or experienced childbirth, your expectations probably consist of what others have told you.

Terms such as exhausting, stressful, exciting, fulfilling, painful, and scary are sometimes used to describe a planned childbirth, one that occurs in the hospital or at home under the supervision of a health-care provider. If you find yourself assisting with the delivery of a baby, however, it is probably not happening in a planned situation. Therefore your feelings, as well as those of the expectant mother, may be intensified by fear of the unexpected or the possibility that something might go wrong.

Take comfort in knowing that things rarely go wrong. Childbirth is a natural process. Thousands of children all over the world are born each day, without complications, in areas where no medical assistance is available during childbirth.

By following a few simple steps, you can effectively assist in the birth process. This chapter will help you better understand the birthing process, how to assist with the delivery of a baby, how to provide care for both the mother and newborn, how to recognize complications, and what complications could require more advanced care.

◆ PREGNANCY

Pregnancy begins when an egg (ovum) is fertilized by a sperm, forming an **embryo.** The embryo implants itself within the mother's ***uterus,*** a pear-shaped organ that lies at the top center of the pelvis. The embryo is surrounded by the ***amniotic sac.*** This is a fluid-filled sac, also called the "bag of waters." The fluid is constantly renewed and helps protect the baby from injury and infection.

As the embryo grows, its organs and body parts develop. After about 8 weeks, the embryo is called a **fetus.** To continue to develop properly, the fetus must receive nutrients. The fetus receives these nutrients from the mother through a specialized organ attached to the uterus called the ***placenta.*** The placenta is attached to the fetus by a flexible structure called the ***umbilical cord.*** The fetus usually will continue to develop for approximately 32 weeks, at which time the birth process will normally begin (Fig. 17-1).

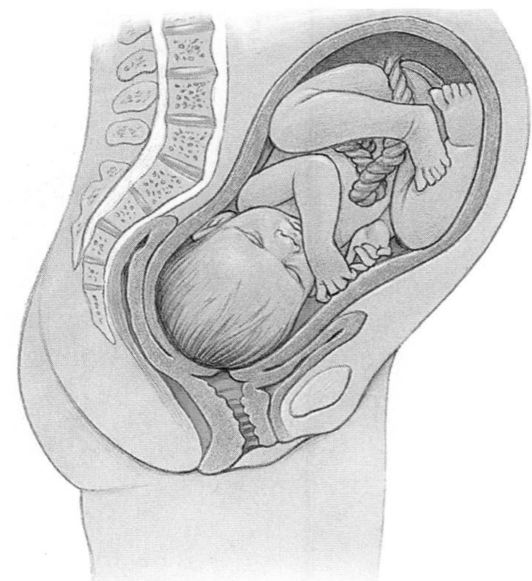

Figure 17-1 Mother and Fetus at 40 Weeks

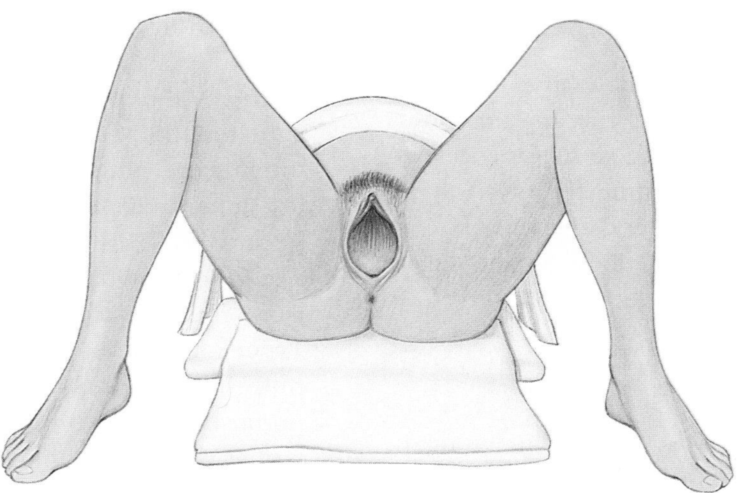

Figure 17-2 When crowning begins, birth is imminent.

◆ THE BIRTH PROCESS

The birth process begins with the onset of labor. ***Labor*** is the final phase of pregnancy. It is a process in which many systems work together to bring about birth. Labor begins with a rhythmic contraction of the uterus. As these contractions continue, they dilate the ***cervix***—a short tube of muscle at the upper end of the ***birth canal,*** the passageway from the uterus to the vaginal opening. When the cervix is sufficiently dilated, it allows the baby to travel from the uterus through the birth canal or **vagina.** The baby passes through the birth canal and emerges at the lower end of the canal to the outside world. For first-time mothers, this process normally takes between 12 and 24 hours. Subsequent babies are usually delivered more quickly.

The Labor Process

The labor process has four distinct stages. The length and intensity of each stage vary.

Stage One—Preparation

In the first stage, the mother's body prepares for the birth. This stage covers the time from the first contraction until the cervix is fully dilated. A ***contraction*** is a rhythmic tightening and relaxing of the muscles in the uterus. It is like a wave. It begins gently, rises to a peak of intensity, then drops off and subsides. The muscles then relax, and there is a break before the next contraction starts. As the time for delivery approaches, the contractions become closer together, last longer, and feel stronger. Normally, when contractions are less than 3 minutes apart, childbirth is near.

Stage Two—Delivery of the Baby

The second stage of labor involves the actual delivery of the baby. It begins once the cervix is completely dilated and ends with the birth of a baby. In a normal delivery, the baby's head becomes visible as it emerges from the vagina. When the top of the head begins to emerge, it is called ***crowning*** (Fig. 17-2). When crowning occurs, birth is imminent and you must be prepared to receive the baby.

Stage Three—Delivery of the Placenta

Once the baby's body emerges, the third stage of labor begins. During this stage, the placenta usually separates from the wall of the uterus and exits from the birth canal. This process normally occurs within 30 minutes of the delivery of the baby.

Stage Four—Stabilization

The final stage of labor involves the initial recovery and stabilization of the mother after childbirth. Normally, this stage lasts for approximately 1 hour. During this time, the uterus contracts to control bleeding and the mother begins to recover from the physical and emotional stress that occurred during childbirth.

Assessing Labor

If you are called to assist a pregnant woman, you will want to determine whether she is in labor. If she is in labor, you should determine how far along she is in the birth process and whether she expects any complications. You can determine these factors by asking a few key questions and making some quick observations. Ask the following:

- What is the due date? Near the end of the pregnancy, the mother can have contractions that are not true signs of labor.
- Is there a chance of a multiple birth? Labor does not usually last as long in a multiple birth. Also, if you know it may be a multiple birth, you can prepare ahead what you will need to help in the delivery of more than one baby. Additional information on multiple births is presented in the Enrichment section of this chapter.
- Is this the first pregnancy? The first stage of labor normally takes longer with first pregnancies than with subsequent ones.
- Has the amniotic sac ruptured? When this happens, fluid flows from the vagina in a sudden gush or a trickle. Some women think they have lost control of their bladder. The breaking of the sac usually signals the beginning of labor. People often describe the rupture of the sac as "the water breaking."
- What are the contractions like? Are they very close together? Are they strong? The length and intensity of the contractions will give you valuable information about the progress of labor. As labor progresses, contractions become stronger, last longer, and are closer together.
- Is there a bloody discharge? This pink or light red, thick discharge from the vagina is the mucous plug that falls from the cervix as it begins to dilate, which also signals the onset of labor. This discharge is also referred to as a ***bloody show.***
- Does she have an urge to bear down? If the expectant mother expresses a strong urge to push, labor is far along.
- Is the baby crowning? If the baby's head is visible, the baby is about to be born.

◆ PREPARING FOR DELIVERY

There comes a time when you realize that you are about to assist with childbirth. Though this realization is often exciting, it is rarely comforting.

Preparing Yourself

Childbirth is messy. It involves a discharge of watery, sometimes bloody, fluid at stages one and two of labor and what appears to be a rather large loss of blood after stage two. Fluid discharge sometimes creates splashes, and it is important for the first responder to practice body substance isolation (BSI) precautions (see Chapter 3). Try not to be alarmed at the loss of blood. It is a normal part of the birth process. Only bleeding that cannot be controlled after the baby is born is a problem. Take a deep breath and try to relax. Remember that you are only assisting in the process; the expectant mother is doing all the work.

Helping the Mother Cope With Labor and Delivery

Explain to the expectant mother that the baby is about to be born. Be calm and reassuring. A woman having her first child often feels fear and apprehension about the pain and the condition of the baby. Labor pain ranges from discomfort similar to menstrual cramps to intense pressure or pain. Many women experience something in between. Factors that can increase pain and discomfort during the first stage of labor include —

- Irregular breathing.
- Tensing up because of fear.
- Not knowing what to expect.
- Feeling alone and unsupported.

You can help the expectant mother cope with the discomfort and pain of labor. Begin by reassuring her that you are there to help. Explain what to expect as labor progresses. Suggest specific physical activities that she can do to relax, such as regulating her breathing. Ask her to breathe in slowly and deeply through the nose and out through the mouth. Ask her to try to focus on one object in the room while regulating her breathing. By staying calm, firm, and confident and offering encouragement, you can help reduce her fear and apprehension. Reducing fear will aid in reducing her pain and discomfort.

Breathing slowly and deeply in through the nose and out through the mouth during labor can help the expectant mother in several ways:

- Aids muscle relaxation
- Offers a distraction from the pain of strong contractions as labor progresses
- Ensures adequate oxygen to both the mother and the baby during labor

Taking childbirth classes, usually offered at local hospitals, can help you become more competent in techniques to help an expectant mother relax.

◆ ASSISTING WITH DELIVERY

It is difficult to predict how much time you have before the baby is delivered. However, if the expectant mother says that she feels the need to push or feels as if she has to have a bowel movement, delivery is near.

You should time the expectant mother's contractions from the beginning of one contraction to the beginning of the next. If they are less than 3 minutes apart, prepare to help with the delivery of the baby.

Assisting with the delivery is often a simple process. The expectant mother is doing all the work. Your job is to create a clean environment and to help guide the baby from the birth canal, minimizing injury to the mother and baby. Begin by positioning the mother. She should be lying on her back, with her head and upper back raised, not lying flat. Her legs should be bent, with the knees drawn up and apart (Fig. 17-3, *A*). Positioning the mother in this way will make her more comfortable.

Next, establish a clean environment for delivery. Since it is unlikely that you will have sterile supplies, use items such as clean sheets, blankets, towels, or even clothes. To make the area around the mother as sanitary as possible, place these items over the mother's abdomen and under her buttocks and legs (Fig. 17-3, *B*). Keep a clean, warm towel or blanket handy to wrap the newborn. Because you will be coming in contact with the mother's and baby's body fluids, be sure to wear disposable gloves. Wear protective eyeware and a disposable gown, if they are available, to protect yourself from splashing.

Other items that can be helpful if available include a bulb syringe to suction secretions from the infant's nose and mouth, gauze pads or sanitary pads to help absorb secretions and vaginal bleeding, a large plastic bag or towel to hold the placenta after delivery, and oxygen.

As crowning occurs, place a hand on the top of the baby's head and apply light pressure (Fig. 17-4). By doing so, you allow the head to emerge slowly, not forcefully. Gradual emergence will help prevent tearing of the vagina and injury to the baby. At this point, the expectant mother should stop pushing. Instruct the mother to concentrate on her breathing tech-

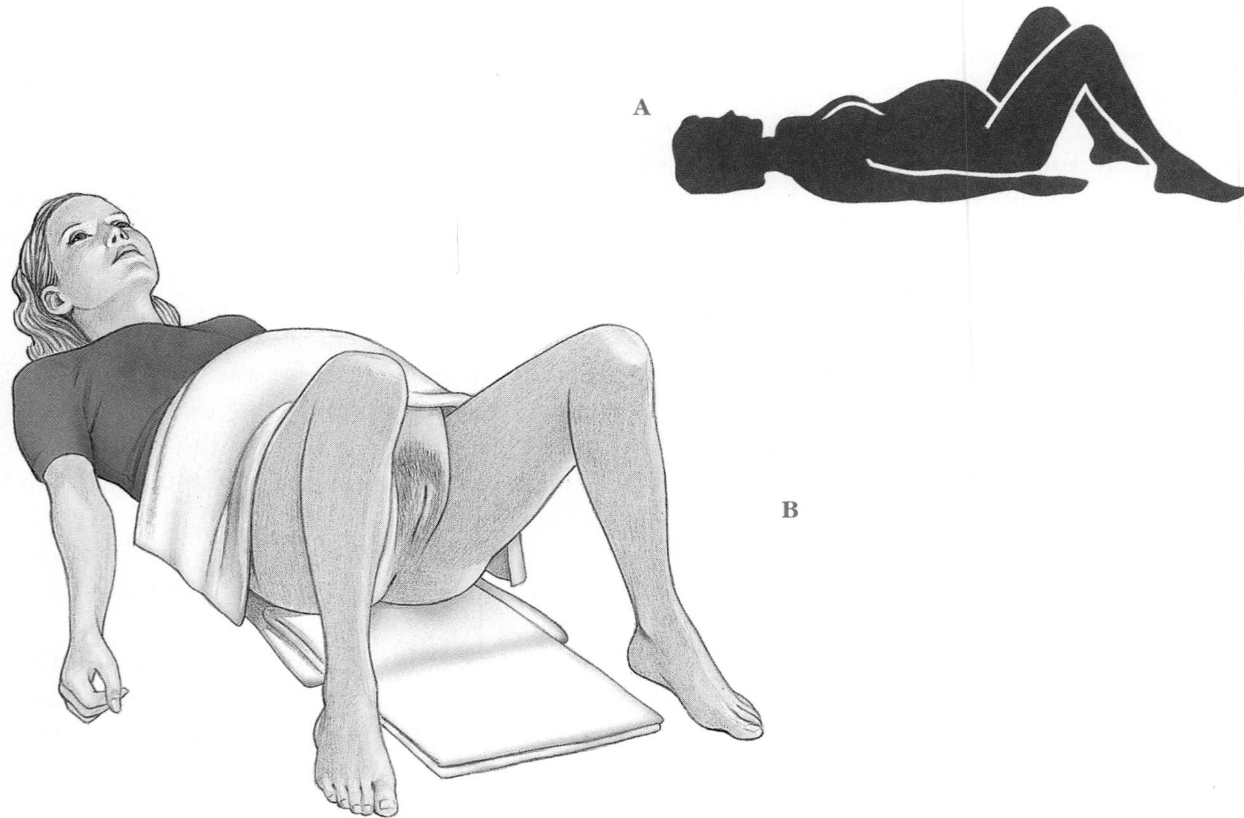

Figure 17-3 **A**, Position the mother with her legs bent and knees drawn up and apart. **B**, Place clean sheets, blankets, towels, or even clothes under the mother.

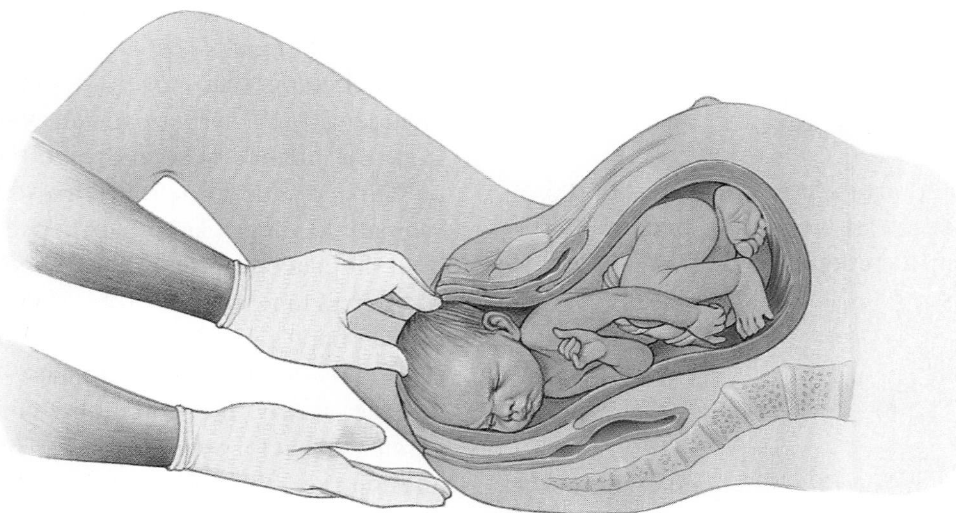

Figure 17-4 Place your hand on top of the baby's head and apply light pressure.

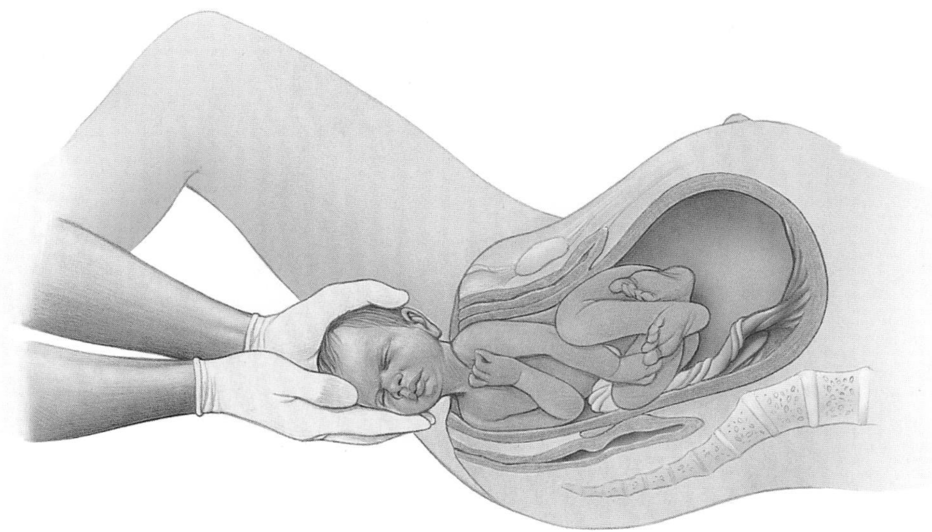

Figure 17-5 As the infant emerges, support the head.

niques. Have her pant. This technique will help her stop pushing and help prevent a forceful birth.

As the head emerges, the baby will turn to one side (Fig. 17-5), which enables the shoulders and the rest of the body to pass through the birth canal. Check to see if the umbilical cord is looped around the baby's neck. If it is, gently slip it over the baby's head. If you cannot slip it over the head, slip it over the baby's shoulders as they emerge. The baby can slide through the loop.

Guide one shoulder out at a time. Do not pull the baby. As the baby emerges, he or she will be wet and slippery. Use a clean towel to catch the baby. Place the baby on its side, between the mother and you. By doing so, you can provide initial care without fear of dropping the newborn. If possible, note the time the baby was born.

◆ CARING FOR THE NEWBORN AND MOTHER

After the baby is delivered, you must focus your care on the newborn and the mother. It is important to make sure the newborn is doing well, while you are also providing care and comfort to the mother.

Caring for the Newborn

The first few minutes of the baby's life are a difficult transition from life inside the mother's uterus to life outside. You have two priorities at this point. Your first is to see that the baby's airway is open and clear. Since a newborn baby breathes primarily through the nose, it is important to immediately clear the nasal passages and mouth thoroughly. You can do this by using your finger, a gauze pad, or a bulb syringe (Fig. 17-6).

Most babies begin crying and breathing spontaneously. If the baby has not made any sounds, stimulate the baby to cry by flicking your fingers on the soles of the baby's feet. Crying helps clear the baby's airway of fluids and promotes breathing. If the baby does not begin breathing on his or her own within the first minute after birth, begin rescue breathing. If the baby does not have a pulse, begin CPR.

If the baby is having difficulty breathing, additional oxygen would be beneficial. If you have oxygen available and are trained to use it, you can attach a section of tubing to the flowmeter

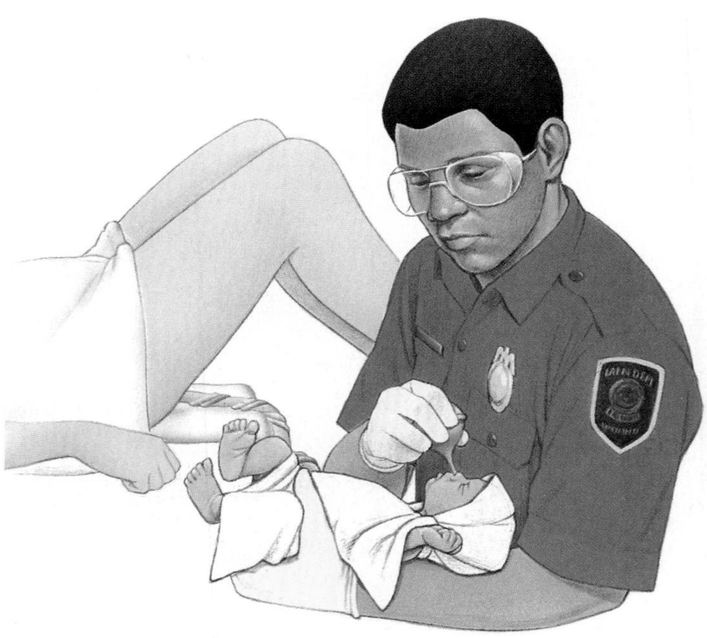

Figure 17-6 A bulb syringe can be used to clear the newborn baby's mouth and nose of any secretions.

and deliver oxygen at 4 liters per minute to the newborn by holding the other end of the tubing near the infant's face (Fig. 17-7).

Your second responsibility is to maintain normal body temperature. Newborns lose heat quickly; therefore it is important to keep him or her warm. Dry the newborn and wrap him or her in a clean, warm towel or blanket. If possible, record a first set of vital signs. Most important are breathing, heart rate, and skin color.

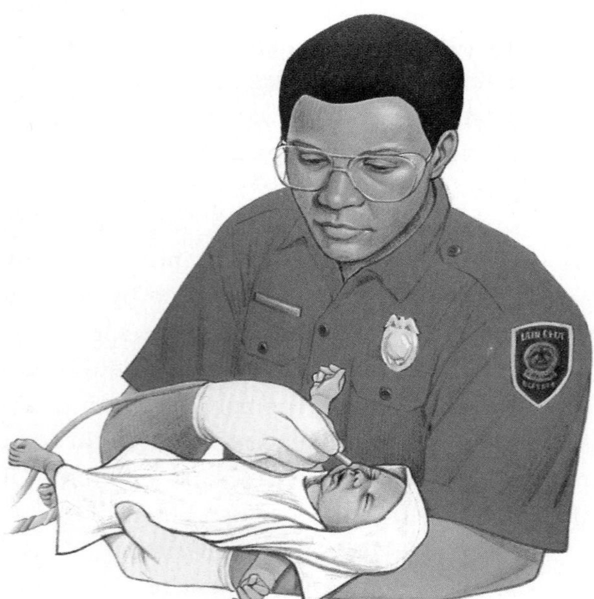

Figure 17-7 Deliver oxygen to a newborn by holding the end of the oxygen tube near the newborn's face.

Caring for the Mother

You can continue to meet the needs of the newborn while caring for the mother. Allow the mother to begin nursing the newborn. Nursing will stimulate the uterus to contract and helps slow bleeding. The placenta will still be in the uterus, attached to the baby by the umbilical cord. Contractions of the uterus usually expel the placenta within 30 minutes of delivery. Catch the placenta in a clean towel or container. When the umbilical cord stops pulsating, tie it with gauze in two places between the mother and the newborn. Place the infant on the mother's abdomen, leave the placenta attached to the newborn, and place it in a plastic bag or wrap it in a towel for transport to the hospital.

Expect some additional vaginal bleeding when the placenta is delivered. Using gauze pads or clean towels, gently clean the mother.

Place a sanitary pad or towel over the vagina. Do not insert anything inside the vagina. Have the mother place her legs together. Feel for a grapefruit-sized mass in the lower abdomen. This is the uterus. Gently massage the lower portion of the abdomen. Massage will help eliminate any large blood clots within the uterus, cause the uterus to contract, and slow bleeding.

Many new mothers experience shocklike signs or symptoms, such as cool, pale or ashen, moist skin, shivering, and slight dizziness, after childbirth. Keep the mother positioned on her back. Administer oxygen if it is available and you are trained to do so. Maintain normal body temperature and monitor vital signs.

◆ SUMMARY

Ideally, childbirth should occur in a controlled environment under the guidance of health-care professionals trained in delivery. In this situation, the necessary medical care is immediately available for mother and baby should any problem arise. However, unexpected deliveries do occur outside of the controlled environment that may require your assistance. By understanding the four stages of labor and knowing how to prepare the expectant mother for delivery, assist in the delivery, and provide proper care for the mother and baby, you will be able to successfully assist in bringing a new child into the world.

Use the activities in Unit 17 of the workbook to review the material in this chapter.

You Are the Responder

1. A 32-year-old woman believes she is in labor. She says that this will be her third child. The amniotic sac ruptured about 1 hour ago. She says she feels a need to move her bowels. Contractions are frequent, about 2 minutes apart. What steps would you take to prepare for delivery of the baby?
2. The same woman screams that she feels the need to push. When you examine her, you see the baby's head crowning. What steps would you take to assist in the delivery of the baby?

ENRICHMENT

◆ SPECIAL SITUATIONS

Most deliveries are fairly routine, with few, if any, surprises or problems. However, you need to be aware of certain special situations or complications that can occur.

Complications During Pregnancy

Complications during pregnancy are rare. One such complication is a ***miscarriage,*** or ***spontaneous abortion***. Since the nature and extent of most complications can only be determined by medical professionals during or after an examination, you should not be concerned with trying to "diagnose" a particular problem. Instead, concern yourself with recognizing signs and symptoms that suggest a serious complication. You should be concerned with two important signs and symptoms—vaginal bleeding and abdominal pain. Any persistent or profuse vaginal bleeding, or bleeding in which tissue passes through the vagina during pregnancy, is abnormal, as is any abdominal pain.

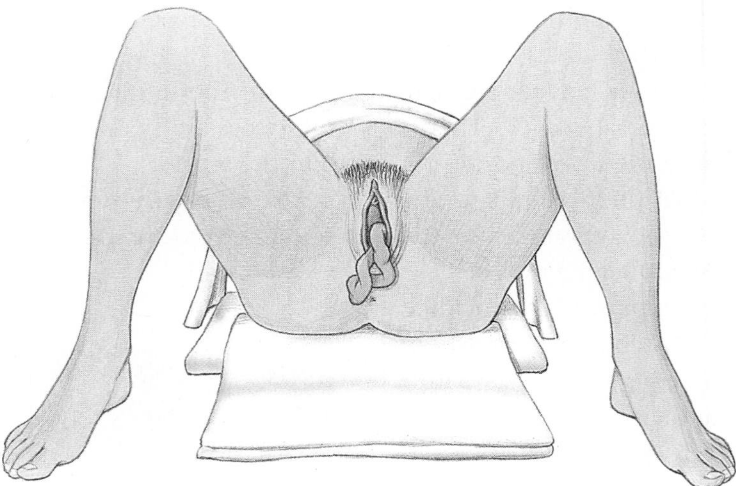

Figure 17-8 Prolapsed Cord

An expectant mother exhibiting these signs and symptoms needs to receive advanced medical care quickly. While waiting for an ambulance, take steps to minimize shock. These include—

- Helping the woman into the most comfortable position.
- Controlling bleeding.
- Keeping the woman from getting chilled or overheated.
- Administering oxygen if it is available and you are trained to do so.

Complications During Childbirth

The vast majority of all births occur without complication. However, this is only reassuring if the one you are assisting with is not complicated. For the few births that do have complications, delivery can be stressful and even life threatening for the expectant mother and the baby. All require the help of more advanced medical personnel.

The most common complication of childbirth is persistent vaginal bleeding. Besides seeking more advanced medical care, you should take steps to minimize shock. Other childbirth complications include a prolapsed cord, breech birth, and multiple births.

Prolapsed Cord

A ***prolapsed cord*** occurs when a loop of the umbilical cord protrudes from the vaginal opening while the baby is still in the birth canal (Fig. 17-8). A prolapsed cord can threaten the baby's life. As the baby moves through the birth canal, the cord will be compressed against the unborn child and the birth canal, and blood flow to the baby will stop. Without this blood flow, the baby will die within a few minutes from lack of oxygen. If you notice a prolapsed cord, have the expectant mother assume a knee-chest position as shown in Figure 17-9. This will help take the pressure off the cord. Administer oxygen to the mother if it is available and you are trained to do so. Summon more advanced medical personnel, if they have not been contacted already.

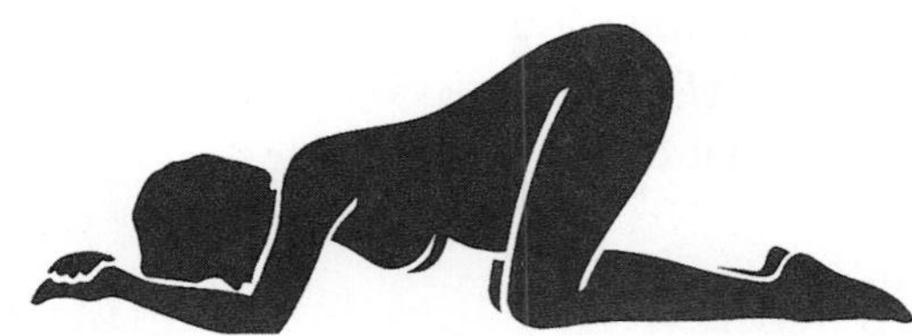

Figure 17-9 The knee-chest position will take pressure off the cord.

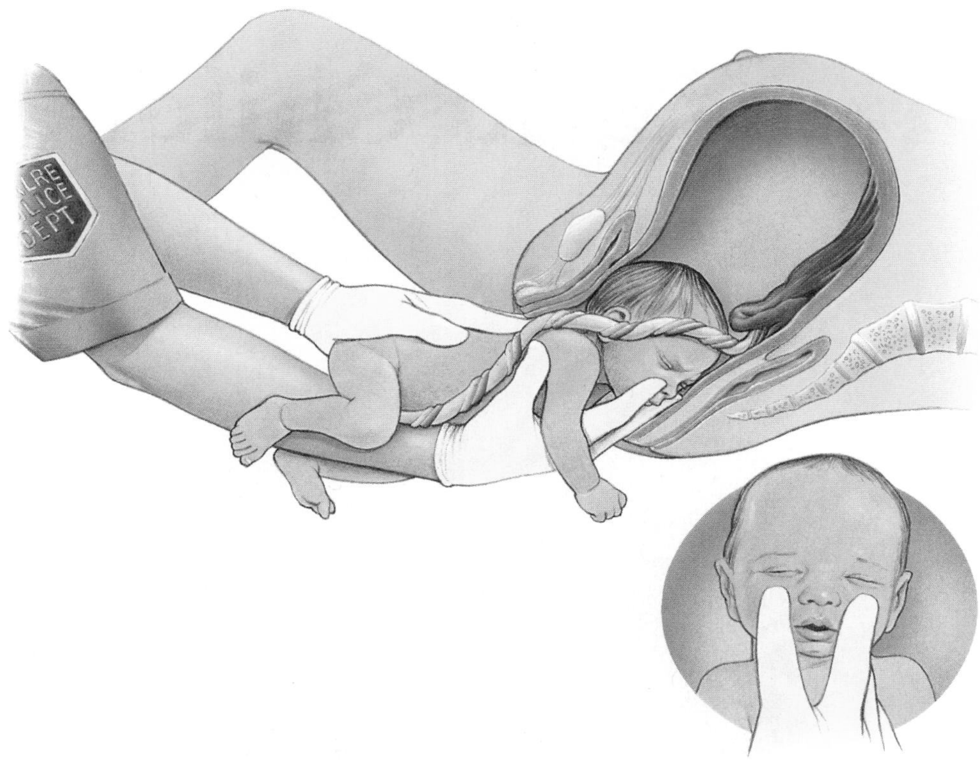

Figure 17-10 During a breech birth, position your index and middle fingers to allow air to enter the baby's mouth and nose.

Breech Birth

Most babies are born head first. However, on rare occasions, the baby is delivered feet or buttocks first. This condition is commonly called ***breech birth.*** If you encounter a breech delivery, support the baby's body as it exits the birth canal while you are waiting for the head to deliver. Do not pull on the baby's body. Pulling will not help to deliver the head.

If, after about 3 minutes, the head has not delivered, you will need to help create an airway for the baby to breathe. Because the weight of the baby's head lodged in the birth canal will reduce or stop blood flow by compressing the cord, the baby will be unable to get any oxygen. Should the baby try to take a spontaneous breath, he or she will also be unable to breathe because the face is pressed against the wall of the birth canal.

To help with a breech delivery, place the index and middle fingers of your gloved hand into the vagina next to the baby's mouth and nose. Spread your fingers to form a V (Fig. 17-10). Though this will not lessen the compression on the umbilical cord, it may allow air to enter the baby's mouth and nose. You must maintain this position until the baby's head is delivered. Administer oxygen to the mother if it is available and you are trained to do so. Summon more advanced medical personnel, if they have not already been contacted.

Multiple Births

Although most births involve only a single baby, a few will involve delivery of more than one. If the mother has had proper prenatal care, she will probably be aware that she is going to have more than one baby. Multiple births should be handled in the same manner as single births. The mother will have a separate set of contractions for each child being born. There may also be a separate placenta for each child, though this is not always the case.

Infants and Children

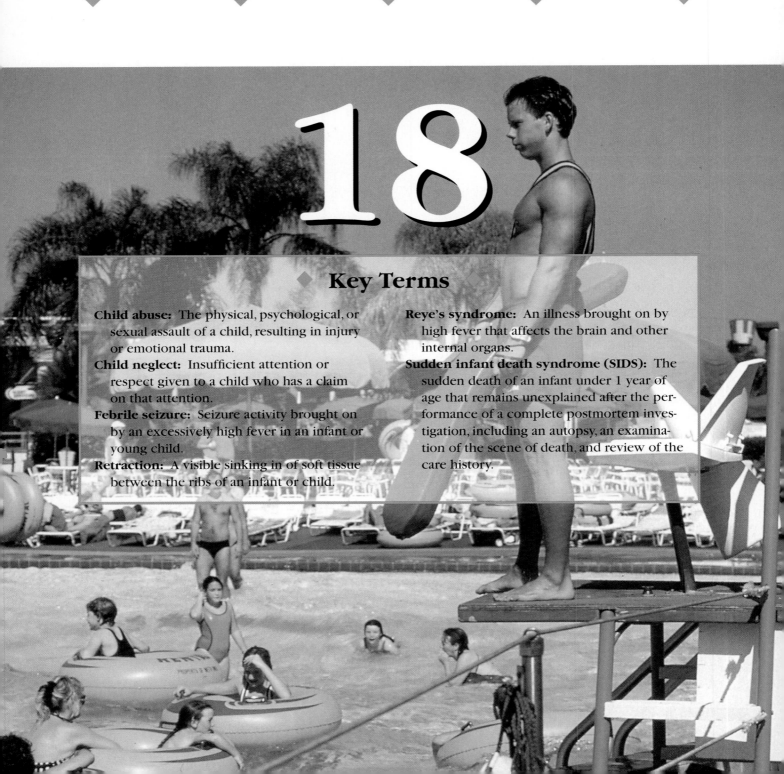

18

Key Terms

Child abuse: The physical, psychological, or sexual assault of a child, resulting in injury or emotional trauma.

Child neglect: Insufficient attention or respect given to a child who has a claim on that attention.

Febrile seizure: Seizure activity brought on by an excessively high fever in an infant or young child.

Retraction: A visible sinking in of soft tissue between the ribs of an infant or child.

Reye's syndrome: An illness brought on by high fever that affects the brain and other internal organs.

Sudden infant death syndrome (SIDS): The sudden death of an infant under 1 year of age that remains unexplained after the performance of a complete postmortem investigation, including an autopsy, an examination of the scene of death, and review of the care history.

◆ Knowledge Objectives ◆

After reading this chapter and completing the class activities, you should be able to—

- Discuss the developmental characteristics of infants and children.
- Describe differences in the anatomy and physiology of an infant, child, and adult.
- Describe the assessment of an infant or child.
- List various causes of respiratory emergencies in infants and children.
- Summarize emergency medical care for respiratory distress and arrest in infants and children.
- List common causes of seizures in infants and children.
- Describe the emergency medical care of infant and child trauma victims.
- Summarize the signs and symptoms of possible child abuse and neglect.
- Describe the medical and legal responsibilities of the first responder who suspects child abuse.

◆ Attitude Objectives ◆

After reading this chapter and completing the class activities, you should be able to—

- Recognize the importance of understanding the various stages of child development.
- Recognize your emotional response to caring for ill or injured infants and children.
- Advocate the need for first responder debriefing after providing care in a difficult situation involving an infant or child.

◆ Skill Objectives ◆

After reading this chapter and completing the class activities, you should be able to—

- Demonstrate how to assess an infant and a child.

◆ INTRODUCTION

In an emergency, you should be aware of the special needs and considerations of infants and children. Knowing these needs and considerations will help you better understand the nature of the emergency and give appropriate care. A young child may be terrified. Being able to communicate with and reassure infants and children can be crucial to your ability to care for them effectively.

◆ INFANTS AND CHILDREN

Infants and children have unique needs and require special care. Assessing a conscious infant's or child's condition can be difficult, especially if he or she does not know you. At certain ages, infants and children do not readily accept strangers. Furthermore, infants and very young children cannot tell you what is wrong.

Communicating With an Ill or Injured Child

We tend to react strongly and emotionally to a child who is in pain or terror. You will need to try exceptionally hard to control your emotions and your facial expressions. Doing so will be helpful to both the child and any concerned adults. To help an ill or injured child, you also need to try to imagine how the child feels. A child is afraid of the unknown. He or she is afraid of being ill or hurt, being touched by strangers, and being separated from his or her parents or other caregiving adults.

How you interact with an ill or injured infant or child is very important. You need to reduce the child's anxiety and panic and gain the child's trust and cooperation, if possible. Move in slowly. The sudden appearance of a stranger may upset the child. Get as close to the infant's or child's eye level as you can, and keep your voice calm (Fig. 18-1). Smile at the child. Ask the child's name, and use it when you talk to him or her. Talk slowly and distinctly, and use words and terms the child will easily understand. Ask questions the child will be able to answer easily. Explain to the child and the parents or caregiver what you are going to do. Reassure a child that you are there to help.

Checking Infants and Children

To be able to effectively check infants and children, it is useful to be aware of certain characteristics of children in specific age groups.

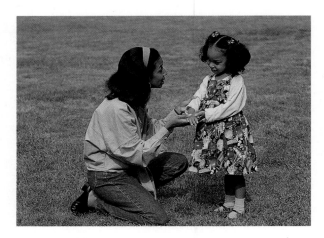

Figure 18-1 To communicate with a child, get as close to eye level as you can.

Children up to 1 year of age are commonly referred to as infants. Infants less than 6 months old are relatively easy to approach and are unlikely to be afraid of you. Older infants, often exhibit "stranger anxiety." They may turn away from you, cry, and cling to their parent or caregiver. If a family member or the caregiver is calm and cooperative, ask that person to help you. Try to check the infant in the parent's or caregiver's lap or arms.

Children age 1 and 2 years are often referred to as toddlers. Toddlers may not cooperate with your attempts to check them. They are usually very concerned about being separated from a parent or caregiver. If you reassure the toddler that he or she will not be separated from a parent or caregiver, the toddler may be comforted. If possible, give the toddler a few minutes to get used to you before attempting to check him or her and check the toddler in the parent's or caregiver's lap. A toddler may also respond to praise or be comforted by holding a special toy or blanket (Fig. 18-2).

Children ages 3, 4, and 5 are commonly referred to as preschoolers. Children in this age group are usually easy to check if you use their natural curiosity. Allow them to inspect items such as bandages. Opportunities to explore can quiet many fears and be a helpful distraction. Reassure the child that you are going to

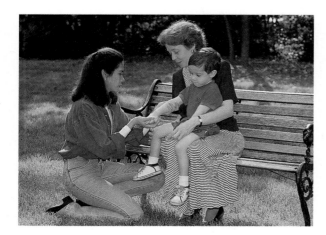

Figure 18-2 Allow a parent to hold the child while you check him or her.

help and will not leave him or her. Sometimes you can demonstrate what you are going to do on a stuffed animal or a doll (Fig. 18-3). The child may be upset by seeing his or her cut or other injury, so cover it with a dressing as soon as possible.

School-age children are between 6 and 12 years of age. They are usually cooperative and can be a good source of information about what happened. You can usually talk readily with school-age children. Do not let the child's general chronological age influence you to expect an injured or ill child to behave in a way consistent with that age. An injured 11-year-old, for example, may behave more like a 7-year-old. Be especially careful not to talk down to these children. Let them know if you are going to do anything that may be painful. Children in this age group are becoming conscious of their bodies and may not like exposure. Respect their modesty.

Adolescents are between 13 and 18 years of age and are typically more adult than child. Direct your questions to an adolescent victim rather than to a parent or guardian. Allow input from a parent or guardian, however. Occasionally, if a parent or guardian is present, you may not be able to get an accurate idea of what happened or what is wrong. Adolescents often respond better to a rescuer of the same gender.

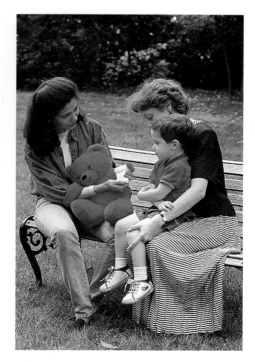

Figure 18-3 Demonstrating first aid steps on a stuffed animal or doll helps a toddler understand how you will care for him or her.

◆ ANATOMICAL AND PHYSIOLOGICAL CONCERNS

The most significant anatomical and physiological differences between infants and young children and adults have to do with the airway. The tongue fills up a large part of the mouth and throat area and is large in relation to the jaw. The tongue can also block the airway in an unresponsive infant or child.

Positioning the airway is done somewhat differently with infants and children than with adults. The first responder must remember not to **hyperextend** (extend as far as possible) the neck, because doing so may block the airway. Properly using the head-tilt/chin-lift or the jaw-thrust maneuver can help to overcome this problem. Take care to not push in on the soft tissue under the jaw.

Infants normally breathe through their nose. When their nose is blocked, they do not readily breathe through their mouth. Suctioning secre-

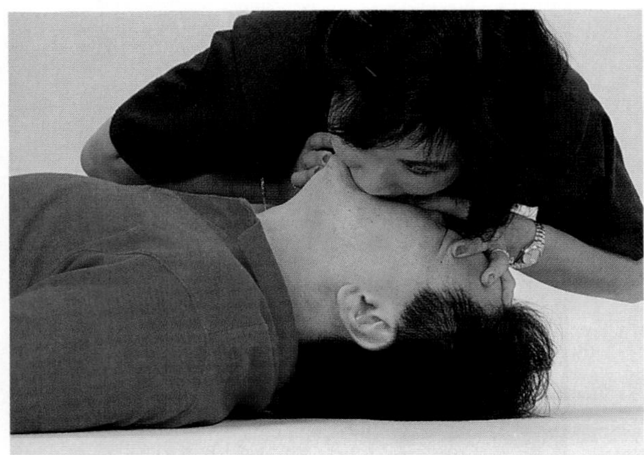

Figure 18-4 To give rescue breathing, tilt the head back, lift the chin, and pinch the nose shut. Breathe into the victim's mouth.

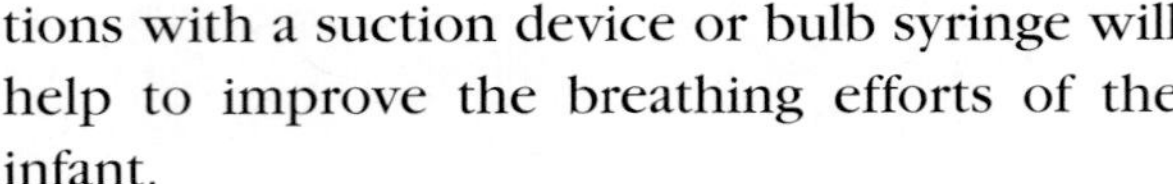

tions with a suction device or bulb syringe will help to improve the breathing efforts of the infant.

When children experience difficulty breathing, their bodies can easily compensate for a short time by increasing the rate and effort of breathing. Increasing the effort uses up a lot of energy, and they will soon get tired. As a result of respiratory and general muscle fatigue, their breathing rate will slow and they will begin to experience respiratory failure. You should watch for signs of respiratory failure and changing levels of consciousness. You should also assist any attempts to breathe that the child may make by using a bag-valve-mask.

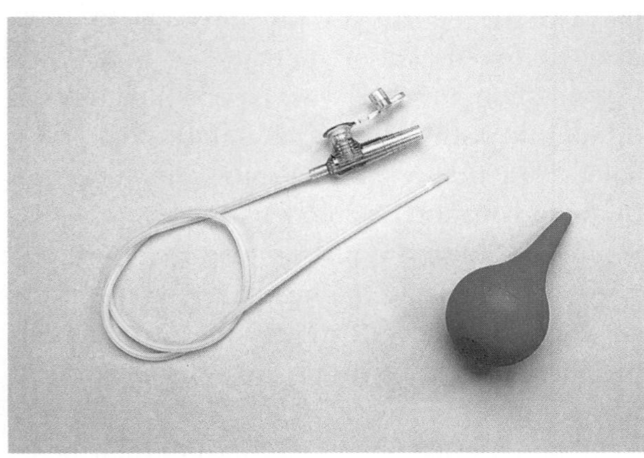

Figure 18-6 A Soft-Tipped Suction Catheter and Bulb Syringe

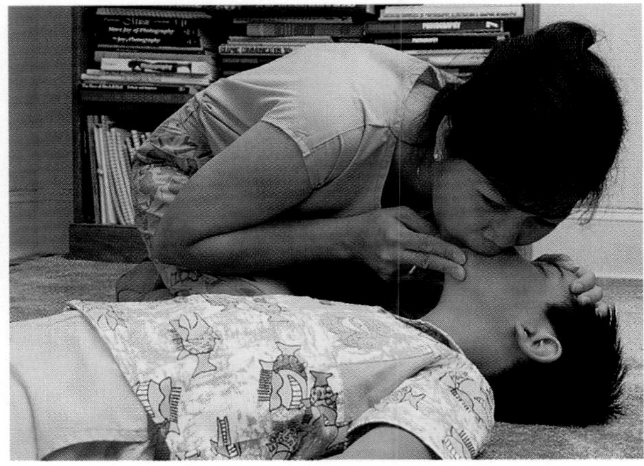

Figure 18-5 Tilt the head gently back, only far enough to allow your breaths to go in.

◆ OPENING THE AIRWAY

In Chapter 8, you learned how to open a victim's airway. When a victim becomes unconscious, all the muscles in the body relax and the tongue may fall back and block the airway. Because of the way the tongue and jaw are connected, the airway can easily be opened by lifting up the lower jaw. You can lift the lower jaw by the head-tilt/chin-lift (Fig. 18-4) or by using the jaw-thrust maneuver when head, neck, or back injury is suspected (Fig. 18-5).

When you are opening the airway of an infant or a child, tilt the head back only enough to have the victim's nose pointing straight up.

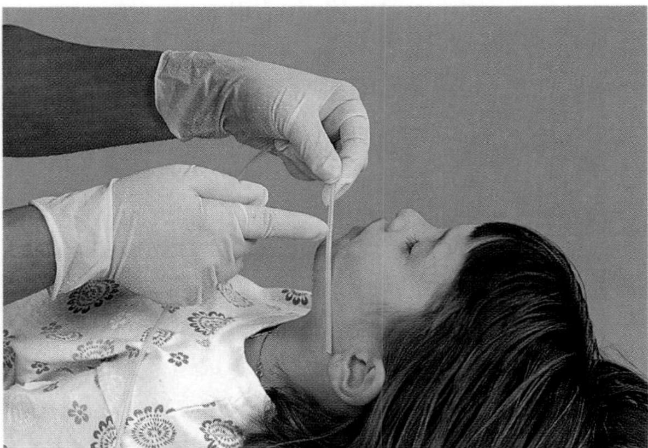

Figure 18-7 Place your finger on the catheter to mark the proper length.

A

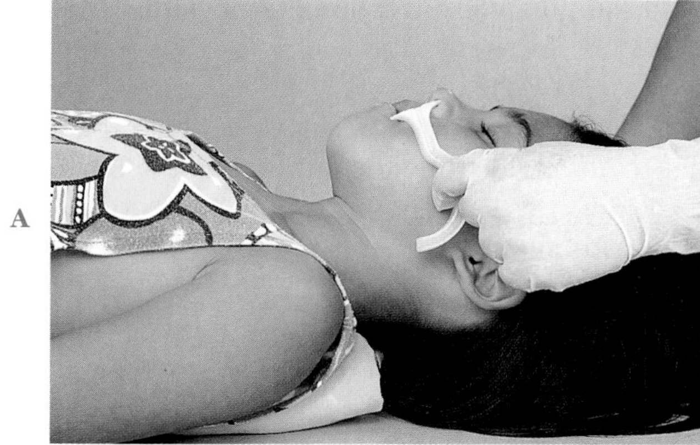

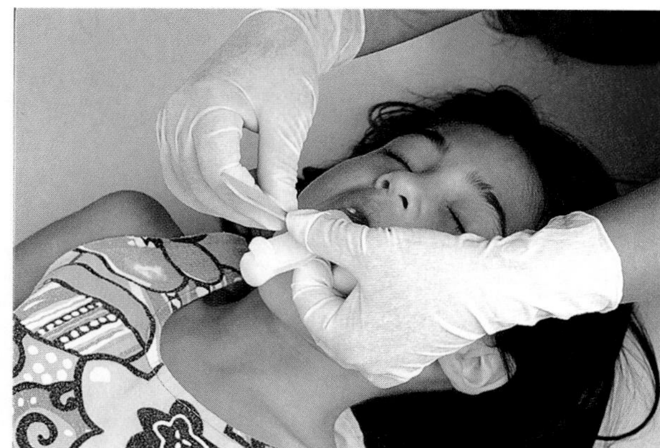

B

C

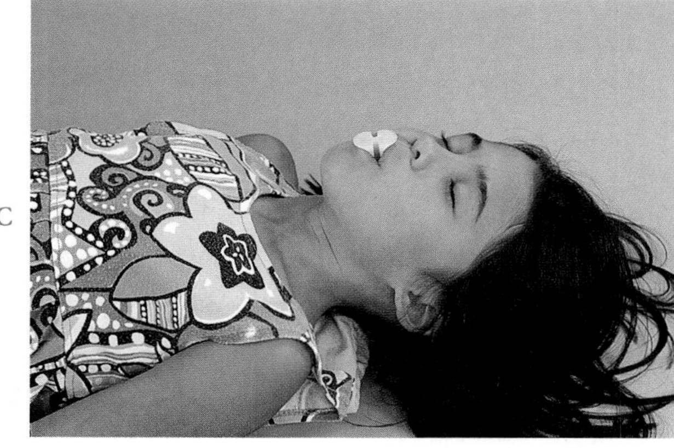

Figure 18-8 **A,** When inserting an oral airway, measure from the earlobe to the corner of the mouth. **B,** Using a tongue depressor, hold the tongue down and slide the airway into place. **C,** The flange should rest on the lips.

Placing a folded towel under the shoulders of an infant or small child will help to maintain good airway position. An oral airway can be used to help maintain an open airway in infants and children if the head-tilt/chin-lift or jaw-thrust maneuver is not effective.

Be prepared to suction the child or infant, if necessary. You should use soft-tipped suction catheters sized for infant and child victims. Bulb syringes can also be used to suction the airway of an infant or small child (Fig. 18-6). When using a soft catheter to suction the airway, measure from the corner of the mouth to the ear lobe. Place your finger on the catheter to mark the proper length (Fig. 18-7). Make sure to insert the catheter only as far as you can see (Fig. 18-8, *A-C*). If the catheter is inserted too far, you may stimulate the back of the victim's throat. This stimulation can cause a gag reflex or vomiting and dramatically slow the victim's heart rate. Suction for no longer than 15 seconds. Review suctioning procedures in Chapter 9.

For an adult, an oral airway is normally inserted with the tip pointing to the roof of the mouth and then rotated into position. In an infant or a child, the airway is inserted with the tip of the device pointing toward the back of the tongue and the throat in the same position it will rest in after insertion. Be careful not to push the tongue toward the back of the throat when you insert the airway.

◆ ASSESSMENT

When you have an ill or injured infant or child, you have an ill or injured family. If the family is excited or agitated, the child is likely to be

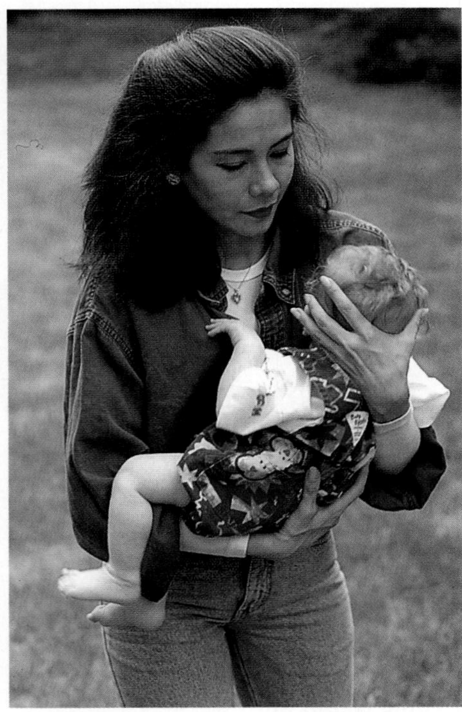

Figure 18-9 Support the head of an infant when picking up him or her.

too. When you can calm the family, the child will often calm down as well. Any concerned adults need your support, so behave as calmly as possible. Remember to get consent from any adult responsible for the child when possible.

You can obtain information by observing the infant or child before actually touching him or her. Look for signs that indicate changes in the level of consciousness, any difficulty breathing, and any apparent injuries and conditions. Realize that the situation may change as soon as you touch the child because he or she may become anxious or upset. Do not separate the infant or child from loved ones. Often a parent, guardian, or caregiver will be holding a crying infant or child. In this case, you can check the child while the adult continues to hold him or her. Unlike some ill or injured adults, an infant or child is unlikely to try to cover up or deny how he or she feels. An infant or child in pain, for example, will generally let you know that he or she hurts and the source of the pain as well as he or she can.

Whenever possible, begin your check of a conscious child at the toe rather than the head. Checking this way is less threatening to the child and allows him or her to watch what is going on and take part in it. Ask a young child to point to any place that hurts. An older child can tell you the location of painful areas. If you need to hold an infant, always support the head when you pick him or her up (Fig. 18-9).

◆ COMMON PROBLEMS IN INFANTS AND CHILDREN

Certain problems are unique to children, such as specific kinds of injury and illness. The following sections discuss some of these concerns.

Airway Obstructions

Some of the most common airway problems the first responder may encounter with infants or small children are airway obstructions. Airway obstructions are divided into two categories: partial airway obstructions and complete airway obstructions. Signs of partial airway obstruction in an infant or child who is alert, responsive, and sitting up are —

- Abnormal, high-pitched musical sounds, crowing, or noisy respirations.
- ***Retractions***, visible sinking in of the tissues around and between the ribs, on breathing in.
- Drooling.
- Frequent coughing.

Keep the infant or child in a position of comfort, probably sitting on the parent's lap.

A complete airway obstruction is a life-threatening situation. A partial airway obstruction in an infant or a child who is showing signs of cyanosis should be treated as a complete airway obstruction. Signs of a complete airway obstruction include—

- Inability to cough, cry, or speak.
- Cyanosis.
- Loss of consciousness.
- Altered mental status.

Care includes clearing the airway and attempting ventilation using the mouth-to-mask technique. For more information on clearing airway obstructions in infants and children, follow the guidelines for foreign body airway obstructions in the infant and child, covered in Chapter 8.

Breathing Emergencies

Respiratory distress is indicated when the infant or child begins to experience difficulty breathing. If uncorrected, respiratory distress can lead to respiratory failure. Respiratory distress preceding respiratory failure is indicated by any of the following:

- Infants: respiratory rate >60 per minute
- Children: respiratory rate >30 per minute
- Flaring of the nostrils
- Use of neck muscles and muscles between and below the margin of the ribs to aid in breathing
- Abnormal high-pitched sounds when breathing
- Cyanosis
- Altered mental status
- Grunting

Signs of respiratory failure or arrest include—

- Infants: respiratory rate <10 per minute.
- Children: respiratory rate <20 per minute.
- Limp muscle tone.
- Unresponsive.
- Slow or absent heart rate.
- Weak or absent pulses.
- Cyanosis.

The importance of recognizing early signs of respiratory distress cannot be emphasized enough. Early recognition of respiratory emergencies can make the life or death difference. More information on the recognition and care of breathing emergencies can be found in Chapter 8.

Circulatory Failure

As with adult victims, undetected and uncorrected circulatory failure in infants and children can cause cardiac arrest. Signs and symptoms of circulatory failure include—

- Increased heart rate.
- Poor skin circulation.
- Changes in mental status.

Care for circulatory failure includes identifying the problem through assessment, assisting attempts to breathe, and observing for signs of cardiac arrest. More information on the identification and care for circulatory failure can be found in Chapters 7 and 10.

Seizures and Fever

Certain signs and symptoms in an infant or child can indicate specific problems. Often these problems are not life threatening, but some can be. A high fever in a child often indicates some form of infection. In a young child, even a minor infection can result in a rather high fever, which is often defined as a temperature above 103 degrees F. Rapidly rising or excessively high fever can result in what is called a ***febrile seizure***. A febrile seizure may have some or all of the following signs and symptoms:

- A sudden rise in body temperature
- A change in consciousness
- Rhythmic jerking of the head and limbs
- Confusion
- Drowsiness
- Crying out
- Becoming rigid

- Holding the breath
- Upward rolling of the eyes

Your initial care for a child with a high fever is to gently cool the child. Care for an infant or child who experiences a febrile seizure is much the same as for any other seizure victim. Most febrile seizures last less than 5 minutes and are not life threatening. However, immediately after a febrile seizure, it is important to cool the body. Remove excessive clothing or blankets, and sponge the child with lukewarm water. Be careful not to cool the infant or child too much, since this could bring on another seizure. Call for more advanced medical help at once. *Do not give the infant or child aspirin*. For an infant or child, taking aspirin, especially if the child is feverish, may result in an extremely serious medical condition called ***Reye's syndrome***. Reye's syndrome is an illness that affects the brain and other internal organs. Ask the parents what medications they may have given the child so that you can inform more advanced medical personnel.

Poisoning

Poisoning is the fifth largest cause of unintentional death in the United States for people ages 1 to 24. For the youngest of these victims, mainly children under 5 years of age, poisoning often occurs from ingesting household products or medications. Care for poisoning is discussed in Chapter 16.

Altered Mental Status

Altered mental status in infants and children is another medical condition that you may encounter. Low blood sugar, poisonings, seizures, infection, trauma, decreased levels of oxygen, and the onset of shock can alter mental status. When assessing altered mental status, use the AVPU scale, which is covered in Chapter 7.

It is not important to try to figure out what specific condition is causing the altered mental status. It is important to support the victim by maintaining an open airway, giving oxygen if it is available and you are trained to use it, and placing the victim in the recovery position if there is no suspicion of head, neck, or back injury. Any information you can gather about the condition will help others to care for the victim.

◆ SUDDEN INFANT DEATH SYNDROME (SIDS)

Sudden infant death syndrome (SIDS) is a disorder that causes seemingly healthy infants to die, almost always while they sleep. SIDS is a leading cause of death for infants between 1 month and 1 year of age. This condition does not seem to be linked to any disease. SIDS is sometimes mistaken for child abuse because of the unexplained death of an otherwise normal child and the bruiselike blotches that are sometimes present on the victim's body. However, SIDS is not related to child abuse. It is also not believed to be hereditary, but does tend to recur in families. What causes SIDS is not yet clear. By the time the infant's condition is discovered, he or she will be in cardiac arrest. Make sure someone has called more advanced medical personnel or call yourself. Give the infant CPR until EMS personnel arrive.

◆ TRAUMA

Injury is the number one cause of death for children in the United States. Many of these deaths are the result of motor vehicle crashes. The greatest dangers to a child involved in a motor vehicle incident are airway obstruction and bleeding. The first responder can help ensure an open airway by using the jaw-thrust maneuver. Severe bleeding must be controlled as quickly as possible. A relatively small amount of blood lost by an adult is a large amount for an infant or child. Because a child's head is

SIDS

"For the first few months, I would lie awake in bed at night and wonder if she was still breathing. I mean you just never know. I couldn't get to sleep until I checked on her at least once." This is how one mother described her first experience with parenting.

Sudden Infant Death Syndrome (SIDS) is the sudden, unexpected, and unexplained death of apparently healthy babies. It is the major cause of death for infants between the ages of 1 month and 1 year. In the United States, SIDS, sometimes called crib death, is responsible for the death of about 7000 infants each year.

Because it cannot be predicted or prevented, SIDS causes many new parents to feel anxious. With no warning signs or symptoms, a sleeping infant can stop breathing and never wake up again. Parents and other family members of SIDS victims often have trouble dealing with this traumatic event. Along with the stress of mourning their loss, they endure tremendous feelings of guilt, believing that they should have been able to prevent the child's death.

Researchers are working to find the cause(s) of SIDS. Several risk factors—characteristics that occur more often in SIDS victims than in normal babies—have been discovered. Yet these risk factors are not causes and cannot be used to predict which infants will die. For example, 95 percent of SIDS deaths occur in infants between 2 and 4 months of age, so being in this age group is a risk factor. Other risk factors for SIDS include smoking by the mother during pregnancy, first pregnancy when the mother is under 20 years of age, several children already born to the mother, a baby with a low birth weight, and a baby with a low growth rate during the mother's pregnancy.

The best prevention for SIDS, as well as many other infant diseases, is for pregnant women to practice healthy behaviors while pregnant. They should get proper prenatal care, eat a balanced diet, not smoke or drink alcoholic beverages, and get adequate rest and exercise.

Some basic facts about SIDS:

- 90 percent of SIDS deaths occur while the infant is asleep.
- SIDS deaths can occur between the ages of 2 weeks and 18 months. Ninety-five percent of SIDS deaths occur between 2 and 4 months of age.
- The majority of SIDS deaths occur in fall and winter.
- Between 30 and 50 percent of SIDS victims have minor respiratory or gastrointestinal infections at the time of death.
- SIDS occurs slightly more often in boys than in girls.

For more information, call the National SIDS Resource Center at (703) 821-8955, ext. 249 or 474.

Sources:

1. National SIDS Resources Center (formerly National SIDS Clearinghouse): *Fact sheets: SIDS information for the EMT*, Mclean, VA, 1990.
2. Department of Health and Human Services, Health Resources and Services Administration, Maternal and Child Health Bureau: *Information exchange: newsletter of the national SIDS clearinghouse*, IE32, July 1991.

large and heavy in proportion to the rest of its body, the head is the most frequently injured part of the child's body. A child injured as the result of force or a blow may also have damage to the organs in the abdomen and chest. Because children have very soft, pliable ribs, such damage can cause severe internal bleeding. Care for a victim with a chest injury involves keeping an open airway, assessing the chest for rise and fall, and supplying oxygen if it is available and you are trained to do so. In a car crash, a child secured only by a lap belt may have serious abdominal or spinal injuries. Try to find out what happened because a severely injured child may not immediately show signs of injury.

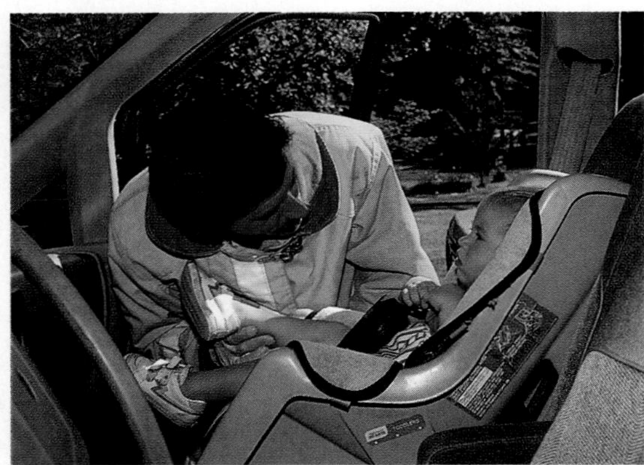

Figure 18-10 A child involved in a motor vehicle crash and found in a car seat should be left in the car seat if the device has not been damaged.

To stop some of the needless deaths of children associated with motor vehicle crashes, laws have been enacted requiring that children ride in safety seats or wear safety belts. As a result, more children's lives are saved. You may have to check and care for an injured infant or child while he or she is in a safety seat (Fig. 18-10). A safety seat does not normally pose any problems while you are checking an infant or child. Leave the infant or child in the seat if the seat has not been damaged. If the infant or child is to be transported to a medical facility for examination, he or she can often be safely secured in the safety seat for transport.

Extremity injuries in the child or infant are cared for in the same way as for adults. If equipment of the proper size is not available, the first responder should manually stabilize extremity injuries until additional help arrives. Information on the general management of extremity injuries can be found in Chapter 13.

When providing care for an injured infant or child, it is important to use equipment of the proper size. As first responders, you may not have this equipment available when responding to a scene. You should try to comfort, calm, and reassure the victim and family members while waiting for additional EMS resources.

◆ CHILD ABUSE AND NEGLECT

At some point, you may encounter a situation involving an injured child in which you have reason to suspect child abuse. ***Child abuse*** is the physical, psychological, or sexual assault of a child resulting in injury and emotional trauma. Child abuse involves an injury or a pattern of injuries that do not result from a mishap. The child's injuries cannot be logically explained, or a caregiver or parent gives an inconsistent or suspicious account of how the injuries occurred.

The signs of child abuse include—

- An injury that does not fit the description of what caused it.
- Patterns of injury that include cigarette burns, whip marks, and hand prints.
- Obvious or suspected fractures in a child less than 2 years of age; any unexplained fractures.
- Injuries in various stages of healing, especially bruises and burns.
- Unexplained lacerations or abrasions, especially to the mouth, lips, and eyes.
- Injuries to the genitalia; pain when the child sits down.
- More injuries than are common for a child of the same age.
- Repeated calls to the same address.

Child neglect is insufficient attention given or respect to a child who has a claim to that attention. Signs and symptoms include—

- Lack of adult supervision.
- A child who appears to be malnourished.
- An unsafe living environment.
- Untreated chronic illness, for example, an asthmatic child with no medications.

When caring for a child who may have been abused, your first priority is to care for the child's injuries or illness. An abused child may be frightened, hysterical, or withdrawn. He or she may be unwilling to talk about the incident in an attempt to protect the abuser. If you suspect abuse, explain your concerns to responding police officers or EMTs, if possible.

If you think you have reasonable cause to believe that abuse has occurred, you can report your suspicions to a community or state agency, such as the Department of Social Services, the Department of Children and Family Services, or Child Protective Services. You may be afraid to report suspected child abuse because you do not wish to get involved or are afraid of getting sued. However, in most states, when you make a report in good faith, you are immune from any civil or criminal liability or penalty, even if you made a mistake. In this instance, "good faith" means that you honestly believe that abuse has occurred or the potential for abuse exists and a prudent and reasonable person in the same position would also honestly believe abuse has occurred or the potential for abuse exists. You do not need to identify yourself when you report child abuse, although your report will have more credibility if you do.

◆ NEED FOR FIRST RESPONDER DEBRIEFING

After a response to an incident involving infants or children, it is helpful to discuss the incident with other first responders or someone to whom you can express your feelings. Scenes involving the severe injury or death of a child or infant can cause tremendous amounts of stress. If you continue to be distressed, seek professional counseling. You need to recognize and understand the feelings brought on by such incidents. Chapter 2 covers more information about the well-being of the first responder and steps to take to help yourself and each other.

◆ SUMMARY

Even when uneventful, calls involving infants and children are some of the more stressful situations for first responders. Some of the anxiety involved is because of the lack of experience that rescuers have in dealing with children. It is important for you to remember that you have learned the skills and information to help you to deal with emergencies, such as airway obstructions, breathing emergencies, circulatory failure, seizures, fever, poisoning, and altered mental status. Most of the principles that you have learned about dealing with adult victims can be applied to infants and children, but you need to remember the differences in the developmental characteristics and anatomy of children.

Use the activities in Unit 18 of the workbook to help you review the material in this section.

You Are the Responder

You respond to a call from a playground where a child has fallen from a piece of climbing equipment. The little boy is about 2 and is lying on the ground crying loudly. A woman who says she is the mother is kneeling next to the child talking to him and he is beginning to calm down. When you walk over to him and he sees you, he begins to shriek. You notice that one arm looks bruised and swollen. What do you do?

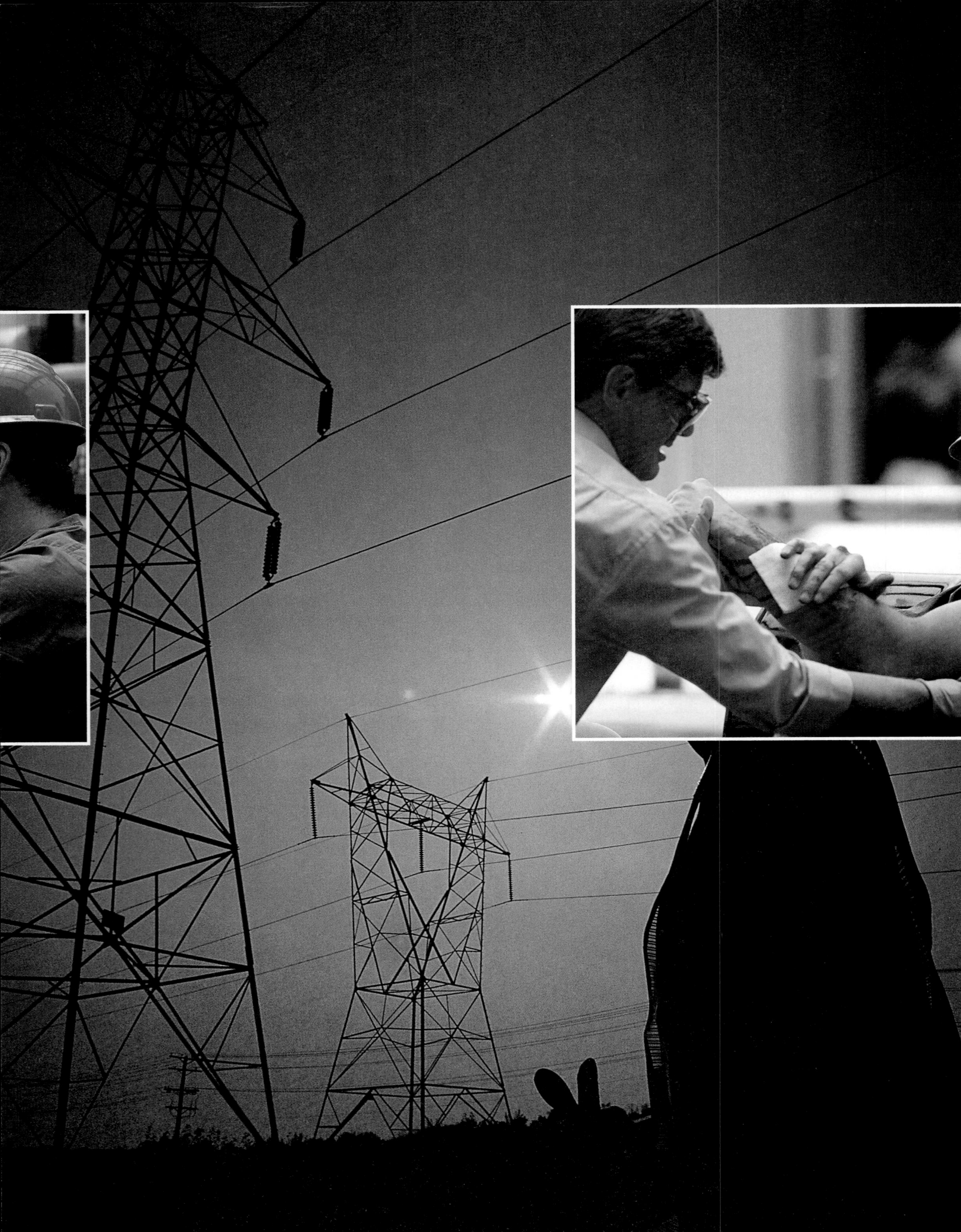

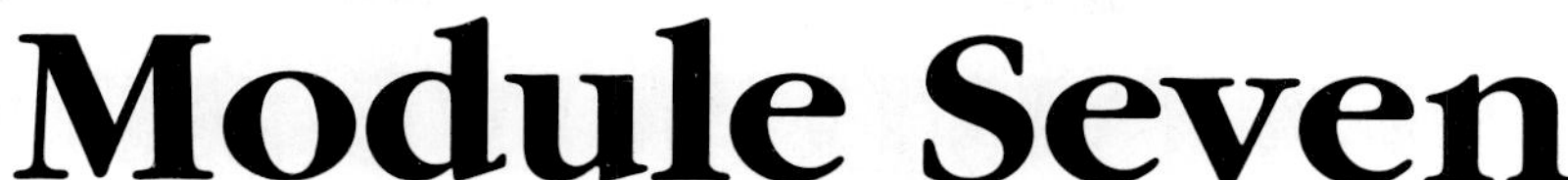

Module Seven

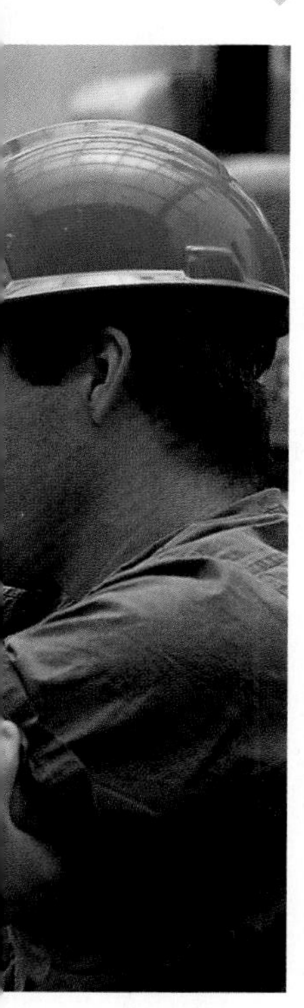

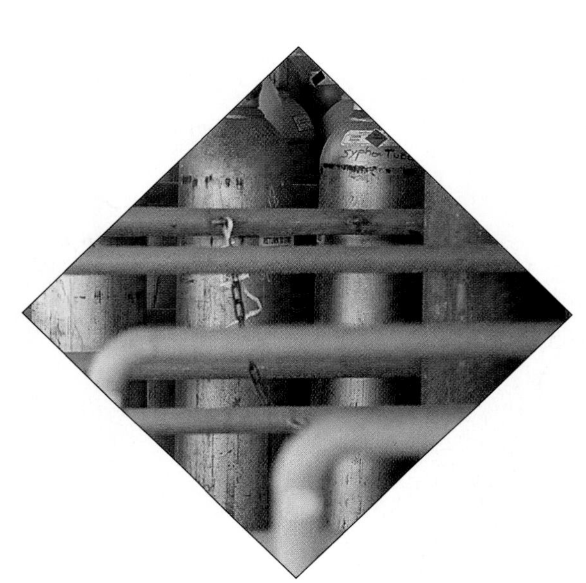

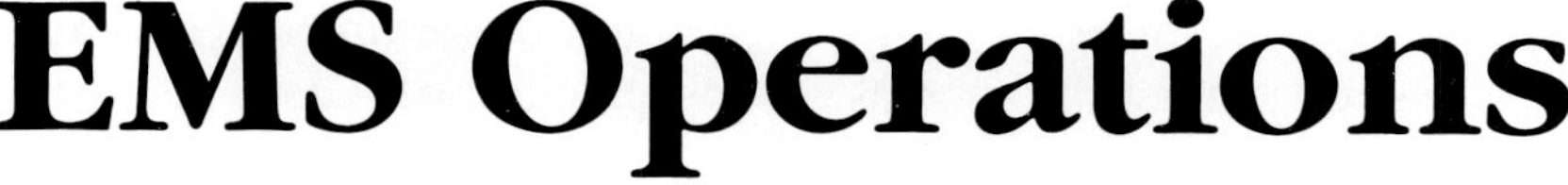

EMS Operations

19

EMS Support and Operations

EMS Support and Operations

19

Key Terms

Active drowning victim: A person exhibiting universal behavior that includes struggling at the surface for 20 to 60 seconds before submerging.

Chocking: The use of items, such as wooden blocks, placed against the wheels of a vehicle to help stabilize the vehicle.

Distressed swimmer: A person capable of staying afloat but likely to need assistance to get to safety.

Drowning: Death by suffocation when submerged in water.

Emergency medical dispatcher (EMD): An emergency medical services employee who has received special training for giving medical instructions to victims or bystanders before the arrival of more advanced medical personnel.

Extrication: The removal of a victim trapped in a motor vehicle or in a dangerous situation.

Hazardous material (HAZMAT): Any chemical substance or material that can pose a threat to health, safety, and property.

Hazardous material incident: Any situation that deals with the unplanned release of hazardous materials.

Incident command system (ICS): A system used to manage resources, such as personnel, equipment, and supplies, at the scene of an emergency.

Multiple casualty incident (MCI): An emergency situation involving two or more victims.

Near-drowning: A situation in which a person who has been submerged in water survives.

Packaging: The steps involved in preparing a victim to be moved and moving the victim onto the device to support the victim during transport.

START (*S*imple *T*riage *A*nd *R*apid *T*reatment) system: A system used at the scene of multiple casualty incidents to quickly assess and prioritize care according to three conditions: breathing, circulation, and level of consciousness.

Triage: The process of sorting and providing care to multiple victims according to the severity of their injuries or illnesses.

Knowledge Objectives

After reading this chapter and completing the class activities you should be able to—

- Describe the medical and non-medical equipment needed to respond to a call.
- List the phases of an out-of-hospital call.
- Describe the information included in the first responder "hand-off" report.
- Describe the role of the first responder in a multiple casualty situation.
- Summarize the components of basic triage.
- Explain the role of the first responder in extrication.
- List various methods of gaining access to the victim.
- Distinguish between simple access and complex access.
- Describe what the first responder should do if there is a hazard at the scene.
- State the role of the first responder at the scene of a hazardous materials incident until appropriately trained personnel arrive.
- List the personal protective equipment necessary for rescue operations and exposure to bloodborne and airborne pathogens.
- *Describe various methods of rescuing a near-drowning victim.

*Signifies an Enrichment section objective.

Attitude Objectives

After reading this chapter and completing the class activities, you should be able to—

- Appreciate the reasons for having an emergency vehicle prepared to respond.

Skill Objectives

After reading this chapter and completing the class activities, you should be able to—

- Use the START system to triage victims, given a scenario of a multiple casualty incident.
- *Demonstrate proper methods of rescuing a near-drowning victim.

*Signifies an Enrichment section objective.

◆ INTRODUCTION

In earlier chapters, you learned how to care for victims of injury and illness when it is safe to do so. Although these skills are important for the first responder to learn, certain non-medical operational skills are just as important. In this chapter, you will learn about EMS support and operations, including phases of an ambulance call, air medical response, and responding to multiple casualty incidents. The chapter also discusses fundamentals of extrication and responding to a hazardous materials scene and gives information on water rescue techniques. As a first responder, you may never be involved in all of these situations, but as a functioning part of the EMS system, you should have a brief overview of some of these aspects of out-of-hospital care.

◆ ROLES OF THE FIRST RESPONDER IN THE EMS SYSTEM

The term first responder can mean different things to different people. In general, a first responder is a person who has been trained to a minimum standard of care. While first responders may function as regular members of an ambulance crew in some states, in other states and areas, first responders have other roles.

Traditional First Responder

When we talk about traditional first responders, we generally refer to people who function in the 9-1-1 systems. These traditional first responders are usually affiliated with a service, such as law enforcement, fire suppression, or sometimes lifeguarding or ski patrolling.

Non-Traditional First Responder

Non-traditional first responders have had the same training as traditional first responders but work in less traditional settings as athletic trainers, trip leaders, and others. You also find these first responders working as members of industrial response teams. Any first responder, traditional or nontraditional, should be familiar with the EMS system and his or her role in it.

◆ PHASES OF A RESPONSE

A typical EMS response has nine phases. They are—

- Preparation for an emergency call.
- Dispatch.
- En-route to the scene.
- Arrival at the scene.
- Transferring the victim to the ambulance.
- En-route to the receiving facility.
- Arrival at the receiving facility.
- En-route to the station.
- Post run.

Preparation for an Emergency Call

To be ready to respond to a scene, it is important to spend some time preparing yourself, your equipment, and in some cases, your vehicle. As a first responder, you have a responsibility to keep yourself physically fit and mentally prepared for the challenges of responding to an emergency. Part of preparing for the call involves the initial training that you received as a first responder. It is important to remember that the end of your first responder training is the beginning of having a duty to respond to emergencies. You have a responsibility to continue your training through refresher and continuing education programs. Some first responders take additional training as an EMT.

In preparing to respond to an emergency, you should have basic medical equipment on hand. First aid kits come in a variety of sizes and shapes and are commercially available, but designing your own can help you be more familiar and comfortable with the contents. When designing your own kit, keep in mind the steps of victim care you will be involved in. Those steps are the initial assessment and the physical exam and history. Most of the care that first responders provide deals with assessing and caring for immediate life-threatening injuries and illnesses. Do not overfill the first aid kit, but at a minimum, include the following medical supplies:

- Airways
- Suction equipment
- Artificial ventilation devices, such as resuscitation mask or bag-valve-mask
- Basic wound supplies, such as dressings and bandages

Some non-medical supplies that the first responder should include are—

- Personal safety equipment, such as gloves and protective eyewear.
- Street maps.
- Scissors.
- Blood pressure cuff and stethoscope (optional—covered in Chapter 7 Enrichment).
- Flashlight.
- Note pad and pen.
- Waterless hand-washing solution.
- Any other equipment required by local or state standards.

In some areas, first responders work in a system in which they may be involved in transporting the victim to the receiving facility. If this is the case, the first responder will have to prepare and inspect the ambulance or transport vehicle before every shift. Local EMS systems and state regulations determine what equipment and supplies must be in the vehicle.

In other areas or circumstances, first responders may be the only emergency personnel responding to a scene. You should review the local policies, rules, and regulations regarding the minimum staffing requirements in your area and of your organization.

Dispatch

In many areas of the country, dispatch centers have central access numbers like 9-1-1 for ambulance, police, or fire personnel. These dispatch centers are often staffed with specially trained personnel known as ***Emergency medical dispatchers (EMDs),*** available on a 24 hours-a-day, 7 days-a-week basis. They assist the caller by taking basic information critical to dispatching the appropriate personnel and are specially trained to help the caller care for victims until emergency personnel arrive.

During the call, the dispatcher will ask the caller specific questions that will help in making the decision about what emergency personnel to dispatch. The dispatcher will want to know the nature of the emergency, the mechanism of injury, or the nature of illness. The dispatcher will ask for the caller's name, location, and call-back number. Additional information, such as the exact location of the victim (e.g., second floor, back apartment), number of victims, and the severity of the injuries, can be relayed to those responding to the emergency after the initial dispatch has been issued. Also, the dispatcher will want the caller to tell him or her about any unusual situations, conditions, or problems at the scene to ensure the appropriate personnel arrive at the scene as quickly and safely as possible.

En-route to the Scene

To help a victim, you must be able to reach the scene safely. The most important skill to use at this time is common sense. Walk, do not run, to any emergency scene or to your vehicle. Pacing yourself allows you to think clearly, survey the area, and plan for arrival at the scene. It also reduces the risk of injuries caused by tripping and falling.

If you are in a vehicle, whether a personal or emergency vehicle, you must always use a safety belt. Some areas require all personnel working in the EMS system to attend an emergency vehicle operator training program. These programs have sessions both in a classroom and on the road. If you function in an EMS system that requires response in a private vehicle, you must become aware of the state and local laws and regulations that govern operations of private vehicles as emergency vehicles in that area. In any and all cases when responding to an emergency, first responders should have appropriate driving behavior involving consideration for the safety of others. The emergency response to the scene does not exempt any emergency personnel from traffic laws. It is the driver's responsibility to make sure that he or she knows the traffic laws that govern the use of lights, sirens, and intersection procedures.

Arrival at the Scene

In this phase of response, you should be slow and cautious in your approach. If you have access to the appropriate equipment, notify the dispatcher of arrival and, if possible, record the time. As you enter the area, use this opportunity to size up the scene and size up the situation. If the scene is not safe, notify dispatch to send whatever agencies are necessary to make it safe. Never endanger your life or the life of anyone else responding or at the scene.

When approaching the scene, you should observe BSI (body substance isolation) before any contact with the victim. Use gloves, gown, mask, and protective eyewear if and when appropriate.

Is the scene safe? Are there any hazards to the rescuers or the victims? What was the mechanism of injury or the nature of illness? How many victims are there? Do you need any additional help? These are questions you should ask yourself whenever you approach a scene. By answering these simple questions, you will be better prepared to handle the different situations in a well-organized, rapid, and efficient manner.

Transferring the Victim to the Ambulance

Though transport is not a traditional role for a first responder, at times you may be part of the ambulance crew or asked to help transfer the victim into the ambulance. By the time the ambulance arrives, you may have done the initial assessment, the physical exam and the history of the victim, and begun care. You even may have recorded the vital signs and started packaging the victim for transfer to the ambulance. ***Packaging*** refers to getting the victim ready to be moved and moving the victim onto the device that will be used to support the victim during transport. Transferring the victim means more than moving the victim to the ambulance. You also have a responsibility to transfer information about the victim and the incident to the EMTs who take over the victim's care.

En-route to the Receiving Facility

Once the victim is loaded into the transport vehicle, all personnel should wear their safety belts, if possible. The dispatch center is notified, and the crew member in charge of caring for the victim determines whether the trip to the receiving facility will be fast, at normal speed, or slow.

The transport crew members provide ongoing care and psychological support for the victim until he or she arrives at the hospital. They also ask additional questions, document the history and care of the victim, and continue to monitor vital signs.

As soon as possible, the transport crew notifies the receiving facility about the victim and the expected time of arrival. The operator is informed if there are any changes in the victim's condition. The driver may have to adjust his or her driving speed to meet what the EMT in charge of the victim says about the victim's needs.

Arrival at the Receiving Facility

During this phase, transport crew members transfer the victim to the care of the nurses and doctors in the receiving facility. Crew members never leave victims unattended during a call or during transfer of care to the hospital. At the hospital, crew members give information about the scene and the victim. They also complete whatever documentation is necessary to meet local or state standards and their organization's protocols. If necessary, crew members begin some of the post-run responsibilities by exchanging or restocking bandages, medications, or IV fluids. The cleaning of the transport vehicle is also done now. Personnel should wear heavy-duty rubber gloves and follow local procedures and body substance isolation (BSI) for disposal of soiled linen and supplies. The ambulance cot should be cleaned and made ready for the next call. Members of the crew should wash their hands thoroughly after every response, paying close attention to the area under the fingernails.

En-route to the Station

When returning to the station, the operator of the vehicle should notify dispatch. During the ride back to quarters, personnel should take the opportunity to review the details of the run and discuss how things could have been done differently or more efficiently. The ride back also provides opportunities for crew members to air any concerns or diffuse any stress that may have developed during the response. Doing these things helps the crew to physically and emotionally prepare for the next response.

Post Run

In this last phase of response, the emergency vehicle should be refueled if necessary and any repairs or adjustments should be made. Crew members should clean and disinfect any equipment that may not have been cleaned earlier. If necessary, they should restock any disposable items to the vehicle's medical supplies. Reports and any unfinished paperwork should be completed and the dispatch center notified that the unit is back in service and ready for another call.

Once back at the station, crew members should also prepare themselves for the next response. Preparation may include removing and laundering contaminated clothing as soon as possible. It is a good idea to have more than one uniform. Uniforms or clothing soiled with the victim's body fluids should not be taken home to be laundered. They should be laundered by a laundry service that deals with contaminated clothing or as specified by the organization's protocols.

◆ AIR-MEDICAL CONSIDERATIONS

In certain situations, it is sometimes best for the victim to be transported to the medical facility by a helicopter or a fixed-wing aircraft. This type of transport enables severely injured or ill victims to be transported quickly to specialty centers and large treatment facilities. Geography and other circumstances play a large role in this type of transport decision, and emergency personnel should follow local and state protocols.

◆ MULTIPLE CASUALTY INCIDENTS

In rush-hour traffic, the driver of a tractor trailer loses control of the vehicle on a rain-slick, four-lane highway. The rig crosses the center line, "jackknifes," and slides into an embankment. Numerous cars and a loaded tour bus try frantically to avoid colliding with the tractor trailer. Two cars collide head on. The bus plunges over an embankment, coming to rest 15 feet below in a ditch. Minor

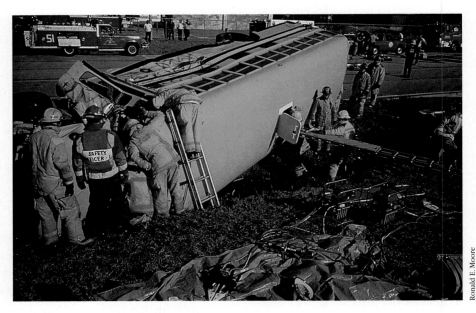

Ronald E. Moore

Figure 19-1 A multiple casualty incident (MCI) involves two or more victims.

collisions occur farther back from the scene. Many people are injured; some are probably dead.

As a first responder, you are likely to be among the first trained individuals nearby or summoned to assist with a serious incident like this. The task of trying to create order out of chaos will initially fall on you. To respond most effectively to an emergency situation with multiple victims, you need a plan of action. This plan must enable you to rapidly determine what additional resources are needed and how best to use them. During a serious incident, it is not uncommon for a first responder to arrive 15 minutes before any other trained personnel. It could be up to an hour before adequate resources are available to care for a large number of victims.

An appropriate initial response by a first responder can eliminate potential problems for arriving personnel and possibly save the lives of one or more injured victims. To respond appropriately, however, you must thoroughly understand your plan of action. Your plan must enable you to take charge. Taking charge includes making the scene safe for you and others to work, delegating responsibilities, managing available resources, identifying and caring for the victims most in need of care, and relinquishing command as more highly trained personnel arrive.

As the term implies, a ***multiple casualty incident (MCI)*** refers to a situation involving two or more victims (Fig. 19-1). You are most likely to encounter small MCIs involving injury to only a few victims, such as a motor vehicle crash involving the driver and a passenger. But MCIs can also be large-scale events, such as those caused by natural, mechanical, or industrial disasters. Examples include —

- Earthquake.
- Tornado.
- Hurricane.
- Flood.
- Fire.
- Explosion.
- Structure collapse.
- Train derailment.
- Airliner crash.
- Hazardous materials incident.

Incidents such as these can result in hundreds or even thousands of injured or ill victims. Whether small or large scale, MCIs can strain the resources of a local community. Coping effectively with an MCI requires a plan to acquire and manage additional personnel, equipment, and supplies.

Organizing Resources

Providing appropriate help to one or more victims in an emergency involves organization. Incidents vary in complexity. MCIs can strain the resources of the first responding personnel and require additional resources from other areas, some far away. The incident command system was developed to ensure that the various resources operate in an orderly, united fashion to accomplish a task.

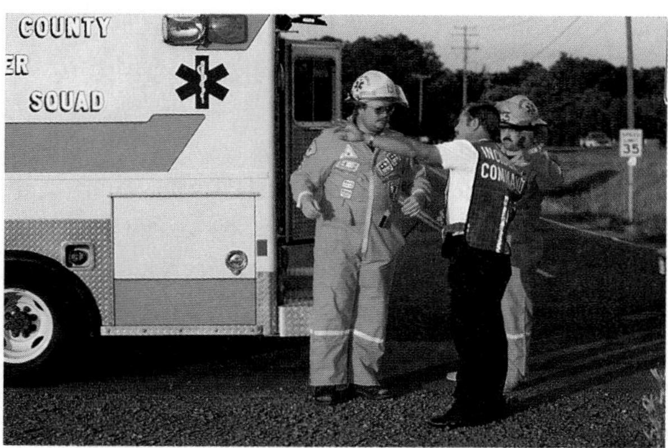

Figure 19-2 The Incident Commander delegates responsibility as the need arises.

Incident Command System

The ***incident command system (ICS)*** is a management system designed to be used for a wide variety of emergencies. It is especially useful in emergencies involving multiple casualties because of its ability to handle several emergency situations at the same time. It is a common system that can be easily understood by different agencies working together at the scene of an emergency.

Originally developed in California to manage the large numbers of fire fighters necessary for major brush and forest fires, the ICS has subsequently been modified across the nation for use in a variety of multiple casualty incidents. To understand the ICS, think of it as an organization. An organization is a group of people working together to achieve a common goal. To do this, the organization must clearly define who is in charge, the scope of authority and responsibility, the goal, and the objectives to accomplish the goal. This same approach applies to the ICS (Fig. 19-2). The advantages of the ICS for use in numerous situations include —

- Terms commonly understood by those taking part.
- One "boss" with the absolute authority to do what is necessary to accomplish the goal.
- One unified command structure with well-established divisions, all working to accomplish the same goal.
- An integrated communications system.
- Easily managed units normally consisting of not more than four people.

Leadership Positions

For the system to work, people must fill various leadership positions. The number of positions that are filled will be based on the magnitude of the incident. Typically, the initial leadership positions are —

- Incident commander.
- Operations section officer.
- Planning section officer.
- Logistics section officer.

The **incident commander** is the person ultimately responsible for managing and directing the response. The incident commander makes initial decisions about the severity of the situation and what resources will be needed. He or she appoints section officers as the need arises. The incident commander may use the sections officers (operations, planning, and logistics) to formulate the overall strategy. For example, in a small-scale incident, there is usually no need to appoint any section officers. For an incident slightly larger in scale, one section officer may be appointed to assist the incident commander and perform multiple functions. As the magnitude of the incident increases, the incident commander will appoint additional officers.

The **operations section officer** is responsible for developing the tactics to carry out the strategy—in other words, putting a plan together that works. For example, in a situation involving a fire that is rapidly engulfing a section of a building where people are trapped, the strategy would be to contain the fire. The tactics refer to the plan developed to get the job done. This plan could include intercepting the path of the fire and establishing safe areas in which to care for any injured persons. The operations section officer coordinates the actions of other leaders under his or her authority, including fire, rescue, and law enforcement personnel.

The **planning section officer** is responsible for keeping the incident commander updated on the status of the incident. Update is done by gathering and analyzing information, such as damage estimates and the status of personnel, equipment, and supplies. The planning section officer coordinates with the logistics section officer and the incident commander on issues such as the need for additional personnel, equipment, and supplies.

The **logistics section officer** is responsible for establishing communication, coordinating crowd control efforts, and evaluating the scene if necessary. The logistics section officer is responsible for getting any additional resources, such as personnel, equipment, and supplies. These resources could include utility personnel, food, water, shelter, and transportation.

The strength of the incident command system is its flexibility. It can be used in whatever manner the incident commander deems necessary to fit the situation. It is similar to a tool box in which many specialized tools are available to the user. The incident commander can select the tool(s) needed for the specific situation. In a large-scale incident in which more resources are needed, more positions can be created. In small incidents or at the conclusion of an incident, fewer resources and positions are needed and the incident commander can reduce resources in an organized manner.

Using the incident command system

A state trooper trained as a first responder is dispatched to a motor vehicle crash. When she arrives, she sees two cars involved in a head-on collision and what appear to be four victims with varying injuries. Since she is the first trained person to arrive at the scene, she assumes the role of incident commander, sizes up the scene, and takes measures to ensure that the scene will be safe for her, the victims, bystanders, and other rescuers when they arrive. During her scene size-up, she identifies the need for other resources including fire/rescue unit, and other troopers to help secure the roadway and radios the request in. After securing the scene by placing flares, the trooper begins to assess the needs of the victims in the two cars. Just as she begins, another car pulls up. The driver identifies himself as a fire fighter and trained first responder. The trooper maintains her role as incident commander and instructs the fire fighter to begin triage of the victims, using the START system.

After taking BSI precautions, the fire fighter begins to triage the four victims. He notes that the driver of the first vehicle is obviously dead/nonsalvagable. He places a black piece of tape on the victim's exposed arm and moves to the next victim who is lying on the ground unconscious next to the wrecked vehicle. He notices that the victim is not breathing; however, after the fire fighter opens the airway using the jaw-thrust method, the victim, still unconscious, begins to breathe. The fire fighter inserts a properly sized oral airway, places red (immediate) tape on the victim's upper arm, and moves to the next vehicle. The victims in the next vehicle are both conscious and breathing, however the driver is complaining of a painful forearm, has a good radial pulse, and is alert and responsive to questions. The fire fighter applies a piece of green tape to this victim, and moves to the final victim who is bleeding severely from the head. He administers direct pressure with some gauze pads, instructs the victim to maintain the pressure, and applies a piece of yellow (delayed) tape to the victim's upper arm as the fire/rescue units arrive.

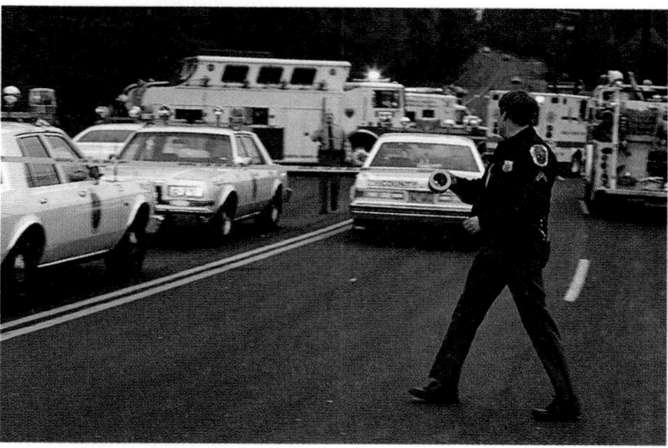

Figure 19-3 When you arrive on the scene, you may be asked to aid in crowd or traffic control.

In this situation, the resources needed were minimal. But what if the car had struck a utility pole and knocked down an electrical wire, the victim had been trapped in a crushed vehicle, or there had been multiple victims? As the incident commander, the police officer would have notified the dispatcher of the situation and requested additional resources. The power company would have been summoned for the downed wire. If a person had been trapped in the vehicle, resources like the fire department or specialized rescue squad personnel would have been sent to the scene.

As these personnel arrived, the police officer could have continued to act as the incident commander, or command could have been turned over to other more experienced personnel. These decisions are often based on the type of emergency and local protocols. If the incident is beyond your scope, you should only act as incident commander until a more experienced person or authority arrives. At this point, he or she will assume command.

At other times, you may be responding to a large-scale MCI because it requires additional personnel. Where you are placed and how your services are used will be based on your expertise and the needs at the time. This could include assisting medical personnel, aiding in crowd or traffic control, helping to maintain scene security, or helping to establish temporary shelter (Fig. 19-3). By using the ICS in numerous emergencies, the tasks of reaching, caring for, and transporting victims are performed more effectively, thereby saving more lives. Since there are variations in the ICS throughout the country, you should become familiar with the ICS for your local community.

Caring for the Ill or Injured Victims

In the previous chapters, you learned how to conduct a systematic assessment of a victim by doing an initial assessment and a physical exam and history. This enabled you to care for life-threatening emergencies before minor injuries. You will recall that the initial assessment has three steps: checking the victim's airway, breathing, and circulation. You will also recall that the physical exam and history have steps that include doing a physical examination, interviewing the victim, and checking vital signs.

Though this approach is appropriate for one victim, it is not effective when there are fewer rescuers than victims. If you took the time to completely conduct each of these steps and to correct all problems that you found, your entire time could be spent with only one victim. A victim who is unconscious and not breathing, simply because the tongue is blocking the airway, could be overlooked and die while your attention is given to caring for someone with a less severe injury, such as a broken arm.

In a multiple casualty incident, you must modify your technique for checking victims. Doing so requires you to understand your priorities. It also requires that you accept death and dying, because some victims, such as those in cardiac arrest who would normally receive CPR and be high-priority victims, will be beyond your ability to help in this situation.

To identify which victims require urgent care in a multiple casualty incident, you use a process known as triage. ***Triage*** is a French term meaning "to sort," which was first used to refer to the sorting and treatment of those injured in battle. Today, the triage process is used any time there are more victims than rescuers. Its common definition is the process of sorting multiple victims according to the severity of their injuries or illnesses.

The START System

Over the years, a number of systems have been used to triage victims. Most, however, required you to diagnose the exact extent of injury or illness. Diagnosing was often time-consuming and resulted in delays in assessment and care for victims in multiple casualty incidents. As a result, the ***START system*** was created. START stands for ***S***imple ***T***riage ***A***nd ***R***apid ***T***reatment. It is a simple way to quickly assess and prioritize victims. The START system requires you to check only three items: breathing, circulation (including bleeding), and level of consciousness. As you check these items, you will classify victims into one of three levels that reflect the severity of injury or illness and need for care. These levels are "immediate," "delayed," and "dead/nonsalvageable."

Using the START system requires that the first rescuers on the scene clear the area of all victims with only minor problems. These are sometimes called the "walking wounded." If a person is able to walk from the site of the incident, allow him or her to walk to a designated area for evaluation by arriving medical personnel (Fig. 19-4). This first action is critical to the success of START. It enables you to move people to safety, ensures higher-level medical care, and reduces the number of remaining victims that you need to check.

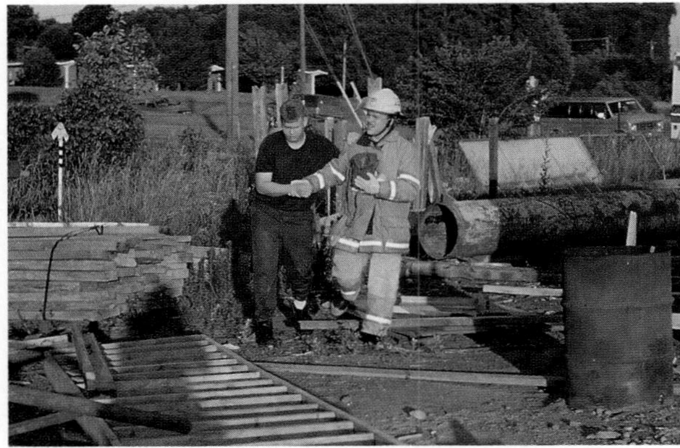

Figure 19-4 Victims who are able to move away from the scene on their own should walk to a designated area.

Next, move quickly among the remaining victims, assessing the severity of the problems. As you do so, you are attempting to classify each victim into one of three or four categories for care.

The first of these categories is "immediate care." This categorization means that the victim needs immediate care and transport to a medical facility. An example of an immediate victim is one who needs the airway cleared to enable breathing to continue.

The second category is "delayed care." This category is assigned to a person who is breathing and has pulse and level of consciousness within normal limits who may not be able to move because of a broken leg or back injury. Some systems use a third category ("minor") to indicate victims with minor injuries.

The final category is "dead/nonsalvageable." This category is assigned to those individuals obviously dead. Victims who are found not breathing and who fail to breathe after attempts to open and clear the airway are classified as dead/nonsalvageable. This classification is also applied to obvious mortal injury, such as decapitation.

As you classify each victim into one of these three or four categories, you need to mark the victim in some distinguishing manner so that rescuers coming behind you will be able to begin care for and remove the most critical

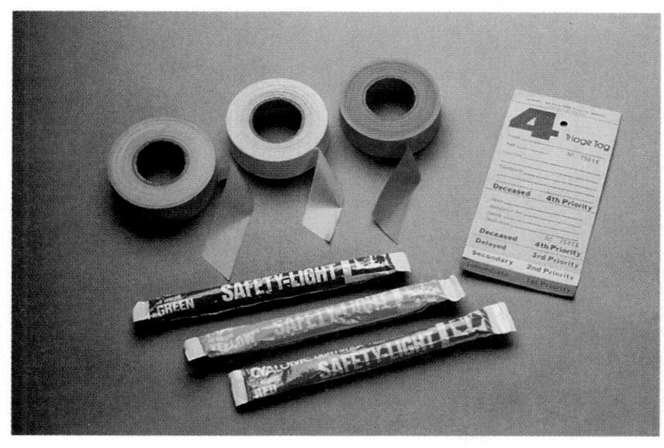

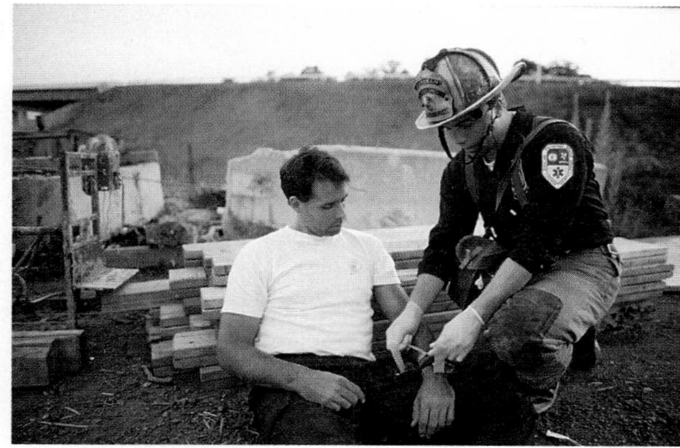

Figure 19-5 Triage markers are used to label victims.

victims first. This process of labeling victims is easily done with commercial triage markers or multicolored tape, which should be fastened to the victim in an easily noticeable area, such as around the wrist (Fig. 19-5, A-B). Color codes are as follows:

- Immediate — red
- Delay — yellow
- Minor — green (if your system uses four categories)
- Dead/nonsalvageable — black or gray

To make these decisions, take the following steps:

Step one: Check breathing. When you locate a victim, begin by assessing whether he or she is breathing. If the victim is not breathing, clear the mouth of any foreign object and make sure the airway is open. If the victim does not begin breathing on his or her own, even with the airway open, the victim is classified as "dead/nonsalvageable." There is no need to check the pulse. Place a black or gray marker on the victim and move on.

On the other hand, if the victim does begin to breathe on his or her own when you open the airway, this person should be classified as needing immediate care. Any individual who needs help maintaining an open airway is a high priority. Position the person in a way that will maintain an open airway, place a red tag on the victim, and move on to the next victim. *Once triage of all victims is complete, you may be able to come back and assist with the care of the victims.*

If the victim is breathing when you arrive, you must check the rate of the victim's breathing. A person breathing more than 30 times a minute should be classified "immediate." A person breathing less than 30 times a minute should be further evaluated. This requires you to move to the next check—circulation.

Step two: Check circulation. The next step is to evaluate the breathing victim's pulse. You do this by checking the radial pulse. You are only checking for *the presence* of the radial pulse (brachial for infants). If you cannot find the radial pulse at either wrist, then the victim's blood pressure is substantially low. Control any severe bleeding by using direct pressure, elevation, and applying a pressure bandage. Classify the victim as one requiring immediate care and move on to the next victim. If the pulse is present and no severe bleeding is evident, conduct the final check—level of consciousness.

Step three: Check level of consciousness. At this point, you know the following about the victim:

1. Breathing is normal (less than 30 times per minute).
2. Pulse is present. (Severe bleeding may or may not be present.)

This final check will serve to classify this victim. You determine the victim's level of consciousness by using the AVPU scale you learned in Chapter 7. You give a person who is alert and responds appropriately to verbal stimuli a final classification of "delayed." This person has some injury that prevents him or her from moving to safety, but his or her present condition is not life threatening. A person who remains unconscious, responds only to painful

Table 19-1 START Classification System

Immediate (red)	Delayed/minor (Yellow/green)	Dead/nonsalvageable (Black/grey)
Breathing more than 20 times a minute	Breathing normal, radial pulse present, and level of consciousness normal	Not breathing
Breathing normal, but radial pulse absent.		
Breathing normal, radial pulse present, but level of consciousness abnormal		

stimuli, or responds inappropriately to verbal stimuli is classified as "immediate."

By using the START system, you will be able to move quickly among victims, assessing and classifying them (Fig. 19-6). Remember, your role is not to provide extensive care for the victim. Instead, you are expected to get to as many victims as possible. You should not at any time stop triaging victims to begin CPR on one of them. This person is dead, and if you start CPR, you will need to continue. As a result, others who might have lived if you had done your job properly could now die as a result of delay. The likelihood that a trauma victim in cardiac arrest will survive is extremely rare. Table 19-1 provides a simple overview of the START classification system.

◆ FUNDAMENTALS OF EXTRICATION AND RESCUE OPERATIONS

One of your primary responsibilities as a first responder is to provide care for an ill or injured victim. Sometimes, however, providing care is not possible because you cannot reach the victim. One example is a situation in which someone is able to call 9-1-1 or another local emergency number for help but is unable to unlock the door of the home or office to let in the responders. This situation also occurs in a large number of motor vehicle collisions. Vehicle doors are sometimes locked or crushed, windows may be tightly rolled up, or the vehicle may be unstable. In other instances, fire, water, or other elements may prevent you from reaching the victim.

In these cases, you must immediately begin to think of how to safely gain access to the victim. If you cannot reach the victim, you cannot help him or her. But remember, when attempting to reach a victim, your safety is the most important consideration. Protect yourself and the victim by doing only what you are trained to do and by using equipment and clothing appropriate for the situation. Items such as helmets, face shields, protective eyewear, heavy duty gloves, heavy clothing, blankets, reflective markers or flares, and flashlights will help keep you safe as you attempt to gain access to a trapped victim. Simple tools, such as a screwdriver, hammer, pocketknife, axe, spare tire, vehicle jack, rope, chains, coat hanger, slim-jim, or center punch, can also be helpful.

Role of the First Responder

Extrication is the safe and appropriate removal of a victim who is trapped in a motor vehicle or a dangerous situation. At times, a first responder may be called upon to help care for

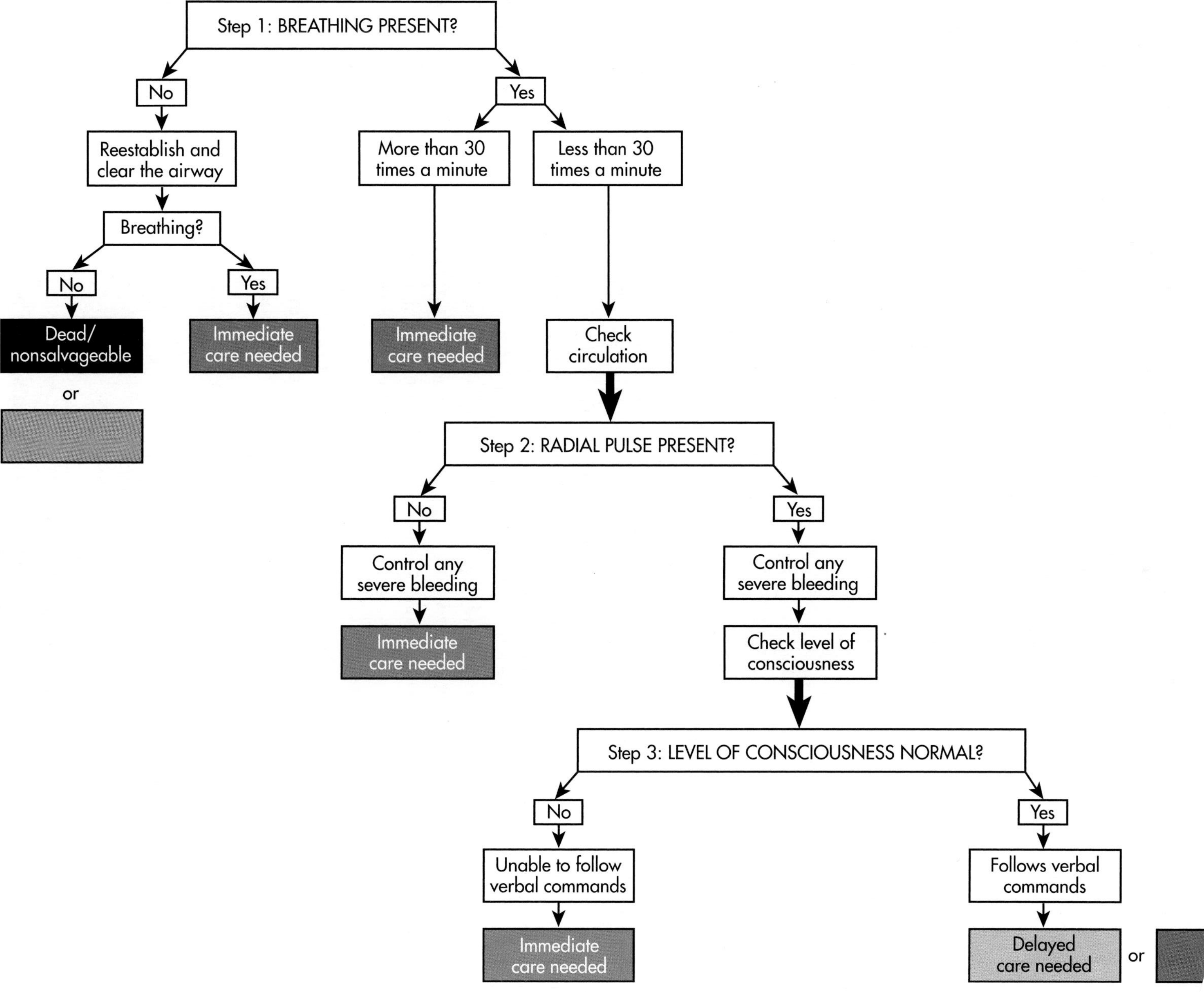
Step 1: BREATHING PRESENT?
No
Yes
Reestablish and clear the airway
Breathing?
No
Yes
Dead/ nonsalvageable
or
Immediate care needed
More than 30 times a minute
Less than 30 times a minute
Immediate care needed
Check circulation
Step 2: RADIAL PULSE PRESENT?
No
Yes
Control any severe bleeding
Immediate care needed
Control any severe bleeding
Check level of consciousness
Step 3: LEVEL OF CONSCIOUSNESS NORMAL?
No
Yes
Unable to follow verbal commands
Immediate care needed
Follows verbal commands
Delayed care needed
or

Figure 19-6 The Three Essentials of START

Recommended Equipment and Clothing for Rescuers

Warning devices

- Flares
- Reflective markers
- Flashlights

Unlocking windows and doors

- Coat hanger or copper tubing, tubing with fishline
- Slim-jim
- Pry bar
- Center punch
- Screwdriver
- Hammer or hatchet

Protective items

- Helmets
- Eyewear
- Face shields
- Gloves
- Heavy clothing

a victim in this type of a situation. It will be your role to administer the necessary care to the victim before extrication and ensure the victim is removed in a way to minimize further injury. Providing lifesaving care for the victim will come before the extrication process unless delaying extrication would endanger the life of the victim or the rescuer.

Although most extrication procedures will be performed by EMTs and other specially trained personnel, when first responders are involved in this type of a rescue, they should work closely with other rescuers to protect the victim. A chain of command should also be established to ensure that the scene is well-managed and the victim's care remains a priority.

Equipment

Your personal safety and the safety of other rescuers and the victim must always be a top priority. Ensuring that you have the proper safety equipment, such as **turnout gear** (puncture- and flame-resistant outerwear), protective eyewear, gloves, and a helmet for the task at hand will help prevent injuries from occurring during a rescue operation.

Personal Safety

All personnel involved in the scene should wear protective clothing and follow the guidelines set up by state and local protocols. The National Fire Protection Association (NFPA) and OSHA have guidelines for you to follow when considering the purchase of safety clothing. At a minimum, when responding to a motor vehicle crash or other extrication, first responders should have the following equipment:

- Protective helmet with chin strap
- Protective eyewear
- Puncture- and flame-resistant outerwear (turnout gear)
- Heavy protective gloves
- Boots with steel toes and steel insoles

Victim Safety

Victims will require protection from the debris of the extrication process. They should be covered with tarps or blankets to protect them from broken glass, sharp metal, and other hazards, including the environment. Their fears can be lessened if you explain to them what will be done and any noise that may occur in the process.

Bystanders in the area should be cautioned to stay away from the scene. Their presence can cause additional confusion and increase the risk of injury.

Gaining Access

Gaining access to the victim may be simple or complex.

Simple Access

The term **simple access** describes the process of getting to the victim without the use of equipment. Although simple access does not require the use of equipment, the first responder should remember to wear protective equipment and use BSI (body substance isolation) as appropriate. Methods of simple access include —

- Trying to open each door.
- Trying to open the windows.
- Having the victim(s) unlock doors or open and roll down windows

When you arrive on the scene, if specialized equipment and personnel are needed to access the victims, call for them. If after accessing the victims you realize that the additional personnel and equipment are not needed, they can easily be canceled.

Complex Access

Complex access describes the process of using specialized tools or equipment to gain access to the victim. Several types of rescue training courses are available that deal with vehicle and ropes rescue. Other types of programs provide training in trench, high angle, and water rescue. If you are interested in any of this specialized training, contact your local EMS system for help in locating these courses. As a first responder, however, you may encounter situations in which you will use basic equipment and techniques to gain access to a victim.

Motor vehicles

As with any emergency situation, begin by sizing up the scene to see if it is safe. If it is not safe, determine whether you can make it safe so that you can attempt to gain access to the victim. Well-intentioned first responders and others are injured or killed each year while attempting to help victims of motor vehicle collisions. Often, these rescuers are struck by oncoming vehicles. Such unfortunate instances can be prevented by taking adequate measures to make the scene safe before trying to gain access and provide care.

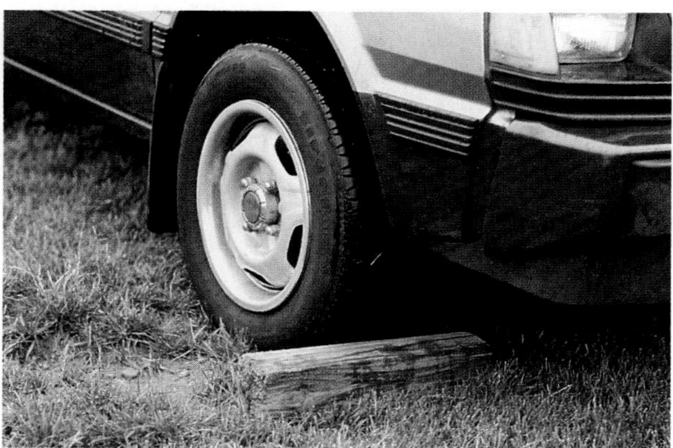

Figure 19-7 Chocking is used to stabilize a vehicle.

Upright vehicles

Fortunately, most motor vehicle collisions you encounter will involve upright, stable vehicles. These vehicles are unlikely to move while you attempt to help their occupants. However, at times the vehicle will not be stable. Environmental factors can influence the stability of the vehicle. Vehicles on slippery surfaces, such as ice, water, or snow, or on inclined surfaces need to be stabilized. In addition, vehicles positioned where oil has been spilled should also be stabilized.

Stabilizing an upright vehicle is a simple task. Placing blocks or wedges against the wheels of the vehicle will greatly reduce the chance of the vehicle moving. This process is called ***chocking*** (Fig. 19-7). You can use items such as rocks, logs, wooden blocks, and spare tires. If strong rope or chain is available, it can be attached to the frame of the car and then secured to strong anchor points, such as large trees, guard rails, or another vehicle. Letting the air out of the car's tires also reduces the possibility of movement.

Once you are certain the vehicle is stable, you should attempt to enter it. Begin by checking all of the doors to see if they are unlocked. Though it may seem obvious to check the doors, sometimes in the excitement it is easy to forget this simple, time-saving step. If the doors are locked, the victim(s) inside might be able

Disaster on I-75

Imagine a highway disaster so catastrophic that authorities do not know for days how many vehicles—or victims—were involved.

Imagine you arrive on the scene to hear the moans and cries of the injured begging to be rescued. But before you even can begin helping, you hear deafening crashes, screeches, and the pounding of metal as more vehicles slam into each other. Most horrifying of all, you cannot see your hand in front of your face.

This was the terrifying scenario on December 11, 1990, as rescuers responded in a shroud of fog to a massive pileup on Interstate 75 near Calhoun, Tennessee. Twelve people died. Fifty-one were injured. Seven rescue workers were hurt, three in a vehicle collision while responding. A total of 99 vehicles were involved in 27 separate collisions in both the southbound and northbound lanes of I-75 at the Calhoun exit. At least six tractor-trailers burst into flames, spreading fire across two miles of the clogged road.

The massive rescue effort, involving several jurisdictions, was a classic example of first responders doing what they were trained to do. Responders from Bradley County worked with those from McMinn County.

The response began shortly after 9:00 AM when a Bradley County sheriff's deputy was dispatched to check on a report of a collision. The caller did not know whether there were injuries. Once word came back as to the possible magnitude of the situation, Bradley County sent a mobile command center—actually a converted school bus equipped with several agencies' radios—to the scene.

"First reports sounded as though the caller was making a dramatic overkill when he reported 75 to 100 vehicles involved," said Russ Newman, director of the Tennessee Emergency Management Agency's eastern region. "The numbers were so incredible that they were discounted to a degree, and in my mind's eye I could visualize an excited deputy escalating his estimates with a generous dose of adrenalin."

Once on the scene, Newman changed his mind. "When I arrived, I saw a scene of carnage reminiscent of wartime," he stated. Mangled, crushed, demolished cars and light trucks were intermingled with other debris and burning tractor-trailers over more than a mile of interstate highway. Most sat as they had abruptly stopped—end-to-end—some literally welded together by collision, the force attesting to the high-speed nature of the multiple crashes.

Benny Waller, the Emergency Medical Services chief for McMinn County, remembers not being able to see his feet in the thick fog when he arrived on the scene. Later, when rescuers conducted their critique of the incident, Dr. Jerry DeVane, McMinn County's Emergency Medical Director, commented that the thick fog—a fairly regular occurrence along that stretch of road—may actually have been a blessing of sorts. DeVane, who helped manage the triage operation, said if rescuers had been able to see the enormity of their task, they might have become overwhelmed.

But instead of being overwhelmed by the problems, rescuers improvised. Inefficient communications was one of the first problems they had to overcome. With everyone trying to transmit at one time, radio communications become a jumble of words. At this point, an order was issued for every one on the EMS channel to stop transmitting unless they had a life-threatening emergency.

The second major problem was determining how many were injured. Benny Waller stated, "Any time you pull up on a scene, your number one job is to assess the problem—whether there are access problems and hazards—and count the number of patients. All this is based on visual assessment, but if you cannot see, you do not know what you have got. At this point, it was necessary to conduct an inch-by-inch reconnaissance. We found patients two ways—one way was going to where screams and cries for help were. They were trapped in vehicles or in groups, yelling as loud as they could. The other way we found them was by literally tripping over them."

One federal investigator called the incident one of the worst highway accidents in U.S. history. If rescue personnel from the two counties had not planned and rehearsed for trouble together, the disaster could have been even more appalling. "It had the potential for being a real tough situation, but fortunately, our people were not overwhelmed," said Joe Wilson of the Bradley County Emergency Management Agency. "They just came in and did their jobs."

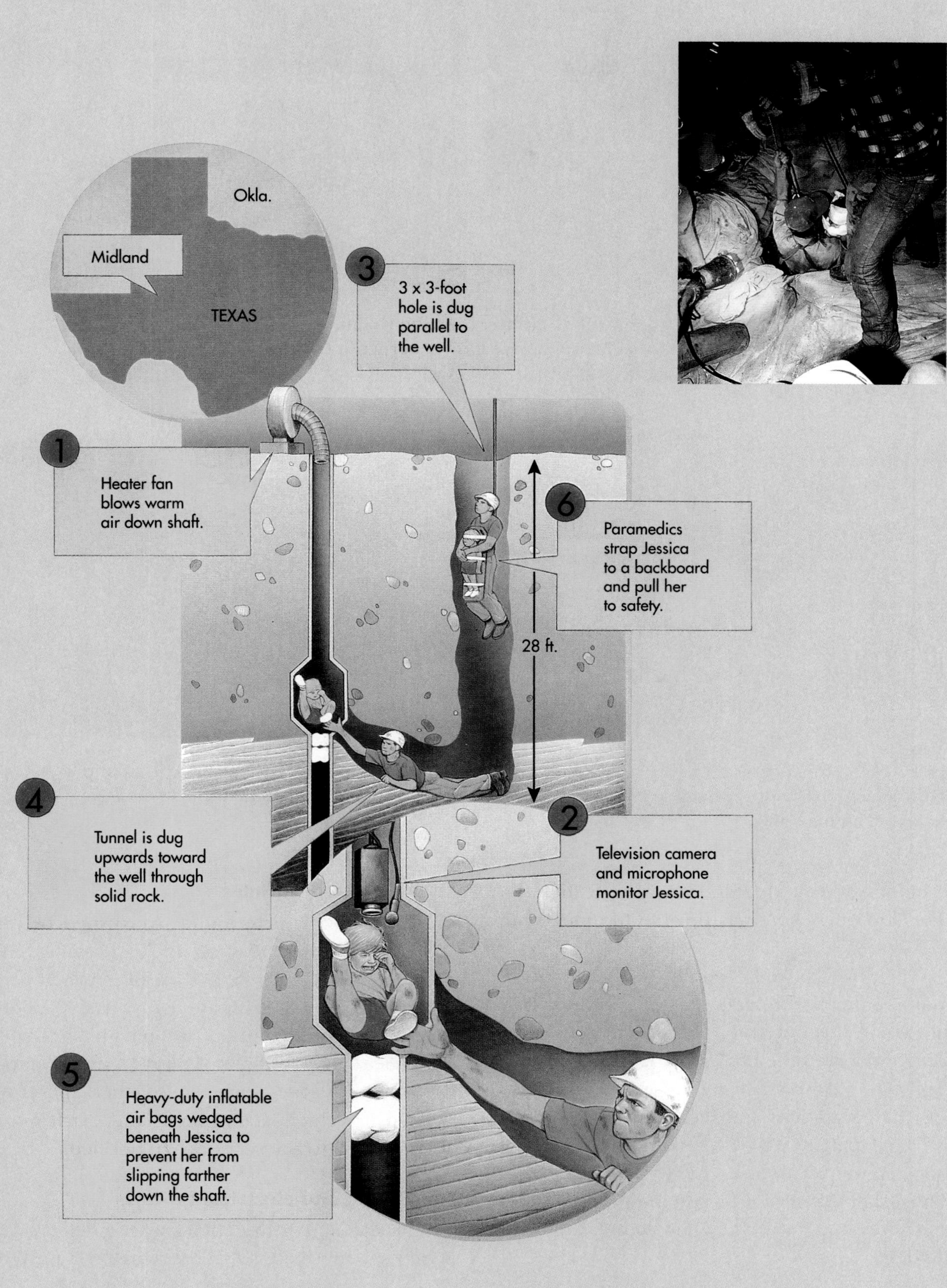

Okla.
Midland
TEXAS
1
Heater fan blows warm air down shaft.
2
Television camera and microphone monitor Jessica.
3
3 x 3-foot hole is dug parallel to the well.
4
Tunnel is dug upwards toward the well through solid rock.
5
Heavy-duty inflatable air bags wedged beneath Jessica to prevent her from slipping farther down the shaft.
6
Paramedics strap Jessica to a backboard and pull her to safety.
28 ft.

A 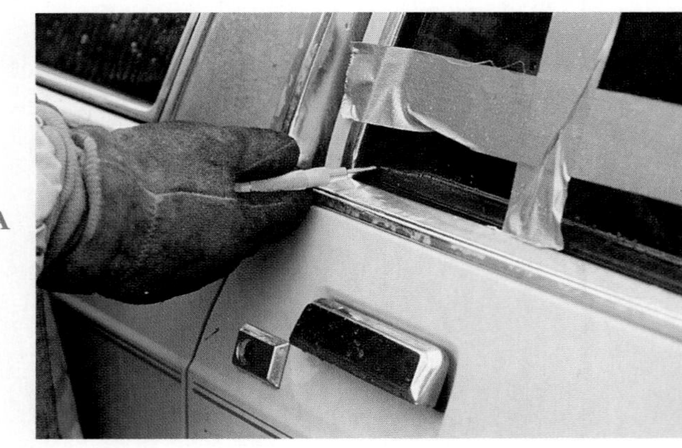 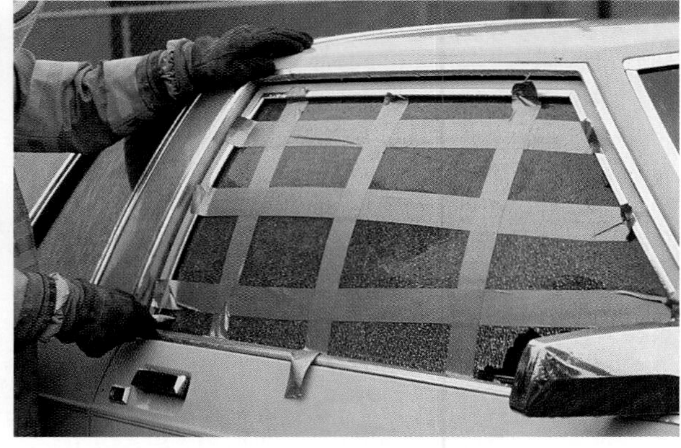 B

Figure 19-8 **A**, Locate the window farthest from the victim. Tape it to avoid flying glass. Position the spring-loaded center punch at a lower corner of the window. **B**, When the punch is pressed against the window, the glass will shatter.

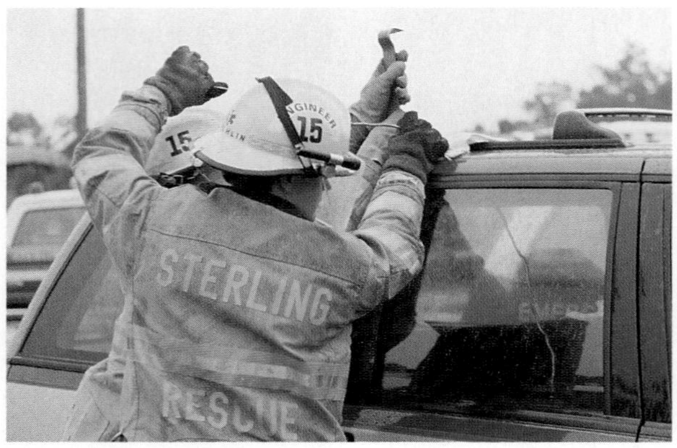

Figure 19-9 To use a wire and pry bar, pry the door frame with the pry bar and insert the wire. Lift the lock with the wire.

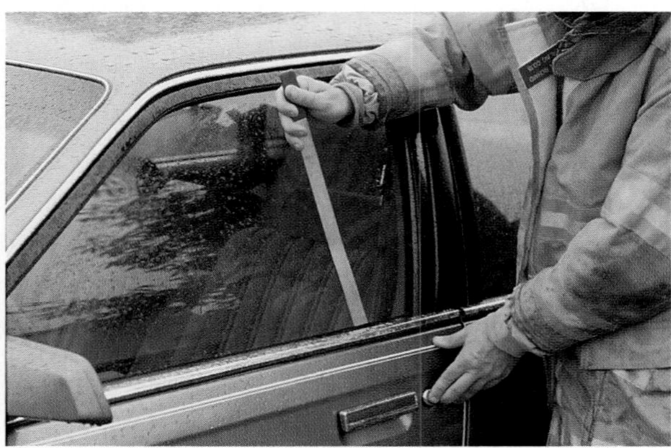

Figure 19-10 A Slim-jim can be used to release the locking mechanism in the vehicle door.

to unlock at least one door for you. If the windows are open, you may be able to unlock the door yourself.

Sometimes locked or jammed doors require you to enter the vehicle through a window. If the window is open or can be rolled down by someone inside the car, entering is not a problem. If the window is rolled up, you can use specific equipment and techniques to get into the car. Figures 19-8 to 19-10 show three common techniques. Once inside the vehicle, you can further stabilize it by placing the vehicle in "park," turning off the key, and setting the parking brake.

Overturned vehicles

Consider any vehicle found overturned or on its side in either position to be unstable. Although a vehicle on its side or overturned can be stabilized by using spare tires, jacks, wooden blocks, or other items, it is unlikely that you can adequately stabilize it. Local fire department and rescue squad personnel specially trained in vehicle stabilization and extrication will respond to the scene when notified.

Vehicles and electrical hazards

When a vehicle is in contact with an electrical wire, you must consider the wire to be ener-

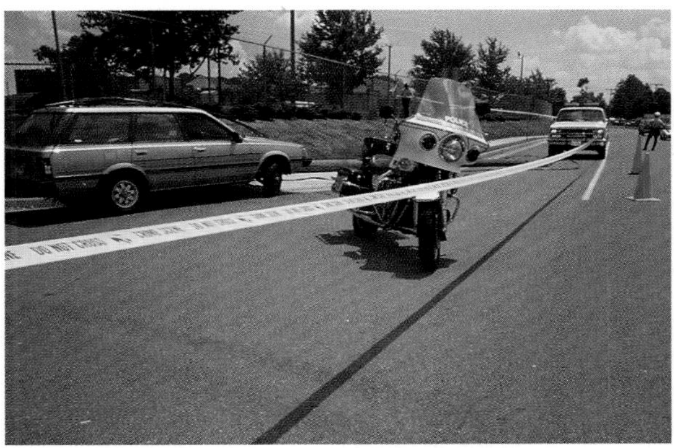

Figure 19-11 Establish a safety area around a downed electrical wire.

gized (live) until you know otherwise. When you arrive on the scene, your first priority is to ensure your safety and that of others in the immediate area. A safety area should be established at a point twice the length of the span (distance between the poles) of the wire (Fig. 19-11). Attempt to reach and move victims *only* after the power company has been notified and has removed any electrical current from the downed wire. Do *not* touch any metal fence, metal structure, or body of water in contact with the downed wire. Tell people inside the vehicle to remain in the vehicle. You can tell them how to provide care for any injured victims in the vehicle. Do *not* attempt to deal with electrical hazards unless you are specifically trained to do so and have the proper equipment.

Once the current has been removed from the wire, you can safely approach the vehicle. Since the vehicle and possibly the victim(s) were in contact with the current, electrical injury is possible. Signs and symptoms of electrical injury include—

- Burns.
- Unconsciousness or dazed, confused behavior.
- Respiratory distress or arrest.
- Abnormality in the pulse rate and quality.

Victim Removal

Once you have gained access to the victim, you should follow the procedures you learned in Chapter 14 that deal with suspected head, neck, or back injuries. As a first responder, you will eventually be working under the supervision and direction of EMS personnel. During and after the extrication you should help with the process of maintaining spinal stabilization, completing the initial assessment, and providing critical care.

◆ HAZARDOUS MATERIALS

As a first responder, you may find yourself involved in a situation in which there are chemical or other harmful or toxic substances. First responders must be trained to quickly identify such situations and activate specially trained personnel to deal with the situation.

Common Problems

A ***hazardous material (HAZMAT)*** is any chemical substance or material that can pose a threat to the health, safety, and property of an individual. ***A hazardous material incident*** is any situation that deals with the release of hazardous material. When dealing with a HAZMAT situation, you work within a structured system that provides guidance in managing this type of scene.

If you work as part of an EMS system, you should receive a First Responder Awareness Level Hazardous Materials training program. This program provides training in recognizing a HAZMAT scene and approaching it safely.

Dealing with the Unknown

The possibility of being involved in a hazardous materials incident should be an everyday concern of all personnel involved in the EMS system. Most people think that a HAZMAT situation only involves train and truck crashes, but hazardous materials can also be found in the home, school, industry, and various public places. Whenever there is any leaking or spilling of chemicals, the potential of a HAZMAT incident exists.

Safety

Unless you have received special training in handling hazardous materials and have the necessary equipment to do so without danger, *you should stay well away from the area.* While en-route to a potential HAZMAT scene, obtain as much pre-arrival information as possible from dispatch. Stay out of low areas where vapors and liquids may collect. Stay upwind and uphill of the scene. Be alert for wind changes that could cause vapors to blow toward you. Do not attempt to be a hero. It is not uncommon for responding ambulance crews approaching the scene to recognize a hazardous materials placard and to immediately move to a safe area and summon more advanced help.

Many fire departments have specially trained teams to handle incidents involving hazardous materials. While awaiting help, keep people away from the danger zone. One easy method to determine the danger zone area is called "the rule of thumb." To be safe, you should position yourself far enough away from the scene so that your thumb, pointing up at arm's length, covers the hazardous area from your view. Binoculars can sometimes be used to help identify the substance involved from a safe distance.

Approaching the Scene

When approaching any scene, you should be aware of dangers involving chemicals. Whether a motor vehicle collision or an industrial emergency is involved, you should be able to recognize clues that indicate the presence of hazardous materials. These include—

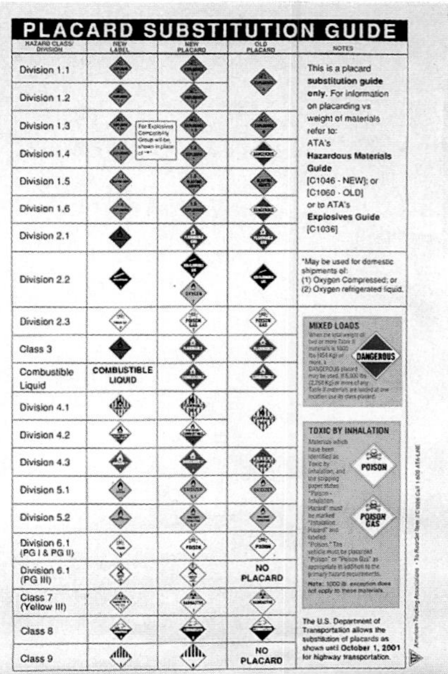

Figure 19-12 American Trucking Association Placard Substitution Guide for Existing Hazardous Materials Placards

- Signs (placards) on vehicles or storage facilities identifying the presence of hazardous materials.
- Spilled liquids or solids.
- Unusual odors.
- Clouds of vapor.
- Leaking containers.

Placards, or signs, are required by federal law to be placed on any vehicles that contain specific quantities of hazardous materials. In addition, manufacturers and others associated with the production and distribution of these materials are required by law to display the appropriate placard. Placards often clearly identify the danger of the substance. Terms such as "explosive," "flammable," "corrosive," and "radioactive" are frequently used. Universally recognized symbols are also used. Figure 19-12 shows some common labels and placards for identifying hazardous materials.

Available Resources and Regulatory Requirements

First responders should review the OSHA and NFPA HAZMAT requirements for EMS providers. Several books available from the U.S. Department of Transportation help identify hazardous materials and appropriate care for victims. One reference book is called *Hazardous Material, The Emergency Response Guidebook.* Further information and guidance on hazardous materials can be obtained from the Chemical Transportation Emergency Center (CHEMTREC). The CHEMTREC toll-free phone number is 1-800-424-9300.

Some hazardous materials, such as natural gas, are flammable and can cause an explosion. Even turning on a light switch or using a telephone or radio may create a spark that sets off an explosion. When you call for help, use a telephone or radio well clear of the scene.

◆ SUMMARY

Depending on the setting in which they work, first responders may or may not have a role in all the nine stages of the EMS response. It is important, however to understand each phase:

- Preparation
- Dispatch
- En-route to the scene
- Arrival at the scene
- Transferring the victim to the ambulance
- En-route to the receiving facility
- Arrival at the receiving facility
- En-route to the station
- Post run

The first responder may be called to or arrive at a multiple casualty incident (MCI). A multiple casualty incident is usually managed by an incident commander, who appoints other rescuers on the scene to assist in various roles. If many victims are injured, rescue personnel may use triage.

At some emergency scenes, victims are trapped in vehicles, and the first responder must gain access to provide care. A first responder who is required to extricate a victim from a vehicle should wear protective equipment, ensure the vehicle is stabilized, and always try the simple means of gaining access. Tell victims trapped in vehicles in contact with downed electric wires to remain in the vehicle. Do not approach the vehicle until you know the power has been turned off.

A hazardous materials incident is one in which dangerous chemicals have somehow been released and pose a threat to life. The first responder must stay at a safe distance until the scene is safe to enter.

Use the activities in Unit 19 of the workbook to help you review the material in this section.

You Are the Responder

Concrete has recently been poured on the uppermost floor of a three-level parking garage under construction. Suddenly, the floor buckles and a portion of the structure crashes down—floor after floor. Thirty workers are in the structure at the time of the collapse. Half of the workers escape injury. The remaining 15 are unaccounted for. Some are probably trapped or crushed under the debris. Others, however, jumped from the structure as it collapsed and are injured. You are the first to respond. Using the principles of the incident command system and triage, describe how you would handle this situation.

ENRICHMENT

◆ WATER EMERGENCIES

In some instances, you may find yourself having to help rescue a person that may be struggling in the water. You should not attempt a swimming rescue unless you are trained to do so.

Reaching and Moving Victims in the Water

People may drown who never intended to be in the water. They may have simply slipped in and not known what to do. Small children can even drown in a bucket of water.

Children under 5 years old and young adults from ages 15 to 24 have the highest rates of drowning. Children with seizure disorders are four times more likely to drown than those without such disorders. Most young children drown in home pools. In Los Angeles, half of all drownings occur in home pools and almost 90 percent of these drownings involve toddlers. Drowning rates are highest in the western and southern United States, in part because of the number of home pools in those regions. But children can also drown in many other kinds of water. In rural areas, for example, drainage canals and irrigation ditches near the home have been the sites of many drownings.

If someone is in trouble in the water, some basic skills can help. Always remember to stay safe. If there is any chance that you cannot safely and easily help the person in trouble, call for rescue personnel.

Recognizing an Emergency

An emergency can happen to anyone in or around the water, regardless of how good a swimmer the person is or what he or she is doing at the time. A strong swimmer can get into trouble in the water because of sudden illness. A nonswimmer playing in shallow water can be swept into deep water by a sudden wave.

Use all of your senses when observing others in and around the water. You may see that a swimmer is acting oddly, or you may hear a scream or sudden splash. Pay attention to anything that seems unusual.

Being able to recognize a person who is having trouble in the water may help save that person's life. Most drowning people cannot or do not call for help. They spend their energy trying to keep their head above water to breathe. They might slip underwater quickly and never resurface. There are two kinds of water emergency situations—a swimmer in distress and a drowning person. Each kind poses a different danger and can be recognized by different behaviors.

A ***distressed swimmer*** may be too tired to get to shore or to the side of the pool but is able to stay afloat and breathe and may be calling for help. The person may be floating, treading water, or clinging to a line for support. Someone who is trying to swim but making little or no forward progress may be in distress (Fig. 19-13). If not helped, a person in distress may lose the ability to float and become a drowning victim.

An ***active drowning victim*** is vertical in the water but has no supporting kick and is unable to move forward or tread water. The victim's arms are at the victim's sides, pressing down in an instinctive attempt to keep the head above water to breathe (Fig. 19-14.) All energy is going into the struggle to breathe, and the person cannot call out for help. A *passive drowning victim* is not moving and will be floating facedown on the bottom or near the surface of the water (Fig. 19-15). Table 19-2 shows characteristics of drowning persons.

An Icy Rescue

Rescuers who pulled Michelle Funk from an icy creek near her home thought she was gone. The child's eyes stared dully ahead, her body was chilled and blue, and her heart had stopped beating. The 2½-year-old had been under the icy water for more than an hour. By all basic measurements of life, she was dead.

Years ago, Michelle's family would have prepared for her funeral. Instead, paramedics performed CPR on Michelle's still body as they rushed her to a children's medical center, where Dr. Robert G. Bolte took over care. Bolte had been reading about a rewarming technique used on adult hypothermia victims, and he thought it would work on Michelle. Surgeons sometimes intentionally cool a patient when preparing for surgery and use heart-lung machines to rewarm the patient's blood after surgery. This cooling helps keep oxygen in the blood longer. Bolte ordered Michelle to the heart-lung machine, which provided oxygen and removed carbon dioxide, in addition to warming the blood. When Michelle's temperature reached 77° F, the comatose child gasped. Soon her heart was pumping on its own.

Doctors once believed the brain could not survive more than five to seven minutes without oxygen, but miraculous survivals like Michelle's have changed opinions. Ironically, researchers have determined that freezing water actually helps to protect the body from drowning.

In icy water, a person's body temperature begins to drop almost as soon as the body hits the water. The body loses heat in water 32 times faster than it does in the air. Swallowing water accelerates this cooling. As the body's core temperature drops, the metabolic rate drops. Activity in the cells comes to almost a standstill, and they require very little oxygen. Any oxygen left in the blood is diverted from other parts of the body to the brain and heart.

This state of suspended animation allows humans to survive underwater four to five times as long as doctors once believed was possible. Nearly 20 cases of miraculous survivals have been documented in medical journals, although unsuccessful cases are rarely described. Most cases involve children who were 15 minutes or longer in water temperatures of 41° F or less. Children survive better because their bodies cool faster than adult bodies.

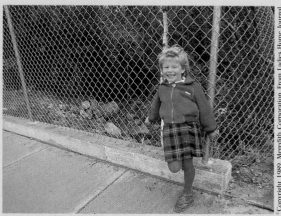

©Copyright 1989, Meredith Corporation. From Ladies Home Journal Magazine.

Researchers once theorized that the physiological responses were caused by a "mammalian dive reflex" similar to a response found in whales and seals. They believed the same dive mechanism that allowed whales and seals to stay underwater for long periods of time was triggered in drowning humans. But experiments have failed to support the idea. Many researchers now say the best explanation for the slowdown is simply the body's response to extreme cold.

After being attached to the heart-lung machine for nearly an hour, Michelle was moved into an intensive care unit. She stayed in a coma for more than a week. She was blind for a short period, and doctors weren't sure she would recover. But slowly she began to respond. First she smiled when her parents came into the room, and soon she was talking like a 2½-year-old again. After she left the hospital, she suffered a tremor from nerve damage. But Michelle was one of the lucky ones — eventually she regained her sight, full balance, and coordination.

Although breakthroughs have saved many lives, parents still must be vigilant around their children when near water. Most near-drowning victims are not as lucky as Michelle. One of every three survivors suffers neurological damage. There is no substitute for close supervision.

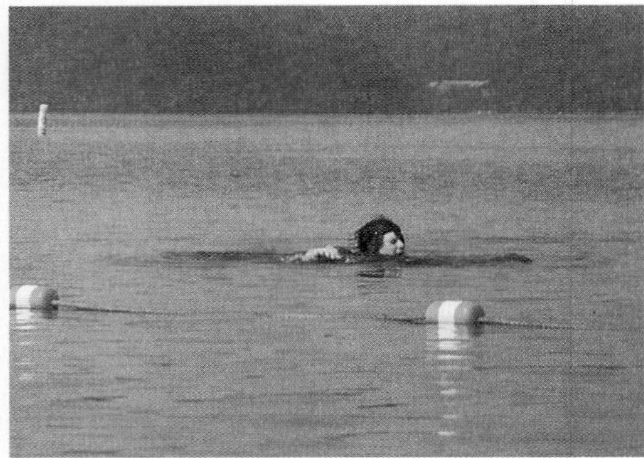

Figure 19-13 A distressed swimmer can stay afloat and usually call for help.

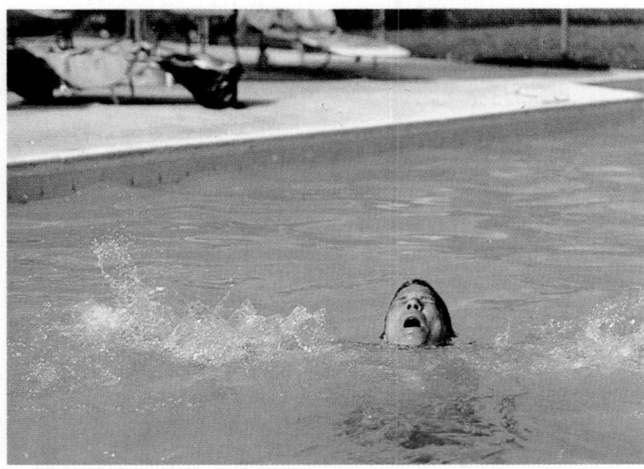

Figure 19-14 An active drowning victim struggles to stay afloat and is unable to callout for help.

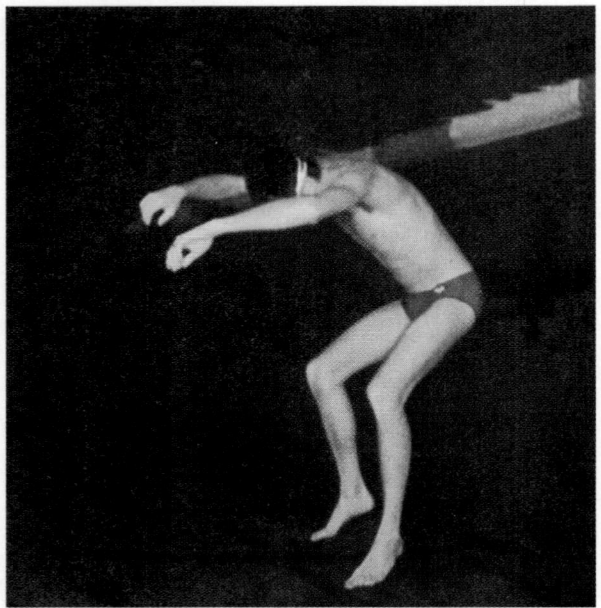

Figure 19-15 A passive drowning victim can be found floating near the surface or submerged on the bottom of the pool.

Once you recognize that there is an emergency, you need to decide how to proceed.

As in any emergency situation, proceed safely. Make sure the scene is safe. If the person is in the water, decide first whether he or she needs help getting out, and then act based on your training. Look for any other victims. Look for bystanders who can help you give first aid or call for help.

If the victim is in the water, your first goal is to stay safe. Rushing into the water to help a victim may lead to you becoming a victim, too. Once you ensure your own safety, your goal is to help get the person out of the water. If the person is unconscious, send someone else to call more advanced medical personnel while you start the rescue. If the person is conscious, you can first act to get the person out of the water and then determine whether more advanced medical personnel are needed.

Out-of-Water Assists

You can help a person in trouble in the water by using reaching and throwing assists. Whenever possible, start the rescue by talking to the person. Let the person know help is coming. If noise is a problem or if the person is too far away to hear you, use gestures. Tell the person what you want him or her to do to help with the rescue, such as grasping a line, rescue buoy, or any other object that floats. Ask the person to move toward you by kicking or stroking. Some people have reached safety by themselves with the calm and encouraging assistance of someone calling to them.

Table 19-2 Characteristics of Distressed Swimmers and Drowning Victims as Compared to Swimmers

	Swimmer	Distressed Swimmer	Active Drowning Swimmer	Passive Drowning Swimmer
Breathing	Rhythmic Breathing	Can continue breathing and call for help	Struggles to breathe; cannot call out for help	Not breathing
Arm and leg action	Relatively coordinated movement	Floating, sculling, or treading water: can wave for help	Arms to sides, pressing down; no supporting kick	None
Body Position	Horizontal or diagonal, depending on means of support	Horizontal, vertical, submerged or near surface	Vertical	Facedown;
Locomotion	Recognizable progress	Little or no forward progress; less and less able to support self	None; has only 20 -60 seconds before submerging	None

Reaching Assists

If the person is close enough, you can use a reaching assist to help him or her out of the water. Firmly brace yourself on a pool deck or pier and reach out to the person with any object that will extend your reach, such as a pole, an oar or paddle, a tree branch, a shirt, a belt, or a towel (Fig. 19-16). Community pools and recreational areas, as well as hotel and motel pools, often have reaching equipment beside the water, such as a **shepherd's crook** (an aluminum or fiberglass pole with a large hook on one end) (Fig. 19-17). When the person grasps the object, slowly and carefully pull him or her to safety. To prevent yourself from being pulled into the water, keep your body low and lean back as you pull the victim.

If you are using a shepherd's crook and the person cannot grasp it, use the hook to encircle the person's body. Keep yourself firmly braced, put the hook around the person's chest under the armpits, and carefully pull him or her to safety. Be careful not to injure the person with the point of the hook as you do this. For a person on the bottom of a pool, try to reach him or her with the hook. Try to encircle the person's body and pull the person to the surface. Then bring the person to the edge and turn him or her face up.

If you have no object for reaching, lie flat on the pool deck or pier and reach with your arm. If you are already in the water, hold onto the pool ladder, overflow trough, piling, or other secure object with one hand and extend your free hand or one of your legs to the victim (Fig. 19-18, *A-B*). Do not release your grasp at the edge, and do not swim out into the water.

Throwing Assists

An effective way to rescue someone beyond your reach is to throw to the victim a floating object with a line attached. The person can

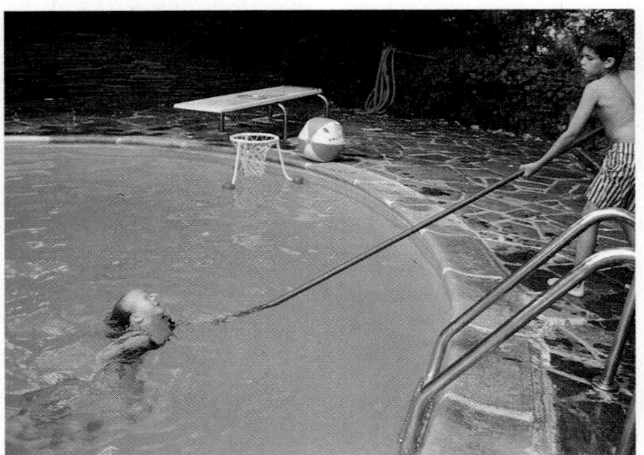

Figure 19-16 With a reaching assist, you remain safe while reaching out to the victim.

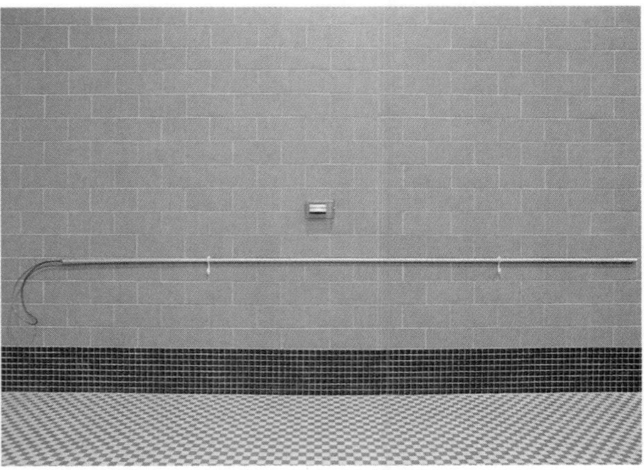

Figure 19-17 A shepherd's crook can be found at most public swimming facilities.

A

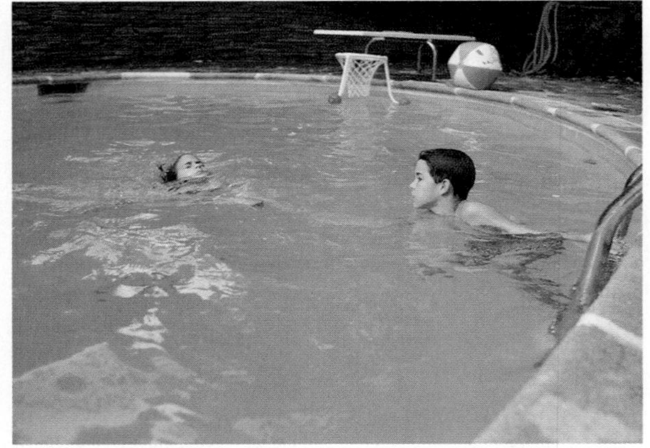

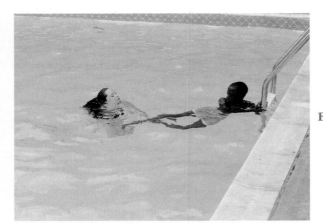

B

Figure 19-18 When no object is available to extend to the victim, try to extend your **A**, hand or **B**, foot to the victim.

grasp the object so that you can pull him or her to safety. Objects you can throw include a **heaving line,** ring buoy, throw bag, rescue tube, or homemade device (Fig. 19-19). You can use any object at hand that will float, such as a picnic jug or tire. Safety equipment for throwing may be in plain view in swimming areas at community pools, hotel and motel pools, and public waterfronts. Recreation and aquatic supply stores sell this equipment for residential pools. You can use certain types of equipment for throwing assists.

A **ring buoy** is made of buoyant cork, **kapok,** cellular foam, or plastic-covered material and weighs about 2 pounds. It should have a towline or lightweight line with an object or knot at the end to keep the line from slipping out from under your foot when you throw it. The buoy and coiled line should be kept on a post where anyone can quickly grasp it to throw to someone in trouble. Hold the underside of the ring with your fingers and throw it underhand (Fig. 19-20).

The **throw bag** is a small but useful rescue device. It is a nylon bag containing 50 to 75 feet of coiled floating line. A foam disk in the

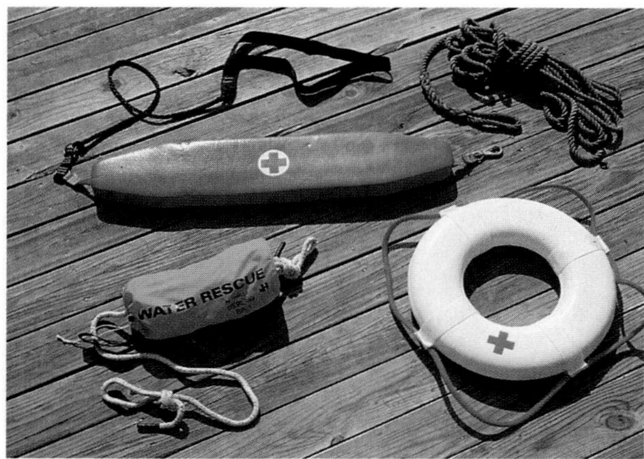

Figure 19-19 Throwing Devices

Figure 19-20 A ring buoy is another piece of rescue equipment that is commonly found at public swimming facilities.

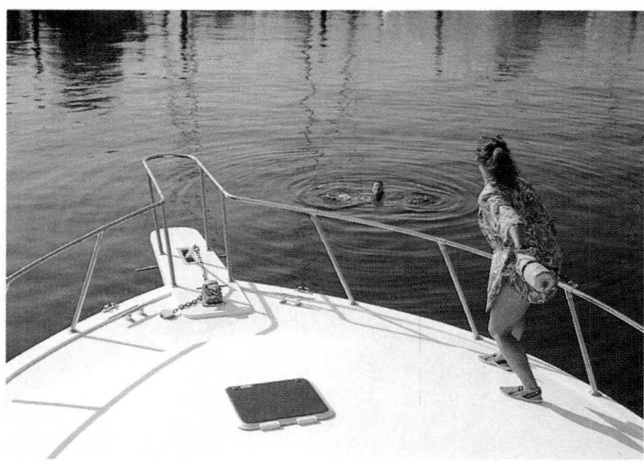

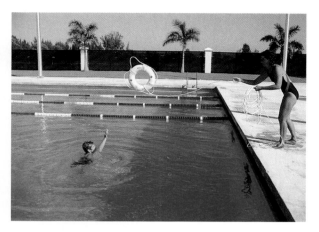

Figure 19-21 A throw bag is a compact rescue device that can be thrown to a victim.

bag gives it shape and keeps it from sinking. Throw bags are often used in canoes and other boats. Hold the end of the line with one hand and throw the bag with your other hand, using an underhand swing (Fig. 19-21).

To perform a throwing assist, follow these guidelines:

1. Get into a stride position (with the leg opposite that of your throwing arm in front of the other leg). This position lets you keep your balance when you throw the equipment.
2. Bend your knees.
3. Step on your end of the line with your forward foot.
4. Try to throw the device just beyond the victim but within reach.
5. Throw the device so that any wind or current will bring it back to the victim.
6. When the victim has grasped the device, slowly pull him or her to safety. Lean back away from the victim as you pull.

If the throwing assist does not work and the water is shallow enough for wading, try a wading assist with equipment.

In-Water Assists

In some situations, you may need to enter the water to rescue a victim. You should only enter water that you are able to stand in.

Wading Assist with Equipment

If you know the water is shallow enough that you can stand with your head out of the water, wade into the water to assist the person. Take a buoyant object and extend it to the victim. Use a rescue tube, a ring buoy, a buoyant cushion, a kickboard, or a life jacket. You may also reach with a ring buoy, tree branch, pole, air mattress, plastic cooler, or paddle (Fig. 19-22, *A-B*). If a

A 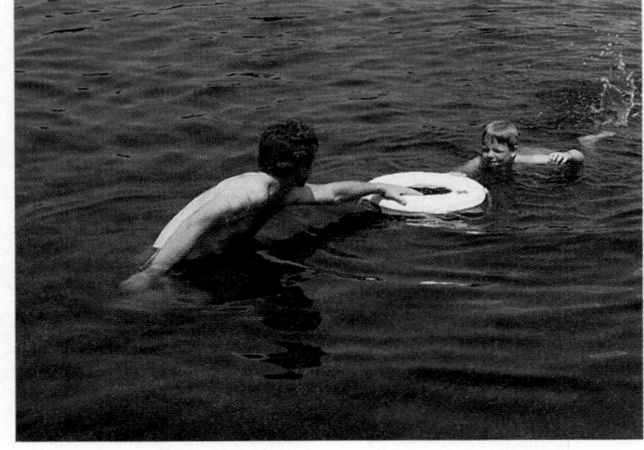

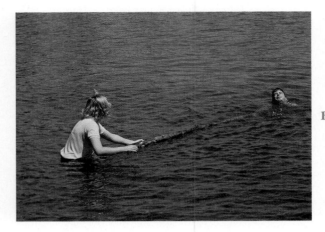 B

Figure 19-22 If you can enter the water without endangering yourself, wade in and reach to the victim. If possible, extend your reach with a A, ring buoy, B, tree branch, or similar object.

current or soft bottom makes wading dangerous, do not enter the water.

Once the person grasps the object, either pull the person to safety or, if it is a buoyant object, let it go and tell the person to kick toward safety using it for support. Always keep the object between you and the person to help prevent the person from grasping and endangering you.

A victim who has been lying motionless and facedown in the water for several seconds is probably unconscious. If the water is not over your head, wade into the water carefully with some kind of flotation equipment and turn the person face up. Bring the victim to the side of the pool or to the shoreline, and then remove him or her from the water.

Walking Assist

If the person is in shallow water where he or she can stand, he or she may be able to walk with some support. Follow these guidelines to perform a walking assist.

1. Place one of the person's arms around your neck and across your shoulder.
2. Grasp the wrist of the arm that is across your shoulder, and wrap your free arm around the person's back or waist.

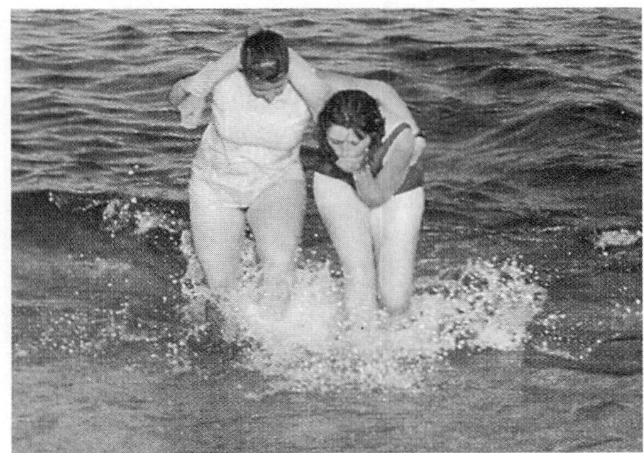

Figure 19-23 When performing a walking assist, maintain a firm grasp on the victim while walking out of the water.

3. Maintain a firm grasp, and help the person walk out of the water (Fig. 19-23).

Beach Drag

You may use the beach drag with a person in shallow water on a sloping shore or beach. This method works well with a heavy or unconscious person.

1. Stand behind the person, and grasp him or her under the armpits, supporting the person's head with your forearms.

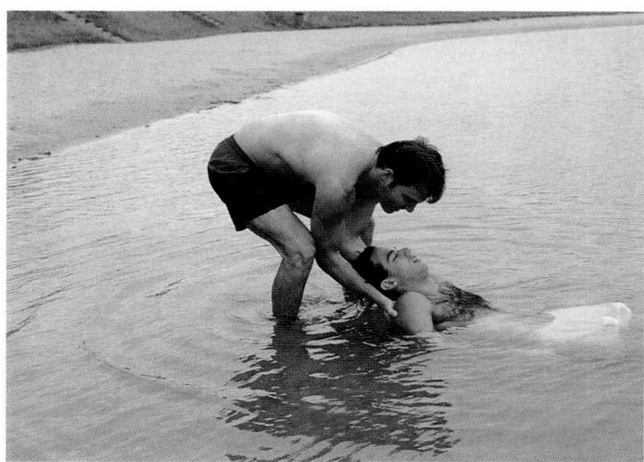

Figure 19-24 When performing a beach drag, walk backward slowly while dragging the victim toward shore.

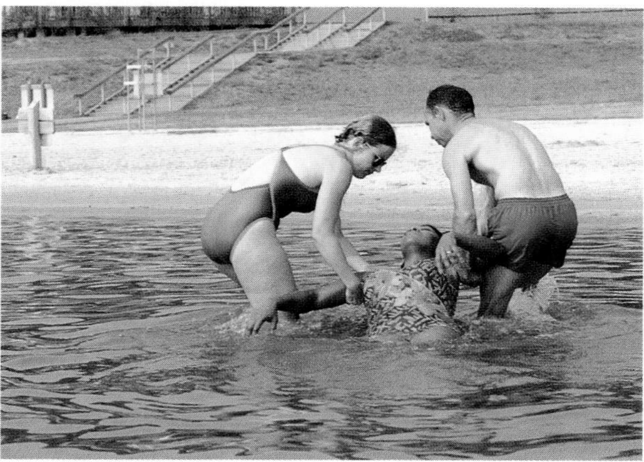

Figure 19-25 If another person is available, have him or her help you.

2. While walking backward slowly, drag the person toward the shore (Fig. 19-24).
3. Remove the person completely from the water or at least to a point where the head and shoulders are out of the water.

You may use a two-person drag if another person is present to help you (Fig. 19-25).

APPENDIX

A

Automated External Defibrillation (AED)

Key Terms

Asystole: The absence of any electrical activity in the heart.

Automated external defibrillator (AED): An automatic or semi-automatic device that recognizes a heart rhythm that requires a shock and either delivers the shock or prompts the rescuer to deliver it.

Atrioventricular (AV) node: A point along the heart's electrical pathway midway between the atria and ventricles that sends electrical impulses to the ventricles.

Defibrillation: An electric shock delivered to the heart to correct certain life-threatening heart rhythms.

Electrocardiogram (ECG): A graphic record produced by a device that records the electrical activity of the heart from the chest.

Normal sinus rhythm: A regular heart rhythm that occurs within a normal rate, 60 to 100 beats per minute (bpm), and without unusual variations.

Sinoatrial (SA) node: The origin of the heart's electric impulse.

Ventricular fibrillation: A life-threatening heart rhythm; a state of totally disorganized electrical activity in the heart.

Ventricular tachycardia: A life-threatening heart rhythm in which there is very rapid contraction of the ventricles.

Knowledge Objectives

After reading this appendix, you should be able to—

- Describe the rationale for early defibrillation.
- Explain when defibrillation is appropriate.
- Describe how defibrillation works.
- Identify the general steps for the use of an automated external defibrillator (AED).

Attitude Objectives

After reading this appendix, you should be able to—

- Value the importance of rapid defibrillation in cardiac arrest situations.
- Serve as a role model for other first responders when you assess and provide care for a victim of cardiac arrest.

Skill Objectives

After reading this appendix and completing the class activities, you should be able to—

- Demonstrate how to use an AED.

INTRODUCTION

Each year, approximately 500,000 Americans die as a result of coronary disease. The majority of these deaths occur suddenly, from cardiac arrest. Most of these arrests occur away from a hospital, where the care needed to immediately correct the cardiac arrest condition is not readily available. CPR, started promptly, can help. However, CPR by itself is insufficient to correct the underlying heart problem. What is needed to correct the problem, in more than two thirds of all cardiac arrests, is an electric shock. And the sooner the shock is administered, the greater the likelihood of the victim's survival.

In the out-of-hospital setting, this shock, known as ***defibrillation***, has typically been administered only by paramedics. Paramedics are rarely the first to arrive on the emergency scene. Often, basic EMTs and first responders, such as fire fighters and law enforcement personnel, arrive first. But without the capability to defibrillate victims of cardiac arrest, they are limited to performing CPR while awaiting the arrival of more advanced personnel. This delay

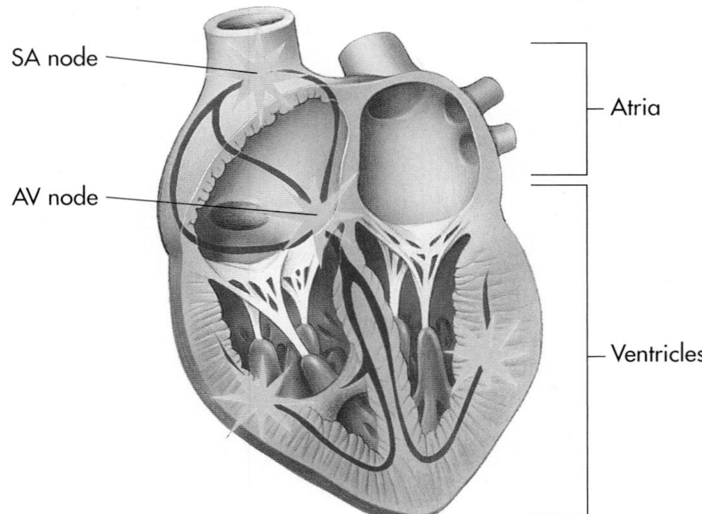

Figure AA-1 The Conduction System of the Heart

in defibrillation is believed to be a major contributing factor to the low survival rate associated with out-of-hospital cardiac arrest.

As a result of this low survival rate, the medical community is focusing efforts on providing earlier defibrillation to cardiac arrest victims. To make earlier defibrillation possible, both the defibrillator and the skills needed to properly operate it have been simplified. Simplification has resulted in more individuals being able to defibrillate cardiac arrest victims and more victims of cardiac arrest being saved. This appendix has been developed to help orient first responders to the need for early defibrillation programs and the basic principles of how automated external defibrillators work.

◆ THE HEART'S ELECTRICAL SYSTEM

To better understand both the limitations of CPR and how defibrillation works, it is helpful to understand how the heart's electrical system functions. This electrical system determines the pumping action of the heart. Under normal conditions, specialized cells of the heart initiate and carry on electrical activity. These cells make up what is commonly called the conduction system. Think of the conduction system as the pathway or road that electrical impulses must travel. This pathway originates in the upper chambers of the heart, known as the **atria.** It ends in the lower chambers of the heart, known as the ***ventricles*** (Fig. AA-1).

The exact point of origin of the electric impulse is the ***sinoatrial node (SA)***. Approximately every second of an adult's life, a new electrical impulse is generated from the SA node. This impulse travels down the pathway of cells to a point midway between the atria and ventricles. This point is the ***atrioventricular node (AV)***.

Below the AV node, the pathway divides, like a fork in a road, into two branches. The electrical impulse travels by way of these right and left bundle branches to its final destination, the right and left ventricles.

These right and left bundle branches become a vast network of microscopic fibers, called Purkinje fibers, which spread electrical impulses across the heart. Under normal conditions, this impulse reaches the muscular walls of the ventricles and causes the ventricles to contract. The strong contraction of the ventricles forces blood out of the heart to circulate through the body. The contraction of the left ventricle results in a pulse. The pauses be-

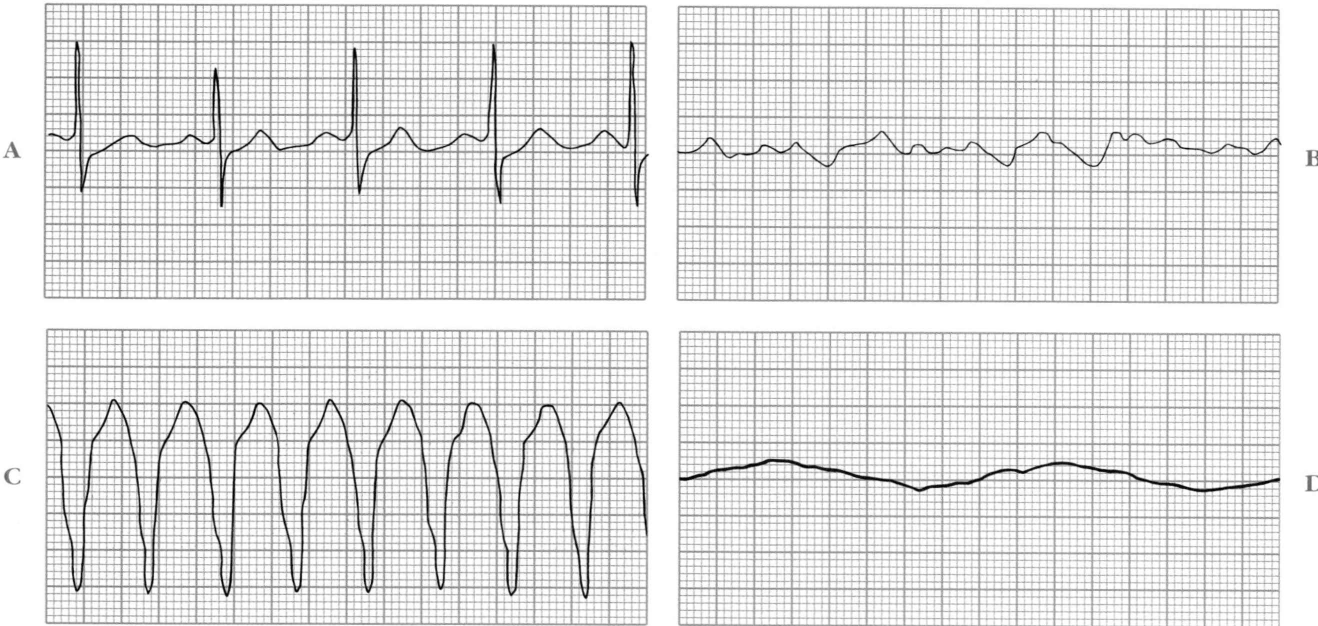

Figure AA-2 **A,** Normal Sinus Rhythm **B,** Ventricular Fibrillation (V-fib) **C,** Ventricular Tachycardia (V-tach) **D,** Asystole

tween the pulse beats you feel are the periods between contractions.

Through the timing of these electrical impulses, the chambers of the heart are able to contract and relax. When they contract, blood is forced out of the heart. When they relax, blood refills the chambers.

The electrical activity of the heart can be evaluated by a cardiac monitor, or **electrocardiograph**. A cardiac monitor has electrodes that usually are attached to the chest. The electrodes pick up the electrical impulse and transmit it to the monitor. The movement of the electrical impulse down the pathway appears as a graphic record on the monitor. This graphic record is referred to as an ***electrocardiogram (ECG).*** A regular rhythm that occurs within a normal rate, 60 to 100 beats per minute (bpm), and without unusual variations, is called a ***normal sinus rhythm***. This rhythm appears on an ECG as a series of regularly spaced and sized peaks and valleys (Fig. AA-2, *A*).

◆ WHEN THE HEART FAILS

Any damage to the heart, caused either by disease or injury, can disrupt the conduction system. This disruption can result in an abnormal heart rhythm that can stop circulation. The two most common abnormal rhythms, present initially in cardiac arrest victims, are ventricular tachycardia (V-tach or VT) and ventricular fibrillation (V-fib or VF). ***Ventricular fibrillation*** is a state of totally disorganized electrical activity in the heart (Fig. AA-2, *B*). It results in the fibrillation, or quivering, of the ventricles. This fibrillation is not adequate for the ventricles to pump blood. Consequently, there is no pulse.

Ventricular tachycardia refers to a very rapid contraction of the ventricles. Though there is electrical activity resulting in a regular rhythm, the rate is often so fast that the heart is unable to pump blood properly (Fig. AA-2, *C*). As with VF, when blood flow is severely impaired, there will not be a pulse.

Defibrillation

In many cases, these two abnormal rhythms can be corrected by early defibrillation. During defibrillation, an electrical shock is delivered to the heart. This shock is not intended to start a dead heart, one without any electrical activity. Instead, it is intended to disrupt abnormal electrical activity, such as that of VF and VT, long enough to allow the heart to spontaneously develop an effective rhythm on its own.

If not interrupted, these rhythms will deteriorate to the point where all electrical activity will cease, a condition known as ***asystole*** (Fig. AA-2, *D*). Asystole is not corrected by defibrillation and indicates a dead heart, which is extremely unlikely to be resuscitated.

CPR, begun immediately and continued until defibrillation is available, helps maintain a low level of circulation in the body until the abnormal rhythms are corrected by defibrillation. In addition, CPR performed during this period appears to contribute to preserving brain function. However, CPR cannot maintain this low level circulation indefinitely and cannot convert VF to a normal sinus rhythm. The major factor determining survival for a person in VF is the time until defibrillation. The longer the wait, the poorer the outcome. For this reason, programs teaching and promoting early defibrillation to more emergency care providers, such as first responders, are encouraged by the EMS community.

◆ AUTOMATED EXTERNAL DEFIBRILLATORS: IMPROVING SURVIVAL OF CARDIAC ARREST

The use of the traditional manual defibrillator requires specialized training that includes learning how to recognize abnormal rhythms on a monitor and how to deliver a shock with hand-held paddles. The process demands extensive training, and the manual defibrillators are expensive. It is impractical to train first responders in their use.

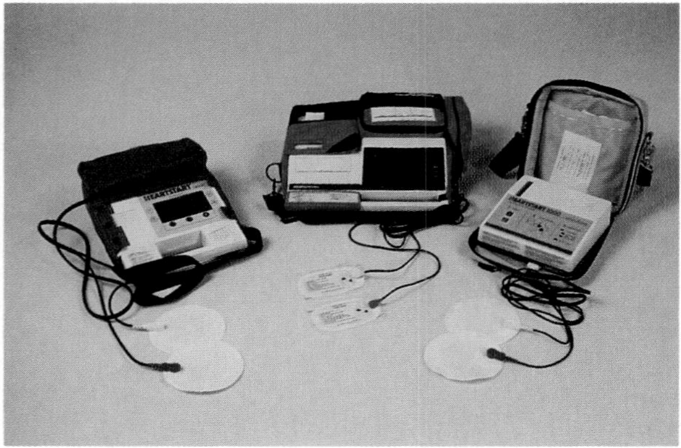

Figure AA-3 Automated External Defibrillators

Instead, the answer to the problem of how to get timely, lifesaving defibrillation to cardiac arrest victims as soon as possible lies with ***automated external defibrillators (AEDs)*** (Fig. AA-3). As the name implies, the AED is an automatic device capable of automatically recognizing a heart rhythm that requires a shock. It can then charge itself and deliver a shock to the victim or request the first responder to do so.

Not only are AEDs simple to operate, they are extremely reliable. Studies have shown that AEDs analyze the victim's heart rhythm several times before identifying it as one for which a shock is indicated.

Using an Automated External Defibrillator (AED)

In a situation involving cardiac arrest, an AED should be put to use as soon as it is available. Other skills, such as CPR already in progress, must be stopped once the AED is applied. All AEDs can be operated by following five simple steps:

1. Confirm cardiac arrest. Check for unresponsiveness and the absence of breathing and pulse.
2. Turn on the AED.

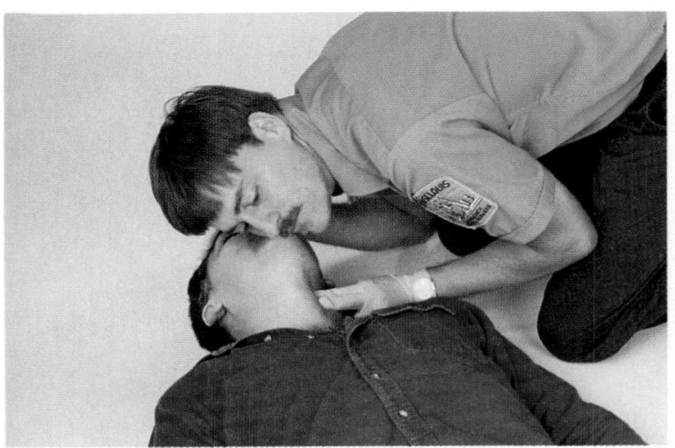

Figure AA-4 Confirm cardiac arrest before applying AED.

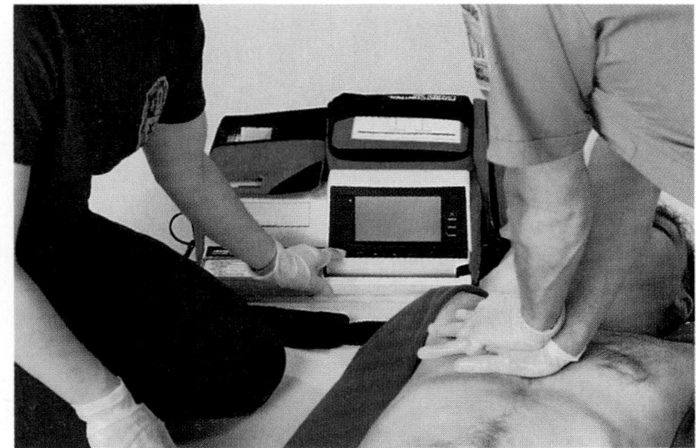

Figure AA-5 After you have confirmed that the victim is in cardiac arrest, turn on AED.

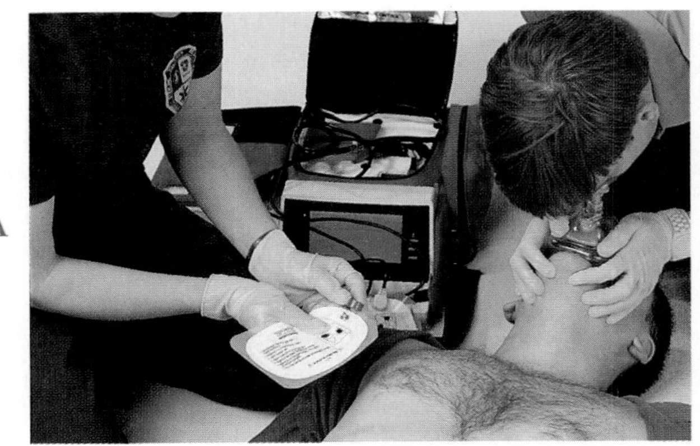

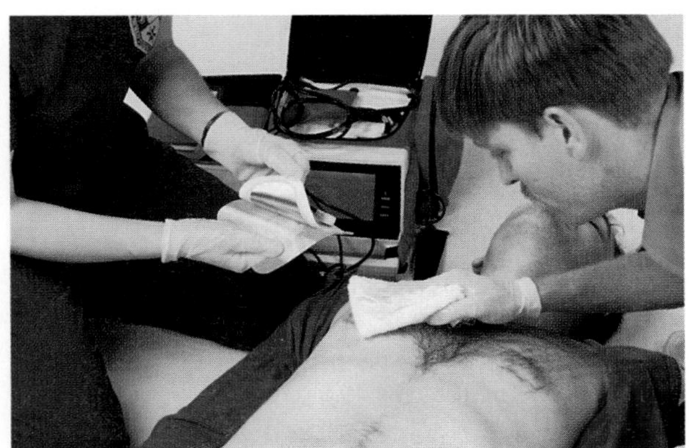

A B

Figure AA-6 **A,** Connect the two cables from the AED to the pads. **B,** Peel away the protective backing from the pads.

3. Attach the AED to large defibrillator electrode pads and apply the pads to the victim's chest.
4. Let the AED analyze the rhythm (or push the button marked "analyze").
5. Deliver a shock, if indicated.

Whether you are the first person to arrive on the scene or arrive after CPR has been started, you should check the victim's pulse to determine that the victim is actually in cardiac arrest before attaching the AED (Fig. AA-4). The absence of a pulse confirms cardiac arrest. When you establish the absence of a pulse, you should turn on the AED (Fig. AA-5). Once turned on, AEDs are capable of recording the events surrounding the care of the victim. If the AED you are using has a voice recording mechanism, you can briefly give a verbal report for the recording. It should include—

- Your identity and location.
- Assessment findings.
- Any significant events that have occurred (drowning incident, trauma, and so on).

Next, prepare to attach the necessary equipment to the victim. Attaching the device to the victim requires that you apply two adhesive pads to the victim's chest. To do this, the victim's chest must be bare and wiped dry.

- Remove the pads from their packaging.
- If needed, connect the two cables from the AED to the pads (Fig. AA-6, *A*). Peel away the

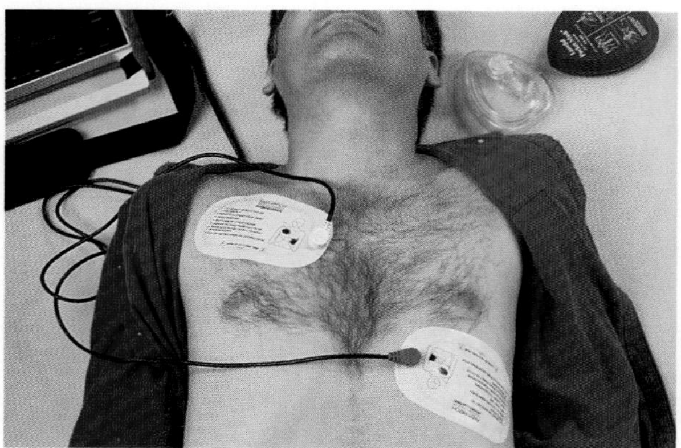

Figure AA-7 Place the pads connected to the white cable on the right side of the chest between the nipple and collarbone. Place the pad connected to the red cable on the left side of the chest below the nipple.

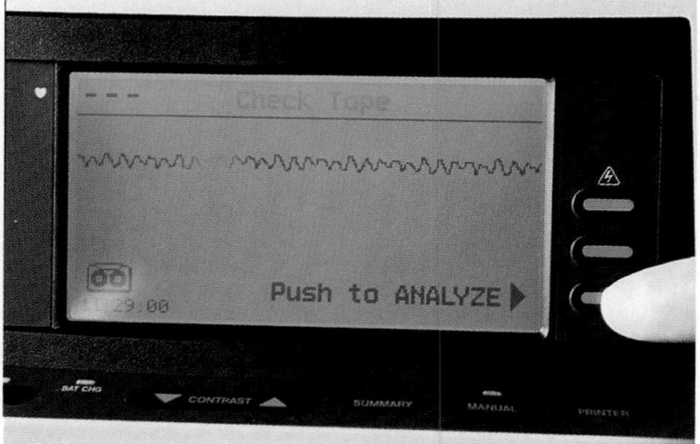

Figure AA-8 Analyze the heart rhythm by depressing the appropriate button.

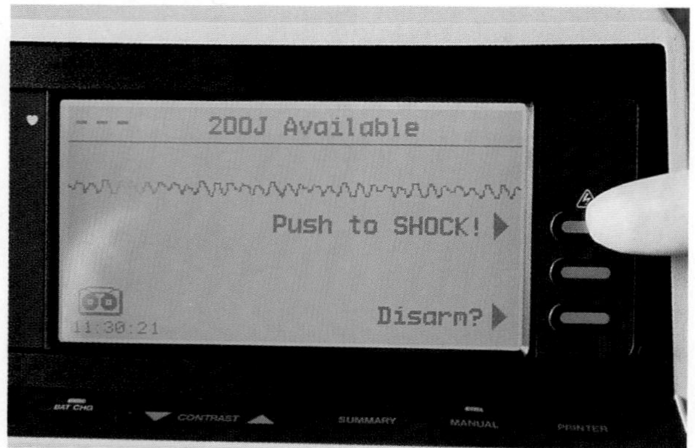

Figure AA-9 The AED will prompt you when to administer the shock

protective plastic backing from the pads (Fig. AA-6, *B*).

- Place the pads, adhesive-side down, on the victim's chest.
- Place one pad on the upper right side of the victim's chest, between the nipple and the collarbone.
- Place the other pad on the lower left side of the victim's chest, below the nipple (Fig. AA-7).

If you are confused about which pad goes where, remember the phrase "white goes upper right." This means that the pad attached to the white cable is applied to the upper right side of the victim's chest.

If the pads are not securely attached to the chest or if the cables are not fastened properly, you will receive an "error" or "check electrodes" message from the AED. This message may appear in print on the small screen on the front of the machine or in voice prompt. If you receive such a message, check to see that the pads and cables are attached properly. In all cases, you should follow the manufacturer's instructions, since AEDs differ in the type of cables and adhesive pads used.

At this point, the device is ready to analyze the heart rhythm. Some devices require the first responder to press the button marked "analyze" to have the machine examine the heart rhythm (Fig. AA-8). Other, newer models, will automatically analyze the heart rhythm. If the AED identifies a rhythm that should be defibrillated, it will prompt you with either an on-screen message or by voice message. This prompt often states, "shock advised," followed by "press to shock," indicating that you need to press a button to defibrillate the victim (Fig. AA-9). The fully automatic AED will analyze the heart rhythm, charge to the appropriate energy level, advise you that a shock is needed, and deliver a shock of the correct intensity automatically.

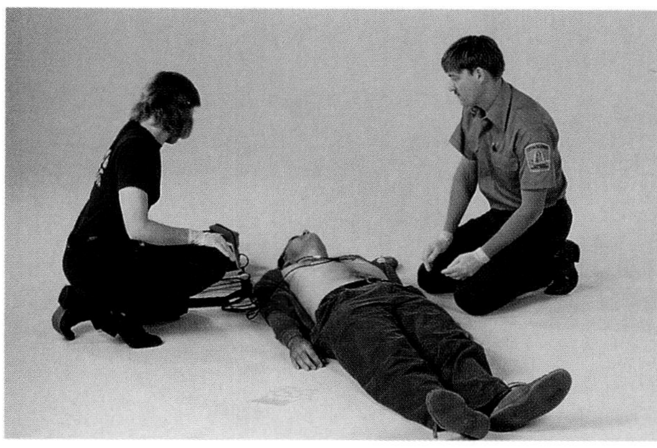

Figure AA-10 Everyone must "stand clear" when the AED is analyzing the rhythm, charging the machine, or administering a shock.

You will also be instructed by a voice message within the AED to "stand clear" before administering a shock. This is an important measure that you and others present must follow. Any time an AED is analyzing the rhythm, charging to a specific energy level, or administering a shock, *you and others must not be in contact with the victim* (Fig. AA-10). It is the responsibility of the operator to move rescuers away from contact with the victim before analyzing and before depressing the shock button. This can be done by shouting "stand clear."

The number of shocks the AED administers and the energy level for each shock is often preset by the manufacturers. These energy levels range upward from 200 to 360 joules. However, the local medical director can modify the device and will establish local operating protocols. The American Heart Association has established guidelines to follow when using the AED. These guidelines include how CPR is to be used as part of the protocol.

In some instances, the heart will *not* require defibrillation. In this case, the device will inform you that no shock is needed. You should recheck the victim's pulse. If it is still absent, resume CPR. If a pulse is present, recheck breathing. If the victim is still not breathing, continue breathing for the victim and monitoring the pulse.

Recommended AED Protocol

Check Pulse
If no pulse . . .
Do CPR until AED is attached.

Analyze Rhythm
If shock advised . . .
Defibrillate at 200 joules.

Analyze Rhythm
If shock advised . . .
Defibrillate at 200-300 joules.

Analyze Rhythm
If shock advised . . .
Defibrillate at 360 joules.

Recheck Pulse
If no pulse . . .
Do 1 minute of CPR and recheck pulse.
If still no pulse . . . Repeat analysis and set of 3 shocks at 360 joules as indicated.

Recheck Pulse
If no pulse . . .
Do 1 minute of CPR and recheck pulse.
If still no pulse . . . Repeat analysis and set of 3 shocks at 360 joules as indicated.

Recheck Pulse
If still no pulse . . .
Continue CPR and prepare to transport.

Note: As long as the pulse is absent and the AED still indicates a need to shock, continue repeating sets of 3 shocks to a maximum of 9 total shocks, with 1 minute of CPR between each set. You should be thoroughly familiar with your local operating procedures, which may vary slightly from this table.

Precautions

You need to take the following precautions when using an AED:

- Do not use alcohol pads to clean the chest before attaching the pads.
- Stand clear of the victim while analyzing and defibrillating.
- Do not analyze the rhythm or defibrillate in a moving vehicle.

- Do not defibrillate a victim who is in water. Move victims away from puddles of water (such as around a swimming pool) before defibrillating.
- Do not defibrillate a victim lying on a surface, such as sheet metal, that is likely to transfer the electrical energy to others on or in contact with the same surface.
- Do not defibrillate a victim who is less than 12 years old or weighs less than 90 pounds.
- Do not defibrillate a victim while he or she is wearing a nitroglycerin patch on the chest. Remove any patch from the chest and wipe the area clean before attaching the device.
- Do not defibrillate someone in the presence of flammable materials, such as gasoline.

◆ ESTABLISHING AN EARLY DEFIBRILLATION PROGRAM

An early defibrillation program must take into account many variables to be fully successful. These variables include—

- The size, age, and location of the populations to be served.
- The number of first responders being trained.
- The response times of both first responders and more advanced personnel.
- The number of AEDs available.
- Where the AEDs are placed within the community.
- The commitment to the program from the local medical director and EMS personnel.
- State requirements for certification in automated defibrillation.

When these variables are examined, the programs established can better suit the community. For example, if an extremely large number of older adults live in the northeast section of your community, this section is where the AED should be placed. This is the area where cardiac arrests are most likely to occur. If you have several AEDs, they should be strategically placed throughout the community so that response times can be reduced and access to defibrillation can be increased, thereby saving more lives.

◆ SUMMARY

Automated external defibrillators (AEDs) show great promise in saving the lives of victims of cardiac arrest. To defibrillate a victim of cardiac arrest by using an AED, take the following basic steps:

1. Confirm cardiac arrest.
2. Turn on the AED.
3. Attach the AED to large defibrillator electrode pads and apply the pads to the victim's chest.
4. Let the AED analyze the heart rhythm (or push the button marked "analyze").
5. Deliver a shock if one is indicated.

You must follow local protocols that establish how many shocks are delivered, the energy setting of each shock, and how CPR and other lifesaving measures are used.

AEDs are easy to operate and require minimal training and retraining. Strategically placed in a community where the first persons to arrive on the scene are trained in their use, AEDs are a highly valuable emergency resource of great promise in saving the lives of cardiac arrest victims.

Using an Automated External Defibrillator (AED)

Skill Summary

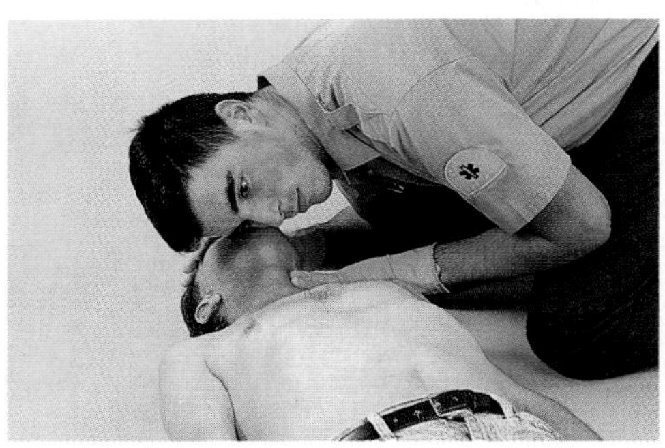

1. Confirm cardiac arrest.

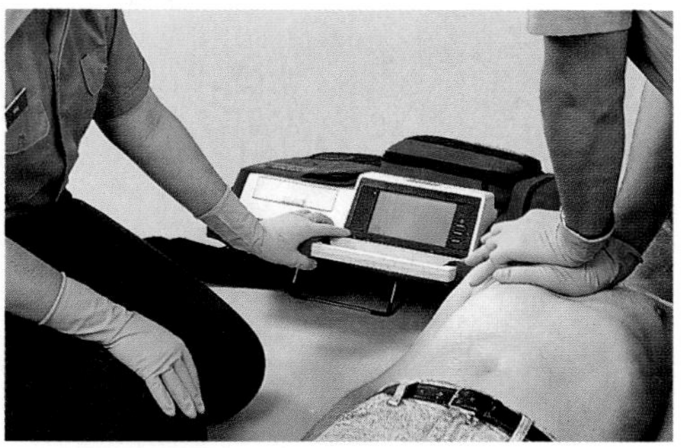

2. Turn on AED.

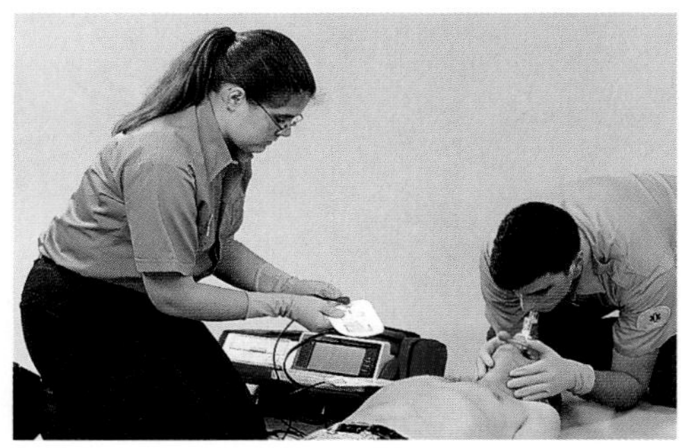

3. Connect AED cables to pads.

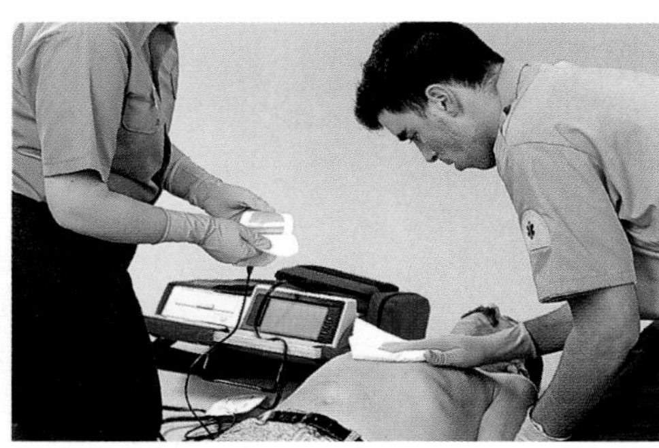

4. Peel away backing from pads and dry chest.

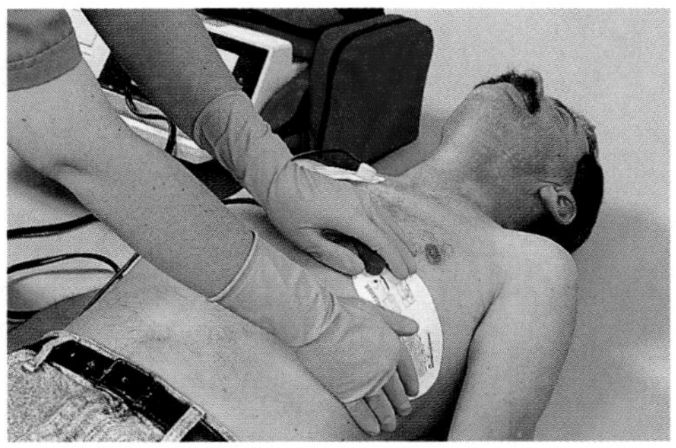

5. Place pads on chest.

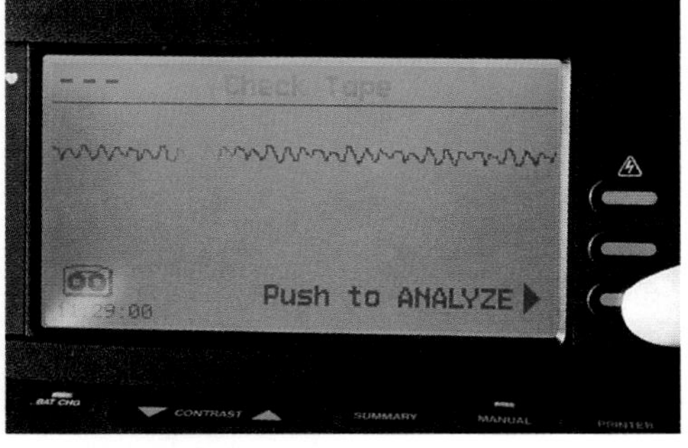

6. Press the "analyze" button.

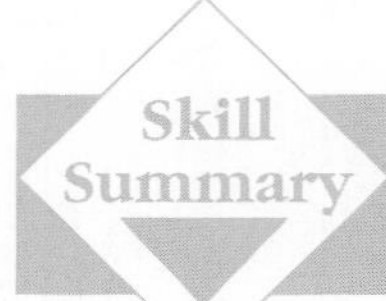

Using an Automated External Defibrillator (AED)—cond'd

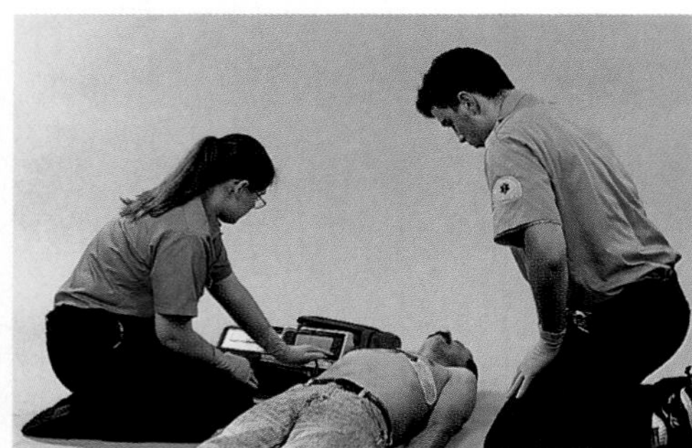

7. Tell everyone "stand clear" while AED is analyzing rhythm or shock is being administered.

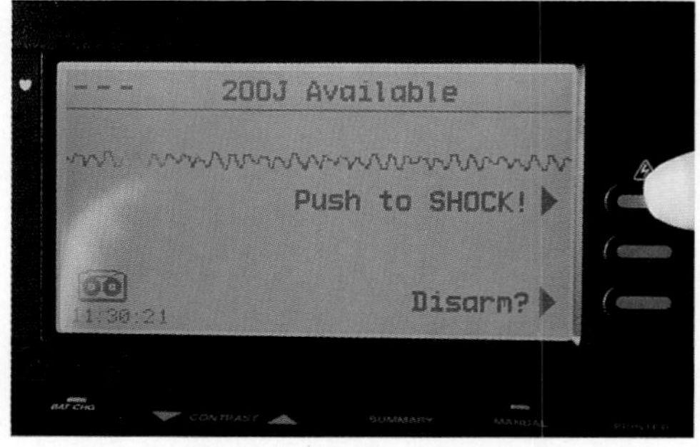

8. Press "shock" button if prompted by AED.

APPENDIX

B

Healthy Lifestyles Awareness Inventory

A healthy lifestyle is a combination of positive beliefs and practices. Following safe practices at home, at work, during recreation, and while traveling in a motor vehicle can prevent events that often lead to disabling injuries. What you eat, how you exercise, and how you manage stress, both on and off the job, also contribute to a healthy lifestyle.

How healthy is your lifestyle? What do your habits say about the life you lead? Complete the following inventory and see how your habits add up. Mark the response that best describes your behavior. Total your points after each section of the survey. Add these subtotals and check your score with the corresponding feedback at the end of each section. The feedback provides a broad interpretation of how your behavior relates to a healthy lifestyle. It will help you focus on the areas of your lifestyle that may need improvement. Record your subtotals and totals on the scorecard on p. 484.

◆ CARING FOR YOUR BODY

	Always (3)	Often (2)	Rarely (1)	Never (−1)	N/A (0)
Part I: Nutrition					
1. I eat a balanced diet.	☐	☐	☐	☐	☐
2. I limit my intake of saturated fats and cholesterol.	☐	☐	☐	☐	☐
3. I limit my intake of salt.	☐	☐	☐	☐	☐
4. I bake, broil, or grill foods rather than frying them.	☐	☐	☐	☐	☐
5. I eat fruits, vegetables, and low-fat yogurt when snacking rather than "junk" food.	☐	☐	☐	☐	☐
6. I read labels for information about the nutritional quality of food.	☐	☐	☐	☐	☐
7. I maintain an appropriate weight.	☐	☐	☐	☐	☐
8. If I need to lose weight, I avoid fad, starvation, or miracle diets that are harmful to my health.	☐	☐	☐	☐	☐
Part I: Subtotal					
Part II: Exercise					
9. I participate in continuous, vigorous physical activity for 20 to 30 minutes or more at least 3 times per week.	☐	☐	☐	☐	☐
10. I follow an exercise program appropriate for my level of fitness.	☐	☐	☐	☐	☐
11. I warm up properly before vigorous activity and cool down afterwards.	☐	☐	☐	☐	☐
12. I use exercise equipment properly and safely.	☐	☐	☐	☐	☐
13. I swim only when others are present.	☐	☐	☐	☐	☐
14. I wear highly visible clothing when exercising outdoors, such as walking, running, or biking.	☐	☐	☐	☐	☐
Part II: Subtotal					

	Always (3)	Often (2)	Rarely (1)	Never (−1)	N/A (0)
Part III: Managing Stress					
15. I schedule my day to allow time for leisure activity.	☐	☐	☐	☐	☐
16. I get an adequate amount of sleep.	☐	☐	☐	☐	☐
17. I express feelings of anger or worry openly and constructively.	☐	☐	☐	☐	☐
18. I say "no" without feeling guilty.	☐	☐	☐	☐	☐
19. I make decisions with a minimum of stress and worry.	☐	☐	☐	☐	☐
20. I set realistic goals for myself.	☐	☐	☐	☐	☐
21. I accept responsibility for my actions.	☐	☐	☐	☐	☐
22. I seek professional help when stress becomes too difficult to manage.	☐	☐	☐	☐	☐
23. I allow myself to cry.	☐	☐	☐	☐	☐
24. I manage stress so that it does not affect my physical well-being.	☐	☐	☐	☐	☐
25. I discuss problems with friends, co-workers, my supervisor, or relatives.	☐	☐	☐	☐	☐
Part II: Subtotal ☐					
Part IV: Work					
26. Work is a place I like to go.	☐	☐	☐	☐	☐
27. I like my supervisors and co-workers.	☐	☐	☐	☐	☐
28. I take advantage of learning opportunities at work.	☐	☐	☐	☐	☐
29. I take advantage of opportunities for advancement at work.	☐	☐	☐	☐	☐
30. I am satisfied with my balance of work and leisure time.	☐	☐	☐	☐	☐
31. I take all my annual vacation in a given year.	☐	☐	☐	☐	☐
Part IV: Subtotal ☐					

	Always (3)	Often (2)	Rarely (1)	Never (−1)	N/A (0)
Part V: Tobacco, Alcohol, and Other Substances					
32. I avoid smoking cigarettes, cigars, pipes, or using other forms of tobacco, such as chewing tobacco or snuff.	☐	☐	☐	☐	☐
33. I try to avoid inhaling the smoke of others.	☐	☐	☐	☐	☐
34. I avoid using illegal substances, such as marijuana, uppers, and crack.	☐	☐	☐	☐	☐
35. I drink fewer than five alcoholic beverages per week.	☐	☐	☐	☐	☐
36. I avoid driving a car or other motor vehicle or operating a boat while under the influence of alcohol or other substances that impair judgment or reactions.	☐	☐	☐	☐	☐
37. I avoid riding in cars, in other motor vehicles, or in boats with people under the influence of alcohol or other substances that impair judgment or reactions.	☐	☐	☐	☐	☐
38. If necessary, I avoid using alcoholic beverages or other substances while taking prescription or over-the-counter medications.	☐	☐	☐	☐	☐
39. I keep my health-care providers informed of medications I am taking to avoid harmfully combining medications.	☐	☐	☐	☐	☐
40. When taking prescription medication, I follow my doctor's instructions.	☐	☐	☐	☐	☐
41. When taking over-the-counter medications, I follow the instructions on the label.	☐	☐	☐	☐	☐

Part V: Subtotal ☐

	Always (3)	Often (2)	Rarely (1)	Never (−1)	N/A (0)
Part VI: Medical Care					
42. I seek appropriate care or cut back on activities, as necessary, when I feel unwell or tired.	☐	☐	☐	☐	☐
43. I maintain an accurate, written, current personal health history.	☐	☐	☐	☐	☐
44. I brush my teeth at least once a day.	☐	☐	☐	☐	☐
45. I floss my teeth at least once a day.	☐	☐	☐	☐	☐
46. I ask questions of health care providers.	☐	☐	☐	☐	☐
47. I use a sunscreen with sufficient ultraviolet (UV) protection when spending time in the sun.	☐	☐	☐	☐	☐
48. I wear sunglasses with UV protection when out in the sun.	☐	☐	☐	☐	☐
49. I use adequate measures to protect myself and my partner(s) from sexually transmitted diseases.	☐	☐	☐	☐	☐
50. I practice good personal hygiene by bathing daily and washing my hands frequently.	☐	☐	☐	☐	☐
51. I have regular medical checkups.	☐	☐	☐	☐	☐
52. I have regular dental checkups.	☐	☐	☐	☐	☐
53. I have regular eye examinations.	☐	☐	☐	☐	☐
54. I routinely examine my testicles/breasts for the pressence of masses or other unusual signs.	☐	☐	☐	☐	☐
55. I maintain adequate health insurance coverage.	☐	☐	☐	☐	☐

Part VI: Subtotal ☐

Add subtotals I to VI to determine your total score.

Total: CARING FOR YOUR BODY

Caring for Your Body: Feedback

> 110 = You are taking excellent care of your body. Keep up the good work. Take note of the behaviors for which you scored 1 or less and make them regular habits in your life.

92 to 110 = Although you are taking adequate care of your body, some behaviors still need improvement. Check your answers and note the behaviors with a score of 2 or less. To perform at your maximum potential and minimize the risks of illnesses that may develop later in life, make these behaviors a more frequent part of your life.

55 to 91 = Several areas indicate you are at risk. Although you may be taking moderate care of your body, some areas require your attention. Any behaviors for which you scored 2 or less need improvement. Consult your doctor or other specialist for advice on how to better care for your body. Incorporating healthy behaviors into your daily life will enable you to perform at your maximum potential and minimize the risks of illnesses that may develop later in life.

< 55 = Apparently, taking care of your body is not a priority. Sooner or later, your body will begin to show and feel signs of neglect. To perform at your maximum potential and minimize the risks of illnesses that may develop later in life, you must start caring for your body now. Your goal is to change habits in order to improve the quality of your daily life. Perhaps you are unaware of how to care for your body. If you are unsure about how to change your habits and take better care of yourself, consult a professional health-care provider.

If you scored low in these sections, remember that there are many ways to change how you care for your body. Each of the areas addressed in the inventory so far has an impact on your health. Changes you make in one area frequently will be beneficial in another area as well.

Proper nutrition combined with exercise and adequate rest and relaxation will help keep your body in peak form. This will enable your body to respond and react most efficiently to demands placed on it. Eating a balanced diet also helps prevent disease.

Exercise helps relieve stress, increases your cardiovascular efficiency, and helps you maintain your desired weight. All of these benefits serve to lower your risks of cardiovascular disease, high blood pressure, and stroke. Consult your physician if you have any questions or concerns about nutrition or exercise. You may also refer to Chapter 8 for specific nutrition information.Do not forget relaxation. It is an important part of a healthy lifestyle. Try to manage stress. Prioritizing daily activities, making time for yourself each day, and exercising are three ways to help do so.

If you scored low in Part IV, the work section, remember that every job has its ups and downs. It may be necessary to evaluate your situation. Make a list of problems and possible solutions. By taking advantage of opportunities at work, you may be able to move into a job role that is more satisfying. This is important, since most adults spend at least 8 hours a day at work. Career counselors are one source of help available to you.

If you scored low in Part V, the tobacco, alcohol, and other substances section, you need to think seriously about the consequences of your actions. For example, when you choose to drink and drive, your actions affect other people. The same is true of smoking or using other substances. Give serious consideration to the outcomes of these behaviors. Not only are these actions detrimental to your health, they are potentially dangerous for others also. Consult your doctor or other health care specialist for advice. Other sources are listed in the telephone directory.

If you scored low in Part VI, the medical care section, remember that preventing disease is much more effective and less expensive in the long run than treating it. Look at the items with a score of 2 or less, and make a commitment to correct them. Taking care of yourself now is the first step toward preventing illness and disease.

◆ OCCUPANT AND RECREATIONAL SAFETY

	Always (3)	Often (2)	Rarely (1)	Never (–1)	N/A (0)
Part VII: Occupant Safety					
56. I wear a safety belt when driving or riding in a motor vehicle.	☐	☐	☐	☐	☐
57. I obey traffic laws.	☐	☐	☐	☐	☐
58. I honor pedestrian crosswalks.	☐	☐	☐	☐	☐
59. I drive anticipating the errors of others.	☐	☐	☐	☐	☐
60. I wear a helmet when I operate or ride on an open-motor vehicle such as a motorcycle or all-terrain vehicle (ATV).	☐	☐	☐	☐	☐
61. When going out, if I believe alcohol will be served, I make sure there is a designated driver.	☐	☐	☐	☐	☐
62. I ride only with a driver who is not under the influence of alcohol or other substances that impair judgment or reactions.	☐	☐	☐	☐	☐
63. I use turn indicators when turning or changing lanes.	☐	☐	☐	☐	☐
64. When driving, I try to leave adequate room between my car and the car in front of me.	☐	☐	☐	☐	☐
65. I obey traffic laws when cycling.	☐	☐	☐	☐	☐
66. I keep my vehicle in good working order and have it inspected regularly.	☐	☐	☐	☐	☐
Part VII: Subtotal ☐					
Part VIII: Recreational Safety					
67. I keep recreational equipment in good working condition.	☐	☐	☐	☐	☐
68. I wear a helmet when cycling.	☐	☐	☐	☐	☐
69. I wear protective equipment to prevent injury when participating in certain recreational activities.	☐	☐	☐	☐	☐

	Always (3)	Often (2)	Rarely (1)	Never (–1)	N/A (0)
70. I wear goggles when participating in sports such as racquetball, squash, or handball.	☐	☐	☐	☐	☐
71. I wear a life jacket (personal flotation device-PFD) when participating in water activities such as boating, fishing, and waterskiing.	☐	☐	☐	☐	☐
72. I make sure life jackets (PFDs) are worn by everyone on the boat.	☐	☐	☐	☐	☐
73. I know and follow the rules that govern my recreational activity.	☐	☐	☐	☐	☐
74. I participate in recreational activities at a level appropriate to my skills.	☐	☐	☐	☐	☐
75. I avoid swimming or diving after consuming alcoholic beverages or other substances that impair judgment or reactions.	☐	☐	☐	☐	☐

Part VIII: Subtotal ______

Add subtotals VII and VIII to determine your total score.

Total: OCCUPANT AND RECREATIONAL SAFETY

Occupant and Recreational Safety: Feedback

> **42** = You are actively tuned in to dangers on the road and at play. Pay attention to those behaviors for which you scored 2 or less. Turn these behaviors into healthy habits.

35 to 42 = You can benefit by paying more attention to safety on the road and at play. Focus on those behaviors for which you scored 2 or less. Decrease your chances of injury by making these behaviors a part of your healthy lifestyle.

21 to 34 = While you do pay attention to a few safety aspects on the road and at play, your current habits invite trouble. Safety procedures were designed to protect you. Improve any behaviors for which you scored 2 or less.

< **21** = Make a strong effort to incorporate safer habits into your lifestyle. Pay attention to all behaviors with a score of 2 or less.

If you scored low, you are putting yourself and those around you at unnecessary risk. Take measures now to correct those items scored 2 or less. Your local Department of Motor Vehicles or Public Safety and your insurance company should also be able to provide you with information about occupant safety.

If you scored low in Part VIII, the recreational safety section, remember that injury-prevention measures taken now can affect the rest of your life. In a split-second, an innocent mistake, such as not wearing the appropriate safety gear or not following the rules, can result in an injury that causes a lifelong disability. Consult your activity's rule book for rules to follow during participation. Ask a coach or reputable sporting goods dealer, or contact the organization that regulates your activity to find out about recommended protective gear, equipment, and conditioning exercises.

◆ HOME AND WORK SAFETY

	True (2)	False (−1)	N/A (0)
Part IX: Home Safety			
76. I post the local emergency number(s) near my telephone(s).	☐	☐	☐
77. I routinely maintain battery-operated smoke detectors where I live.	☐	☐	☐
78. The stairs where I live are equipped with handrails.	☐	☐	☐
79. All passageways where I live, including staircases, are adequately lighted.	☐	☐	☐
80. I keep all medicines safely and securely stored out of the reach of children.	☐	☐	☐
81. I make sure that all medicines are secured with childproof packaging and caps securely in place.	☐	☐	☐
82. I keep cleansers and other poisonous material safely and securely out of the reach of children and separate from medicines and foods.	☐	☐	☐
83. The heating and cooling systems where I live are kept in good working order.	☐	☐	☐
84. I read the manufacturer's instructions for tools and electrically operated appliances before operating.	☐	☐	☐
Part IX: Subtotal ☐			
Part X: Work Safety			
85. I follow safety procedures at work.	☐	☐	☐
86. I know fire evacuation procedures at work.	☐	☐	☐
87. I know the location of the nearest fire extinguisher at work.	☐	☐	☐
88. I can quickly obtain first aid supplies at work if necessary.	☐	☐	☐

	True (2)	False (−1)	N/A (0)
89. I know how to get professional medical help in the event of an emergency at work.	☐	☐	☐
90. I am aware of safety hazards that exist at work.	☐	☐	☐
91. I wear recommended safety equipment at work, such as protective shoes, hard hats, gloves, and goggles,and use proper barriers when giving emergency care.	☐	☐	☐
92. When lifting objects, I use proper lifting techniques.	☐	☐	☐
93. To obtain high, out-of-reach objects, I use a sturdy stool or stepladder.	☐	☐	☐
Part X: Subtotal ☐			

In parts IX and X, if you marked more than three responses N/A, give yourself 1 point for each N/A.

Add subtotals IX and X to determine your total score.

Total: HOME AND WORK SAFETY

Home and Work Safety: Feedback

> **28** = By following recommended safety practices, it looks as if you have made your home and workplace safe. A safe environment can prevent many mishaps. However, do not be lax. Change any behaviors with a score of less than 2 and try to anticipate the unexpected. Your awareness of safety is a positive example for those with whom you live and work.

13 to 28 = You have taken your first steps toward making your home and work environments safe. Give behaviors for which you scored less than 2 serious consideration. Then make changes to ensure a safe environment.

< **13** = Improving your safety practices at home and work would benefit your well-being as well as that of others around you. Changes you make to correct any behaviors with a score of less than 2 will help prevent disabling injuries or sudden illnesses.

If you scored low in Part IX, the home safety section, you should be able to immediately identify areas for improvement. Practicing home safety is critical to your well-being as well as to the well-being of those around you. If you have questions about specific ways to make your home safer, consult your phone directory for local resources or ask a librarian to direct you to information that may help you.

Work-related injuries are a major cause of death and permanent disability costing billions of dollars annually. Of the disabling work injuries, injuries to the back occur most frequently, according to state labor department reports.

If you scored low in Part X, the work safety section, you need to take steps to make your workplace safer. For your safety and the safety of others, know and follow your employer's regulations and recommendations.

SCORE CARD

Healthy Lifestyles Awareness Inventory

CARING FOR YOUR BODY

Part I: Nutrition	
Part II: Exercise	
Part III: Managing Stress	
Part IV: Work	
Part V: Alcohol, Tobacco, and Other Drugs	
Part VI: Medical Care	
Subtotal:	

OCCUPANT AND RECREATIONAL SAFETY

Part VII: Occupant Safety	
Part VIII: Recreational Safety	
Subtotal:	

HOME AND WORK SAFETY

Part IX: Home Safety	
Part X: Work Safety	
Subtotal:	
TOTAL SCORE:	

APPENDIX

C

Removing Gloves

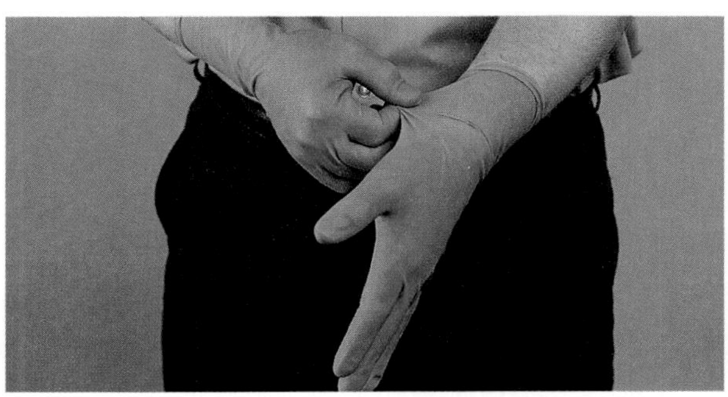

C-1. Pinch the glove at the wrist, being careful to touch only the glove's outside surface.

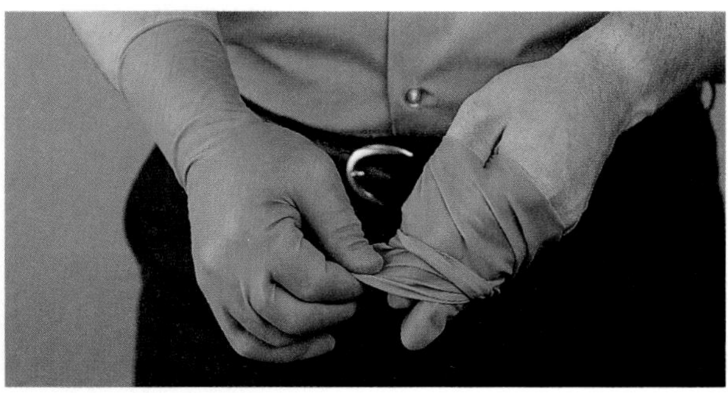

C-2. Pull the glove toward the fingertips without completely removing it.

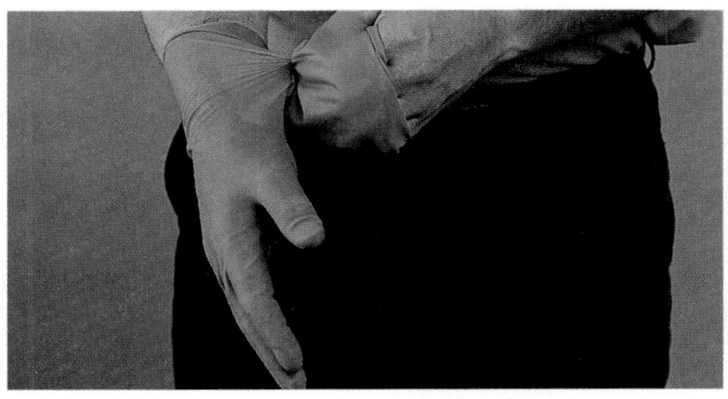

C-3. Pinch the exterior of the second glove at the wrist.

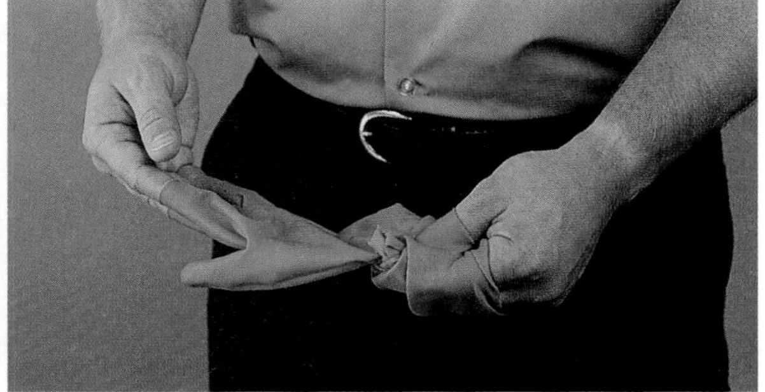

C-4. Pull the second glove toward the fingertips, then remove it completely.

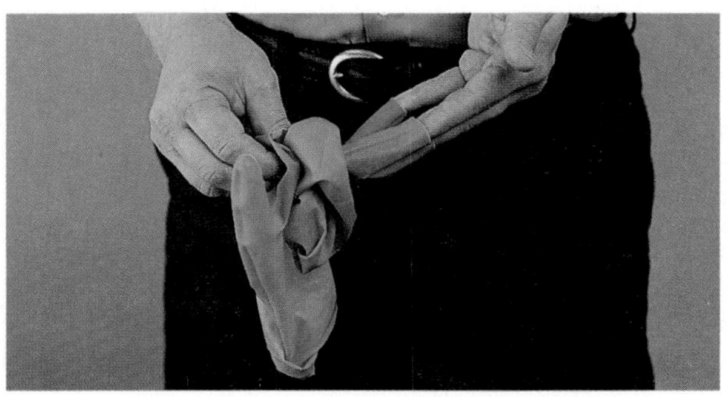

C-5. Finish removing both gloves.

Glossary

Pronunciation Guide

The accented syllable in a word is shown in capital letters.

river = RIV er

An unmarked vowel that ends a syllable or comprises a syllable has a long sound.

silent = SI lent

A long vowel in a syllable ending in a consonant is marked ¯.

snowflake = SNO flāk

An unmarked vowel in a syllable that ends with a consonant has a short sound.

sister = SIS ter

A *short vowel that comprises a syllable or ends a syllable is marked* ˘.

decimal = DES ĭmal

The sound of the letter **a** *in an unaccented syllable is spelled* **ah**.

ahea = ah HED

Abandonment: Ending the care of an ill or injured person without that person's consent or without ensuring that someone with equal or greater training will continue that care.

Abdomen: The part of the trunk below the ribs and above the pelvis.

Abdominal cavity: An area located in the trunk that contains the liver, pancreas, intestine, stomach and spleen; not protected by any bones.

Abdominal thrusts: A technique for unblocking an obstructed airway by forcefully pushing on the victim's abdomen.

Abrasion (ah BRA zhun): A wound characterized by skin that has been scraped or rubbed away.

Absorbed poison: A poison that enters the body through the skin.

Activated charcoal: A substance that prevents the absorption of poison into the body.

Active drowning victim: A person exhibiting

universal behavior that includes struggling at the surface for 20 to 60 seconds before submerging.

Active listening: A process that helps you more fully communicate with a victim by focusing on what the victim is saying.

Addiction: The compulsive need to use a substance. Stopping use would cause the user to suffer mental, physical, and emotional distress.

Advance directives: Written instructions from a physician that protect a victim's rights to refuse efforts to resuscitate him or her. *(See also do not resuscitate orders.)*

Advanced cardiac life support (ACLS): Techniques and treatments designed for use with victims of cardiac emergencies.

AIDS (acquired immunodeficiency syndrome): A result of infection caused by the human immunodeficiency virus (HIV).

Airborne transmission: The transmission of a disease by inhaling infected droplets that become airborne when an infected person coughs or sneezes.

Airway: The pathway for air from the mouth and nose to the lungs.

Airway obstruction: A blockage of the airway that prevents air from reaching a person's lungs.

Alveoli (al VE oli): Tiny air sacs in the lungs where gases and waste are exchanged between the lungs and the blood.

Alzheimer's disease: A progressive, degenerative disease that affects the brain. It results in impaired memory, thinking, and behavior.

Amniotic (am n̅e̅ OT ik) sac: A fluid-filled sac that encloses, bathes, and protects the developing baby; commonly called the bag of waters.

Amputation: The complete removal or severing of a body part.

Anaphylaxis (an ah fĭ LAK sis): A severe allergic reaction in which air passages may swell and restrict breathing; a form of shock.

Anaphylaxis kit: A container that holds the medication and any necessary equipment used to prevent or counteract anaphylactic shock.

Anatomical obstruction: The blockage of the airway by a bodily structure such as the tongue.

Anatomical position: A posture in which the body is standing, arms at the side, palms facing forward. All medical terms that refer to the body are based on this stance.

Anatomical splint: A splint that uses an uninjured body part to immobilize an injured body part.

Angina (an JI nah) pectoris: Chest pain that comes and goes at different times; commonly associated with cardiovascular disease.

Angulated: Bent at an unusual angle.

Angulation (AN gu lay shun): An angular shape.

Anorexia nervosa: A disorder characterized by a long-term refusal to eat food with sufficient nutrients and calories.

Anterior: Toward the front of the body.

Antibiotic: A medicine used to help the body fight bacterial infection.

Antibodies (AN tĭ bod ēz): Infection-fighting proteins released by white blood cells.

Antihistamines: Drugs used to treat the signs and symptoms of allergic reactions.

Antiinflammatory drugs: Substances used to reduce heat, swelling, redness, and pain in a body area.

Antiseptic: A substance that inhibits the growth and reproduction of microorganisms, or germs.

Arm: The upper extremity from the shoulder to the wrist.

Arteries (AR ter ez): The large blood vessels that carry oxygen-rich blood from the heart to all parts of the body, except for the pulmonary arteries, which carry oxygen-poor blood to the lungs from the heart.

Arthritis (ar THRI tis): An inflamed condition of the joints, causing pain and swelling and sometimes limiting motion.

Ashen: A grayish color that darker skin becomes when it turns pale.

Aspiration (as pĭ RA shun): Taking blood, vomit, saliva, or other foreign material into the lungs.

Assault: The threat of actual abuse, either physical or sexual, resulting in injury and often emotional crisis.

Asthma: A condition that narrows the air passages and makes breathing difficult.

Atherosclerosis (ath er o sklĕ RO sis): A form of cardiovascular disease marked by a narrowing of the arteries in the heart and other parts of the body.

Atrioventricular (AV) node: A point along the heart's electrical pathway midway between the atria and ventricles that sends electrical impulses to the ventricles.

Aura: An unusual sensation or feeling a person may experience before an epileptic seizure; it may be a visual hallucination; a strange sound, taste, or smell; or an urgent need to get to safety.

Auscultation (aws kul TA shun): The process of using a blood pressure cuff and a stethoscope to listen for characteristic blood pressure sounds.

Automated external defibrillator (AED): An automatic device used to recognize a heart rhythm that requires a shock and either delivers the shock or prompts the rescuer to deliver it.

Avulsion (ah VUL shun): A wound in which a portion of the skin, and sometimes other soft tissue, is partially or completely torn away.

Bacteria (bac TE rē ah): One-celled microorganisms capable of causing infections.

Bag-valve-mask (BVM) resuscitator: A hand-held breathing device, consisting of a self-inflating bag, a one-way valve, and a face mask; can be used with or without supplemental oxygen.

Bandage: Material used to wrap or cover a part of the body, commonly used to hold a dressing or splint in place.

Bandage compress: A thick gauze dressing attached to a gauze bandage.

Behavioral emergency: A situation in which a victim exhibits abnormal behavior that is unacceptable or intolerable.

Biohazard: A substance that may be contaminated by disease-causing organisms.

Biological death: The irreversible damage caused by the death of brain cells.

Birth canal: The passageway from the uterus to the vaginal opening through which a baby passes during birth.

Bladder: An organ in the pelvis in which urine is stored until released from the body.

Blanket drag: An emergency move in which the rescuer positions the victim on a blanket and walks backwards, pulling the blanket.

Blood pressure (BP): The force exerted by blood against the blood vessel walls as it travels through the body.

Blood pressure cuff: A device used to measure a person's blood pressure.

Blood volume: The total amount of blood circulating within the body.

Bloodborne pathogens: Bacteria and viruses present in human blood and other body fluids that can cause disease in humans.

Bloody show: Light vaginal bleeding that occurs during labor; sometimes signifies the onset of labor.

Body cavity: A hollow place in the body that contains organs, glands, blood vessels, and nerves.

Body substance isolation (BSI): An infection control concept that approaches all body substances as potentially infectious.

Body system: A group of organs and other structures working together to carry out specific functions.

Bone: Hard, dense tissue that forms the skeleton.

Brachial (BRA kē al) arteries: Large arteries located in the upper portion of each arm.

Brain: The center of the nervous system that controls all body functions.

Breathing devices: Equipment used to help with ventilation.

Breathing emergency: An emergency in which breathing is so impaired that life can be threatened; also called a respiratory emergency.

Breech birth: The delivery of a baby feet or buttocks first.

Bronchi (BRONG kī): The air passages that lead from the trachea to the lungs.

Bulimia: A condition in which victims gorge themselves with food, then purge by vomiting or using laxatives.

Burn: An injury to the skin or other body tissues caused by heat, chemicals, electricity, or radiation.

Cannabis products: Substances, such as marijuana and hashish, that are derived from the ***Cannabis sativa*** plant; can produce feelings of elation, distorted perceptions of time and space, and impaired motor coordination and judgment.

Capillaries (KAP ĭ ler ēz): Tiny blood vessels linking arteries and veins that transfer oxygen and other nutrients from the blood to all body cells and remove waste products.

Capillary refill: A technique for estimating how the body is reacting to illness or injury by checking the ability of the capillaries to fill with blood; an estimate of the amount of blood flowing through the capillary beds.

Carbon dioxide: A colorless, odorless gas; a waste product of respiration.

Carbon monoxide (CO): A colorless, odorless gas.

Cardiac arrest: A condition in which the heart has stopped or beats too irregularly or weakly to pump blood effectively.

Cardiac emergencies: Sudden illnesses involving the heart.

Cardiologist: A physician specializing in the diagnosis and treatment of heart disorders.

Cardiopulmonary resuscitation (kar de o PUL mo ner e) (re sus ĭ TA shun) (CPR): A technique that combines rescue breathing and chest compressions for a victim whose breathing and heart have stopped.

Cardiovascular (kar de o VAS ku lar) disease: A disease of the heart and blood vessels; commonly known as heart disease.

Carotid arteries: Arteries located in the neck that supply blood to the head and neck.

Carpals: Bones of the wrist.

Cartilage: An elastic tissue that acts as a shock absorber when a person is running, walking, or jumping.

Case law: A law based on judicial decisions (cases) rather than statutes, which are enacted by legislatures.

CAT scan: Computerized Axial Tomography; an x-ray technique that produces a film representing a detailed cross section of tissue structure.

Caustic: Eating away or destroying.

Cells: The basic units of all living tissue.

Cerebrospinal fluid (CSF): Fluid that circulates around the brain and spinal cord to cushion the brain.

Cervical collar: A ridged device positioned around the neck to limit movement of the head and neck.

Cervix: The upper part of the birth canal; the opening of the uterus.

Chain of survival: A basic principle of the emergency medical services system in which assistance begins with the recognition that an emergency exists.

Chemical burn: A burn caused by caustic chemicals, such as strong acids or alkalis.

Chest: The upper part of the trunk, containing the heart, major blood vessels, and lungs.

Chest thrusts: Forceful pushes on the chest delivered to a person with an obstructed airway in an attempt to expel any foreign object blocking the airway.

Child abuse: The physical, psychological, or sexual assault of a child, resulting in injury or emotional trauma.

Child neglect: Insufficient attention or respect given to a child who has a claim on that attention.

Chocking: The use of items, such as wooden blocks, placed against the wheels of the vehicle to help stabilize the vehicle.

Cholesterol (ko LES ter ol): A fatty substance made by the body and found in certain foods. Diets high in cholesterol contribute to the risk of heart disease.

Circulatory cycle: The flow of blood in the body; oxygen-rich blood flows through arteries and oxygen-poor blood flows in the veins.

Circulatory (SIR ku lă tor e) system: A group of organs and other structures that carries oxygen-rich blood and other nutrients throughout the body and removes waste.

Citizen responder: Someone who recognizes an emergency and decides to help; the first link in the emergency medical services (EMS) system.

Clavicle (KLAV ǐ kl): See collarbone.

Clinical death: The condition when the heart stops beating and breathing stops.

Closed bone injury: An injury that leaves the skin unbroken.

Closed wound: A wound in which soft tissue damage occurs beneath the skin and the skin is not broken.

Clotting: The process by which blood thickens at a wound site to seal an opening in a blood vessel and stop bleeding.

Collarbone: A horizontal bone that connects with the sternum and the shoulder; also called the clavicle.

Communicable disease: Disease capable of being transmitted, or passed, from people, objects, animals, or insects, directly or indirectly.

Competence: The victim's ability to understand the questions of the first responder and to understand the implications of decisions made.

Complete airway obstruction: A completely blocked airway.

Complex access: The process of using specialized tools or equipment to gain access to the victim.

Concussion: An injury to the brain caused by a violent blow to the head, followed by a temporary impairment of brain function, usually without permanent damage to the brain.

Confidentiality: Protecting a victim's privacy by not revealing any personal information you learn about the victim except to law enforcement personnel or EMS personnel caring for the victim.

Consciousness: The state of being aware of one's self and one's surroundings.

Consent: Permission to provide care, given by an ill or injured person to a rescuer.

Contraction: The pumping action of the heart; the rhythmic tightening of muscles in the uterus during labor.

Coronary arteries: Blood vessels that supply the heart muscle with oxygen-rich blood.

Corrosive substance: A substance that eats away or destroys, such as a acid.

Corticosteroid: A hormone, made synthetically or in the body, that is used in antiinflamatory medications.

Cranial cavity: An area in the head that contains the brain and is protected by the skull.

Cravat: A triangular bandage folded to form a long, narrow strip.

Critical burn: Any burn that is potentially life-threatening, disabling, or disfiguring; a burn that requires medical attention.

Critical Incident Stress Debriefing (CISD): A process by which emergency personnel are offered the support necessary to reduce stress after a significant incident.

Croup: A respiratory infection that occurs mainly in children and infants.

Crowning: The time in labor when the baby's head is seen at the opening of the vagina.

Cumulative stress: An accumulation of stress over a period of time.

Cyanosis (si ah NO sis): A blue discoloration of the skin and mucous membranes of the mouth and eyes, resulting from a lack of oxygen in the blood.

Defibrillation: An electric shock delivered to

the heart to correct certain life-threatening heart rhythms.

Defibrillator (de FIB rĭ la tor): A device that sends an electric shock through the chest to the heart.

Dehydration: An abnormal depletion of body fluids.

Dentures: A set of false teeth.

Dependency: The desire or need to continually use a substance.

Depressants: Substances that affect the central nervous system to slow physical and mental activity.

Dermis (DER mis): The deeper of the two layers of skin.

Designated officer: An employer representative responsible for maintaining records and monitoring exposure incidents.

Designer drug: A potent and illegal street drug formed from a medicinal substance whose chemical composition has been modified (designed).

Developmentally disabled: A term referring to a person with impaired mental function, resulting from injury or genetics.

Diabetic (di ah BET Ik): A person with the condition called diabetes mellitus, which causes a body to produce insufficient amounts of the hormone insulin.

Diabetic coma: A life-threatening emergency in which the body needs insulin.

Diabetic emergency: A situation in which a person becomes ill because of an imbalance of insulin and sugar in the bloodstream.

Diastolic (di as TOL ik) blood pressure: The pressure in the arteries when the heart is at rest.

Digestive system: A group of organs and other structures that work together to break down food, absorb nutrients, and eliminate wastes.

Direct carry: A move in which two rescuers supporting the victim's head, shoulders, waist, and hips lift and move the victim from a bed to a stretcher.

Direct contact transmission: The transmission of a disease from touching an infected person's body fluids or other agents, such as chemicals, drugs, or toxins.

Direct lift: An emergency move in which three rescuers lift and move the victim.

Direct medical control: A type of medical oversight, also called "on-line," "base-station," "immediate," or " concurrent medical control. The physician speaks directly with emergency care providers at the scene of an emergency.

Direct pressure: The pressure applied on a wound to control bleeding.

Disease transmission: The passage of a disease from one person to another.

Disks: Flat, circular, cushions of cartilage between the vertebrae.

Dislocation: The displacement of a bone from its normal position at a joint.

Disoriented: A state of mental confusion; not knowing place, identity, or what happened.

Distal: Away from the trunk of the body.

Distressed swimmer: A person capable of staying afloat but likely to need assistance to get to safety.

Do Not Resuscitate (DNR) order: A physician's order, issued after consulting with a patient or surrogate decision maker, to withhold resuscitation efforts.

Draw sheet: A method of transferring a victim from a stretcher to a bed by moving the victim on a sheet.

Dressing: A pad placed directly over a wound to absorb blood and other body fluids and to prevent infection.

Drowning: Death by suffocation when submerged in water.

Drug: Any substance other than food intended to affect the functions of the body.

Drug paraphernalia: Devices used to contain or administer drugs.

Duty to act: A legal responsibility of some individuals to provide a reasonable standard of emergency care that may be required by case law, statute, or job description.

Elastic bandage: A stretchable bandage used to

maintain continuous pressure on a body part.

Electrical burn: A burn caused by an electrical source, such as an electrical appliance or lightning.

Electrocardiogram (ECG): A graphic record produced by a device that records the electrical activity of the heart from the chest.

Electrocardiograph: A device used to record the electric activity of the heart; a cardiac monitor.

Embedded object: A foreign body that remains in an open wound.

Embolism: An abnormal circulatory condition in which a clot or other material, such as fat or air, becomes lodged in a blood vessel.

Embryo (EM bre o): The early stages of a developing ovum; characterized by the rapid growth and development of body systems.

Emergency medical dispatcher (EMD): An employee who has received special training for giving medical instructions to victims or bystanders before the arrival of more advanced medical personnel.

Emergency medical services (EMS) system: A network of community resources and medical personnel that provides emergency care to victims of injury or sudden illness.

Emergency medical technician (EMT): Someone who successfully completed a state-approved Emergency Medical Technician training program. The different levels of EMTs include paramedics at the highest level.

Emergency move: Transferring a victim before completing care if the victim is in immediate danger.

Emotional crisis: A highly distressed state resulting from stress, often involving a significant event in a person's life, such as death of a loved one.

Emphysema: A disease in which the lungs lose their ability to exchange carbon dioxide and oxygen effectively.

Endocrine (EN do krin) system: A group of organs and other structures that regulates and coordinates the activities of other systems by producing chemicals that influence tissue activity.

Engineering controls: Safeguards intended to isolate or remove a hazard from the workplace.

Enhanced 9-1-1 (E-911) system: A state-of-the art emergency call-taking system that displays information on a computer screen showing the name, address, and phone number where the call for help originated.

Epidermis (ep ĭ DER mis): The outer layer of skin.

Epiglottis (ep ĭ GLOT is): The flap of tissue that covers the trachea to keep food and liquid out of the lungs.

Epilepsy (EP ĭ lep se): A chronic condition characterized by seizures that vary in type and duration; usually can be controlled by medication.

Esophagus (e SOF ah gus): The tube leading from the mouth to the stomach.

Exhale: To breathe air out of the lungs.

Exposure control plan The method by which an employer creates a system to protect its employees from infection.

Expressed consent: *see informed consent.*

External bleeding: Visible bleeding.

Extremity lift: An emergency move in which two rescuers place their arms under the arms and knees of the victim and lift and move the victim.

Extrication: The removal of a victim trapped in a motor vehicle or in a dangerous situation.

Fainting: A loss of consciousness resulting from a temporary reduction of blood flow to the brain.

Febrile seizure: Seizure activity brought on by an excessively high fever in an infant or young child.

Femoral (FEM or al) artery: The large artery that supplies the leg with oxygen-rich blood.

Femur (FE mur): The thigh bone.

Fetus (FE tus): The developing unborn offspring after the embryonic period.

Fibula (FIB u lah): One of the bones in the lower leg.

Finger sweep: A technique used to remove foreign material from a victim's airway.

Fire fighter's carry: An emergency move used to quickly move a victim, carried across the rescuer's shoulders, from a dangerous situation; not appropriate for victims with a suspected head, spine, or abdominal injury.

First responder: A person trained in emergency care who may be called on to provide such care as a routine part of his or her job, paid or volunteer; often the first trained professional to respond to emergencies.

Flail chest: An injury involving fractured ribs that do not move normally with the rest of the chest during breathing.

Flow rate: The rate that oxygen is administered to a victim, measured in liters per minute (lpm).

Flowmeter: A device used to regulate in liters per minute (lpm) the amount of oxygen administered to a person.

Foot drag: An emergency move in which the rescuer grasps the victim's ankles and pulls the victim.

Forearm: The upper extremity from the elbow to the wrist.

Fracture: A break or disruption in bone tissue.

Full-thickness burn: A burn injury involving both layers of skin and underlying tissues; skin may be brown or charred, and underlying tissues may appear white, also referred to as a third-degree burn.

Fumes: An often noxious suspension of particles in a gas.

Gag reflex: Contraction of the throat muscles and retraction of the tongue brought on by touching the back of the throat.

Gastric distention: Air in the stomach.

Genitalia: The external reproductive organs.

Genitourinary (jeni to U ri ner e) system: A group of organs and other structures that eliminates waste and enables reproduction.

Glands: Organs that release fluid and other substances into the blood or on the skin.

Glucose: A simple sugar found in certain foods, especially fruits, and a major source of energy occurring in human and animal body fluids.

Good Samaritan laws: Laws that protect people who willingly give emergency care without accepting anything in return.

Hallucinogens (hah LU sǐ no jenz): Substances that affect mood, sensation, thought, emotion, and self-awareness; alter perceptions of time and space; and produce delusions.

Hazardous material (HAZMAT): Any chemical substance or material that can pose a threat to health, safety, and property.

Hazardous material incident: Any situation that deals with the unplanned release of hazardous material.

Head-tilt/chin-lift: A technique for opening the airway in which the forehead is tilted back and the chin is lifted.

Hearing impaired: A nonspecific term applied to a person who is either deaf or partially deaf.

Heart: A fist-sized muscular organ that pumps blood throughout the body.

Heart attack: A sudden illness resulting from death of heart muscle tissue when it does not receive enough oxygen-rich blood.

Heaving line: Floating rope, white, yellow, or some other highly visible color, used for water rescue.

Heimlich maneuver: A technique used to clear the airway of a choking victim; see *Abdominal thrusts.*

Hemorrhage (HEM or ij): A loss of a large amount of blood in a short time.

Hepatitis (hep ah TI tis): An inflammation of the liver.

Herpes (HER pēz) simplex: A viral simplex infection that causes eruptions of the skin and mucous membranes.

HIV (human immunodeficiency virus): A virus that destroys the body's ability to fight infection. A result of HIV infection is referred to as AIDS.

Hormone: A substance that circulates in body

fluids and has a specific effect on cell activity.

Humerus (HU mer us): The bone of the upper arm.

Hyperextend: To extend as far as possible.

Hyperglycemia (hi per gli SE me ah): A condition in which too much sugar is in the bloodstream.

Hypertension: High blood pressure.

Hyperventilation: Breathing that is faster than normal.

Hypoglycemia (hi po gli SE me ah): A condition in which too little sugar is in the bloodstream.

Hypoperfusion: A condition in which the circulatory system fails to adequately circulate oxygen-rich blood to all parts of the body. See also *shock.*

Hypoxia (hy POK se ah): A condition in which insufficient oxygen reaches the cells, resulting in cyanosis and in changes in consciousness and in breathing and heart rates.

Immobilize: To use a splint or other method to keep an injured body part from moving.

Immune system: The body's group of responses for fighting disease.

Immunization (im u nǐ ZA shun): A specific substance containing weakened or killed pathogens introduced into the body to build resistance to specific infection.

Implied consent: A legal concept assuming that persons who are unconscious, or so severely injured or ill that they cannot respond, would consent to receive emergency care.

In-line stabilization: A technique used to minimize movement of the victim's head and neck.

Incident command system (ICS): A system used to manage resources, such as personnel, equipment, and supplies, at the scene of an emergency.

Incident commander: The person in the incident command system ultimately responsible for managing and directing an emergency response.

Indirect contact transmission: The spreading of a disease by touching a contaminated object.

Indirect medical control: A type of medical oversight, also called "off-line," "retrospective," or "prospective" medical control. Indirect medical control includes education, protocol review, and quality improvement of emergency care providers.

Infection: A condition caused by disease-producing microorganisms, called pathogens or germs, in the body.

Infectious disease: Disease caused by the invasion of the body by a pathogen, such as a bacterium, virus, fungus, or parasite.

Inferior: Toward the feet.

Informed (actual) consent: Permission the victim, parent, or guardian gives the rescuer to provide care. This consent requires the rescuer to explain his or her level of training, what the rescuer thinks is wrong, and the care the rescuer intends to give.

Ingested poison: A poison that is swallowed.

Inhalants: Substances, such as a medication, that a person inhales to counteract or prevent a specific condition; substances inhaled to produce a mood-altering effect.

Inhale: To breathe in.

Inhaled poison: A poison breathed into the lungs.

Initial assessment: A check for conditions that are an immediate threat to a victim's life.

Injected poison: A poison that enters the body through a bite, sting, or syringe.

Insulin: A hormone produced in the pancreas that enables the body to use sugar (glucose) for energy; frequently used to treat diabetes.

Insulin reaction: A potentially life-threatening condition in which too much sugar is in the bloodstream.

Integumentary (in teg u MEN tar e) system: A group of organs and other structures that protects the body, retains fluids, and helps to prevent infection. It consists of the skin, hair, and nails.

Internal bleeding: Bleeding inside the body.

Involuntary muscles: Body structures like the heart and intestines that are automatically controlled by the brain.

Jaw thrust: A technique for opening the airway in which the rescuer places the fingers behind the angle of the jaw and brings the jaw forward.

Job burnout: A condition in which a person may feel frustrated, overwhelmed, or unhappy about continuing in his or her present employment.

Joint: A structure where two or more bones are joined.

Kapok: A fiber used to fill life jackets and other floating devices.

Ketoacidosis: An increased acidity level in the blood.

Kidney: An organ that filters waste from the blood to form urine.

Labor: The birth process; beginning with the contraction of the uterus and dilation of the cervix and ending with the birth of the baby; followed by the stabilization of the mother.

Laceration (las e RA shun): A cut, usually from a sharp object; may have jagged or smooth edges.

Larynx (LAR ingks): A part of the airway connecting the pharynx with the trachea; commonly called the "voice box."

Lateral: Away from the midline.

Left atrium: The upper left chamber of the heart, where oxygen-rich blood returns from the lungs.

Left ventricle: The lower left chamber of the heart, where oxygen-rich blood is pumped to all parts of the body.

Leg: The lower extremity.

Level of consciousness (LOC): A person's state of awareness, ranging from being fully alert to unconscious; also referred to as mental status.

Ligament (LIG ah ment): A fibrous band that holds bones together at a joint.

Liver: An organ located in the abdomen that has many functions, such as causing important changes in many substances in the blood.

Lividity: Following death, a large pooling of blood in the trunk resulting in discoloration.

Logistics section officer: A leadership position in the incident command system; this person is responsible for establishing communication, coordinating crowd control, and evaluating the scene if necessary

Lower leg: The lower extremity between the knee and the ankle.

Lungs: A pair of organs in the chest that provides the mechanism for taking oxygen in and removing carbon dioxide during breathing.

Lyme disease: An illness transmitted by a certain kind of infectious tick; victims may or may not develop a rash.

Mania: Excitement shown by mental and physical hyperactivity.

Mechanical obstruction: The blockage of the airway by a foreign object, such as food, a toy, or fluids.

Mechanism of injury: The force or energy that causes a traumatic injury.

Medial: Closer to the midline.

Medical director: A physician who assumes the responsibility for care given in the out-of-hospital setting to ill or injured victims.

Medical oversight: The monitoring of care given by out-of-hospital providers to ill or injured victims; usually done by the medical director.

Medication: A drug given to prevent or correct the effects of a disease or condition or otherwise enhance mental or physical welfare.

Meningitis (men in JI tis): An inflammation of the brain or spinal cord caused by a viral or bacterial infection.

Mentally disabled: A term referring to a person who has an impairment of mental function that interferes with normal activity.

Metabolism: The process by which all cells convert nutrients to energy.

Metacarpal: Bones of the hand and fingers.

Metatarsals: Bones of the foot and toes.

Microorganism (mi kro OR gah nǐzm): A bacterium, virus, or other microscopic organism that may enter the body. Those that cause an infection or disease are called germs.

Midline: An imaginary line that runs down the middle of the body from the head to the ground, dividing the body into left and right halves.

Minors: People who not reached legal age.

Miscarriage (spontaneous abortion): A spontaneous end to pregnancy before the twentieth week; usually because of defects of the fetus or placenta.

Multiple casualty incident (MCI): An emergency situation involving two or more victims.

Muscle: A tissue that lengthens and shortens to create movement.

Musculoskeletal (mus Ku lo SKEL ĕ tal) system: A group of tissues and other structures that supports the body, protects internal organs, allows movement, stores minerals, manufactures blood cells, and creates heat.

Narcotics: Powerful depressant substances used to reduce pain.

Nasal airway: A soft, flexible tube inserted into a nostril and positioned at the back of the throat to keep the tongue from blocking the airway; also called a nasopharyngeal airway.

Nasal cannula: A device used to administer oxygen through the nostrils to a breathing person.

Nature of illness: The type of medical condition or complaint a victim has.

Near-drowning: A situation in which a person who has been submerged in water survives.

Negligence: The failure to provide the level of care a person of similar training would provide, thereby causing injury or damage to another.

Nerve: A part of the nervous system that send impulses to and from the brain and all other body parts.

Nervous system: A group of organs and other structures that regulates all body function.

Neurosurgeon: A physician who performs operations on the brain, spinal cord, or peripheral nerves.

Nonrebreather mask: A type of oxygen mask used to administer high concentrations of oxygen to a breathing person.

Nonverbal communication: Expressing oneself through body actions, such as assuming a non-threatening posture or using hand gestures.

Normal sinus rhythm: A regular heart rhythm that occurs within a normal rate, 60 to 100 beats per minute (bpm), and without usual variations.

Occlusive (o KLOO siv) dressing: A dressing that does not allow air to pass through it.

Ongoing assessment: The process of repeating the initial assessment and physical exam while awaiting the arrival of more highly trained personnel.

Open bone injury: An injury that causes a break in the continuity of the skin.

Open wound: A wound resulting in a break in the skin surface.

Operations section officer: The person in the incident command system responsible for developing the tactics to carry out the strategy.

Opportunistic infections: Infections that strike people whose immune systems are weakened by HIV or other infections.

Oral airway: A curved plastic tube inserted into the mouth and positioned at the back of the throat to keep the tongue from blocking the airway, also called an oropharyngeal airway.

Organ: A collection of similar tissues acting together to perform specific body functions.

Orthopedic surgeon: A physician specializing in the diagnosis and treatment of musculoskeletal injuries.

Osteoporosis (os te o po RO sis): The progressive weakening of bone.

Out-of-hospital care: A term used interchangeably with "prehospital care," treatment given before the victim arrives at a hospital.

Overdose: The use of an excessive amount of a substance, resulting in adverse reactions ranging from mania (physical and mental hyperactivity) and hysteria to coma and death.

Oxygen: A tasteless, colorless, odorless gas necessary to sustain life.

Oxygen cylinder: A steel or alloy container that holds 100 percent oxygen under high pressure.

Oxygen delivery devices: Apparatus of various types used to administer oxygen from a cylinder to either a breathing or nonbreathing person.

Pack-strap carry: An emergency move in which the victim is supported by the rescuer's back that can be used on both conscious or unconscious victims; leaves one hand free.

Packaging: The steps involved in preparing a victim to be moved and moving the victim onto the device to support the victim during transport.

Painful, swollen, deformed extremities (PSD extremity): All injuries to the extremities caused by a force.

Palpate: To feel.

Palpation (pal PA shun): A technique requiring you to feel with your hand for the radial pulse when taking a person's blood pressure.

Paralysis: A loss of muscle control; a permanent loss of feeling and movement.

Paramedics (EMT-P): Highly trained EMTs who are authorized to administer medications and intravenous fluids and deliver advanced care for breathing problems and abnormal heart rhythms. They serve as the out-of-hospital extension of the emergency physician.

Paraphernalia: Devices; articles of equipment.

Paraprofessionals: Workers who are not members of a profession but who assist professionals.

Partial airway obstruction: An incomplete blockage of the airway.

Partial-thickness burn: A burn injury involving both layers of skin characterized by red, wet skin and blisters; also referred to as a second-degree burn.

Patella (pah TEL ah): The kneecap.

Pathogen (PATH o jen): A disease-causing agent; also called a microorganism or germ.

Pelvic cavity: The lowest part of the trunk that contains the bladder, rectum, and the reproductive organs in females.

Pericardial fluid: Fluid that lubricates the thin membrane surrounding the heart.

Peritoneal fluid: Fluid in the abdominal cavity that lubricates surfaces between organs.

Phalanges: Bones of the fingers.

Pharynx (FAR ingks): A part of the airway formed by the back of the nose and throat.

Physical assault: Abuse that may result in bodily injury.

Physical exam: Examination performed after the initial assessment; used to gather additional information and identify signs and symptoms of injury and illness.

Physically disabled: A term referring to a person who sustains a serious injury that results in the loss of body function or someone who is born with an impairment that interferes with normal activity.

Placards: Posters; signs.

Placenta (plah SEN tah): An organ attached to the uterus and unborn child through which nutrients are delivered to the fetus; expelled after the baby is delivered.

Planning section officer: A leadership position in the incident command system This person is responsible for keeping the incident commander updated as to the status of the incident.

Plasma: The liquid part of the blood.

Platelets: Disk-shaped structures in the blood that are made of cell fragments; help stop bleeding by forming blood clots at wound sites.

Pleural fluid: Fluid that acts as a lubricant as the lungs expand and contract during breathing.

Poison: Any substance that causes injury, illness, or death when introduced into the body.

Poison control center (PCC): A specialized health center that provides information in poisoning or suspected poisoning emergencies.

Posterior: Toward the back of the body.

Pregnancy: A condition in which the egg (ovum) of the female is fertilized by the sperm of the male, forming an embryo.

Pressure bandage: A bandage applied snugly to create pressure on a wound to aid in controlling bleeding.

Pressure points: Sites on the body where pressure can be applied to major arteries to slow the flow of blood to a body part.

Pressure regulator: A device attached to an oxygen cylinder that reduces the delivery pressure of oxygen to a safe level.

Prolapsed cord: A complication of childbirth in which a loop of umbilical cord protrudes through the vaginal opening before the delivery of the baby.

Protocols: Standardized procedures to be followed when providing care to victims of illness or injury.

Proximal: Closer to the trunk of the body.

Public safety personnel: People employed in a governmental system who are required to respond to and assist with a medical emergency. These typically include police officers, fire fighters, and ambulance crew members.

Pulse: The beat felt in arteries with each contraction of the heart.

Puncture: A wound that results when the skin is pierced with a pointed object, such as a nail, a piece of glass, or a knife.

Rabies: A disease transmitted through the saliva and urine of diseased mammals.

Radial pulse: The pulse felt in the wrist.

Radiation burn: A burn caused by rays, energy, or electromagnetic waves.

Radius: One of the bones of the forearm, lying parallel to the ulna.

Rape: A crime of violence or one committed under threat of violence involving a sexual attack.

Reasonable force: The minimal force necessary to keep a victim from injuring himself or herself and you or others.

Recovery position: A posture used to help maintain a clear airway in a victim with a decreased level of consciousness who has not sustained traumatic injuries and is breathing.

Refusal of care: The declining of care by a victim. A victim has the right to refuse the care of anyone who responds to an emergency scene.

Rehabilitation: The final link in the chain of survival, in which a victim of illness or injury is restored to normal or near normal health.

Reproductive system: A group of organs and other structures that enables sexual reproduction.

Rescue breathing: A technique of breathing for a nonbreathing victim.

Respiration: The breathing process.

Respiratory arrest: A condition in which breathing has stopped.

Respiratory distress: A condition in which breathing is difficult.

Respiratory (re SPI rah to re or RES pah rah tor e) system: A group of organs and other structures that brings air into the body and removes wastes through a process called breathing, or respiration.

Resuscitation mask: A pliable, dome-shaped device that fits over the nose and mouth; used to administer oxygen and assist with rescue breathing.

Retraction: A visible sinking in of soft tissue between the ribs of an infant or child.

Reye's syndrome: An illness brought on by high fever that affects the brain and other internal organs.

Ribs: Bones that attach to the spine and sternum and protect the heart and lungs.

Right atrium: The upper right chamber of the heart, which receives oxygen-depleted blood from the veins of the body.

Right ventricle: The lower right chamber of the heart, which pumps oxygen-depleted blood to the lungs where waste products are removed and oxygen absorbed.

Rigid splints: A splint made of boards, metal strips, and folded magazines or newspaper.

Rigor mortis: The rigid stiffening of heart and skeletal muscle after death.

Ring buoy: A rescue device made of buoyant

cork, kapok, or plastic-covered material attached to a line with an object or knot at the end to keep the line from slipping out from under your foot when you throw the buoy.

Risk factors: Conditions or behaviors that increase the chance that a person will develop a disease.

Rocky Mountain spotted fever (RMSF): A disease transmitted by a certain kind of infected tick; victims develop a spotted rash.

Roller bandage: A bandage usually made of gauze or gauzelike material used to wrap around a dressing.

Salmonella: A common cause of food poisoning, caused by a bacteria most commonly found in poultry or raw eggs.

SAMPLE history: A victim's history, comprised of Signs and symptoms, Allergies, Medications, Pertinent past history, Last oral intake, and Events leading to the incident.

Saturated fat: Fat derived from animal products; a solid at room temperature.

Scapula (SKAP u lah): *See shoulder blade.*

Scope of practice: The range of duties and skills a first responder is allowed and expected to perform when necessary.

Seizure (SE zhur): A disorder in the brain's electrical activity, usually marked by loss of consciousness and often uncontrollable muscle movement.

Septum: The wall of tissue that separates the nostrils.

Sexual assault: Forcing another person to take part in a sexual act.

Shepherd's crook: A aluminum or fiberglass pole with a large hook on one end.

Shock: The failure of the circulatory system to provide adequate oxygen-rich blood to all parts of the body. *See also hypoperfusion.*

Shoulder blade: A large, flat , triangular bone at the back of the shoulder in the upper part of the back; also called the scapula.

Shoulder drag: An emergency move in which the rescuer reaches under the victim's armpits, grasps the victim's forearms, and pulls the victim.

Signs: Any observable evidence of injury or illness, such as bleeding or unusual skin color.

Sinoatrial (SA) node: The origin of the heart's electric impulse.

Simple access: The process of gaining access to a victim without the use of equipment.

Skeletal muscles: Muscles that attach to bones.

Skeleton: The 206 bones of the body that protect vital organs and other soft tissue.

Sling: A bandage or device used to hold or support an injured part of the body; often used to support an injured arm.

Soft tissues: Body structures that include the layers of skin, fat, and muscles.

Spasm: Contract abnormally.

Spinal column: The series of vertebrae extending from the base of the skull to the tip of the tailbone (coccyx).

Spinal cavity: An area that extends from the bottom of the skull to the lower back that contains the spinal cord and is protected by the bones of the spine.

Spinal cord: A cylindrical structure extending from the base of the skull to the lower back, consisting mainly of nerve cells and protected by the spinal column.

Spine: A strong, flexible column of vertebrae, extending from the base of the skull to the tip of the tailbone.

Spleen: An organ in the abdomen, one function is to store blood.

Splint: A device used to immobilize body parts; to support or immobilize a body part using a device or part of the body.

Spontaneous abortion: The spontaneous termination of pregnancy before the fetus is born.

Sprain: The excessive stretching and tearing of ligaments and other soft tissue structures at a joint.

Standard of care: The criterion established for the extent and quality of a first responder's care.

Standard precautions: Safety measures, such as body substance isolation, taken to prevent occupational-risk exposure to blood or other potentially infectious materials, such as body fluids containing visible blood.

Standing orders: Protocols issued by the medical director that allow specific skills to be performed or specific medications administered in certain situations.

START (Simple Triage and Rapid Treatment) system: A system used at the scene of multiple casualty incidents to quickly assess and prioritize care according to three conditions: breathing, circulation, and level of consciousness.

Starting blocks: Platforms competitve swimmers dive from to start a race.

Statute: A written law; a law enacted by a legislature.

Sternum: The long, flat bone in the middle of the front of the rib cage; also called the breastbone.

Stethoscope (STETH o skōp): An instrument used to hear heart and lung sounds and to determine the systolic and diastolic blood pressure.

Stimulants: Substances that affect the central nervous system to speed up physical and mental activity.

Stoma: An opening in the front of the neck through which a person whose larynx has been removed breathes.

Stomach: One of the main organs of digestion, located in the abdomen.

Strain: The excessive stretching and tearing of muscles and tendons.

Stress: The body's normal response to any situation that changes a person's existing mental, physical, or emotional balance.

Stroke: A disruption of blood flow to a part of the brain that causes permanent damage; also called a cerebrovascular accident (CVA) or TIA. *See transient ischemic attack.*

Substance abuse: The deliberate, persistent, excessive use of a substance without regard to health concerns or accepted medical practices.

Substance misuse: The use of a substance for unintended purpose or for intended purposes but in improper amounts or doses.

Sucking chest wound: An injury in which the chest cavity is punctured, allowing air to pass freely in and out.

Suction tip: A rigid or flexible tubing attached to the end of a suction device and placed in the mouth of a person to remove foreign matter.

Suctioning: The process of removing matter such as saliva, vomit, or blood from a person's mouth and throat by means of a mechanical or manual device.

Sudden death: Death resulting from unforeseen cardiac arrest.

Sudden infant death syndrome (SIDS): The sudden death of an infant under 1 year of age that remains unexplained after the performance of a complete postmortem investigation, including an autopsy, an examination of the scene of death, and review of the care history.

Suicide: Self-inflicted death.

Superficial burn: A burn injury involving only the top layer of skin, characterized by red, dry skin, also referred to as a first-degree burn.

Superior: Toward the head of the body.

Supplemental oxygen: Additional oxygen provided to help resuscitate a person.

Symptoms: What the victim tell you about his or her condition, such as pain, nausea, headache, or shortness of breath.

Synergistic effect: A heightened or exaggerated effect produced when two or more substances are used at the same time.

Synovial fluid: A transparent, viscous fluid secreted by synovial membranes that lubricates many joints, bursae, and tendons. It resembles the white of an egg.

Syrup of ipecac: An expectorant used to induce vomiting.

Systolic (sis TOL ik) blood pressure: The pressure in the arteries when the heart is contracting.

Tarsals: Bones of the foot.

Tendon (TEN don): A fibrous band of tissue that attaches muscle to bone.

Tetanus: An acute infectious disease caused by

a bacteria that produces a powerful poison; can occur in puncture wounds, such as human and animal bites; also called lockjaw.

Thigh: The lower extremity between the pelvis and the knee.

Thoracic (tho RAS ik) cavity: An area in the body that contains the heart and lungs and is protected by the rib cage and upper portion of the spine.

Thrombus: A collection of blood components that forms in the heart vessels, obstructing blood flow.

Throw bag: A water rescue device composed of a nylon bag with 50 to 75 feet of coiled, floating line and a foam disk to keep the bag from sinking.

Tibia (TIB e ah): One of the bones in the lower leg.

Tissue: A collection of similar cells acting together to perform specific body functions.

Tolerance: A condition in which the effects of an substance or the body decreases as a result of continual use.

Tourniquet (TOOR ni ket): A tight band placed around an arm or leg to constrict blood vessels to stop the flow of blood to a wound.

Toxic: Relating to or caused by a poison.

Toxins: Poisonous substances produced by certain living organisms.

Trachea (TRA ke ah): A tube leading from the upper airway to the lungs; also called the windpipe.

Traction splint: A special type of splinting device used primarily to immobilize fractures of the thigh.

Transient ischemic (Tranz e ent is KE mik) attack (TIA): A temporary disruption of blood flow to the brain; sometimes called a ministroke.

Trauma: Physical injury caused by shock, pressure, or violence.

Trauma surgeon: A physician who performs operations on patients who have suffered serious, unexpected injuries.

Triage: The process of sorting and providing care to multiple victims according to the severity of their unjuries or illnesses.

Triangular bandage: A bandage that can be used as a sling or to hold a dressing or splint in place.

Tuberculosis (tu ber Ku LO sis): A disease, commonly respiratory, caused by a bacterium.

Turnout gear: Puncture and flame-resistant outerwear.

Two-person seat carry: A method for moving a victim that requires a second rescuer; should not be used on a victim with suspected head or spine injury.

Ulna: The bone on the medial, or little finger, side of the forearm, lying parallel to the radius.

Umbilical (um BIL ǐ kal) cord: A flexible structure that attaches the placenta to the unborn child, allowing for the passage of blood, nutrients, and waste.

Universal dressing: A bulky dressing used to cover large wounds or multiple wounds in one area.

Upper arm: The upper extremity between the shoulder and the elbow.

Upper extremities: The arms and hands.

Urinary system: A group of organs and other structures that eliminates waste products from the blood.

Uterus (U ter us): A pear-shaped organ in a woman's pelvis in which an embryo is formed and develops into a baby.

Vagina (vah JI nah): *See Birth canal.*

Vapors: Diffused matter (as smoke or fog) suspended floating in the air.

Vector transmission: The transmission of a disease by an animal or insect bite through exposure to blood or other body fluids.

Veins: Blood vessels that carry oxygen-poor blood from all parts of the body to the heart, except for the pulmonary veins, which carry oxygen-rich blood to the heart from the lungs.

Ventilation: The process of providing oxygen to the lungs.

Ventricles (VEN tri kelz): The two lower chambers of the heart.

Ventricular fibrillation: A life-threatening

heart rhythm; a state of totally disorganized electrical activity in the heart.

Ventricular tachycardia: A life-threatening heart rhythm in which there is a very rapid contraction of the ventricles.

Vertebrae (VER tĕ bra): The 33 bones of the spinal column.

Vertebral column: *See spinal column.*

Viruses (VI rus ez): Disease-causing agents, or pathogens. Unlike bacteria, they require another organism to live and reproduce.

Visually impaired: A nonspecific term applied to a person who is either blind or partially blind.

Vital organs: Organs whose functions are essential to life, including the brain, heart, and lungs.

Vital signs: Important information about the victim's condition, obtained by checking consciousness, breathing, and circulation, including pulse and skin characteristics.

Voluntary muscles: Tissues, such as those in arms and legs, that are under a person's conscious control.

Walking assist: A basic method of helping a victim who needs assistance to walk to safety.

Withdrawal: The condition of mental and physical discomfort produced when a person stops using or abusing a substance to which he or she is addicted.

Work practice controls: Employee and employer behaviors that reduce the likelihood of exposure to a hazard at the job site.

Wound: An injury to the soft tissues.

Xiphoid (ZI foid): An arrow-shaped piece of hard tissue at the lowest point of the sternum.

References

American Academy of Orthopaedic Surgeons: *Basic rescue and emergency care*, Park Ridge, IL, 1990, American Academy of Orthopaedic Surgeons.

American Academy of Orthopaedic Surgeons: *Rural rescue and emergency care*, Park Ridge, IL, 1990, American Academy of Orthopaedic Surgeons.

American Academy of Orthopaedic Surgeons: *Your first response in emergency care*, Park Ridge, IL, 1990, American Academy of Orthopaedic Surgeons.

American Heart Association: *Heart and stroke facts*, 1992.

American Liver Foundation: *Hepatitis C Fact Sheet*, Cedar Grove, NJ, 1996.

American Lyme Disease Foundation: *A quick guide to Lyme disease*, 1995.

American Red Cross: *Emergency response*, ed 1, St Louis, 1990, Mosby.

American Red Cross: *First aid—responding to emergencies*, ed 2, St Louis, 1995, Mosby Lifeline.

American Red Cross: *Head lifeguard*, ed 1, St Louis, 1994, Mosby Lifeline.

American Red Cross: *Lifeguarding today*, ed 1, St Louis, 1994, Mosby Lifeline.

Anderson K: *Mosby's medical, nursing, and allied health dictionary*, ed 4, St Louis, 1994, Mosby.

Anspaugh DJ, Hamrick MH, Rosato AA: *Wellness: concepts and applications*, ed 2, St Louis, 1994, Mosby.

Associated Press: *The New York Times*, p 87, January 31, 1989.

Auerbach PS: *Wilderness medicine: management of wilderness and environmental emergencies*, ed 3, St Louis, 1995, Mosby.

Bergeron D, Bizjak G: *First responder*, 1996, Brady.

Berkow R: *The Merck manual of diagnosis and therapy*, ed 17, Rahway, NJ, 1993, Regents/Prentice Hall.

Beyette B: Stigma of SIDS, *LA Times*, ed 1, January 12, 1990.

Bogert J, DDS, Executive Director, American Academy of Pediatric Dentists: *Interview*, April 1990.

Canadian Red Cross Society: *The vital link*, St Louis, 1994, Mosby Lifeline.

Centers for Disease Control: Alcohol-related mortality and years of potential life lost—United States, 1987, *MMWR* 39(11):173, 1990.

Cohn AH: *It shouldn't hurt to be a child*, Chicago, 1987, National Committee for Prevention of Child Abuse.

Dallas Times Herald, Dallas Morning News, People Weekly, Midland Police Department Cpl. Jim White.

Division of Medical Sciences, National Academy of Sciences—National Research Council: *Accidental death and disability: the neglected disease of modern society*, Washington, DC, September 1966.

Dorsman J: *How to quit drinking without AA: a complete self-help guide*, ed 2, Rocklin, CA, 1994, Prima Pub.

Driesbach RH, Robertson WO: *Handbook of poisoning*, ed 12, East Norwalk, CT, 1987, Appleton and Lange.

Emergency Cardiac Care Committee and Subcommittees, American Heart Association: Guidelines for cardiopulmonary resuscitation and emergency cardiac care, *JAMA* 268:2172-2183, 1992.

Excerpt from Department of Health and Human Services, Public Health Services: *A curriculum guide for public-safety and emergency-response workers: prevention of transmission of human immunodeficiency virus and hepatitis B virus*, Atlanta, 1989, Department of Health and Human Services, Public Health Services, Centers for Disease Control.

Federal Register: *Rules and regulations*, vol 56, No 235, December 6, 1991.

Getchell B, Pippin R, Varnes J: *Health*, Boston, 1989, Houghton Mifflin.

Goldin S, Director of Biochemistry, Cambridge NeuroScience Research Inc, 1 Kendall Square, Cambridge, MA 02139: *Interview*, April 1990.

Graves JR, Austin D Jr, Cummins RO: *Rapid zap: automated defibrillation*, Englewood Cliffs, NJ, 1989, Prentice-Hall.

Green M, editor: *Bright futures: guidelines for health supervision of infants, children, and adolescents*, Arlington, VA, 1994, National Center for Education in Maternal and Child Health.

Guthrie HA, Picciano MF: *Human nutrition*, St Louis, 1995, Mosby.

Hafen BO, Karren KJ: *First aid for colleges and universities*, ed 5, Englewood Cliffs, NJ, 1993, Regents/Prentice Hall.

Hahn DB, Payne WA: *Focus on health*, ed 2, St Louis, 1994, Mosby.

Hauser WA, Hesdorffer DC: *Facts about epilepsy*, 1994, Epilepsy Foundation of America.

Hoekelman RA, Friedman SB, Nelson NM, et al.: *Primary pediatric care*, St Louis, 1992, Mosby.

Instant health boost: stop smoking, *Glamour* May 1995, p 48.

Isaac J, Goth P: *Wilderness first aid handbook*, New York, 1991, Lyons & Burford.

Major R MD: *A history of medicine*, Springfield, Ill, 1954, Charles C Thomas.

Marnell T: *Drug identification bible,* ed 1, Denver, 1993, Drug Identification Bible.

Merenstein GB, Kaplan DW, Rosenberg AA: *Handbook of pediatrics*, ed 17, East Norwalk, CT, 1994, Appleton and Lange.

National Capital Poison Center, Georgetown University Hospital, 3800 Reservoir Rd, NW, Washington, DC.

National Clearinghouse for Alcohol and Drug Information: *The fact is . . . , OSAP responds to national crisis,* Rockville, MD, Summer 1990.

National Committee for Injury Prevention and Control: *Injury prevention: meeting the challenge,* New York, 1989, Oxford University Press as a supplement to the American Journal of Preventive Medicine, 5:3, 1989.

National Emergency Number Association: *Nine one one 9-1-1 (what's it all about?).*

National Fire Protection Association. *NFPA 1561 standard on fire department incident management system*, Current edition, Quincy, MA, National Fire Protection Association.

National Fire Service Incident Mangement System Consortium, Model Procedures Commmittee: *Model procedures guide for structural firefighting*, Current edition, Stillwater, OK, Fire Protection Services.

National Institutes on Drug Abuse: *Anabolic steroids: a threat to body and mind,* National Institutes of Health, No 94-3721, 1994.

National Safety Council: *Accident facts*, Chicago, 1995, National Safety Council.

National Safety Council, Thygerson AL, editors: *First aid essentials*, Boston, 1989, Jones and Bartlett.

Payne WA, Hahn WB: *Understanding your health*, St Louis, 1989, Mosby.

Randall T: 50 million volts may crash through a lightning victim, *The Chicago Tribune*, 2D, August 13, 1989.

Rice DP, MacKenzie EJ, et al.: *Cost of injury in the United States: a report to Congress 1989*, San Francisco, 1989, Institute for Health and Aging, University of California, and Injury Prevention Center, The Johns Hopkins University.

Rideing WH: Hospital life in New York, *Harper's New Monthly Magazine* 57:171, 1878.

Rob C: *The caregiver's guide: helping elderly relatives cope with health and safety problems*, Boston, 1991, Houghton Mifflin.

Rodwell SR: *Basic nutrition and diet and therapy*, ed 10, St Louis, 1995, Mosby.

Safety IQ: a quiz for the whole family, *Geico Direct*, pp 7-10, K.L Publications, Spring, 1995.

Schimelpfenig T, Lindsey I: *NOLS wilderness first aid*, Lander WY, 1991, NOLS Publications.

Seeley RR, Stevens TD, Tate P: *Anatomy and physiology*, ed 3, St Louis, 1995, Mosby.

Simon JE , Goldberg AT: *Prehospital pediatric life support*, St Louis, 1989, Mosby.

Spence WR: *Substance abuse identification guide,* Waco, TX, 1991, Health Edco.

Stanton W, Executive Director, National Emergency Number Association: *Interview,* Feb 13, 1990.

Strauss RH, editor: *Sports medicine*, Philadelphia, 1984, WB Saunders.

Turkington C: *Poisons and antidotes*, New York, 1994, Facts on File.

Twardzik D, PhD, Affiliate Professor of Medicine, University of Washington School of Medicine; Research Fellow, Oncogen/Bristol Myers/Squibb: *Interview,* April 1990, Seattle, Wash.

U.S. Department of Health and Human Services; Public Health Service; Alcohol, Drug Abuse, and Mental Health Administration; and National Institute on Alcohol Abuse and Alcoholism: *Seventh special report to the U.S. Congress on alcohol and health*, Alexandria, VA, January, 1990, Editorial Experts.

United States Department of Labor News, USDL: 92-436, July 6, 1992.

Wardlaw GM, Insel PM: *Perspectives in nutrition*, St Louis, 1990, Mosby.

Wardlaw GM, Insel PM, Seyler MF: *Contemporary nutrition: issues and insights*, ed 2, St Louis, 1994, Mosby.

Weil A, Rosen W: *From chocolate to morphine: everything you need to know about mind-altering drugs,* ed 2, New York, 1993, Houghton-Mifflin.

West KH: *OSHA Bloodborne pathogens & tuberculosis curriculum guide*, Springfield, VA, 1992, Infection Control/Emerging Concepts.

White House: *National drug control strategy*, September 1989.

Williams SR: B*asic nutrition and diet therapy*, ed 10, St Louis, 1995, Mosby.

Wyllie I: *The treatment of epilepsy: principles and practice*, Philadelphia, 1993, Lea and Febeger.

Index

D

I

N

O

S

T

U